Surgical Anatomy of the Cervical Plexus and its Branches

Surgical Anatomy of the Cervical Plexus and its Branches

Edited by

R. SHANE TUBBS, MS, PA-C, PHD

MARIOS LOUKAS, MD, PHD

MALCON ANDREI MARTINEZ-PEREIRA, SR., PHD

CLAUDIA CEJAS, MD

C.J. BUI, MD

MIGUEL ANGEL REINA, MD, PHD

JOE IWANAGA, DDS, PHD

ELSEVIER

Surgical Anatomy of the Cervical Plexus and its Branches   ISBN: 978-0-323-83132-1
Copyright © 2022 Elsevier Inc. All rights reserved.

Notices

Publisher: Cathleen Sether
Acquisitions Editor: Humayra Khan
Editorial Project Manager: Tracy I. Tufaga
Production Project Manager: Kiruthika Govindaraju
Cover Designer: Miles Hitchen

3251 Riverport Lane
St. Louis, Missouri 63043

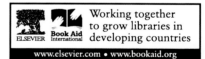

Working together
to grow libraries in
developing countries

www.elsevier.com • www.bookaid.org

List of Contributors

André P. Boezaart, MD, PhD
Professor of Anesthesiology
Department of Anesthesiology and Department of
    Orthopaedic Surgery University of Florida College
    of Medicine
Gainesville, Florida, United States
The Alon P. Winnie Research Institute
Gainesville, FL, United States
The Alon P. Winnie Research Institute
Still Bay, South Africa

Stephen J. Bordes, Jr., MD
Department of Surgery
Louisiana State University Health Sciences Center
New Orleans, LA, United States

C.J. Bui, MD
Chairman
Department of Neurosurgery
Ochsner Health System
New Orleans, LA, United States

Anna Carrera, MD, PhD
Professor of Human Anatomy
Neuroscience, Embryology and Clinical Anatomy
    Research Group (NEOMA)
Department of Medical Sciences (Human Anatomy and
    Embryology Unit) School of Medicine
University of Girona
Girona, Spain

Claudia Cejas, MD
Head of Radiology Department
Head of MRI Division
Fundación para la Lucha de Enfermedades
    Neurológicas (Fleni)
Montañeses
CABA, Buenos Aires, Argentina

Tess Decater, MD
Department of Anatomical, Sciences
St. George's University
St. George's, Grenada, West Indies

Graham Dupont, BS
Tulane University School of Medicine
New Orleans, LA, United States

Paloma Fernández, BS, PhD
Histology Unit
Institute of Applied Molecular Medicine
School of Medicine
CEU-San Pablo University
Madrid, Spain

Virginia García-García, TCH
Tech, Histology Unit
Institute of Applied Molecular Medicine
School of Medicine
CEU-San Pablo University
Madrid, Spain

Joe Iwanaga, DDS, PhD
Associate Professor
Department of Neurosurgery
Clinical Neuroscience Research Center (CNRC)
Tulane University School of Medicine
New Orleans, LA, United States

Skyler Jenkins, MD
Department of Neurosurgery
Tulane University School of Medicine
New Orleans, LA, United States

Shogo Kikuta, DDS, PhD
Assistant Professor
Dental and Oral Medical Center
Kurume University School of Medicine
Kurume, Fukuoka, Japan

Mitchell D. Kilgore, BS
Tulane University School of Medicine
New Orleans, LA, United States

Jin-Soo Kim, MD, PhD
Department of Anesthesiology and Pain Medicine
Ajou UniversitySchool of Medicine
Suwon, Gyeonggi-do, South Korea

Ha Yeon Kim, MD
Department of Anesthesiology and Pain Medicine
Ajou UniversitySchool of Medicine
Suwon, Gyeonggi-do, South Korea

Marios Loukas, MD, PhD
Professor and Dean
St. George's University School of Medicine
St. George's, Grenada

Department of Anatomy
University of Warmia and Mazury
Olsztyn, Poland

Malcon Andrei Martinez-Pereira, Sr., PhD
Veterinary Doctor
Professor
Animal Anatomy and Histology
Embryology and Neurology
Center of Rural Sciences
Federal University of Santa Catarina
Curitibanos, Santa Catarina, Brazil

Mansour Mathkour, MD
Tulane University & Ochsner Clinic
Neurosurgery Program
Tulane University School of Medicine
New Orleans, LA, United States

Ana V. Montaña, DVM, PhD
Department of Human Anatomy
School of Medicine
Francisco de Vitoria University
Madrid, Spain

Javier Moratinos-Delgado, TCH
Histology Unit
Institute of Applied Molecular Medicine
School of Medicine
CEU-San Pablo University
Madrid, Spain

Miguel Angel Reina, MD, PhD
Professor of Anesthesiology
Department of Clinical Medical Sciences and Applied
    Molecular Medicine Institute
CEU San Pablo University School of Medicine
Madrid, Madrid, Spain

Department of Anesthesiology
University of Florida College of Medicine
Gainesville, Florida, United States

Francisco Reina, MD, PhD
Professor of Human Anatomy
Neuroscience
Embryology and Clinical Anatomy Research Group
    (NEOMA)
Department of Medical Sciences (Human Anatomy and
    Embryology Unit)
School of Medicine
University of Girona, Girona, Spain

Irene Riquelme, MD
Pain Clinic Unit
Hospital Universitario Sanitas La Moraleja
Madrid, Spain

Xavier Sala-Blanch, MD
Associate Professor of Human Anatomy
Department of Human Anatomy and Embryology
Faculty of Medicine
Universitat of Barcelona
Barcelona, Spain

Department of Anesthesiology
Hospital Clínic
Universitat de Barcelona
Barcelona, Spain

Emilia Osa Sanz, MD
MRI Division
Fundación para la Lucha de Enfermedades
    Neurológicas (Fleni)
Montañeses
CABA, Buenos Aires, Argentina

R. Shane Tubbs, MS, PA-C, PhD
Professor
Departments of Neurosurgery, Neurology, Surgery, and
    Structural and Cellular Biology
Tulane University School of Medicine
New Orleans, LA, United States

Department of Neurosurgery and Ochsner
   Neuroscience Institute
Ochsner Health System
New Orleans, LA, United States

Department of Anatomical Sciences
St. George's University
St. George's, Grenada

Enrique Verdú, PhD
Professor of Human Physiology
Neuroscience
Embryology and Clinical Anatomy Research Group
   (NEOMA)
Department of Medical Sciences (Human Physiology
   Unit) School of Medicine
University of Girona
Girona, Spain

Tyler Warner, MD
Researcher
Department of Anatomical Sciences
St. George's University
St. George's, Grenada

Cassidy Werner, MD
Tulane University School of Medicine
New Orleans, LA, United States

Contents

CHAPTER 1

An Overview of the Cervical Plexus

R. SHANE TUBBS • MARIOS LOUKAS • JOE IWANAGA •
MALCON ANDREI MARTINEZ-PEREIRA, SR. • CLAUDIA CEJAS • C.J. BUI •
MIGUEL ANGEL REINA

The anatomy of the cervical plexus (Figs. 1.1 and 1.2) often receives less attention than the other main plexuses of the body such as the brachial and lumbosacral plexuses. However, important nerves emanate and are related to this plexus formed by the upper cervical ventral rami (Figs. 1.3−1.6). Moreover, its branches

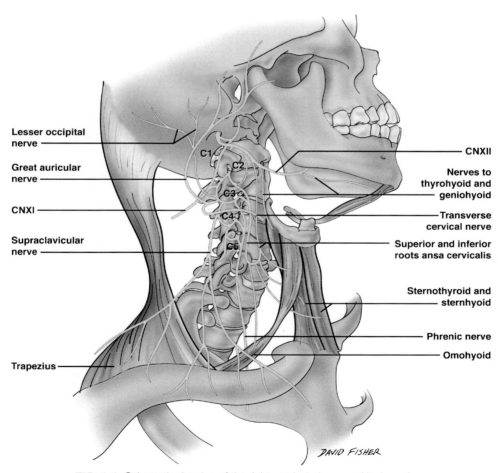

FIG. 1.1 Schematic drawing of the right cervical plexus and its branches.

Surgical Anatomy of the Cervical Plexus and its Branches. https://doi.org/10.1016/B978-0-323-83132-1.00017-2

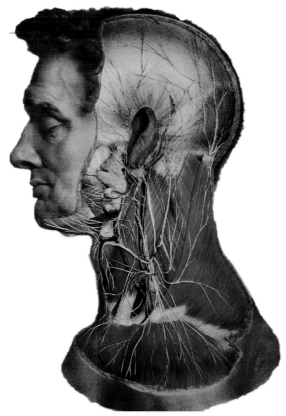

FIG. 1.2 Drawing of the left cervical plexus and its branches (after Bougery).

have relationships with cranial nerves (e.g., spinal accessory, hypoglossal, facial nerves) and other important neurovascular structures of the neck.

Shearer, in his book (1937) on human dissection, described the overall anatomy of the cervical plexus well. He said, "This is a looped nerve plexus (Fig. 1.7) derived from the anterior rami of the first four cervical nerves; it lies under cover of the upper part of the sterno(cleido)mastoid muscle. The anterior ramus of the first cervical nerve is small and difficult to expose. It emerges above the transverse process of the atlas and turns downward in front of that process to join the second nerve. The second, third, and fourth nerves are each successively larger and enter the present area of dissection by passing laterally and downward from between the anterior and posterior tubercles of the transverse processes of the corresponding cervical vertebrae. The plexus proper takes the form of three loops. The first is that already noted between the first and second

nerves, and lies in front of the transverse process of the atlas. The second loop is formed by the second and third nerves, and the third by the third and fourth nerves. These loops are longer and more laterally directed, and rest against the levator scapulae and scalenus medius. The cutaneous branches of the cervical plexus, which have already been seen in the dissection of the posterior triangle, should now be traced back to their origins. The less occipital, great auricular, and cervical cutaneous nerves all arise from the loop between the second and third nerves. Anterior, middle, and posterior supraclavicular nerves arise from the lower loop, usually by a common stem. From this loop are also derived muscular twigs, which cross the posterior triangle to reach the deep surface of the trapezius. Muscular branches arise also from the roots of the cervical plexus. The largest of these is the phrenic nerve. This nerve is derived principally from the fourth cervical and passes downward and medially on the anterior surface of the scalenus anterior, to enter the thoracic cavity behind the innominate (brachiocephalic) vein. It usually receives a twig from the fifth cervical nerves, and often one from the third. From the second and third nerves arise the two roots of the descendens cervicalis (superior root of ansa cervicalis), whose part in the formation of the ansa hypoglossi (ansa cervicalis) has already been seen. The first cervical gives rise to a branch that passes forward deep to the internal jugular vein to join the hypoglossal nerves under cover of the posterior belly of the digastric. The remaining branches of the cervical plexus are small muscular twigs that pass from the second, third, and fourth nerves directly into the longus colli, longus capitis, and scalenus medius, for the supply of those muscles."

Anteriorly, many of the more familiar cutaneous nerve branches of the cervical plexus originate from a said "nerve point" (not to be confused with Erb's point—see below) located at the junction of the upper 2/5's and lower 3/5's of the sternocleidomastoid muscle and inferior to the spinal accessory nerve's emergence from the lateral margin of this same muscle. This nerve point is approximated by the hyoid bone, which is approximately at the level of the C3 vertebral body. Additionally, this point is located approximately 6 cm inferior to the mastoid process. Some have also stated that this area is approximated by the midpoint of the posterior border of the sternocleidomastoid muscle. The position of the main superficial nerves of the cervical region can also be found by six lines all drawn from the middle of the posterior border of the sternocleidomastoid muscle. First, a line drawn forwards from this spot to cross the sternocleidomastoid at right angles

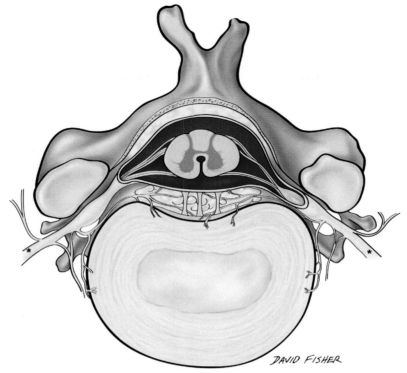

FIG. 1.3 Drawing of an axial section through the cervical spine and noting the left and right cervical ventral rami (*).

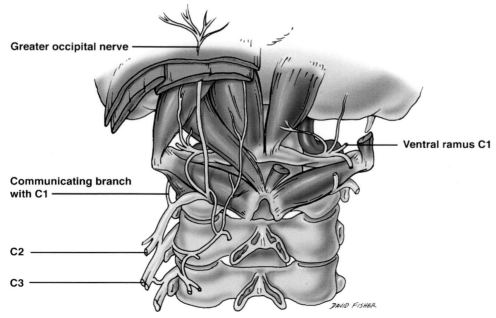

FIG. 1.4 Posterior view of the upper ventral and dorsal cervical rami.

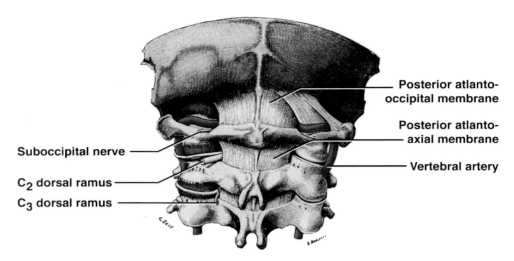

FIG. 1.5 Posterior view of the upper cervical nerves branching into the dorsal and ventral rami. Note the course of the ventral rami anteriorly along the vertebral column (after Piersol).

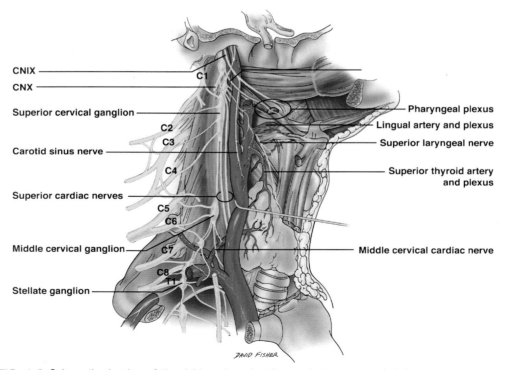

FIG. 1.6 Schematic drawing of the right neck noting the cervical nerves and their connections to the sympathetic trunk. Please note the sympathetic trunk connecting the superior and middle cervical ganglia.

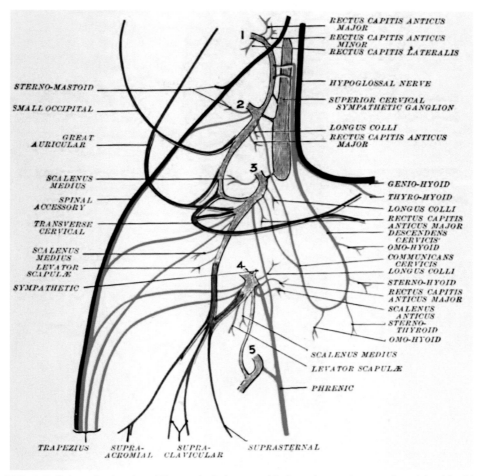

FIG. 1.7 Schematic drawing of the cervical plexus and its branches and connections (after Morris).

to its long axis corresponds to the transverse cervical nerve. A second line drawn up across the muscle to the posterior auricle to run parallel with the external jugular vein corresponds to the great auricular nerve. Third, a line running along the posterior border of the sternocleidomastoid muscle to the scalp marks the course of the lesser occipital nerve. These lines continued inferiorly to cross the sternum, the middle of the clavicle, and the acromion will indicate the branches of the supraclavicular nerves respectively. The transverse cervical nerve may cross anterior or posterior to the external jugular vein. It does so at the midpoint of this vessel. The great auricular nerve travels parallel with the external jugular vein and just posterior to this vessel. The external jugular vein may be visible through the skin across the sternocleidomastoid muscle and hence used to localize the great auricular nerve. The

lesser occipital nerve follows approximately the posterior border of the sternocleidomastoid muscle as it approaches the skin of the lateral occiput and ear. The supraclavicular nerves supply the skin of the deltoid and pectoralis major inferiorly to approximately the second rib and lie deep to the platysma muscle.

Anatomically, Erb described a superficial point 2−3 cm superior to the clavicle, "somewhat outside of the posterior border of the sternomastoid" and at the level of the carotid tubercle that when stimulated resulted in the contraction of such muscles as the deltoid, biceps brachii, and brachialis. Many have misidentified Erb's point as the so-called nerve point or punctum nervosum located approximately at the midpoint of the posterior border of the sternocleidomastoid muscle. This point marks the general region where the cutaneous branches (i.e., lesser occipital, greater auricular, transverse cervical, and supraclavicular nerves) of the cervical plexus emerge into the subcutaneous tissues of the neck. Some have also defined the nerve point as being found at the posterior border of the sternocleidomastoid muscle at the junction between its superior and middle thirds. The nerve point can be further localized as lying at the approximate level of the hyoid bone (approximately the level of the C3 vertebrae) and roughly 6 cm inferior to the tip of the mastoid process of the temporal bone. Regardless, the nerve point (C3 vertebral level) is superior to Erb's point (approximately the C6 vertebral level) and hugs the posterior border of the sternocleidomastoid muscle.

In this collection of chapters, we seek to highlight the surgical anatomy of the cervical plexus and all of its branches with the hopes that a better understanding of their morphology will lead to better patient outcomes in regard to diagnoses and treatments.

REFERENCES

Shearer, E.M., 1937. Manual of Human Dissection. P. Blakiston's Son & Co., Inc., Philadelphia.

FURTHER READING

Tubbs, R.S., Loukas, M., Salter, E.G., Oakes, W.J., 2007. Wilhelm Erb and Erb's point. Clin. Anat. 20, 486–488.

CHAPTER 2

The Lesser Occipital Nerve

SKYLER JENKINS • R. SHANE TUBBS

ANATOMY

The lesser occipital nerve (LON) (Fig. 2.1) is a cutaneous nerve of the cervical plexus that innervates most of the ear and an area of the scalp posterior to the ear. It is approximately 1.2 ± 1.6 mm in diameter and is derived primarily from the ventral rami of the second cervical spinal nerve, with some contributions from the third cervical spinal nerve (Ducic et al., 2009). The LON traverses rostrally and dorsally, looping around the inferior border of the spinal accessory nerve.

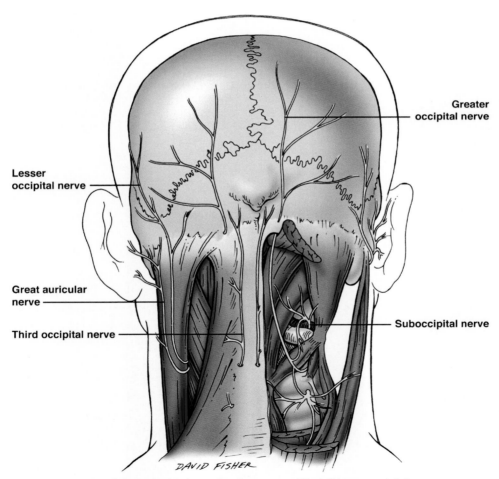

FIG. 2.1 Schematic drawing noting the course of the left lesser occipital nerve.

Surgical Anatomy of the Cervical Plexus and its Branches. https://doi.org/10.1016/B978-0-323-83132-1.00002-0

It then emerges posterior to the sternocleidomastoid (SCM) muscle superior to the great auricular nerve and ascends along the posterior margin of the SCM toward the mastoid process (Schaeffer, 1953). In a minority of cases, the LON pierces the SCM or travels deep to it (Dash et al., 2005; Fujimaki et al., 2007). It most often travels over the SCM muscle's fascia, running between that fascia and the superficial musculoaponeurotic system (Pantaloni and Sullivan, 2000). However, it has also been shown to cross the splenius and levator scapulae muscle fasciae (Pantaloni and Sullivan, 2000). It then pierces the deep cervical fascia at the level of the cranium and travels into the superficial fascia of the scalp (Schaeffer, 1953). The main nerve trunk is found on average 70 mm lateral to the external occipital protuberance (Cesmebasi et al., 2014). The nerve then trifurcates into auricular, occipital, and mastoid branches. The auricular branch, coursing anterosuperiorly, supplies the upper medial aspect of the auricle and communicates with the posterior branch of the great auricular nerve (Schaeffer, 1953; Standring, 2008). However, the auricular branch sometimes arises from the greater occipital nerve (Standring, 2008). The occipital branch terminates and supplies the skin above the mastoid process, whereas the mastoid branch provides innervation to

the skin overlying the mastoid process (Schaeffer, 1953). This nerve travels approximately 2.5 cm lateral to the occipital artery over the occiput (Fig. 2.2).

Tubbs et al. (2016a) showed that the LON has two types, of course, type I and type II. Type I nerves travel along the posterior border of the SCM muscle, staying within 10 mm of it throughout their full length, continuing on to the occiput after the muscle insertion at the skull with a small deviation toward the posterior pinna (Tubbs et al., 2016a). However, some type I nerves cross anterior to the SCM near the mastoid process (Tubbs et al., 2016a). These nerves were found at a point one-third of the distance along a line drawn from the mastoid process to the external occipital protuberance (Tubbs et al., 2016a). Type II nerves, in contrast, leave the posterior border of the SCM and course medially (up to 45 mm posterior to the posterior border of the SCM) over the nuchal region as they ascend over the occiput (Tubbs et al., 2016a). This type of nerve is found at a point midway between the mastoid process and the external occipital protuberance (Tubbs et al., 2016a).

The location and course of the LON are somewhat variable. Lucas et al. (1994) discovered a variation in which one of the loops of the C2 ventral rami encircles the levator scapulae or anterior scalene. Tubbs et al.

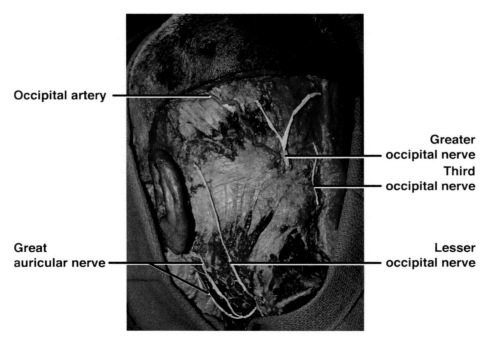

FIG. 2.2 Cadaveric dissection of the left occiput. From left to right, note the great auricular, lesser occipital, greater occipital, and third occipital nerves. The occipital artery is seen medial to the lesser occipital nerve.

(2007) found that the LON branched into medial and lateral components at approximately the midpoint between a horizontal line drawn through the external occipital protuberance and the intermastoid line. Other sources have reported duplication of the nerve where the lateral nerve supplies the retroauricular region and the medial nerve supplies the adjacent scalp (Lucas et al., 1994). The LON can arise from the accessory nerve and can communicate with the posterior auricular branch of the facial nerve (Baumel, 1974; Nageris et al., 2000; Tubbs et al., 2016b).

In one case report, three distinct LONs were observed, named LON-I, LON-II, and LON-III (Madhavi and Holla, 2004). LON-I hooked around the posterior border of the SCM and coursed cranially, superficial to the muscle (Madhavi and Holla, 2004). LON-II arose from the supraclavicular nerve trunk branch to the trapezius and ascended along the posterior border of the SCM parallel to LON-I (Madhavi and Holla, 2004). LON-III emerged from the posterior border of SCM, most cranially, and passed superomedially deep to the trapezius, piercing the fascia 35 mm inferior to the superior nuchal line and lateral to the midline before dividing into medial and lateral branches (Madhavi and Holla, 2004) with the former usually communicating with the greater occipital nerve (Fig. 2.3).

Ravindra et al. (2014) showed a path of the LON resembling LON-III; however, it pierced the fascia of the trapezius 75 mm below the superior nuchal line.

Other common variations that include the LON may be very small and distributed only to the skin of the neck. In such cases, the greater occipital nerve supplies the areas usually supplied by the LON. In some cases instead of its usual dorsal and upward course beneath the deep fascia along the posterior border of the sternocleidomastoid muscle, the LON passes directly backward, piercing the trapezius muscle near its upper border before reaching the scalp. The auricular branch of the LON may be derived from the greater occipital nerve. It usually arises from the second and third cervical nerves or from the second and third cervical nerves or from the loop between them.

CLINICAL

An understanding of the anatomy, variability, and cutaneous innervation of the LON allows for clinical diagnosis and treatment options. The main clinical implication of the LON arises from its role in occipital neuralgia, cervicogenic headaches, and occipitoparietal headaches. Most treatment options have been performed using external landmarks to find the nerve, but the advent of high-resolution ultrasound (HRUS) has facilitated the identification and increased the precision of these interventions. Coupling anatomical knowledge with HRUS, an experienced technician can find and trace the path of the LON, facilitating visualization of pathology and more focused treatment (Narouze, 2016; Platzgummer et al., 2014).

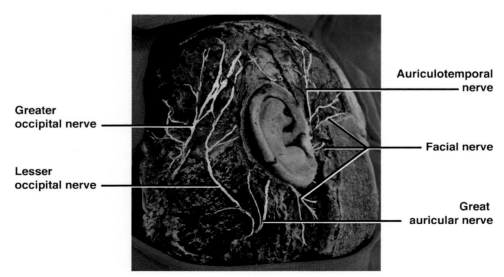

FIG. 2.3 Cadaveric dissection of the right occiput and face. Note the communication between the lesser and greater occipital nerves.

Occipital neuralgia is a clinical pathology associated with the compression, entrapment, and/or stretching of the occipital nerves. Its symptoms include paroxysmal burning pain in the cutaneous distribution of the nerve involved. LON-related neuralgia is sometimes confused with that caused by the greater occipital nerve, so its manifestations have been underreported. Stretch injuries most often result from forceful, rotational head movements. Lucas et al. (1994) articulated a case where contraction of the inferior oblique muscle stretched the C2 ventral rami that encircled the levator scapulae or anterior scalene, causing pain (Lucas et al., 1994). Their study also revealed a point of stretching as the nerve crossed the lateral atlantoaxial articulation on the posterosuperior articular process of the axis (Lucas et al., 1994). The increased distance the nerve then traveled owing to head rotation potentially caused a stretch injury (Hunter and Mayfield, 1949).

In addition to stretch injuries, the LON can be compressed by various masses. Given its close proximity to the vertebral artery, the C2 ventral ramus can be compressed as it crosses the posterolateral or, less often, the ventral surface (Bogduk, 1981; Lucas et al., 1994). Han et al. (2016) reported compression of the nerve by an intramuscular lipoma within the splenius muscle.

Iatrogenic injury to the nerve is also a common complication of neurosurgical procedures. In retrosigmoid craniotomies, a traditional approach to exposure warrants a lateral incision along a line drawn from the root of the zygoma to the external occipital protuberance, marking the level of the transverse sinus. This incision places type I nerves at risk of injury, potentially leading to chronic occipital headaches. However, Schessel et al. (1993) stated that there was no difference in the incidence and severity of pain between the linear incision and the inverted "U" incision. Other researchers have promoted a "crutch-like" incision to spare the LON (Chen et al., 2018). Occipital neuralgia is the second most common cause of postoperative headache at 16.6% and can be amenable to surgical decompression or excision of the occipital nerve following craniotomy given the significant alleviation of symptoms (Guyuron et al., 2009; Janis et al., 2011; Schankin et al., 2009).

Surgical resection has often been described as the appropriate first-line intervention for occipital neuralgia and chronic headaches related to the LON in view of its smaller, less clinically significant, area of innervation (Lee et al., 2013). Of the three occipital nerves, the LON is located most laterally and can be accessed through an incision, separate from that of the other occipital nerves, 40 mm from the mastoid prominence along the posterior border of the SCM muscle (Khavanin et al., 2018). It can found within 10 mm of this location bilaterally, and the greater auricular nerve and spinal accessory nerve are rarely encountered (Khavanin et al., 2018). After neurectomy, the nerve must be implanted deep within a large muscle, and there is a risk of neuroma formation if it is forced out (Dellon and Mackinnon, 1986; Patrick et al., 2010; Wolfort and Dellon, 2001).

Another option is surgical decompression and neurolysis/neuroplasty, which minimizes the risks associated with neurectomy and preserves optimal sensation to the innervated area. There are three potential areas of compression, termed compression zones. Zone 1 correlates with the emergence of the LON from behind the SCM; zone 2 is the cephalic ascent along the SCM; and zone 3 is the crossing point of the LON and the nuchal line (Peled et al., 2016). Since the branching pattern is highly variable, Peled et al. (2016) recommend that the nerve be dissected with a vertical incision from zones 1 through 3, in addition to the universal fascial band present at the nuchal line for full decompression. However, if decompression of both the greater and lesser occipital nerves is required, Afifi et al. (2019) recommend a transverse incision from 25 mm caudal to the external occipital protuberance along a line connecting the posterior edges of the SCM.

Various approaches have been presented for nonsurgical treatment of cervicogenic headaches or occipitoparietal migraines. Injections of local anesthetic, steroids, or botulinum toxin have all been suggested. One study proposed a point 30 mm in diameter located 65 mm lateral to midline and 53 mm inferior to a line connecting the external auditory canals; another found the main nerve trunk 70 mm lateral to the external occipital protuberance (Dash et al., 2005; Tubbs et al., 2007). This method will give temporary relief and can be used to block the LON alone, or as part of a multiple cranial nerve blockade to treat chronic headaches refractory to greater occipital nerve blocks alone (Miller et al., 2019). Blocking multiple nerves can also provide greater symptomatic relief as the lesser, greater, and third occipital nerves have multiple areas of overlap (Kwon et al., 2018). Occipital nerve stimulation, nerve cryoablation, and pulsed radiofrequency are also being studied as possible treatment options (Kim et al., 2015; Sweet et al., 2015).

Because the LON enters the subcutaneous plane superficial to the SCM fascia, clinical consideration needs to be given so that the nerve is not injured during the creation of a posterior auricular flap during face-lift surgery (Pantaloni and Sullivan, 2000). The flap should be created at a more superficial level to avoid injury to the nerve.

REFERENCES

Afifi, A.M., Carbullido, M.K., Israel, J.S., Sanchez, R.J., Albano, N.J., 2019. Alternative approach for occipital headache surgery: the use of a transverse incision and "w" flaps. Plast. Reconstr. Surg. Glob. Open 7 (4), e2176. https://doi.org/10.1097/GOX.0000000000002176.

Baumel, J.J., 1974. Trigeminal-facial nerve communications. Their function in facial muscle innervation and reinnervation. Arch Otolaryngol. 99, 34–44.

Bogduk, N., 1981. Local anesthetic blocks of the second cervical ganglion: a technique with application in occipital headache. Cephalgia 1, 41–50.

Cesmebasi, A., Muhleman, M.A., Hulsberg, P., Gielecki, J., Matusz, P., Tubbs, R.S., Loukas, M., 2014. Occipital neuralgia: anatomic considerations. Clin. Anat. 28 (1), 101–108. https://doi.org/10.1002/ca.22468.

Chen, F., Wen, J., Li, P., Ying, Y., Wang, W., Yi, Y., Cao, Y., Xie, W., Zhang, G., Wang, X., Ruan, X., 2018. Crutch-like incision along the mastoid groove and above the occipital artery protects the lesser occipital nerve and occipital artery in microvascular decompression surgery. World Neurosurg. 120, e755–e761. https://doi.org/10.1016/j.wneu.2018.08.162.

Dash, K.S., Janis, J.E., Guyuron, B., 2005. The lesser and third occipital nerves and migraine headaches. Plast. Reconstr. Surg. 115, 1752–1758 [discussion 1759–60].

Dellon, A.L., Mackinnon, S.E., 1986. Treatment of the painful neuroma by neuroma resection and muscle implantation. Plast. Reconstr. Surg. 77, 427–438.

Ducic, I., Moriarty, M., Al-Attar, A., 2009. Anatomical variations of the occipital nerves: implications for the treatment of chronic headaches. Plast. Reconstr. Surg. 123 (3), 859–863. https://doi.org/10.1097/prs.0b013e318199f080.

Fujimaki, T., Son, J.H., Takanashi, S., Ishii, T., Furuya, K., Mochizuki, T., et al., 2007. Preservation of the lesser occipital nerve during microvascular decompression for hemifacial spasm. Technical note. J Neurosurg. 107 (6), 1235–1237.

Guyuron, B., Reed, D., Kriegler, J.S., et al., 2009. A placebo-controlled surgical trial of the treatment of migraine headaches. Plast. Reconstr. Surg. 124, 461–468.

Han, H.H., Kim, H.S., Rhie, J.W., Moon, S.H., 2016. Intramuscular lipoma-induced occipital neuralgia on the lesser occipital nerve. J. Craniofac. Surg. 27 (4), e350–e352. https://doi.org/10.1097/scs.0000000000002516.

Hunter, C.R., Mayfield, F.H., 1949. Role of the upper cervical roots in the production of pain in the head. Am. J. Surg. 78, 743–751.

Janis, J.E., Dhanik, A., Howard, J.H., 2011. Validation of the peripheral trigger point theory of migraine headaches: single surgeon experience using botulinum toxin and surgical decompression. Plast. Reconstr. Surg. 128, 123–131.

Khavanin, N., Carl, H., Yang, R., Dorafshar, A., 2018. Surgical "safe zone": rapid anatomical identification of the lesser occipital nerve. J. Reconstr. Microsurg. 35 (5), 341–345. https://doi.org/10.1055/s-0038-1676601.

Kim, C.H., Hu, W., Gao, J., Dragan, K., Whealton, T., Julian, C., 2015. Cryoablation for the treatment of occipital neuralgia. Pain Physician 18, E363–E368.

Kwon, H.J., Kim, H.S., J, O., et al., 2018. Anatomical analysis of the distribution patterns of occipital cutaneous nerves and the clinical implications for pain management. J. Pain. Res. 11, 2023–2031. https://doi.org/10.2147/JPR.S175506.

Lee, M., Lineberry, K., Reed, D., et al., 2013. The role of the third occipital nerve in surgical treatment of occipital migraine headaches. J. Plast. Reconstr. Aesthet. Surg. 66, 1335–1339.

Lucas, G.D.A., Laudanna, A., Chopard, R.P., Raffaelli, E., 1994. Anatomy of the lesser occipital nerve in relation to cervicogenic headache. Clin. Anat. 7, 90–96.

Madhavi, C., Holla, S.J., 2004. Triplication of the lesser occipital nerve. Clin. Anat. 17 (8), 667–671. https://doi.org/10.1002/ca.10252.

Miller, S., Lagrata, S., Matharu, M., 2019. Multiple cranial nerve blocks for the transitional treatment of chronic headaches. Cephalalgia 39 (12), 1488–1499. https://doi.org/10.1177/0333102419848121.

Nageris, B., Braverman, I., Kalmanowitz, M., Segal, K., Frenkiel, S., 2000. Connections of the facial and vestibular nerves: an anatomic study. J. Otolaryngol. 29, 159–161.

Narouze, S., 2016. Occipital neuralgia diagnosis and treatment: the role of ultrasound. Headache 56 (4), 801–807. https://doi.org/10.1111/head.12790.

Pantaloni, M., Sullivan, P., 2000. Relevance of the lesser occipital nerve in facial rejuvenation surgery. Plast. Reconstr. Surg. 105 (7), 2594–2599. https://doi.org/10.1097/00006534-200006000-00051.

Patrick, J., Frank, W., Theodora, M., et al., 2010. The pedicled serratus anterior muscle wrap-around flap: a treatment option in the management of post-traumatic axillary neuroma and neuropathic pain. Ann. Plast. Surg. 65, 170–173.

Peled, Z.M., Pietramaggiori, G., Scherer, S., 2016. Anatomic and compression topography of the lesser occipital nerve. Plast. Reconstr. Surg. Glob. Open 4 (3), e639. https://doi.org/10.1097/gox.0000000000000654.

Platzgummer, H., Moritz, T., Gruber, G.M., Pivec, C., Wöber, C., Bodner, G., Lieba-Samal, D., 2014. The lesser occipital nerve visualized by high-resolution sonography—normal and initial suspect findings. Cephalalgia 35 (9), 816–824. https://doi.org/10.1177/0333102414559293.

Ravindra, S.S., Sirasanagandla, S.R., Nayak, S.B., Rao, K.M., Patil, J., 2014. An anatomical variation of the lesser occipital nerve in the "carefree part" of the posterior triangle. J. Clin. Diagn. Res. 8 (4), AD05–AD06. https://doi.org/10.7860/JCDR/2014/7423.4276.

Schaeffer, J.P., 1953. The Nervous System, Morris' Human Anatomy, eleventh ed. McGraw Hill, New York, pp. 1126–1133. Section 9.

Schankin, C.J., Gall, C., Straube, A., 2009. Headache syndromes after acoustic neuroma surgery and their implications for quality of life. Cephalalgia 29, 760–771.

Schessel, D.A., Rowed, D.W., Nedzelski, J.M., et al., 1993. Postoperative pain following excision of acoustic neuroma by the suboccipital approach: observations on possible cause and potential amelioration. Am. J. Otol. 14, 491–494.

Standring, S., 2008. Gray's Anatomy. Elsevier, Philadelphia.

Sweet, J.A., Mitchell, L.S., Narouze, S., Sharan, A.D., Falowski, S.M., Schwalb, J.M., Machado, A., Rosenow, J.M., Petersen, E.A., Hayek, S.M., Arle, J.E., Pilitsis, J.G., 2015. Occipital nerve stimulation for the treatment of patients with medically refractory occipital neuralgia. Neurosurgery 77 (3), 332–341. https://doi.org/10.1227/neu.0000000000000872.

Tubbs, R.S., Salter, E.G., Wellons, J.C., Blount, J.P., Oakes, W.J., 2007. Landmarks for the identification of the cutaneous nerves of the occiput and nuchal regions. Clin. Anat. 20, 235–238.

Tubbs, R.S., Fries, F.N., Kulwin, C., Mortazavi, M.M., Loukas, M., 2016a. Modified skin incision for avoiding the lesser occipital nerve and occipital artery during retrosigmoid craniotomy: potential applications for enhancing operative working distance and angles while minimizing the risk of postoperative neuralgias and intraoperative hemorrhage. J. Clin. Neurosci. 32, 83–87. https://doi.org/10.1016/j.jocn.2016.03.015.

Tubbs, R.S., Ajayi, O.O., Fries, F.N., Spinner, R.J., 2016b. Variations of the accessory nerve: anatomical study including previously undocumented findings-expanding our misunderstanding of this nerve. Br. J. Neurosurg. 31 (1), 113–115. https://doi.org/10.1080/02688697.2016.1187253.

Wolfort, S.F., Dellon, A.L., 2001. Treatment of recurrent neuroma of the interdigital nerve by implantation of the proximal nerve into muscle in the arch of the foot. J. Foot Ankle. Surg. 40, 404–410.

FURTHER READING

Manolitsis, N., Elahi, F., 2014. Pulsed radiofrequency for occipital neuralgia. Pain Physician 17 (6), E709–E717.

CHAPTER 3

The Great Auricular Nerve

STEPHEN J. BORDES, JR. • R. SHANE TUBBS

ANATOMY

Formed from the ventral rami of the second and third cervical spinal nerves, the great auricular nerve (GAN) is the largest sensory branch of the cervical plexus (Altafulla et al., 2019; Raikos et al., 2017; Tayebi Meybodi et al., 2018). It emerges at the nerve point in the posterior triangle of the neck (Figs. 3.1 and 3.2) (Raikos et al., 2017; Brown and Dellon, 2018). It first courses beneath the platysma and sternocleidomastoid muscle (SCM) between deep and superficial layers of cervical fascia before wrapping around the posterior border of the SCM, at which point it perforates the muscle's investing fascia (Altafulla et al., 2019; Raikos et al., 2017; Tayebi

Meybodi et al., 2018; Ozturk et al., 2014; Ella et al., 2015; Iwanaga et al., 2019). It then travels along the anterior superior one-third of the SCM toward the ear, parallel and posterior to the external jugular vein (EJV) (Altafulla et al., 2019; Raikos et al., 2017; Ozturk et al., 2014; Ella et al., 2015; Iwanaga et al., 2019). After reaching its most superficial position, the GAN divides into two cutaneous branches, anterior and posterior, at the inferior margin of the parotid gland (Altafulla et al., 2019; Raikos et al., 2017; Ozturk et al., 2014; Lefkowitz et al., 2013). The anterior branch, which continues between the SCM and parotid gland, further divides into superficial and deep branches, which

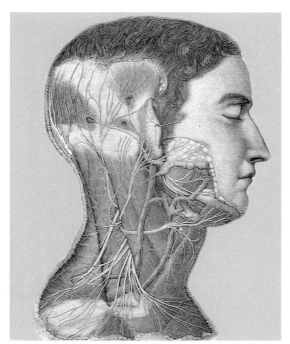

FIG. 3.1 Schematic drawing of the superficial branches of the cervical plexus with the course of the great auricular nerve in yellow (after E. Salle).

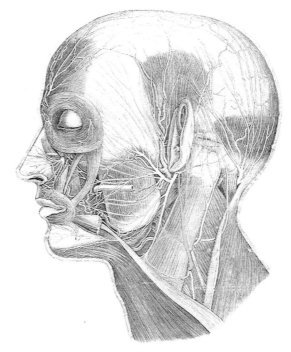

FIG. 3.2 Schematic drawing of the superficial branches of the cervical plexus with the course of the great auricular nerve in yellow (after Arnold).

Surgical Anatomy of the Cervical Plexus and its Branches. https://doi.org/10.1016/B978-0-323-83132-1.00009-3

provide sensory innervation to the skin in the preauricular, parotid gland, and mandibular regions (Fig. 3.3) (Raikos et al., 2017; Tayebi Meybodi et al., 2018; Lefkowitz et al., 2013; Peuker and Filler, 2002). Branches of the anterior division have been seen to penetrate the parotid gland and, in some cases, communicate with branches of the facial nerve (Raikos et al., 2017; Tayebi Meybodi et al., 2018; Zohar et al., 2002). There are variations in which the anterior division communicates with the marginal mandibular or cervical branches of the facial nerve; some have even demonstrated innervation of the platysma by the anterior branch of the GAN (Brennan et al., 2008). The posterior branch of the GAN, which continues superiorly along the anterior surface of the SCM toward the mastoid process, innervates skin overlying the mastoid process and the dorsal inferior one-third of the auricle (Altafulla et al., 2019; Tayebi Meybodi et al., 2018; Lefkowitz et al., 2013; Peuker and Filler, 2002). Additional variations include the mastoid branch may arise independently from the cervical plexus, in which case it passes upward between the lesser occipital and great auricular nerves to reach its destination and the GAN may arise solely from the third or from the third and fourth cervical nerves.

TOPOGRAPHICAL LANDMARKS

The nerve point (see Chapter 1) of the neck, or punctum nervosum, is an important landmark for identifying the GAN and spinal accessory nerve, which is usually found 1 cm superior to the GAN (Raikos et al., 2017; Ella et al., 2015; Tubbs et al., 2007; Rohrich et al., 2011). The nerve point is located approximately at the level of the C3 vertebra at the posterior border of the SCM, at which point the lesser occipital, great auricular, transverse cervical, and supraclavicular nerves of the cervical plexus emerge and wrap around the belly of the SCM (Ella et al., 2015; Tubbs et al., 2007). Other terms have been used as synonyms for "nerve point," such as Erb's point and McKinney's point; however, those terms are not interchangeable and remain anatomically distinct (Raikos et al., 2017). Erb's point was first described as a superficial point 2–3 cm superior to the clavicle and at the level of the carotid tubercle, placing it approximately at the level of the C6 vertebra (Tubbs et al., 2007). The term great auricular point has also been used in the literature, though less commonly, to define the point of GAN emergence; however, descriptions of this point are similar to, if not the same as, that of the nerve point (Raikos et al., 2017).

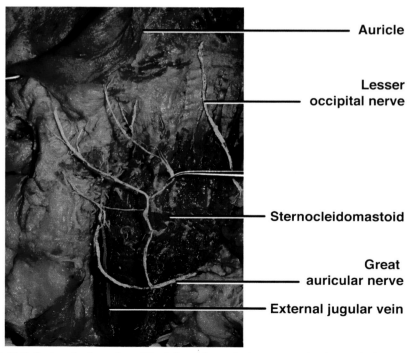

— Auricle

— Lesser occipital nerve

— Sternocleidomastoid

— Great auricular nerve

— External jugular vein

FIG. 3.3 Cadaveric dissection of the left greater auricular nerve noting its terminal branches.

The external acoustic meatus (EAM) is used to identify McKinney's point, which is typically the GAN's point of greatest vulnerability owing to its superficial location (Rohrich et al., 2011; McKinney and Katrana, 1980). McKinney's point is typically found over the belly of the upper one-third of the SCM, 6.5 cm inferior to the EAM (McKinney and Katrana, 1980). This point is roughly lateral to the superior margin of the cricoid cartilage and remains important during cosmetic surgery and anesthetic block (Raikos et al., 2017).

Studies of bony landmarks, including the clavicle, mastoid process, angle of the mandible, and EAM, show that the mastoid process, located slightly posterior and inferior to the EAM, could be a more reliable and less variable landmark for identifying the GAN's course (Raikos et al., 2017). The GAN may have a mastoid branch that is, on average, 9 cm lateral to the inion. On average, this branch is 1 cm superior to the mastoid tip.

The EJV is another widely-used landmark in addition to the bony prominences. The GAN typically travels parallel and approximately 0.5—1.0 cm lateral to the middle and upper thirds of the EJV (Lefkowitz et al., 2013; McKinney and Katrana, 1980).

HISTOLOGY AND PATHOLOGY

The GAN is an ideal nerve for grafting owing to its size, large cross-sectional area, and superficial course (Yang et al., 2015). It closely resembles the composition of the inferior alveolar nerve, lingual nerve, and facial nerve especially, as it has a similar number of fascicles (Tayebi Meybodi et al., 2018). Iwanaga et al. found the mean length of the GAN to be 74.86 ± 20.99 mm and its mean diameter 1.51 ± 0.23 mm distally, 1.38 ± 0.34 mm centrally, and 1.58 ± 0.26 mm proximally (Iwanaga et al., 2019). When it was harvested proximally from the nerve point to a distal point before the division into anterior and posterior branches, Yang et al. found that the fascicles increased in number from proximal to distal (mean 2.5 vs. 5.0) while their cross-sectional area decreased (0.57 vs. 12 mm^2) (Yang et al., 2015).

The GAN can be enlarged in patients with leprosy, as demonstrated in case reports (Gupta et al., 2019; Maurya et al., 2016). While leprosy typically affects the radial, ulnar, common peroneal, and posterior tibial nerves, the condition can be suspected in cases of cordlike swelling along the anterior SCM with sensory loss in the GAN distribution (Maurya et al., 2016). Histology in such cases would show enlarged fascicles with epithelioid granulomas (Maurya et al., 2016).

The GAN is easily identified externally using high-resolution imaging and if widening is noted, clinical suspicion for such pathology can be increased (Noto et al., 2015).

IMAGING

The GAN is easily identified by ultrasound and is a common target during peripheral nerve block for various surgical procedures and pain conditions that require cutaneous anesthesia in the regions of the mandibular angle, parotid gland, inferior helix, lobule, and antitragus (Thallaj et al., 2010; Ritchie et al., 2016). The GAN can first be identified where it lies medial and deep to the SCM. Using an oblique transducer angle, it can be visualized both deep and superficial to the SCM, as it wraps around the SCM's posterior border (Thallaj et al., 2010). GAN blocks are typically administered using this view. Studies have also shown that transcutaneous nerve stimulation can make the GAN easier to identify, especially in cases of variable anatomy (Christ et al., 2012).

CLINICAL AND SURGICAL APPLICATIONS

The GAN is the most commonly injured and sacrificed nerve during parotidectomy and rhytidectomy, more commonly known as a face-lift, with complications reported in up to 6% in both cases (Brown and Dellon, 2018; Ozturk et al., 2014; Lefkowitz et al., 2013; Rohrich et al., 2011; Barbour et al., 2014). The nerve can also be placed at risk of injury by cervical lymph node dissection, carotid endarterectomy, and submandibular gland resection (Duvall et al., 2020). It has been suggested that minimally invasive cervical approaches such as short-scar rhytidectomy increase the rate of complications because surgical field visibility is decreased (Barbour et al., 2014). GAN paresthesia and transient neuropraxia is common postoperatively owing to edema and can be treated expectantly (Brown and Dellon, 2018; Barbour et al., 2014). Neuromas can develop if the GAN or its branches are completely transected and reattach to scar tissue or a skin flap (Yang et al., 2015; Barbour et al., 2014). Such complications can result in trigger points that induce migraine-type pain along the lateral face or neck that can be induced by Tinel's test (Brown and Dellon, 2018; Barbour et al., 2014). In such cases, wide release and decompression is indicated (Barbour et al., 2014). If found, neuromas should be resected and the proximal portion of the GAN should be attached to the SCM or nearby muscle to avoid reattachment to a skin flap (Brown and

Dellon, 2018; Barbour et al., 2014). To avoid GAN injury during rhytidectomy, it is suggested that skin flap elevation is begun in the cheek, thus extending inferiorly at a 30-degree angle over the SCM, increasing the chance of avoiding the nerve's superior course (Ozturk et al., 2014). To avoid GAN injury during parotidectomy, an approach from a point posterior to the EJV is suggested (Yang et al., 2015). Some studies have highlighted the importance of preserving the posterior branch of the GAN to decrease sensory loss and pain syndromes following parotidectomy, which commonly adds 5–15 min of procedural time; however, other studies show the 6-month outcomes are similar regardless of posterior branch sacrifice or preservation (Min et al., 2007; George et al., 2013).

The GAN is ideal for grafting procedures and repair of nerves such as the trigeminal, facial, submandibular, lingual, inferior alveolar, and recurrent laryngeal (Tayebi Meybodi et al., 2018; Iwanaga et al., 2019). In some cases, the donor nerve can prevent muscle atrophy and restore muscle function, including phonation (Iwanaga et al., 2019). In most cases, the GAN can be harvested from an anterior SCM approach, which decreases the risk of iatrogenic nerve injury and is often closer to the primary surgical field during head and neck procedures (Tayebi Meybodi et al., 2018).

Lastly, invasive vagal stimulation following cardiac surgery reduces postoperative atrial fibrillation, which occurs in up to 40% of patients (Andreas et al., 2019). Recent pilot studies using low-level electrical stimulation of the GAN have shown similar promising results, requiring less invasive methods (Andreas et al., 2019). As a result, future multisite trials could be warranted in this regard (Andreas et al., 2019).

REFERENCES

Altafulla, J., Iwanaga, J., Lachkar, S., et al., 2019. The great auricular nerve: anatomical study with application to nerve grafting procedures. World Neurosurg. 125, e403–e407. https://doi.org/10.1016/j.wneu.2019.01.087.

Andreas, M., Arzl, P., Mitterbauer, A., et al., 2019. Electrical stimulation of the greater auricular nerve to reduce postoperative atrial fibrillation. Circ. Arrhythmia. Electrophysiol. 12 (10), 1–7. https://doi.org/10.1161/CIRCEP.119.007711.

Barbour, J.R., Iorio, M.L., Halpern, D.E., 2014. Surgical decompression of the great auricular nerve: a therapeutic option for neurapraxia following rhytidectomy. Plast. Reconstr. Surg. 133 (2), 255–260. https://doi.org/10.1097/01.prs.0000436861.85892.a1.

Brennan, P.A., Webb, R., Kemidi, F., Spratt, J., Standring, S., 2008. Great auricular communication with the marginal mandibular nerve - a previously unreported anatomical variant. Br. J. Oral Maxillofac. Surg. 46 (6), 492–493. https://doi.org/10.1016/j.bjoms.2007.12.005.

Brown, D.L., Dellon, A.L., 2018. Surgical approach to injuries of the cervical plexus and its peripheral nerve branches. Plast. Reconstr. Surg. 141 (4), 1021–1025. https://doi.org/10.1097/PRS.0000000000004240.

Christ, S., Kaviani, R., Rindfleisch, F., Friederich, P., 2012. Identification of the great auricular nerve by ultrasound imaging and transcutaneous nerve stimulation. Anesth. Analg. 114 (5), 1128–1130. https://doi.org/10.1213/ANE.0b013e3182468cc1.

Duvall, J.R., Garza, I., Kissoon, N.R., Robertson, C.E., 2020. Great auricular neuralgia: case series. Headache 60 (1), 247–258. https://doi.org/10.1111/head.13690.

Ella, B., Langbour, N., Caix, P., Midy, D., Deliac, P., Burbaud, P., 2015. Transverse cervical and great auricular nerve distribution in the mandibular area: a study in human cadavers. Clin. Anat. 28 (1), 109–117. https://doi.org/10.1002/ca.22369.

George, M., Karkos, P.D., Dwivedi, R.C., et al., 2013. Preservation of greater auricular nerve during paroidectomy: sensation, quality of life, and morbidity issues. A systemic review. Head Neck. https://doi.org/10.1002/HED.

Gupta, N., Vinod, K.S., Singh, G., Nischal, N., 2019. Bilateral greater auricular nerve thickening in leprosy. QJM An Int. J. Med. https://doi.org/10.1093/qjmed/hcz287.

Iwanaga, J., Altafulla, J.J., Kikuta, S., Tubbs, R.S., 2019. An anatomical feasibility study using a great auricular nerve graft for ipsilateral inferior alveolar nerve repair. J. Craniofac. Surg. 30 (8), 2625–2627. https://doi.org/10.1097/SCS.0000000000005739.

Lefkowitz, T., Hazani, R., Chowdhry, S., Elston, J., Yaremchuk, M.J., Wilhelmi, B.J., 2013. Anatomical landmarks to avoid injury to the great auricular nerve during rhytidectomy. Aesthetic Surg. J. 33 (1), 19–23. https://doi.org/10.1177/1090820X12469625.

Maurya, P.K., Kazmi, K.I., Kulshreshtha, D., Singh, A.K., Malhotra, K.P., 2016. Isolated thickened greater auricular nerve due to leprosy. Neurol. Sci. 37 (4), 649–650. https://doi.org/10.1007/s10072-015-2452-2.

McKinney, P., Katrana, D., 1980. Prevention of injury to the great auricular nerve during rhytidectomy. Plast. Reconstr. Surg. 675–679.

Min, H.J., Lee, H.S., Lee, Y.S., et al., 2007. Is it necessary to preserve the posterior branch of the great auricular nerve in parotidectomy? Otolaryngol. Head Neck Surg. 137 (4), 636–641. https://doi.org/10.1016/j.otohns.2007.05.061.

Noto, Y.I., Shiga, K., Tsuji, Y., et al., 2015. Nerve ultrasound depicts peripheral nerve enlargement in patients with genetically distinct Charcot-Marie-Tooth disease. J. Neurol. Neurosurg. Psychiatry 86 (4), 378–384. https://doi.org/10.1136/jnnp-2014-308211.

Ozturk, C.N., Ozturk, C., Huettner, F., Drake, R.L., Zins, J.E., 2014. A failsafe method to avoid injury to the great auricular nerve. Aesthetic Surg. J. 34 (1), 16–21. https://doi.org/10.1177/1090820X13515881.

Peuker, E.T., Filler, T.J., 2002. The nerve supply of the human auricle. Clin. Anat. 15 (1), 35–37. https://doi.org/10.1002/ca.1089.

Raikos, A., English, T., Yousif, O.K., Sandhu, M., Stirling, A., 2017. Topographic anatomy of the great auricular point: landmarks for its localization and classification. Surg. Radiol. Anat. 39 (5), 535–540. https://doi.org/10.1007/s00276-016-1758-y.

Ritchie, M.K., Wilson, C.A., Grose, B.W., Ranganathan, P., Howell, S.M., Ellison, M.B., 2016. Ultrasound-guided greater auricular nerve block as sole anesthetic for ear surgery. Clin. Pract. 6 (2) https://doi.org/10.4081/cp.2016.856.

Rohrich, R.J., Taylor, N.S., Ahmad, J., Lu, A., Pessa, J.E., 2011. Great auricular nerve injury, the "subauricular band" phenomenon, and the periauricular adipose compartments. Plast. Reconstr. Surg. 127 (2), 835–843. https://doi.org/10.1097/PRS.0b013e318200aa5a.

Tayebi Meybodi, A., Gandhi, S., Lawton, M.T., Preul, M.C., 2018. Anterior greater auricular point: novel anatomic landmark to facilitate harvesting of the greater auricular nerve. World Neurosurg. 119, e64–e70. https://doi.org/10.1016/j.wneu.2018.07.001.

Thallaj, A., Marhofer, P., Moriggl, B., Delvi, B.M., Kettner, S.C., Almajed, M., 2010. Great auricular nerve blockade using high resolution ultrasound: a volunteer study. Anaesthesia 65 (8), 836–840. https://doi.org/10.1111/j.1365-2044.2010.06443.x.

Tubbs, R.S., Loukas, M., Salter, E.G., Oakes, W.J., 2007. Wilhelm Erb and Erb's point. Clin. Anat. 20 (5), 486–488. https://doi.org/10.1002/ca.20385.

Yang, H.M., Kim, H.J., Hu, K.S., 2015. Anatomic and histological study of great auricular nerve and its clinical implication. J. Plast. Reconstr. Aesthetic Surg. 68 (2), 230–236. https://doi.org/10.1016/j.bjps.2014.10.030.

Zohar, Y., Siegal, A., Siegal, G., Halpern, M., Levy, B., Gal, R., 2002. The great auricular nerve; does it penetrate the parotid gland? An anatomical and microscopical study. J. Cranio-Maxillofacial Surg. 30 (5), 318–321. https://doi.org/10.1054/jcms.2002.0287.

CHAPTER 4

The Transverse Cervical Nerve

TESS DECATER • R. SHANE TUBBS

INTRODUCTION

The transverse cervical nerve (also known historically as the "superficial cervical nerve," the "transverse cutaneous nerve of the neck," or the "cutaneous colli nerve") (Malhotra et al., 2012; Rizzolo et al., 1988) is one branch of the cervical plexus, which is formed from the ventral rami of the cervical spinal nerves. In this paper, the anatomy, variants, and clinical significance of the transverse cervical nerve will be discussed.

ANATOMY

The transverse cervical nerve originates from the cervical plexus (C2–3) (Paul, 2016) and its penetration becomes superficial once it passes the posterior border of the sternocleidomastoid muscle near its middle (Figs. 4.1 and 4.2). It lies obliquely forward beneath the external jugular vein to the anterior border of the muscle. It penetrates the deep cervical fascia and then separates beneath the platysma into ascending and descending branches to provide cutaneous innervation to this area (Rizzolo et al., 1988).

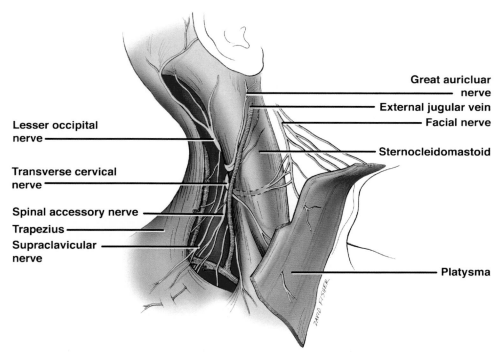

FIG. 4.1 Schematic drawing of the superficial branches of the cervical plexus. Note the course of the transverse cervical nerve and its connections with the facial nerve.

Surgical Anatomy of the Cervical Plexus and its Branches. https://doi.org/10.1016/B978-0-323-83132-1.00005-6

19

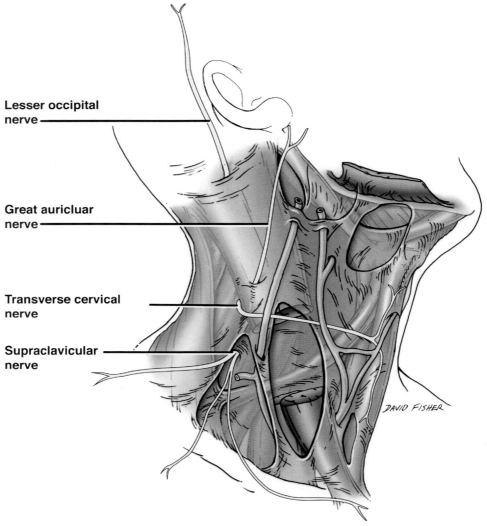

Lesser occipital nerve

Great auricluar nerve

Transverse cervical nerve

Supraclavicular nerve

DAVID FISHER

FIG. 4.2 Schematic drawing of the superficial branches of the cervical plexus. Note the course of the transverse cervical nerve and its relationships to the cervical fasciae and superficial veins of the neck.

The ascending branches travel to the submandibular region to form a plexus with the cervical branch of the facial nerve beneath the platysma muscle (Neil, 2011). The remaining superior branches penetrate the platysma muscle and contribute to the dermatome along the upper and anterior surface of the neck (Fig. 4.3). The ascending communicating branch of these cervical nerves contributes to other cervical nerves, making them wider than the adjacent marginal mandibular branches of the facial nerve. The descending branches penetrate the platysma muscle and contribute to innervating the skin over the anterior

and lateral portion of the neck as far as the sternum (Ziarah and Atkinson, 1981).

ANATOMICAL VARIANTS

The transverse cervical nerve is not always a single nerve; occasionally it comprises two or more nerves branching from the cervical plexus (Tubbs et al., 2016). It has been reported to arise from both C2 and C3 (Paul, 2016), C3 alone, or both C3 and C4 (Tubbs et al., 2016). Anastomosis with the marginal mandibular branch of the facial nerve has been reported (Reuther et al., 2014;

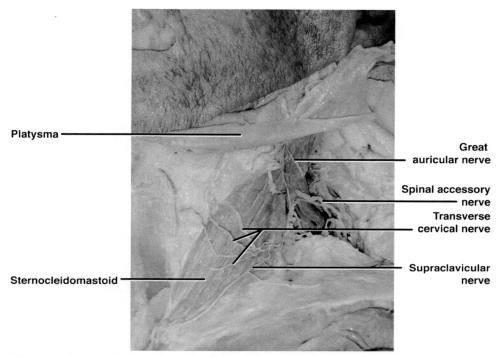

Platysma

Great
auricular nerve

Spinal accessory
nerve

Transverse
cervical nerve

Supraclavicular
nerve

Sternocleidomastoid

FIG. 4.3 Left cadaveric dissection noting the transverse cervical nerve and related nerves of the neck.

Salinas et al., 2009; Ella et al., 2015), although the overall incidence of this anastomosis is not certain (Brennan et al., 2017). To begin this investigation, Brennan et al. (2019) studied 188 cadaver necks and reported an incidence of 2.1%. Anastomosis of the transverse cervical nerve with the cervical branch of the facial nerve is better known, and one cadaveric study by Domet et al. demonstrated this anastomosis in all cases (22/22) (Domet et al., 2005). Communication between those two nerves can either be posterior to the submandibular gland, usually within the parotid gland, or along the inferior border of the submandibular gland (Domet et al., 2005).

Paraskevas et al. reported an aberrant innervation of the sternocleidomastoid (SCM) muscle by the transverse cervical nerve, discovered during a routine cadaveric dissection (Paraskevas et al., 2015). Lin et al. found one cadaveric specimen with the transverse cervical nerve entering the lower border of the posterior mandible (Lin et al., 2013), whereas Rizzolo et al. (1988) found no branches of this nerve entering the mandible.

Kim et al. studied the four cervical cutaneous nerve branches that penetrate the fascia of the posterior border of the SCM muscle: the lesser occipital nerve (L), the great auricular nerve (G), the transverse cervical nerve (T), and the supraclavicular nerves (S). These authors classified them into seven types on the basis of the points at which they emerge. The most common was the separated type (L-G-T-S) with a frequency of 50%, and the second most common was the L-G × T-S type (20.3%), where the great auricular and transverse cervical nerves emerged at the same level on the SCM border.

CLINICAL SIGNIFICANCE

Building a more thorough understanding of the anastomosis between the cervical branch of the facial nerve and the transverse cervical nerve will make it easier to identify a starting point for retrograde facial nerve dissections (Domet et al., 2005). A deeper understanding of the communicating branch of the transverse cervical nerve will also help surgeons to avoid transection of the cervical branch of the facial nerve; numerous common surgical procedures in the area of the submandibular triangle result in its transection (Ziarah and Atkinson, 1981). Patients showed lower lip weakness when the cervical branch of the facial nerve was injured during surgical procedures, presumably because of reduced platysma function (Wildmalm et al., 1985). This was also observed in patients who underwent rhytidectomies during which the cervical branch of the facial nerve was injured (Ella et al., 2015). The anastomosis between the marginal mandibular nerve and the transverse cervical nerve should also be remembered in attempts to lower the risk of postoperative lower lip weakness, as it could be mistaken for the marginal mandibular nerve itself. This becomes especially important when there is limited operative exposure, for instance during submandibular gland removal (Brennan et al., 2019).

One of the major procedures involving encounters of the transverse cervical nerve is carotid endarterectomy. As the transverse cervical nerve travels anteriorly to the SCM muscle, it is often exposed during a standard longitudinal neck incision and its dysfunction is usually due to direct trauma during the procedure, from stretch, retraction, clamping, or transection (Schauber et al., 1997). Dehn and Taylor studied 43 patients undergoing carotid endarterectomy. Among that group, 30 and 27 patients showed clinical evidence of paresthesia over the relevant dermatome at postoperative weeks one and six, respectively (Dehn and Taylor, 1983). Sixty-nine percent of patients experience anesthesia of the transverse cervical nerve 1 week postoperatively, indicating the clinical importance of recognizing this nerve during carotid endarterectomies.

Although communication between the transverse cervical nerve and the cervical branch of the facial nerve has been identified and investigated anatomically, there is surprisingly little mention of it in surgical otolaryngology texts (Gray, 1918; Myers and Carl, 1997).

From the dental perspective, accessory innervation of the posterior part of the mandible by the transverse cervical nerve could account for the failure of anesthesia of the lower teeth, for example, with an inferior alveolar nerve block (Lin et al., 2013). It has been hypothesized that accessory foramina in the mandible provide pathways for branches of the transverse cervical nerve to reach the teeth. However, Rizzolo et al. (1988) found no branches of the transverse cervical nerve entering the mandible. Their conclusion, reported as mirroring those of other studies, was that the supplementary innervation of the mandibular teeth did not involve the transverse cervical nerve. Also, this "supplementary innervation" has no foundation in our knowledge of embryological development. The mandible and mandibular teeth are innervated by the trigeminal complex, the nervous component of the first brachial arch. The skin of the lower border of the mandible, which is derived from the upper cervical segment of the embryo, receives its cutaneous nerve supply from branches of the cervical plexus (Rizzolo et al., 1988).

Pathology

Malhotra et al. reported two cases of bilateral enlargement of the transverse cervical nerve in leprosy patients (Malhotra et al., 2012).

CONCLUSION

Many studies have shown that the branches of the transverse cervical nerve are involved in injury during surgical procedures in the submandibular area, but studies focusing on that nerve are scarce. Further studies on this topic are necessary for helping to avoid minor postoperative side effects.

REFERENCES

Brennan, P.A., Elhamshary, A.S., Alam, P., Anand, R., Ammar, M., 2017. Anastomosis between the transverse cervical nerve and marginal mandibular nerve: how often does it occur? Br. J. Oral Maxillofac. Surg. 55, 293–295.

Brennan, P.A., Mak, J., Massetti, K., Parry, D.A., 2019. Communication between the transverse cervical nerve (C2,3) and marginal mandibular branch of the facial nerve: a cadaveric and clinical study. Br. J. Oral Maxillofac. Surg. 57, 232–235.

Dehn, T.C., Taylor, G.W., 1983. Cranial and cervical nerve damage associated with carotid endarterectomy. Br. J. Surg. 70, 365–368.

Domet, M.A., Connor, N.P., Heisey, D.M., Hartig, G.K., 2005. Anastomoses between the cervical branch of the facial nerve and the transverse cervical cutaneous nerve. Am. J. Otolaryngol. 26, 168–171.

Ella, B., Langbour, N., Caix, P., Midy, D., Deliac, P., Burbaud, P., 2015. Transverse cervical and great auricular nerve distribution in the mandibular area: a study in human cadavers. Clin. Anat. 28, 109–117.

Gray, H., 1918. Anatomy of the Human Body. Lea & Febiger, Philadelphia.

Lin, K., Uzbelger, F.D., Barbe, M.F., 2013. Transverse cervical nerve: implications for dental anesthesia. Clin. Anat. 26, 688–692.

Malhotra, H.S., Garg, R.K., Goel, M.M., 2012. Bilateral enlargement of transverse cervical nerve in two patients of leprosy. Am. J. Trop. Med. Hyg. 86, 382.

Myers, E.N., Carl, H.S., 1997. Operative Otolaryngology Head and Neck Surgery. WB Saunders Company, Philadelphia.

Neil, N., 2011. Netter's Head and Neck Anatomy for Dentistry, second ed. Elsevier/Saunders, Philadelphia.

Paraskevas, G., Lazaridis, N., Spyridakis, I., Koutsouflianiotis, Kitsoulis, P., 2015. Aberrant innervation of the sternocleidomastoid muscle by the transverse cervical nerve: a case report. J. Clin. Diagn. Res. 9, AD01–2.

Paul, R., 2016. Essential Clinically Applied Anatomy of the Peripheral Nervous System in the Head and Neck. Elsevier Inc.

Reuther, W.J., Blythe, J.N., Anand, R., Brennan, P.A., 2014. Communication of the transverse cervical nerve with the marginal mandibular nerve: a previously unreported anatomical variant. Br. J. Oral Maxillofac. Surg. 52, 577–578.

Rizzolo, R.C.J., Madeira, M.C., Bernaba, J.M., de Freitas, V., 1988. Clinical significance of the supplementary innervation of the mandibular teeth: a dissection study of the transverse cervical (cutaneous colli) nerve. Quintessence Int. 19, 167–169.

Salinas, N.L., Jackson, O., Dunham, B., Bartlett, S.P., 2009. Anatomical dissection and modified Sihler stain of the lower branches of the facial nerve. Plast. Reconstr. Surg. 124, 1905–1915.

Schauber, M.D., Fontenelle, L.J., Solomon, J.W., Hanson, T.L., 1997. Cranial/cervical nerve dysfunction after carotid endarterectomy. J. Vasc. Surg. 25, 481–487.

Tubbs, R.S., Shoja, M.M., Loukas, M., 2016. Bergman's Comprehensive Encyclopedia of Human Anatomic Variation. John Wiley & Sons, New Jersey.

Wildmalm, S.E., Nemeth, P.A., Ash Jr., M.M., Lillie, J.H., 1985. The anatomy and electrical activity of the platysma muscle. J. Oral Rehabil. 12, 17–22.

Ziarah, H.A., Atkinson, M.E., 1981. The surgical anatomy of the cervical distribution of the facial nerve. Br. J. Oral Surg. 19, 171–179.

FURTHER READING

Kim, H.J., Koh, K.S., Oh, C.S., Hu, K.S., Kang, J.W., Chung, I.H., 2002. Emerging patterns of the cervical cutaneous nerves in Asians. Int. J. Oral Maxillofac. Surg. 31, 53–56.

Pandit, J.J., Satya-Krishna, R., Gration, P., 2007. Superficial or deep cervical plexus block for carotid endarterectomy: a systematic review of complications. Br. J. Anaesth. 99, 159–169.

CHAPTER 5

The Supraclavicular Nerve

TESS DECATER • R. SHANE TUBBS

INTRODUCTION

The supraclavicular nerve is a sensory branch of the cervical plexus, originating from C3 and C4 spinal nerves (Imada et al., 2017; Giddie et al., 2017; Nathe et al., 2011; Rockwood and Matsen, 2009; Mancall and Brock, 2011) (Figs. 5.1 and 5.2). These nerves travel over the clavicle, then over the pectoralis major and deltoid muscles, and finally, over the upper and posterior shoulder. The medial supraclavicular nerve provides sensation to the anterior neck and clavicle, while the intermediate and lateral nerves provide sensation to the anteromedial shoulder and proximal thorax up to the midline (Nathe et al., 2011; Tubbs et al., 2015). Variations exist in the pathways of these nerves that involve boney tunnels through the clavicle and entrapments caused by other structures such as muscles. This nerve's close relationship to the clavicle makes it vulnerable during clavicular fractures and surgical procedures. In this chapter, the supraclavicular nerve will be reviewed, along with its anatomical variations and clinical significance.

ANATOMY

As mentioned earlier, the supraclavicular nerve is a superficial sensory branch of the cervical plexus (Giddie et al., 2017) and originates from C3 and C4 (Imada et al., 2017; Giddie et al., 2017; Nathe et al., 2011; Rockwood and Matsen, 2009; Mancall and Brock, 2011). The ventral rami of C3 and C4 emerge between the longus colli and longus capitis and scalenus medius (Rockwood and Matsen, 2009) and combine to form a common trunk (Tubbs et al., 2015). This trunk emerges from beneath the sternocleidomastoid (SCM) muscle (Imada et al., 2017) and descends in the posterior cervical triangle of the neck beneath the platysma and deep cervical fascia (Mancall and Brock, 2011) (Fig. 5.3). It then divides into three groups: the medial, intermediate, and lateral supraclavicular nerves (Imada et al., 2017). Finally, these groups pierce the deep cervical fascia and platysma above the clavicle (Giddie et al., 2017; Tubbs et al., 2015) to become cutaneous (Gray, 1918). These three groups are referred to by different names in other texts: the medial supraclavicular is also known as the anterior supraclavicular, the intermediate supraclavicular as the middle supraclavicular, and the lateral supraclavicular as the posterior supraclavicular (Tubbs et al., 2015). Historically, the intermediate supraclavicular nerve was termed the supraclavicular nerve, the lateral supraclavicular nerve the supraacromial nerve, and the medial supraclavicular nerve the suprasternal nerve.

The branches of the medial supraclavicular nerves run inferomedially across the external jugular vein, the medial third of the clavicle, and the sternal head of the SCM. These branches supply the sensory innervation to the skin of the thorax up to the midline and down to the level of the second rib, as well as the sternoclavicular joint (Tubbs et al., 2015). The intermediate nerves cross the middle third of the clavicle to supply the skin over the pectoralis major and deltoid muscles (Tubbs et al., 2015). The intermediate nerves supply structures that are closely related to those supplied by the second intercostal nerve and one study reports that the cutaneous branches of the upper intercostal nerves communicate with the intermediate nerve branches of the supraclavicular nerve (Gray, 1918). However, the extent of overlap and communication between these nerves may be minimal (Tubbs et al., 2015). The lateral supraclavicular nerve descends superficially over the trapezius, the lateral third of the clavicle, and the acromion and innervates the skin of the upper and posterior shoulder down to the level of the second rib (Gray, 1918).

These nerve branches are also responsible for neck or shoulder pain during times of pleural irritation. Referred pain from the central diaphragmatic pleura, as well as the mediastinal pleura, can be referred to these locations through the phrenic nerves (C3-5)

Surgical Anatomy of the Cervical Plexus and its Branches. https://doi.org/10.1016/B978-0-323-83132-1.00006-8

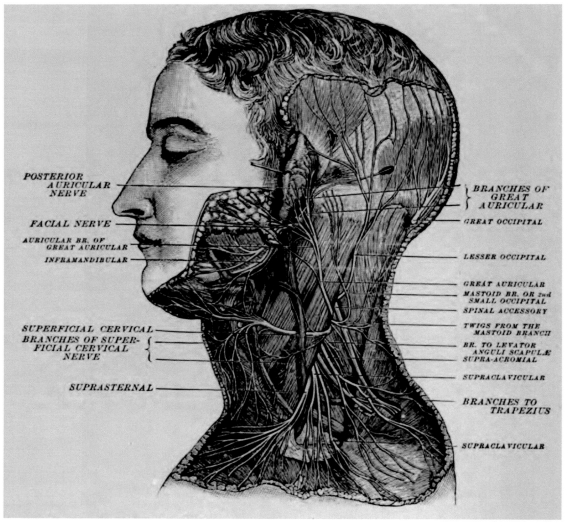

POSTERIOR
AURICULAR
NERVE

FACIAL NERVE

AURICULAR BR. OF
GREAT AURICULAR

INFRAMANDIBULAR

SUPERFICIAL CERVICAL
BRANCHES OF SUPER-
FICIAL CERVICAL
NERVE

SUPRASTERNAL

BRANCHES OF
GREAT
AURICULAR

GREAT OCCIPITAL

LESSER OCCIPITAL

GREAT AURICULAR
MASTOID BR. OR 2nd
SMALL OCCIPITAL
SPINAL ACCESSORY

TWIGS FROM THE
MASTOID BRANCH

BR. TO LEVATOR
ANGULI SCAPULÆ
SUPRA-ACROMIAL

SUPRACLAVICULAR

BRANCHES TO
TRAPEZIUS

SUPRACLAVICULAR

FIG. 5.1 Schematic drawing of the left cervical plexus (after Morris). Note the course of the supraclavicular nerve.

because the supraclavicular nerves (C3-5) are involved in supplying some of the skin at these locations (Singh, 2014).

During a study of 20 healthy subjects and two patients with supraclavicular nerve lesions, it was reported that the mean conduction velocity of the branches of this nerve was 70–78 m/s (SD 8–10 m/s), with an amplitude of 3–4 µV (SD 0.9–1.0 µV). This study also found no side-to-side or sex differences for the supraclavicular nerve (Martinez-Aparicio et al., 2018).

ANATOMICAL VARIANTS

Most of the literature on this nerve reports that it originates from C3 and C4; however, some have stated it arises from C2, C3, and C4 (Chung, 2009). Additionally, most studies describe the pathway of this nerve as being beneath the platysma muscle until its three branches reach the clavicle and pierce through this muscle and the deep cervical fascia. However, one report described this nerve as descending on the superficial surface of the platysma (Rockwood and Matsen, 2009).

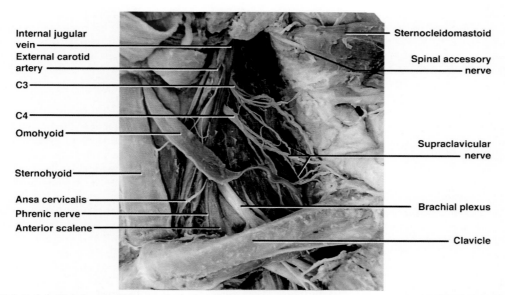

FIG. 5.2 Left cadaveric dissection (embalmed specimen) noting the supraclavicular nerve at its origin from C3 and C4 ventral rami and its relationship to regional nerves.

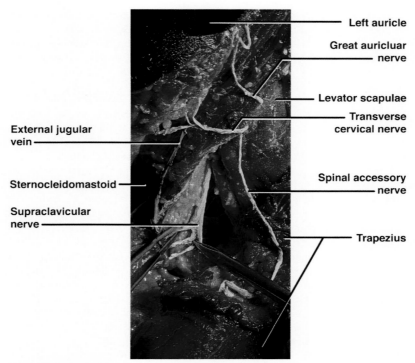

FIG. 5.3 Left cadaveric dissection (fresh frozen specimen) noting the supraclavicular nerve and its relationship to regional nerves.

Different branching patterns and nerve arrangements have also been discovered during investigations of the supraclavicular nerve. One group found that in some subjects, the intermediate and lateral branches emerged from a common trunk behind the SCM, at a mean distance of 96 mm (70–137) from the sternal angle (Havet et al., 2007). The intermediate branch then divided into two or three secondary rami, and the lateral branch divided into two or three rami in eight subjects while not dividing at all in six subjects (Havet et al., 2007). Other studies have found the intermediate branch to be completely absent, with the areas normally supplied by this branch being innervated by the medial and lateral branches (Tubbs et al., 2015).

In a study conducted by Nathe et al., it was found that 97% of their specimens had medial and lateral branches, 49% of specimens had an intermediate branch, and one specimen had only a medial branch (2.7%) (Nathe et al., 2011). This research team then grouped the specimens into two groups: group 1 had medial and lateral nerve branches (49%) and group 2 had medial, intermediate, and lateral nerve branches (49% of specimens). Nathe et al. also found that two or three nerves predictably crossed the clavicle in 97% of their subjects; however, there was considerable variability in the distance from certain landmarks to these nerves. From this observation, they concluded that there is no clinically relevant predictable safe zone between the medial and lateral branches, but small safe zones exist medially and laterally with no medial branches found within 2.7 cm of the sternoclavicular joint and no lateral branches found within 1.9 cm of the acromioclavicular joint (Nathe et al., 2011).

A common variant of the supraclavicular nerve is that in which some of its branches perforate the clavicle. This variant is described as passing through a bony tunnel or groove on the superior surface, making the nerve vulnerable to injury during clavicular fractures or surgical manipulation (Natsis et al., 2019). Some studies have reported that this variant occurs with a frequency of 1%–6.6% (Giddie et al., 2017; Natsis et al., 2019), while in a study conducted by Papadatos, using 254 specimens, the incidence of clavicular tunneling by this nerve was reported as 4%, with 3% of those cases being male (Papadatos, 1980). The formation of interclavicular canals, which can be superficial or deep, has been deduced to occur later than original bone formation, enclosing nerves late in development. Polarizing microscope analysis supports this claim, showing that these canals do not have the same structure as perforating canals of Volkmann (Papadatos, 1980). A study by Giddie et al. further supports this theory by their conclusion that the supraclavicular nerve does not pierce the clavicle, but rather gets enclosed during the late stages of ossification (Giddie et al., 2017).

Investigations into which nerves tunnel through the clavicle have been conflicting. One report on the supraclavicular nerves concluded that it is the medial nerve group that can have an anomalous pattern in which it passes through foramina in the clavicle its way to the anterior chest (Rockwood and Matsen, 2009). However, Tubbs et al. (2006) found that the right intermediate branch pierced the clavicle of a male cadaver, and others have reported that the intermediate branch of the supraclavicular nerve was the most commonly entrapped (Giddie et al., 2017).

A branch to the phrenic nerve may pass down into the thorax over the subclavian artery or vein before joining the phrenic nerve. An additional bundle from the fifth cervical nerve joining this nerve has been reported. A branch to the rhomboid muscles may pass through the trapezius muscle on its way to the skin close to the midline, at the level of the spinous processes of the fifth and sixth thoracic vertebrae (Tubbs et al., 2015).

It is important to note that variations in the pathway of the supraclavicular nerve and its branches near the clavicle are not only due to bony canals in the clavicle but also to abnormal fibrous and muscular structures (Jelev and Surchev, 2007). These become especially important during diagnosis and treatment procedures involving clavicular fractures.

CLINICAL SIGNIFICANCE

The supraclavicular nerves have a close relationship to the clavicle, making it vulnerable to injury in association with clavicular fractures and operative exposure of the clavicle (O'Neill et al., 2012; Jupiter and Leibman, 2007). Procedures used to correct clavicular fractures, such as plate positioning during clavicle fracture fixation, may require division of this nerve for appropriate plate positioning (Giddie et al., 2017), with anterior chest wall numbness commonly occurring postoperatively (Imada et al., 2017). This nerve is also commonly exposed during transverse or vertical incisions along the clavicle, and the frequency of postoperative incisional and proximal chest wall numbness is about 10%–29% (Giddie et al., 2017; Nathe et al., 2011). Notably, vertical incisions have been reported as being less likely to cause postoperative numbness (Giddie et al., 2017).

Symptoms of entrapment syndrome of the supraclavicular nerves (Imada et al., 2017) when they travel through the clavicle are thought to be due to narrowed osseous clavicular tunnels (Raikos et al., 2014; Omokawa et al., 2005). The supraclavicular nerves that tunnel through the clavicle are compressed as a result of overuse of the shoulder joint causing pain in the neck, clavicular, thorax, and shoulder region (Imada et al., 2017). Although this syndrome is considered to be rare (Tubbs et al., 2006; Douchamps et al., 2012), it should be included as a differential during cases of anterior shoulder girdle pain (Giddie et al., 2017; Tubbs et al., 2006; Douchamps et al., 2012). It is also important to remember the possibility of nerve tunnels through the clavicle while studying chest and shoulder radiographs (Natsis et al., 2019).

Other than tunnels in the clavicle, there has been a report of a patient with supraclavicular nerve compression by a cardiac implantable electrical device implantation (Imada et al., 2017). Additionally, entrapment syndrome can be due to other anatomical variations involving bony structures, fibrous bands, muscles, or tendons (Giddie et al., 2017; Tubbs et al., 2006; Jelev and Surchev, 2007). One study found that the entrapment of this nerve was being controlled by a unique location of the supraclavicularis muscle. This unique muscle variant had fibers originating posteriorly on the medial clavicle and then it formed an arch over the supraclavicular nerve (Raikos et al., 2014). All of these possibilities must be considered before choosing a treatment option for surgical decompression.

The supraclavicular nerve has also been noted as being important to preserve as a potential donor for nerve graft material (Chung, 2009). An example of this was shown in a study conducted on trigeminal nerve palsy. Neurotization of the mental nerve with the supraclavicular nerve was shown to restore sensation to the lower lip in patients with dysfunction of the trigeminal nerve (Mucci and Dellon, 1997).

Finally, interscalene brachial plexus blockade and selective supraclavicular nerve blockade (SNB) have been associated with successful outcomes in the treatment of clavicle fractures while avoiding complications commonly associated with cervical plexus blockade (Ozen, 2019), such as phrenic nerve paralysis. Ueshima and Otake (2016) completed a selective supraclavicular nerve blockade rather than a cervical plexus nerve block to anesthetize the supraclavicular nerve. Administering the nerve block at the site of the pectoralis major muscle enabled safety and ease, and it was postulated as being a possible effective alternative for patients with bilateral pneumothorax, hemorrhagic diathesis, low pulmonary reserve (Ozen, 2019), and other severe complications. Other study teams performed an SNB using the supraclavicular approach but found a greater risk of phrenic nerve block if more than required volumes of anesthetic were injected.

CONCLUSION

The supraclavicular nerve is closely associated with the clavicle, making it a clinically significant structure during clavicular injuries and procedures. It is also an important component of differential diagnoses during cases of shoulder girdle pain. The many variations of the supraclavicular nerve are important to recognize and understand before operative procedures or nerve blocks to better avoid nerve injury. Additionally, selective supraclavicular nerve blocks should be investigated further to better understand their efficacy and risk profile in comparison to cervical nerve blocks during treatments of clavicular fractures.

REFERENCES

Chung, K.C. (Ed.), 2009. Hand and Upper Extremity Reconstruction. Saunders Elsevier, p. 249.

Douchamps, F., Courtois, A.C., Bruyère, P.J., Crielaard, J.M., 2012. Supraclavicular nerve entrapment syndrome. Joint Bone Spine 79, 88−89.

Giddie, J., Fisher, R., White, A., 2017. A rare anatomical variant: transosseous supraclavicular nerve identified during clavicle fracture fixation. J. Surg. Case Rep. 2017, rjx230.

Gray, H., 1918. Anatomy of the Human Body, twentieth ed. Lea & Febiger, Philadelphia and New York, p. 928.

Havet, E., Duparc, F., Tobenas-Dujardin, A.C., Muller, J.M., Fréger, P., 2007. Morphometric study of the shoulder and subclavicular innervation by the intermediate and lateral branches of supraclavicular nerves. Surg. Radiol. Anat. 29, 605−610.

Imada, H., Fukuzawa, K., Kichuchi, K., Hirata, K.I., Sato, H., 2017. Experience managing pain associated with supraclavicular nerves compressed by a cardiac implantable electrical device, diagnosed by the local nerve block. J. Arrhythm. 34, 84−86.

Jelev, L., Surchev, L., 2007. Study of variant anatomical structures (bony canals, fibrous bands, and muscles) in relation to potential supraclavicular nerve entrapment. Clin. Anat. 20, 278−285.

Jupiter, J.B., Leibman, M.I., 2007. Supraclavicular nerve entrapment due to clavicular fracture callus. J. Shoulder Elbow Surg. 16, e13−e14.

Mancall, E.L., Brock, D.G., 2011. In: Mancall, E.L., Brock, D.G. (Eds.), Gray's Clinical Neuroanatomy: The Anatomic Bases for Clinical Neuroscience. Elsevier Saunders, Philadelphia, p. 315.

Martinez-Aparicio, C., Jääskeläinen, S.K., Muyor, J.M., Falck, B., 2018. Nerve conduction study of the three supraclavicular nerve branches. Muscle Nerve 58, 300−303.

Mucci, S.J., Dellon, A.L., 1997. Restoration of lower-lip sensation: neurotization of the mental nerve with the supraclavicular nerve. J. Reconstr. Microsurg. 13, 151–155.

Nathe, T., Tseng, S., Yoo, B., 2011. The anatomy of the supraclavicular nerve during surgical approach to the clavicular shaft. Clin. Orthop. Relat. Res. 469, 890–894.

Natsis, K., Totlis, T., Chorti, A., Karanassos, M., Didagelos, M., Lazaridis, N., 2019. Tunnels and grooves for supraclavicular nerves within the clavicle: review of the literature and clinical impact. Surg. Radiol. Anat. 38, 687–691.

O'Neill, K., Stutz, C., Duvernay, M., Schoenecher, J., 2012. Supraclavicular nerve entrapment and clavicular fracture. J. Orthop. Trauma 26, e63–e65.

Omokawa, S., Tanaka, Y., Miyauchi, Y., Komei, T., Takakura, Y., 2005. Traction neuropathy of the supraclavicular nerve attributable to an osseous tunnel of the clavicle. Clin. Orthop. Relat. Res. 238–240.

Ozen, V., 2019. Ultrasound-guided, combined application of selective supraclavicular nerve and low-dose interscalene brachial plexus block in a high-risk patient. Hippokratia 23, 25–27.

Papadatos, D., 1980. Supraclavicular nerves perforating the clavicle. Study of 10 cases. Anat. Anz. 147, 371–381.

Raikos, A., English, T., Agnihotri, A., Yousif, O.K., Sandhu, M., Bennetto, J., Stirling, A., 2014. Supraclavicularis proprius muscle associated with supraclavicular nerve entrapment. Folia Morphol. (Warsz) 73, 527–530.

Rockwood, C.A., Matsen, F.A. (Eds.), 2009. The Shoulder, fourth ed. Saunders Elsevier, Philadelphia, p. 77.

Singh, V., 2014. Textbook of Anatomy: Upper Limb and Thorax, second ed. Reed Elsevier India Private Limited, p. 231.

Tubbs, R.S., Rizk, E., Sohja, M.M., Loukas, M., Barbaro, N., Spinner, R.J. (Eds.), 2015. Nerves and Nerve Injuries Volume 1: History, Embryology, Anatomy, Imagine, and Diagnostics. Elsevier.

Tubbs, R.S., Salter, E.G., Oakes, W.J., 2006. Anomaly of the supraclavicular nerve: case report and review of the literature. Clin. Anat. 19, 599–601.

Ueshima, H., Otake, H., 2016. Successful clavicle fracture surgery performed under selective supraclavicular nerve block using the new subclavian approach. JA Clin. Rep. 2, 34.

CHAPTER 6

The Phrenic Nerve

GRAHAM DUPONT • R. SHANE TUBBS

INTRODUCTION

An important branch of the cervical plexus arising principally off the ventral ramus of C4, also receiving contributions from C3 and C5, is the phrenic nerve (Fig. 6.1). The phrenic nerve continues inferiorly from its origin, through the neck and upper thorax, passing beyond the mediastinum to project fibers into the parietal pleura and fibrous pericardium; the right and left phrenic nerves vary slightly in their path through the mediastinum, and furthermore, pierce and innervate the right and left diaphragmatic domes, respectively, conveying motor and sensory fibers to its recipients.

The anatomy of the phrenic nerve has been appreciated in extensive detail, both in its fluctuating architecture—an accessory phrenic nerve is observed in rare cases to innervate muscles of the neck—and inferior continuations, appropriate for the practicing clinician in the treatment of high cervical spine injury, brachial plexus injuries, and diaphragmatic palsy or paresis (Gu et al., 1989; Bergman et al., 1996; Robaux et al., 2001; Oliver and Zito, 2018). Iatrogenic injury to the phrenic nerve is common in nerve blocks for surgical approaches to the shoulder, in cardiac surgery, and radiofrequency energy delivery (Efthimiou et al., 1991; Bunch et al., 2005). More generally, any lesions to the phrenic nerve risk paralysis of the ipsilateral hemisphere of the diaphragm, which may be potentially life-threatening for infants (Joho-Arreola et al., 2005). Referred pain in the shoulder may often indicate phrenic nerve injury after thoracotomy (Scawn et al., 2001).

Indeed, appreciating the course of the phrenic nerve and its relationship to its flanking viscera in the mediastinum is of great importance for limiting surgical complications. This chapter is dedicated to the phrenic nerve, providing the reader with the detailed organization of this nerve and its neighboring structures, physiology, embryology, studies of interest, surgical relevance and complications, and other salient topics for the practical knowledge of the clinician.

ANATOMY
Origins in the Brainstem

The respiratory system is under two modes of control: voluntary and automatic. For voluntary control of respiration, corticospinal tracts in the dorsolateral spinal cord descend from the forebrain; in automatic control, these axons descend from the ventral and lateral columns of the spinal cord that originate at the pons and medulla. It was proposed that the brainstem contained four respiratory centers: pneumotaxic and apneustic, which have an inhibitory effect on one another; and expiratory and gasping centers (Lumsden, 1923a,b,c). Control centers in the medulla were discovered by Archard and Bucher (1954), Baumgarten et al. (1957), and Merrill (1970), wherein three aggregations of rhythmic respiratory nuclei were uncovered: a dorsal respiratory group related to the nucleus of the tractus solitarius (NTS); and two ventrolateral masses of neurons related to the nucleus ambiguus and nucleus retroambigualis. The pneumotaxic center proposed by Lumsden's model was reported to originate within the nucleus parabrachialis in the dorsolateral rostral pons, and upon electrical stimulation to this area, neurophysiological changes were observed in the phrenic nerve (Mitchell and Berger, 1975). A dorsal respiratory group of neurons near the NTS are responsible for rhythmic excitations to contralateral phrenic motoneurons (Nair et al., 2017).

Origins in the Spinal Cord and Cervical Plexus

These respiratory nuclei send their tracts down the medulla oblongata as it nears the foramen magnum, whereby the brainstem transitions into the spinal cord. The efferent projections of the phrenic nerve exit the upper and midcervical ventral roots. The ventral rami of C1—C4 interdigitate to form the cervical plexus, providing innervation to the infrahyoid muscles, anterolateral skin of the neck, the angle of the mandible, and the diaphragm (Standring, 2016). The phrenic

Surgical Anatomy of the Cervical Plexus and its Branches. https://doi.org/10.1016/B978-0-323-83132-1.00013-5

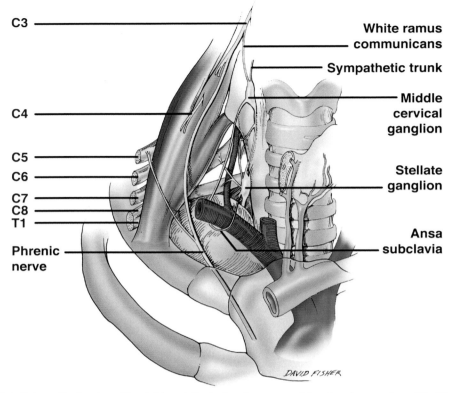

C3

White ramus
communicans

Sympathetic trunk

Middle
cervical
ganglion

C4

C5
C6
C7
C8
T1

Stellate
ganglion

Phrenic
nerve

Ansa
subclavia

DAVID FISHER

FIG. 6.1 Schematic drawing of the right neck illustrating the source of the phrenic nerve from C3—C5 ventral rami.

nerve originates from the ventral rami of C3—C5, conveying motor, sensory, and sympathetic fibers to the diaphragm. The motor branches of the phrenic nerve are conveyed to the diaphragmatic muscle, and the sensory branches to the central tendon. Though primarily consisting of motor axons, the remaining 30%—45% are sensory afferents and sympathetic fibers (Landau et al., 1962; Duron and Caillol, 1973; Frazier and Revelette, 1991; Nair et al., 2017). Of these fibers, 60% are estimated to be myelinated, and 40% unmyelinated (Nair et al., 2017). Langford and Schmidt (1983) noted these myelinated and unmyelinated axons, where the dorsal root ganglion and ventral root contribute 31% and 69% of the myelinated axons of the phrenic nerve, respectively. Furthermore, it was determined that the dorsal root ganglion contributes 59%, cervical sympathetic trunk 24%, and ventral roots 17%, to the unmyelinated axons. The phrenic nerve contains mechanosensitive receptors in the fibrous layer of the pericardium, which were demonstrated to have a

cardiac rhythm as well as exhibiting sensitivity to increasing lung volume (Kostreva and Pontus, 1993a,b). Interestingly, the phrenic nerve afferents rising from the diaphragm have been shown to reflexively contribute to the respiratory rhythm (Frazier and Revelette, 1991). Kostreva and Pontus (1993a,b) also discovered mechanoreceptors in the hepatic veins and parenchyma, and in the inferior vena cava, with phrenic nerve afferents. Bergman et al. (1996) describes a direct communication between the inferior cervical ganglion and the phrenic nerve. Mechanosensitive and nociceptive branches of the phrenic are also provided to the mediastinal surface of the pleura and pericardium (Oliver and Zito, 2018).

Innervation of the Thorax and Diaphragm
In the thorax, the phrenic nerve is contained within the middle mediastinum. The left and right phrenic nerves differ slightly in their course down the mediastinum. The left phrenic nerve descends on the anterior scalene

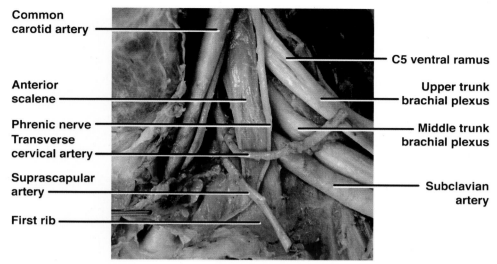

Common carotid artery

Anterior scalene

Phrenic nerve
Transverse cervical artery

Suprascapular artery

First rib

C5 ventral ramus

Upper trunk brachial plexus

Middle trunk brachial plexus

Subclavian artery

FIG. 6.2 Left cadaveric dissection noting the course of the phrenic nerve over the anterior scalene muscle.

muscle and flanks the subclavian artery (Fig. 6.2). The right phrenic courses are superficial to the anterior scalene muscle and second part of the subclavian artery (Fig. 6.3). The phrenic nerves descend bilaterally, anterior to the roots of the lungs between the mediastinal surface of the parietal pleura and fibrous pericardium (Oliver and Zito, 2018) (Fig. 6.4). The right phrenic nerve laterally flanks the right atrium and ventricle to provide innervation to the right diaphragmatic dome. The right phrenic nerve passes through the caval foramen (Bhimji and Burns, 2017). The left phrenic nerve passes anterior to the pericardial sac at the left ventricle to supply the central tendon and left diaphragmatic dome (Fig. 6.5). In the thorax, the right and left phrenic nerves divide into a variable number of branches, ranging from two to seven (Botha, 1957). The diaphragmatic portion of the parietal pleura is also innervated by the phrenic nerve (Goizueta and Bhimji, 2018). Motor innervation of the diaphragm results in contraction of the diaphragm during inspiration, depressing the diaphragm and increasing the pleural space to allow for expansion of the lungs. Exhalation reposes the diaphragm into its normal dome-like shape.

BLOOD SUPPLY

In a historical review of the blood supply of nerves, Adams (1942) articulated the vasa nervorum or "arteries which run in company of nerves." Of these, he described the arteriae comites—vessels that, while chiefly providing blood to neighboring tissues, supply the nerve that they escort. The arteriae comites send branches to cutaneous nerves as well as deeper nerves such as the phrenic nerve. In turn, the phrenic nerve also provides vasomotor innervation to the arteriae comites that supply it. In regards to the diaphragm, the superior phrenic, musculophrenic, inferior phrenic, and pericardiocophrenic, all provide blood to this muscular structure (Bhimji and Burns, 2017; Goizueta and Bhimji, 2018). The superior phrenic arteries issue from the thoracic aorta; the musculophrenic and pericardiacophrenic arteries are branches from the internal thoracic artery, and the inferior phrenic arteries issue from the superior aspect and anterior trunk of the abdominal aorta, atop the celiac artery. The pericardiacophrenic arteries and veins also flank their respective phrenic nerves on their way to be distributed to the diaphragm, also being anastomosed with the musculophrenic and superior phrenic arteries (Drake, 1918).

EMBRYOLOGY

Interestingly, the phrenic nerve is the first nerve whose fibers reach complete development and terminate before any other spinal nerve in the developing embryo (Amin, 1914). The embryological development of the phrenic nerve occurs in tandem with the musculotendinous diaphragm of the human fetus, of which there are

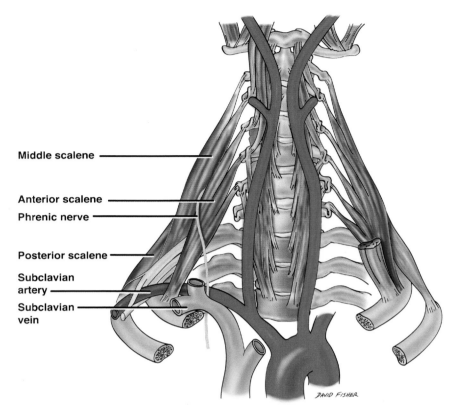

Middle scalene

Anterior scalene

Phrenic nerve

Posterior scalene

Subclavian artery

Subclavian vein

DAVID FISHER

FIG. 6.3 Schematic drawing of the neck illustrating the course of the phrenic nerve as it leaves the neck to enter the thorax.

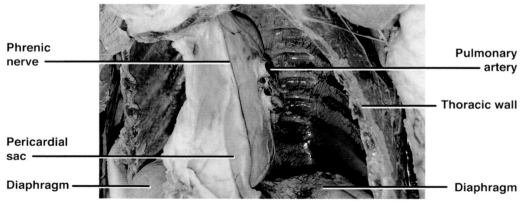

Phrenic nerve

Pericardial sac

Diaphragm

Pulmonary artery

Thoracic wall

Diaphragm

FIG. 6.4 Left cadaveric dissection noting the course of the phrenic nerve over the pericardial sac. Note the pericardiacophrenic vessels traveling with the nerve.

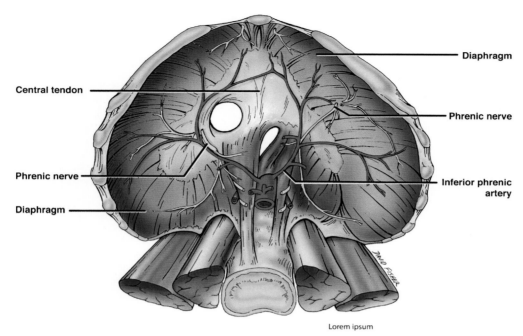

Lorem ipsum

FIG. 6.5 Schematic drawing of the inferior surface of the diaphragm and course of the phrenic nerves.

many gaps in understanding of this phenomenon. Chiefly related to the formation of the phrenic nerves is the septum transversum, which, along with the pleuroperitoneal membranes, dorsal mesentery of the esophagus, and body wall, gives rise to the diaphragm (Schumpelick et al., 2000).

During the fifth week of gestation, as the septum transversum is migrating downward, nerves issue from the fourth and fifth cervical segments and travel through the pleuropericardial folds and into the septum transversum, forming the phrenic nerves. Lateral to each issuing nerve is the remains of a somite. Amin (1914) provides a description of the course of the phrenic nerve starting at the level of the fourth cervical ganglion. The nerve descends, moving ventrally to situate itself behind the anterior cardinal vein, where it then forms a confluence with the fifth cervical nerve. This main trunk then rests in a cup-shaped indention at the ramification of the anterior cardinal and primitive subclavian vein. As it descends further, the nerve comes into contact with the early part of the coelomic cavity, flanked laterally by the anterolateral recess and medially by the pleuropericardial passage. The nerve descends even further, situating lateral to the lung bud and posterior to the pericardium.

The phrenic nerve finds its final location between the pericardium and mediastinal pleura due to the detachment of the pleuroperitoneal folds from the somatopleure; this detachment forms the pericardium (Schumpelick et al., 2000). By the eighth week of gestation, the diaphragm has descended significantly from the level of the thoracic somites (week 6) to the L1 vertebra. The descent of the diaphragm pulls the phrenic nerves inferiorly to reach their adult length.

PHYSIOLOGY

The coordination activation of the respiratory muscles is due to motoneurons that stretch from the respiratory centers in the brainstem through the lumbar levels of the spinal cord. Rhythmic contraction of the diaphragm is overseen by these phrenic motoneurons. Phrenic motoneurons are widely distributed about the C3—C6 levels of the spinal cord, and predominantly concentrated in the C4 and C5 spinal segments. The geometrical configuration of phrenic motoneuron soma is pyramidal or fusiform (Dobbins and Feldman, 1994). The physiological model of generation of breathing has undergone several cosmetic changes, with current advancements favoring the pre-Bötzinger complex in the origin of the respiratory rhythm (Feldman et al., 2013). Phrenic motoneurons also receive input from bulbospinal (second-order) neurons from the rostral ventral respiratory groups within the lateral tegmental field, and dorsal respiratory (third-order) groups of the NTS within the brainstem (Dobbins and Feldman, 1994; Ghali, 2018). Of the premotoneurons in the brainstem, the rostral ventral group is the principal governing population over the phasic activity of the phrenic motoneurons (Dobbins and Feldman, 1994). Ghali (2018) proposed a general model of the phasic activity phrenic motoneurons, wherein phrenic motoneurons receive phasic input during inspiration via the rostral ventral respiratory group and phrenic premotoneurons from C1—C2 spinal cord levels; phasic inhibition may also stem from projections of the Bötzinger complex.

The pre-Bötzinger complex influences respiratory activity via its projections to premotoneurons of the rostral ventral respiratory group and hypoglossal nerve, which then send their projections for inspiratory motor output inferiorly to the diaphragm and intercostal muscles (Feldman et al., 2013). Tonic excitation from below is received from the nucleus gigantocellularis and its pars alpha portion, and median raphe of the medullary reticular formation. Interneurons located in the phrenic nucleus may also display excitatory and inhibitory behavior. A marked decrease in phrenic nerve activity as a result of phrenic motoneuron inhibition is observed before the postinspiratory period, that is, the interval at which inspiration ends, inward airflow ceases, and the expiratory phase begins. Following the expiratory and preinspiratory phases, there is a sharp peak in phrenic nerve activity right before inhalation that slows outward airflow by contracting and lengthening the diaphragm, in preparation for the next phase of the respiratory cycle (Feldman et al., 2013).

VARIATIONS

Variations of the phrenic nerve are not rare and are described in reports in the literature as early as the 19th century (Larkin, 1889). A common variant, the accessory phrenic nerve, whose origins are described by Bergman et al. (1996), may arise from C5, or C5 and C6, passing in front or behind the subclavian vein and joining the inferior continuation of the main phrenic nerve either the neck or the thorax. The reported incidence of this variant is up to 75% (Bergman et al., 1996). The accessory phrenic generally joins the main trunk of the phrenic nerve at the level of the first rib,

but may join lower in the thorax at the pulmonary hilum. In almost all cases, the accessory phrenic nerve courses lateral to the main trunk of the phrenic nerve (Mahan and Spinner, 2016). In a more recent study, Loukas et al. (2006) observed the accessory phrenic nerve in human cadaveric specimens arising from the nerve to the subclavius, from the ansa cervicalis, and nerve to the stylohyoid. A phrenic-accessory phrenic nerve loop was also seen near the subclavian vein (Loukas et al., 2006).

Mendelsohn et al. (2011) also studied variations of the phrenic nerve as it forms from the cervical plexus, assessing the frequency by which C3—C5 contribute to the phrenic. Branching patterns were observed to be the classic three branches from C3—C5; an absent C5 contribution; a lone C4 phrenic nerve; a double contribution from C5; an absent C3 contribution; a double C4 contribution; an accessory phrenic arising from the C3—C5 ventral rami; and a lone C3 phrenic nerve (Mendelsohn et al., 2011). Paviraev and Chernikov (1967) have described branches of the ansa cervicalis joining the phrenic nerve and providing innervation to the heart, pericardium, and diaphragm. The phrenic nerve may also traverse through the belly of the anterior scalene. As described earlier, ganglionic communications to the phrenic nerve generally include the inferior cervical ganglion, but less frequently may issue from the middle cervical ganglion (Irwin et al., 2016). Kocabiyik (2016) mentions that the phrenic nerve may be absent unilaterally, and in extremely rare cases be absent bilaterally. Furthermore, the phrenic nerve may receive branches from the ansa cervicalis, brachial plexus, hypoglossal (CNXII), and the spinal accessory (CNXI) nerves. There are also variations seen where the phrenic nerve does not form a main trunk until more inferior in the thorax. The lengths of the left and right phrenic nerves also differ slightly (Jiang et al., 2011). One case reports a right accessory phrenic nerve originating from the C5 nerve root, then traveling through a fenestrated subclavian vein near the jugulosubclavian junction (Codesido and Guerri-Guttenberg, 2008).

One very interesting case encountered by Paraskevas et al. (2016) mentions an accessory phrenic nerve with an abnormal course. The nerve arose from the supraclavicular nerves and formed a triangular loop that formed a confluence with the phrenic nerve. The loop encircled the superficial cervical artery, which was spiral in form. The ansa cervicalis may also give off branches that supply regions generally innervated by the phrenic nerve (Turner, 1893; Banneheka, 2008). The phrenic nerve may also be pushed laterally by variant vascular structures, as described by Ogami et al. (2016), wherein a variation of the origin of the right thyrocervical trunk pushed the phrenic nerve extremely far laterally resulting in marked diaphragmatic atrophy of the ipsilateral side.

Anatomical Landmarks
The phrenic nerve commences deeply at the side of the neck, about the level of the midpoint of the thyroid cartilage, and runs downward to a point behind the sternal end of the clavicle. About the level of the cricoid cartilage, it lies beneath the sternocleidomastoid about midway between the anterior and posterior borders of the muscle. It is crossed anteriorly by the inferior belly of the omohyoid muscle and transverse cervical and suprascapular arteries. The left nerve is also crossed anteriorly by the thoracic duct. The phrenic nerve crosses the anterior border of the anterior scalene muscle that is approximated by the nerve point. As it crosses this muscle it does so from lateral to medial the accessory phrenic nerve (C5) when present, travels lateral to the phrenic nerve, and also crosses anterior to the anterior scalene muscle. The phrenic nerve travels posterior to the junction between the subclavian and internal jugular veins and anterior to the subclavian artery. Rarely, the accessory or the entire phrenic nerve may travel anterior to the subclavian vein. The phrenic nerve lies posterior to the internal jugular vein.

PHRENIC NERVE INJURY AND ETIOLOGY
Diaphragmatic dysfunction due to brain injury is rare; however, cerebrovascular accidents, schwannoma compressing the phrenic nerve, and amyotrophic lateral sclerosis (ALS) may all result in acute or progressive respiratory dysfunction (Arnulf et al., 2000; Similowski et al., 2000; McCool et al., 2018). Progressive diaphragmatic dysfunction from ALS may also lead to sleep apnea as well as cause general dyspnea. There is also evidence for disorderly breathing during sleep in individuals with unilateral diaphragmatic paralysis (Steier et al., 2008).

Although rare, phrenic nerve injury may also arise in individuals with diabetes as a result of peripheral neuropathy, and is one explanation for unexplained shortness of breath (Wanke et al., 1992; White et al., 1992). In even rarer cases, unilateral diaphragmatic paralysis may be observed (Aslam et al., 2011). Demyelination of phrenic nerve fibers may also cause diaphragmatic dysfunction in individuals with multiple sclerosis (Garland et al., 1996). Individuals with muscular dystrophy may encounter sleep disorders as a result of diaphragmatic dysfunction from phrenic nerve degeneration or decrease in compound motor action potential (Leonardis et al., 2015).

SURGICAL COMPLICATIONS, DIAGNOSIS, AND TREATMENT
Iatrogenic injury to the phrenic nerve is frequent in the clinic. One cause, seen widespread in the literature, is an iatrogenic injury to the phrenic nerve during catheterization of the subclavian or internal jugular vein (Hadeed and Braun, 1988; Ugalde-Fernández et al., 1989; Pleasure and Shashikumar, 1990; Armengaud et al., 1991; Caballero-Noguez et al., 1993; Sakai et al., 1993; Sánchez Castilla et al., 1995; Akata et al., 1997; Rigg et al., 1997; Takasaki and Arai, 2001; Mir and Serdaroglu, 2003; Torres et al., 2007). Many of these cases arise due to miscalculated placement and cannulation that may damage or compress the phrenic nerve; therefore, it is paramount that the clinician be able to understand and anticipate accessory branches of the phrenic nerve, as well as a phrenic nerve that arises from a different origin (variants having the main trunk from C3 or C5). Loukas et al. (2016) noted that the accessory phrenic nerve and phrenic nerve may form a loop around the subclavian vein, reported in 45.5% of specimens. Phrenic nerve injury is also a complication for cardiac intervention or surgery, as it sends branches to the pericardium and parietal pleura. It was noted by Sánchez-Quintana et al. (2005) that both the superior caval vein and right superior pulmonary vein may be found within 2.1 mm of the right phrenic nerve. The left phrenic nerve crosses the obtuse cardiac margin and the left obtuse marginal vein with a very high incidence as well (79%). Thus, performing ablations of tissue of the pericardium and pleura near these structures may result in injury to the phrenic nerve.

Loukas et al. (2006) also clarified the many anatomical variations of the accessory phrenic nerve as it pertains to skeletonizations of the internal thoracic artery, devascularization of the vessels supplying the phrenic nerve, and surgical manipulations of the phrenic nerve. Phrenic nerve injury is well documented in cases of high mobilization of the internal thoracic artery for myocardial revascularization (Landymore and Howell, 1990; Cunningham et al., 1992; Deng et al., 2003). Findings by

Loukas (2016) demonstrate an accessory phrenic nerve-phrenic nerve loop forming around the right or left internal thoracic artery in 38.4% of specimens. Due to the high incidence of this loop, it is recommended that the clinician should carefully consider high internal thoracic artery harvesting in individuals where pulmonary dysfunction is already present. Kessler et al. (2008) also mentioned that the phrenic nerve and the brachial plexus are within 2 mm of each other at the level of the cricoid cartilage. Caution should be taken in approaches to the neck at this level to minimize movement or blunt trauma to the phrenic nerve during surgery.

Temporary paralysis of the ipsilateral diaphragmatic dome may arise following the application of ice to the phrenic nerve during coronary bypass surgery due to topical hypothermia (Benjamin et al., 1982). Incidence of this complication can be decreased by insertion of a cardiac insulation pad or cooling without ice chips or slush (Wheeler et al., 1985). Severe ipsilateral shoulder pain may arise following thoracic surgery (Scawn et al., 2001; Martinez-Barenys et al., 2011). Thoracic epidurals may not significantly decrease this pain; however, Scawn et al. (2001) have shown that infiltration of the phrenic nerve with a local anesthetic may significantly reduce shoulder pain.

Injury to the phrenic nerve may be diagnosed by various imaging methods such as ultrasound, electromyography, and fluoroscopy (Mandoorah and Mead, 2018). Ultrasound provides the highest clarity, as the diaphragm is thick and echogenic. Both hemidiaphragms may be evaluated without issue, the left through the liver window and the right through the splenic window.

In cases of diaphragmatic paralysis due to phrenic nerve injury, paradoxical movement or decreased diaphragmatic displacement on the paralyzed side can be observed (Lloyd et al., 2006). Asymptomatic unilateral diaphragmatic paralysis does not require treatment (Mandoorah and Mead, 2018). However, if bilateral paralysis or other pulmonary dysfunction is discovered, diaphragmatic plication is accepted (Declerck et al., 2013). Phrenic nerve stimulation is also a viable option for treatment (Bellemare and Bigland-Ritchie, 1984). The interscalene brachial plexus nerve block has also been shown to induce diaphragmatic paralysis due to the proximity of the brachial plexus to the phrenic nerve (2 mm) (Bigeleisen, 2003). The cause of this is a transient phrenic nerve blockade—anesthetic solution travels toward the C3−C5 roots or scalenus anterior fascia (Robaux et al., 2001).

PHRENIC NERVE TRANSFER

Lurje (1948) noted that the phrenic nerve can be used as a source of motor axons. Currently, the phrenic nerve, as well as its communicating branches, serves as donor nerves for restoring motor functionality to neighboring structures (Al-Qattan and El-Sayed, 2014; Nair et al., 2017). Restoration of elbow flexion in individuals that have brachial plexus injury requires nerve transfer and possible nerve graft to compensate for a shorter donor nerve (Siqueira and Martins, 2009). In the correction of brachial plexus avulsion, portions of the phrenic nerve are harvested. Gu and Ma (1996) provided substantial evidence for this approach being a viable option, where 84.6% ($n = 180$) of patients had regained threshold bicep strength. It was believed that if further grafting is needed, then one would expect longer recovery times and potentially irreversible muscle atrophy. Xu et al. (2002) demonstrated that full-length phrenic nerve transfer is achievable through minimally invasive video-assisted surgery for treating brachial plexus avulsion injury and that this may decrease recovery time and prevent certain muscular atrophy. In a comparative study between phrenic nerve transfer with and without nerve graft for restoring elbow flexion, Liu et al. (2014) noticed no significant differences between each group. Despite this slight disagreement, phrenic nerve transfer with or without nerve graft is both safe and practical options for recovering biceps function.

Al-Qattan and El-Sayed (2014) demonstrated that an accessory branch of the phrenic nerve arising from C5 may be used for neurotization of the suprascapular nerve. Seemingly, the only risks for nerve transfers involving the phrenic nerve are respiratory problems; however, these are few and far between in cases of brachial plexus reconstruction. Gu and Ma (1996) mentioned one out of 180 patients showing decreased pulmonary capacity within a year after treatment.

Intercostal to phrenic nerve transfer is also a viable option for remedying diaphragmatic paralysis. The phrenic nerve is transected 5 cm proximal to its insertion into the diaphragm and is then anastomosed with the fourth intercostal nerve once after being dissected and mobilized for its entire length (Krieger and Krieger, 2000). Generally, axonal regeneration in this approach takes 3 months, and the time from surgery to diaphragmatic response to electrical stimulation took an average of 9 months.

REFERENCES

Adams, W.E., 1942. The blood supply of nerves: I. Historical review. J. Anat. 76 (Pt 4), 323–341.

Akata, T., Noda, Y., Nagata, T., Noda, E., Kandabashi, T., 1997. Hemidiaphragmatic paralysis following subclavian vein catheterization. Acta Anaesthesiol. Scand. 41 (9), 1223–1225.

Al-Qattan, M.M., El-Sayed, A.A., 2014. The use of the phrenic nerve communicating branch to the fifth cervical root for nerve transfer to the suprascapular nerve in infants with obstetric brachial plexus palsy. Biomed Res. Int. 2014, 153182.

Amin, M., 1914. The course of the phrenic nerve in the embryo. J. Anat. Physiol. 48 (Pt 2), 215–218.

Archard, O., Bucher, V., 1954. Courants d'action bulbaires a rythme respiratoire. Helv. Physiol. Acta. 12, 265.

Armengaud, M.H., Trevoux-Paul, J., Boucherie, J.C., Cousin, M.T., 1991. [Diaphragmatic paralysis after puncture of the internal jugular vein]. Ann. Fr. Anesth. Reanim. 10 (1), 77–80.

Arnulf, I., Similowski, T., Salachas, F., Garma, L., Mehiri, S., Attali, V., Behin-Bellhesen, V., Meininger, V., Derenne, J.P., 2000. Sleep disorders and diaphragmatic function in patients with amyotrophic lateral sclerosis. Am. J. Respir. Crit. Care Med. 161 (3 Pt 1), 849–856.

Aslam, F., Kolpakchi, A., Musher, D., Lu, L., 2011. Unilateral diaphragmatic paralysis in a diabetic patient: a case of trepopnea. J. Gen. Intern. Med. 26 (5), 555–558.

Banneheka, S., 2008. Morphological study of the ansa cervicalis and the phrenic nerve. Anat. Sci. Int. 83 (1), 31–44.

Baumgarten, R., Baumgarten, A., Schaefer, K., 1957. Beitrag zur lokalisationsfrag bulboreticuliirer respiratorischer neurone der katz. Pfliigers Arch. Gesamte Physiol. 264, 217.

Bellemare, F., Bigland-Ritchie, B., 1984. Assessment of human diaphragm strength and activation using phrenic nerve stimulation. Respir. Physiol. 58 (3), 263–277.

Benjamin, J.J., Cascade, P.N., Rubenfire, M., Wajszczuk, W., Kerin, N.Z., 1982. Left lower lobe atelectasis and consolidation following cardiac surgery: the effect of topical cooling on the phrenic nerve. Radiology 142 (1), 11–14.

Bergman, R., Afifi, A., Miyauchi, R., 1996. Phrenic Nerve. Illustrated Encyclopedia of Human Anatomic Variation.

Bhimji, S., Burns, B., 2017. Anatomy, Abdomen, Diaphragm. StatPearls Publishing, Treasure Island (FL).

Bigeleisen, P.E., 2003. Anatomical variations of the phrenic nerve and its clinical implication for supraclavicular block. Br. J. Anaesth. 91 (6), 916–917.

Botha, G., 1957. The anatomy of the phrenic nerve termination and the motor innervation of the diaphragm. Thorax 12, 50–56.

Bunch, T.J., Bruce, G.K., Mahapatra, S., Johnson, S.B., Miller, D.V., Sarabanda, A.V., Milton, M.A., Packer, D.L., 2005. Mechanisms of phrenic nerve injury during radiofrequency ablation at the pulmonary vein orifice. J. Cardiovasc. Electrophysiol. 16 (12), 1318–1325.

Caballero-Noguez, B., Fernández-Corte, M.G., Escobedo-Chávez, E., 1993. [Diaphragmatic paralysis due to a lesion of the phrenic nerve secondary to venesection at the neck for parenteral feeding]. Bol. Med. Hosp. Infant. Mex. 50 (2), 125–128.

Codesido, M., Guerri-Guttenberg, R.A., 2008. Right accessory phrenic nerve passing through an annulus of the subclavian vein. Clin. Anat. 21 (8), 779–780.

Cunningham, J.M., Gharavi, M.A., Fardin, R., Meek, R.A., 1992. Considerations in the skeletonization technique of internal thoracic artery dissection. Ann. Thorac. Surg. 54 (5), 947–950 discussion 951.

Declerck, S., Testelmans, D., Nafteux, P., Coosemans, W., Belge, C., Decramer, M., Buyse, B., 2013. Diaphragm plication for unilateral diaphragm paralysis: a case report and review of the literature. Acta Clin. Belg. 68 (4), 311–315.

Deng, Y., Byth, K., Paterson, H.S., 2003. Phrenic nerve injury associated with high free right internal mammary artery harvesting. Ann. Thorac. Surg. 76 (2), 459–463.

Dobbins, E.G., Feldman, J.L., 1994. Brainstem network controlling descending drive to phrenic motoneurons in rat. J. Comp. Neurol. 347 (1), 64–86.

Drake, R., 1918. Gray's Anatomy for Students. Saunders.

Duron, B., Caillol, M.C., 1973. Investigation of afferent activity in the intact phrenic nerve with bipolar electrodes. Acta Neurobiol. Exp. (Wars) 33 (1), 428–432.

Efthimiou, J., Butler, J., Woodham, C., Benson, M.K., Westaby, S., 1991. Diaphragm paralysis following cardiac surgery: role of phrenic nerve cold injury. Ann. Thorac. Surg. 52 (4), 1005–1008.

Feldman, J.L., Del Negro, C.A., Gray, P.A., 2013. Understanding the rhythm of breathing: so near, yet so far. Annu. Rev. Physiol. 75, 423–452.

Frazier, D.T., Revelette, W.R., 1991. Role of phrenic nerve afferents in the control of breathing. J. Appl. Physiol. (1985) 70 (2), 491–496.

Garland, S.J., Lavoie, B.A., Brown, W.F., 1996. Motor control of the diaphragm in multiple sclerosis. Muscle Nerve 19 (5), 654–656.

Ghali, M.G.Z., 2018. Phrenic motoneurons: output elements of a highly organized intraspinal network. J. Neurophysiol. 119 (3), 1057–1070.

Goizueta, A., Bhimji, S., 2018. Anatomy , Thorax, Lung, Pleura and Mediastinum. StatPearls Publishing, Treasure Island (FL).

Gu, Y.D., Ma, M.K., 1996. Use of the phrenic nerve for brachial plexus reconstruction. Clin. Orthop. Relat. Res. 323, 119–121.

Gu, Y.D., Wu, M.M., Zhen, Y.L., Zhao, J.A., Zhang, G.M., Chen, D.S., Yan, J.G., Cheng, X.M., 1989. Phrenic nerve transfer for brachial plexus motor neurotization. Microsurgery 10 (4), 287–289.

Hadeed, H.A., Braun, T.W., 1988. Paralysis of the hemidiaphragm as a complication of internal jugular vein cannulation: report of a case. J. Oral Maxillofac. Surg. 46 (5), 409–411.

Irwin, P., Tubbs, R., Tubbs, R., 2016. Autonomic nervous system. In: Tubbs, R. (Ed.), Bergman's Comprehensive Atlas of Human Anatomic Variation. John Wiley & Sons, pp. 1050–1055.

Jiang, S., Xu, W.D., Shen, Y.D., Xu, J.G., Gu, Y.D., 2011. An anatomical study of the full-length phrenic nerve and its blood supply: clinical implications for endoscopic dissection. Anat. Sci. Int. 86 (4), 225—231.

Joho-Arreola, A.L., Bauersfeld, U., Stauffer, U.G., Baenziger, O., Bernet, V., 2005. Incidence and treatment of diaphragmatic paralysis after cardiac surgery in children. Eur J. Cardiothorac. Surg. 27 (1), 53—57.

Kessler, J., Schafhalter-Zoppoth, I., Gray, A.T., 2008. An ultrasound study of the phrenic nerve in the posterior cervical triangle: implications for the interscalene brachial plexus block. Reg. Anesth. Pain Med. 33 (6), 545—550.

Kocabiyik, N., 2016. Cervical Plexus. Bergman's Comprehensive Encyclopedia of Human Anatomic Variation. In: Tubbs, R. (Ed.). John Wiley & Sons, pp. 1062—1066.

Kostreva, D.R., Pontus, S.P., 1993a. Hepatic vein, hepatic parenchymal, and inferior vena caval mechanoreceptors with phrenic afferents. Am. J. Physiol. 265 (1 Pt 1), G15—G20.

Kostreva, D.R., Pontus, S.P., 1993b. Pericardial mechanoreceptors with phrenic afferents. Am. J. Physiol. 264 (6 Pt 2), H1836—H1846.

Krieger, L.M., Krieger, A.J., 2000. The intercostal to phrenic nerve transfer: an effective means of reanimating the diaphragm in patients with high cervical spine injury. Plast. Reconstr. Surg. 105 (4), 1255—1261.

Landau, B., Akert, K., Roberts, T., 1962. Studies on the innervation of the diaphragm. J. Comp. Neurol. 119, 1—10.

Landymore, R.W., Howell, F., 1990. Pulmonary complications following myocardial revascularization with the internal mammary artery graft. Eur J. Cardiothorac. Surg. 4 (3), 156—161 discussion 161-152.

Langford, A., Schmidt, R.F., 1983. An electron microscopic analysis of the left phrenic nerve in the rat. Anat. Rec. 205 (2), 207—213.

Larkin, F.C., 1889. Accessory phrenic nerve. J. Anat. Physiol. 23 (Pt 2), 340.

Leonardis, L., Blagus, R., Dolenc Groselj, L., 2015. Sleep and breathing disorders in myotonic dystrophy type 2. Acta Neurol. Scand. 132 (1), 42—48.

Liu, Y., Lao, J., Gao, K., Gu, Y., Zhao, X., 2014. Comparative study of phrenic nerve transfers with and without nerve graft for elbow flexion after global brachial plexus injury. Injury 45 (1), 227—231.

Lloyd, T., Tang, Y.M., Benson, M.D., King, S., 2006. Diaphragmatic paralysis: the use of M mode ultrasound for diagnosis in adults. Spinal Cord 44 (8), 505—508.

Loukas, M., Du Plessis, M., Louis, R.G., 2016. The subdiaphragmatic part of the phrenic nerve - morphometry and connections to autonomic ganglia. Clin. Anat. 29 (1), 120—128.

Loukas, M., Kinsella, C.R., Louis, R.G., Gandhi, S., Curry, B., 2006. Surgical anatomy of the accessory phrenic nerve. Ann. Thorac. Surg. 82 (5), 1870—1875.

Lumsden, T., 1923a. Observations on the respiratory centres. J. Physiol. 57 (6), 354—367.

Lumsden, T., 1923b. Observations on the respiratory centres in the cat. J. Physiol. 57 (3—4), 153—160.

Lumsden, T., 1923c. The regulation of respiration: Part I. J. Physiol. 58 (1), 81—91.

Lurje, A., 1948. Concerning surgical treatment of traumatic injury to the upper division of the brachial plexus (Erb's Type). Ann. Surg. 127 (2), 317—326.

Mahan, M., Spinner, R., 2016. Nerves of the upper extremity. In: Tubbs, R. (Ed.), Bergman's Comprehensive Encyclopedia of Human Anatomic Variation. John Wiley & Sons, pp. 1068—1104.

Mandoorah, S., Mead, T., 2018. Phrenic Nerve Injury. StatPearls Publishing, Treasure Island (FL).

Martinez-Barenys, C., Busquets, J., de Castro, P.E., Garcia-Guasch, R., Perez, J., Fernandez, E., Mesa, M.A., Astudillo, J., 2011. Randomized double-blind comparison of phrenic nerve infiltration and suprascapular nerve block for ipsilateral shoulder pain after thoracic surgery. Eur J. Cardiothorac. Surg. 40 (1), 106—112.

McCool, F.D., Manzoor, K., Minami, T., 2018. Disorders of the Diaphragm. Clin. Chest Med. 39 (2), 345—360.

Mendelsohn, A.H., Deconde, A., Lambert, H.W., Dodson, S.C., Daney, B.T., Stark, M.E., Berke, G.S., Wisco, J.J., 2011. Cervical variations of the phrenic nerve. Laryngoscope 121 (9), 1920—1923.

Merrill, E.G., 1970. The lateral respiratory neurones of the medulla: their associations with nucleus ambiguus, nucleus retroambigualis, the spinal accessory nucleus and the spinal cord. Brain Res. 24 (1), 11—28.

Mir, S., Serdaroglu, E., 2003. An elevated hemidiaphragm 3 months after internal jugular vein hemodialysis catheter placement. Semin. Dial. 16 (3), 281—283.

Mitchell, R.A., Berger, A.J., 1975. Neural regulation of respiration. Am. Rev. Respir. Dis. 111 (2), 206—224.

Nair, J., Streeter, K.A., Turner, S.M.F., Sunshine, M.D., Bolser, D.C., Fox, E.J., Davenport, P.W., Fuller, D.D., 2017. Anatomy and physiology of phrenic afferent neurons. J. Neurophysiol. 118 (6), 2975—2990.

Ogami, K., Saiki, K., Okamoto, K., Wakebe, T., Manabe, Y., Imamura, T., Tsurumoto, T., 2016. Marked lateral deviation of the phrenic nerve due to variant origin and course of the thyrocervical trunk: a cadaveric study. Surg. Radiol. Anat. 38 (4), 485—488.

Oliver, K., Zito, P., 2018. Anatomy, Neck, Nerves, Phrenic. StatPearls Publishing LLC.

Paraskevas, G., Koutsouflianiotis, K., Kitsoulis, P., Spyridakis, I., 2016. Abnormal origin and course of the accessory phrenic nerve: case report. Acta Med. (Hradec Kralove) 59 (2), 70—71.

Paviraev, N., Chernikov, Y., 1967. Anatomy of the ansa cervicalis. Excerpta Med. 21, 219.

Pleasure, J.R., Shashikumar, V.L., 1990. Phrenic nerve damage in the tiny infant during vein cannulation for parenteral nutrition. Am. J. Perinatol. 7 (2), 136—138.

Rigg, A., Hughes, P., Lopez, A., Filshie, J., Cunningham, D., Green, M., 1997. Right phrenic nerve palsy as a complication of indwelling central venous catheters. Thorax 52 (9), 831—833.

Robaux, S., Bouaziz, H., Boisseau, N., Raucoules-Aimé, M., Laxenaire, M.C., S. O. S. R. H. L. Service, 2001. Persistent phrenic nerve paralysis following interscalene brachial plexus block. Anesthesiology 95 (6), 1519—1521.

Sakai, M., Morimoto, M., Tanaka, Y., Hara, N., Hyodo, M., 1993. [A case of right phrenic nerve paralysis as a complication of internal jugular vein cannulation by anterior approach]. Masui 42 (9), 1355–1358.

Scawn, N.D., Pennefather, S.H., Soorae, A., Wang, J.Y., Russell, G.N., 2001. Ipsilateral shoulder pain after thoracotomy with epidural analgesia: the influence of phrenic nerve infiltration with lidocaine. Anesth. Analg. 93 (2), 260–264, 261st contents page.

Schumpelick, V., Steinau, G., Schlüper, I., Prescher, A., 2000. Surgical embryology and anatomy of the diaphragm with surgical applications. Surg. Clin. North Am. 80 (1), 213–239 (xi).

Similowski, T., Attali, V., Bensimon, G., Salachas, F., Mehiri, S., Arnulf, I., Lacomblez, L., Zelter, M., Meininger, V., Derenne, J.P., 2000. Diaphragmatic dysfunction and dyspnoea in amyotrophic lateral sclerosis. Eur. Respir. J. 15 (2), 332–337.

Siqueira, M.G., Martins, R.S., 2009. Phrenic nerve transfer in the restoration of elbow flexion in brachial plexus avulsion injuries: how effective and safe is it? Neurosurgery 65 (4 Suppl. l), A125–A131.

Standring, S., 2016. Gray's Anatomy: The Anatomical Basis for Clinical Practice. Elsevier.

Steier, J., Jolley, C.J., Seymour, J., Kaul, S., Luo, Y.M., Rafferty, G.F., Hart, N., Polkey, M.I., Moxham, J., 2008. Sleep-disordered breathing in unilateral diaphragm paralysis or severe weakness. Eur. Respir. J. 32 (6), 1479–1487.

Sánchez Castilla, M., López Martínez, J., Rodríguez Tato, P., Asuero de Lis, M.S., 1995. [Diaphragmatic paralysis after the catheterization of the internal jugular vein]. Nutr. Hosp. 10 (6), 377–378.

Sánchez-Quintana, D., Cabrera, J.A., Climent, V., Farré, J., Weiglein, A., Ho, S.Y., 2005. How close are the phrenic nerves to cardiac structures? Implications for cardiac interventionalists. J. Cardiovasc. Electrophysiol. 16 (3), 309–313.

Takasaki, Y., Arai, T., 2001. Transient right phrenic nerve palsy associated with central venous catheterization. Br. J. Anaesth. 87 (3), 510–511.

Torres, B., Sotomayor, L., Sanchez-Cazau, D., Vazquez-Torres, O., 2007. Right hemidiaphragm paralysis as a rare complication of a central venous port catheter insertion. Bol. Asoc. Med. P. R. 99 (1), 31–37.

Turner, W., 1893. A phrenic nerve receiving a root of origin from the descendens hypoglossi. J. Anat. Physiol. 27 (Pt 3), 427.

Ugalde-Fernández, J.H., Suárez-Ríos, L.F., Arellano-Cuevas, R., 1989. [Diaphragmatic paralysis caused by a phrenic nerve lesion secondary to internal jugular vein cutdown]. Bol. Med. Hosp. Infant. Mex. 46 (7), 497–499.

Wanke, T., Paternostro-Sluga, T., Grisold, W., Formanek, D., Auinger, M., Zwick, H., Irsigler, K., 1992. Phrenic nerve function in type 1 diabetic patients with diaphragm weakness and peripheral neuropathy. Respiration 59 (4), 233–237.

Wheeler, W.E., Rubis, L.J., Jones, C.W., Harrah, J.D., 1985. Etiology and prevention of topical cardiac hypothermia-induced phrenic nerve injury and left lower lobe atelectasis during cardiac surgery. Chest 88 (5), 680–683.

White, J.E., Bullock, R.E., Hudgson, P., Home, P.D., Gibson, G.J., 1992. Phrenic neuropathy in association with diabetes. Diabet. Med. 9 (10), 954–956.

Xu, W.D., Gu, Y.D., Xu, J.G., Tan, L.J., 2002. Full-length phrenic nerve transfer by means of video-assisted thoracic surgery in treating brachial plexus avulsion injury. Plast. Reconstr. Surg. 110 (1), 104–109 discussion 110-101.

CHAPTER 7

The Ansa Cervicalis

SHOGO KIKUTA • TESS DECATER • R. SHANE TUBBS

INTRODUCTION

The ansa cervicalis (Figs. 7.1–7.3) innervates the infra-hyoid muscles. "Ansa" is Latin for the handle of a cup (Clemente, 1986). It lies deep to the sternocleidomastoid and is a neural loop with two roots consisting of fibers from cervical ventral rami related to the cervical plexus (Fig. 7.1). Generally, fibers arising from the ventral rami of cervical spinal nerves (C1–2) connect to the hypoglossal nerve within 3–4 cm. These then branch from the hypoglossal nerve and descend as the

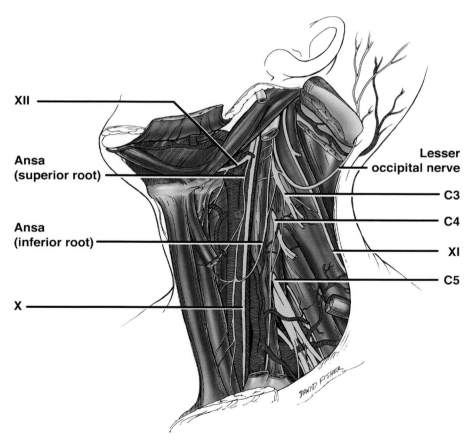

FIG. 7.1 Schematic drawing of the ansa cervicalis in the left neck. The platysma, sternocleidomastoid, omohyoid muscle, all veins have been dissected. X, vagus nerve; XII, hypoglossal nerve.

Surgical Anatomy of the Cervical Plexus and its Branches. https://doi.org/10.1016/B978-0-323-83132-1.00003-2

43

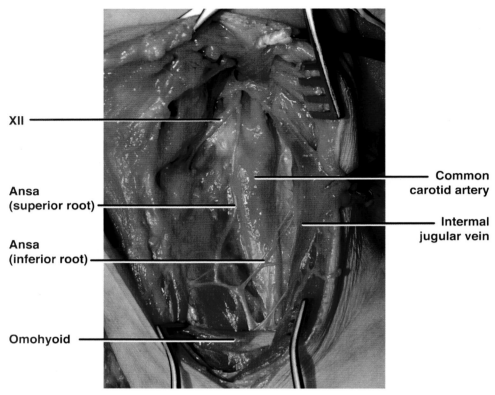

FIG. 7.2 Fresh frozen cadaveric dissection of the left neck noting the ansa cervicalis and related structures.

superior root of the ansa cervicalis; the inferior root comprises nerve fibers arising from ventral rami of C2—C3. These two branches join in the anterior wall of the carotid sheath and form a neural loop. The ansa cervicalis almost always travels anterior to the internal jugular vein (Tubbs et al., 2005). This loop was previously called the "ansa hypoglossi" as it appeared to arise from the hypoglossal nerve and connect to the inferior root stemming from the cervical plexus (Chaurasia, 1980) (Figs. 7.4 and 7.5). The aim of this chapter is to review the anatomy, variations, and pathology of the ansa cervicalis and discuss its clinical applications.

REVIEW
Anatomy
The ansa cervicalis, which innervates the infrahyoid muscles, is a neural complex in the neck formed by the combination of the ventral rami of the first three or four cervical spinal nerves. It comprises superior and inferior roots. The superior root, the ramus descendens hypoglossi, travels with the hypoglossal nerve and descends along the anterior wall of the carotid sheath. It

contains only fibers from the first and second cervical spinal nerves (C1—2), not including the hypoglossal nerve (Olry and Haines, 2002). After the superior root gives rise to a branch to the superior belly of the omohyoid, sternothyroid and sternohyoid muscles, it joins the inferior root arising from C2—3, forming the ansa cervicalis (Chaurasia, 1980). Blythe et al. described a rare case where the descendens hypoglossi (superior root) innervated the lower third of the sternocleidomastoid muscle (Blythe et al., 2015). Chhetri and Berke reviewed the literature about the ansa cervicalis and found that the inferior root arises from the ventral rami of C2—3 in 74% of cases (Chhetri and Berke, 1997). Usually, the ansa cervicalis travels anterior to the internal jugular vein (Tubbs et al., 2005). Its inferior root gives rise to a branch that innervates the inferior belly of the omohyoid muscle, which sometimes branches from the fourth spinal cervical nerve (C4) (Olry and Haines, 2002). Another branch descends into the thorax to join the cardiac or phrenic nerve (Standring, 2016).

The ansa cervicalis is considered an efferent nerve. However, there can be an afferent neural component

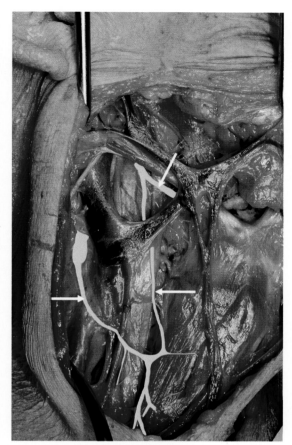

FIG. 7.3 Fresh frozen cadaveric dissection of the right neck noting the ansa cervicalis (indicated at the lower two arrows) and related structures. Note the hypoglossal nerve (upper arrow) giving rise to the superior root of the ansa which here is seen passing deep to the common facial vein.

to the infrahyoid muscles during phonation and deglutition (Chhetri and Berke, 1997). Zapata and Torrealba reported that reflex contraction of the cricothyroid muscle, mediated by afferent fibers, was induced by stimulating the central end of the transected ramus descendens hypoglossi in cats (Zapata and Torrealba, 1988). Previous studies have also reported various connections between the ansa cervicalis and the cervical sympathetic trunk, the descending branch of the ansa cervicalis linking to a branch arising from C4 (Tunner, 1893; Lippmann, 1910; Schaefer et al., 1915; Rodrigues, 1930b; Winckler, 1955; Wischnewsky, 1930).

Variations
Usually, the superior root of the ansa cervicalis travels along the anterior wall of the carotid sheath after leaving the hypoglossal nerve. However, the inferior root has a more varied composition and course, often making the ansa cervicalis asymmetric (Khaki et al., 2006). Caliot et al. found the superior root to be symmetric in almost all cases, but the inferior root was asymmetric in 75% (Caliot et al., 1986). They also described seven forms of ansa cervicalis differing in regard to the inferior roots: a simple classic form (27%), a very short single form (1.2%), a double classic form (40%), a double form with two separate roots (11%), a double short form (7.5), a triple form (8.7%), and a quadruple form (1.2%) (Caliot et al., 1986). In addition, the inferior root was absent 3% of the time (Caliot et al., 1986). Quadros et al. found the "triple form" of ansa cervicalis unilaterally during routine cadaveric dissection of the left neck (Quadros et al., 2015). This case had three inferior roots originating from the accessory nerve and the C1, C2, and C3 spinal nerves. A single inferior root was formed between a branch from the accessory nerve and C1.

The ansa cervicalis has also been classified on the basis of its relationship to the internal jugular vein (IJV) (Olry and Haines, 2002). There are three types: (1) the medial type, where both roots of the ansa cervicalis are located deep to the IJV; (2) the lateral type, in which the inferior root is anterior to the IJV (Kikuchi, 1970); and (3) the mixed type, where the ansa cervicalis has double loops - the upper branch of the inferior root running posterior to the IJV, the lower root traveling anterior to it. Moreover, Banneheka classified different arrangements of the inferior root of the ansa cervicalis into seven groups (Banneheka et al., 2008). In all cases, the superior root was formed by C1–2. Group 1 forms a single loop with the superior root, and the inferior root consists of a single branch from either C2 or C3 ($n = 46$, 22.1%). Group 2 is the most common variation: the inferior root has two branches joining the superior root independently of one another ($n = 86$, 41.3%). In Group 3, the inferior root consists of two branches, but the two branches join the superior root at a single point ($n = 6$, 2.9%). Group 4 shows two branches arising from C2, C3, or C4 joining to form one inferior root that forms a single loop with the superior root ($n = 58$, 27.9%); two branches arose from C2 or C3 in 53 cases and from C3 and C4 in five cases. Group 5 has an inferior root with three branches, which connect to the superior root independently of one another ($n = 6$, 2.9%). Group 6 has an inferior root with three branches similar to Group 5, but these branches join the superior root at a single point ($n = 1$, 0.5%) (Machalek et al., 2009). Group 7 has three branches arising from C2, C3, or C4 joining to form one inferior root, which forms a single loop with the superior root ($n = 5$; 2.4%).

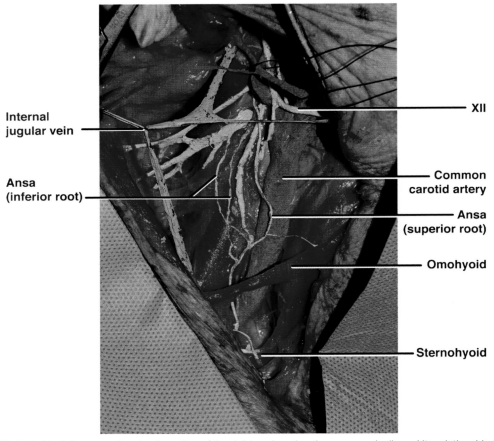

Internal jugular vein

Ansa (inferior root)

XII

Common carotid artery

Ansa (superior root)

Omohyoid

Sternohyoid

FIG. 7.4 Fresh frozen cadaveric dissection of the right neck noting the ansa cervicalis and its relationship to the major vascular structures of the region.

Rodrigues described six types of anastomoses between the descendens cervicalis (i.e., the inferior root of the ansa cervicalis) and the superior cervical ganglion: (I) branches from the superior cervical ganglion [observed in 13 out of 90 cases]; (II) branches from the ramus communicans to C2 [17 cases]; (III) branches from the ramus communicans to C3 [four cases]; (IV) branches from a ramus communicans joining the loop between C2 and C3 [two cases]; (V) filaments joining the loops between the cervical spinal nerves, or joining these nerves, close to the points from which the roots of the descendens cervicalis nerve arise; (VI) the ramus communicans to C2 being so closely associated with one or more roots of the descendens cervicalis arising from C2 that it can be regarded as assisting in their formation [10 cases] (Rodrigues, 1930a).

Jelev classified the ansa cervicalis into five types (Jelev, 2013). It is further classified into three components for different neural communications: C1–2 fibers with the hypoglossal nerve (hypoglossal component), C1–2 fibers with the vagus nerve (vagal component), and separate branches off C2–3 (cervical component). Type I does not form an ansa cervicalis as it has the hypoglossal and cervical components without a connection (Venugopal and Mallula, 2010). Type II is a typical ansa cervicalis (the so-called hypoglosso-cervical ansa). The superior root branches from the hypoglossal component to form a loop with the inferior root from the cervical component. Type III has double loops and comprises the hypoglosso-cervical ansa and vago-cervical ansa (hypoglosso-vago-cervical ansa) (Fig. 7.6) (Rao et al., 2007; Kumar et al., 2014; Sangvichien et al., 2017). Type IV has the hypoglossal component but forms a loop with the vagal and cervical components (vago-cervical ansa) (Sangvichien et al., 2017; Manjunath, 2000; Vollala et al.,

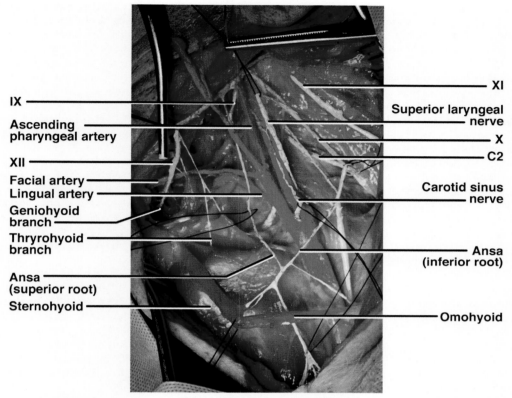

IX

Ascending
pharyngeal artery

XII

Facial artery
Lingual artery

Geniohyoid
branch

Thryrohyoid
branch

Ansa
(superior root)

Sternohyoid

XI

Superior laryngeal
nerve

X

C2

Carotid sinus
nerve

Ansa
(inferior root)

Omohyoid

FIG. 7.5 Fresh frozen cadaveric dissection of the left neck noting the ansa cervicalis and its branches and their relationship to the major neural structures of the region.

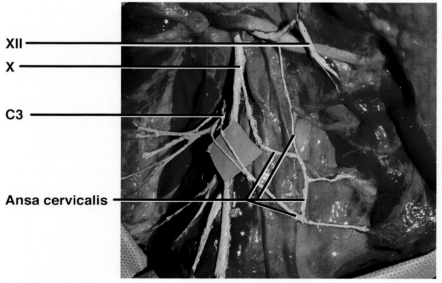

XII

X

C3

Ansa cervicalis

FIG. 7.6 Fresh frozen cadaveric dissection of the right neck noting the ansa cervicalis. Here, the ansa cervicalis is composed of three roots with one arising from the vagus nerve.

2005; D'Souza and Biswabina, 2010; Ayyoubian and Koruji, 2011). Type V has the hypoglossal and vagal components but does not form an ansa cervicalis (Manjunath, 2000; D'Souza and Biswabina, 2010; Rath and Anand, 1994). These authors have reported that with the exception of type II, most variations of the ansa have a frequency of less than 1%.

There are a few reports of unusual forms of the superior root of the ansa cervicalis. Verma et al. described a case where the vagus and hypoglossal nerves were fused immediately after exiting the hypoglossal canal and jugular foramen, respectively (Verma et al., 2005). Branches from the vagus nerve innervated the sternohyoid, sternothyroid, and superior belly of the omohyoid muscles forming the superior root of the ansa cervicalis. Nayak et al. also reported a rare variant of the superior root branching off the vagus and hypoglossal nerves (Nayak et al., 2017). Some variations lack the typical ansa cervical loop, forming the "vagocervical plexus" or "vagocervical complex" (Rath and Anand, 1994; Abu-Hijleh, 2005), a replacement for the ansa cervicalis formed by the vagus nerve and fibers from C1-2. The vagocervical plexus, a unilateral absence of the ansa cervicalis, is very rare (Rath and Anand, 1994). Another rare case has been presented in which the ansa cervicalis was totally absent on both sides but replaced by a vagocervical plexus (Abu-Hijleh, 2005). The descending branch of this plexus entered the superior and inferior belly of the omohyoid, sternothyroid, and sternohyoid muscles, distinguishing it from a pseudo-ansa cervicalis, which does not give rise to branches to the infrahyoid muscles. It could be considered a pseudo-ansa cervicalis if the superior and inferior roots arose from the vagus nerve and the superior cervical sympathetic ganglion, respectively (Indrasingh and Vettivel, 2000).

Shoja et al. reported an anastomosis between the descendens hypoglossi and the vagus nerve that replaced the ansa cervicalis. In their specimen, the C1 contribution to the hypoglossal nerve passed from the suboccipital nerve to the accessory nerve and entered the vagus nerve at the level of the jugular foramen. The fibers then exited the inferior vagal ganglion, joined the hypoglossal nerve, and formed the descendens hypoglossi. The descendens hypoglossi then fused with the vagus nerve again to form a common nerve trunk because the inferior root of the ansa cervicalis, which normally joins the descendens hypoglossi, was absent (Shoja et al., 2015).

Banneheka et al. studied communications between the ansa cervicalis and the vagus nerve using a surgical microscope (Banneheka, 2008a). Two types of communication were observed: (1) false (pseudo) communications, where the two nerves were connected only by connective tissue; and (2) true communications, in which the two nerves were connected by nerve fibers. Most of the ansa-vagal communications were false (pseudo) communications. The authors suggested that ansa—vagal communications result from the close physical relationship between the two nerves and should be considered during certain surgical procedures such as laryngeal reinnervation using the ansa cervicalis.

In another study, Banneheka described the relationship between the ansa cervicalis and the phrenic nerve. The phrenic nerve arises from C3—C5, and C6 when the accessory and secondary phrenic nerves are also considered (Benneheka, 2008b). The origins of the ansa cervicalis and phrenic nerve were arranged into three groups: continuous, overlapped, and discontinuous. Over 80% of the studied cases were grouped as continuous, where C1—C3 gave rise to the ansa cervicalis and C4 ± C5 to the phrenic nerve. When the segmental origins of these nerves were grouped as overlapping, the ansa cervicalis was mostly of the lateral type (statistically significant difference, $P = .005$). When the origins were grouped as discontinuous, the ansa cervicalis was mostly of the medial type (no statistically significant difference, $P = .49$) (Benneheka, 2008b). Additionally, this team found that the contribution of C4 to the phrenic nerve remained constant (100%) irrespective of the type or segmental composition of the ansa cervicalis.

Pathology

Schwannomas of the ansa cervicalis are rare (Hirabayashi et al., 1987; Diego Sastre et al., 1996; Okonkwo et al., 2011; Park et al., 2014; Rath et al., 2015; Righini et al., 2007). Schwannomas, also known as neuromas, neurilemmomas, or neurinomas, are benign nerve sheath tumors composed of Schwann cells (Kang et al., 2007). They are most common in the head and neck regions, arising from the vagus nerve or the sympathetics (Kim et al., 2010). They are usually characterized by a painless mass in the neck and are difficult to diagnose because they are often mistaken for other lesions such as carotid body tumors, enlarged lymph nodes, branchial cysts, or thyroid lesions (Kamal et al., 2007; Zhang et al., 2007). Although Diego Sastre et al. reported a schwannoma of the ansa cervicalis, the preoperative diagnosis was a thyroid tumor (Indrasingh and Vettivel, 2000; Diego Sastre et al., 1996).

Clinical Applications

The ansa cervicalis is an attractive and useful candidate for laryngeal reinnervation in cases of recurrent laryngeal nerve paralysis (RLNP) (Paniello, 2004). RLNP is one of the most serious complications in esophageal cancer surgery. Functional depression of deglutition and phonation induced by RLNP can lead to postoperative malnutrition and degradation of communication (Baba et al., 1998). Moreover, RLNP can cause pneumonia by aspiration, affecting the long-term prognosis after esophageal cancer surgery (Loukas et al., 2007). Frazier first reported laryngeal reinnervation using the ansa cervicalis for nonselective laryngeal reinnervation in 1924 (Frazier, 1924). Which branch of the ansa cervicalis should be used has been debated, many reporting that the superior root gives better surgical outcomes (Frazier, 1924). The collateral branches of the sternothyroid and omohyoid muscles have also been recommended for such operations (Crumley, 1994). Prades et al. recommend the common nerve trunk to the sternothyroid and sternohyoid muscles as the prime choice (Prades et al., 2015). In 80% of cases, it was close to the larynx and corresponded to the size of the recurrent laryngeal nerve. Recently, the application of the common trunk for laryngeal reinnervation was proposed as an easy, safe, and consistent method (Chhetri and Blumin, 2012).

The ansa cervicalis can be injured iatrogenically during surgical procedures such as thyroplasty (Isshiki et al., 1975), arytenoid adduction (Isshiki et al., 1978), Teflon injection (Arnold, 1962), nerve-muscle pedicle implantation (Tucker and Rusnov, 1981), surgery of the parotid gland, removal of the deep cervical lymph nodes (Nayak et al., 2017), reanimation of facial paralysis using the hypoglossal nerve (Yoleri et al., 2000), and during infrahyoid myocutaneous flap reconstruction (Deganello et al., 2005).

CONCLUSION

Comprehensive knowledge of the anatomy, variations, and clinical importance of the ansa cervicalis will allow for greater preoperative and surgical accuracy.

REFERENCES

Abu-Hijleh, M., 2005. Bilateral absence of ansa cervicalis replaced by vagocervical plexus:case report and literature review. Ann. Anat. 187, 121–125.

Arnold, G., 1962. Vocal rehabilitation of paralytic dysphonia, VIII, phoniatric methods of vocal compensation. Arch. Otolaryngo. l76, 76–83.

Ayyoubian, M., Koruji, M., 2011. A rare anatomical variant of ansa cervicalis: case report. Med. J. Islam. Repub. Iran 24, 238–240.

Baba, M., Aikou, T., Natsugoe, S., Kusano, C., Shimada, M., Nakano, S., Fukumoto, T., Yoshinaka, H., 1998. Quality of life following esophagectomy with three-field lymphadenectomy for carcinoma, focusing on its relationship to vocal cord palsy. Dis. Esophagus 11, 28–34.

Banneheka, S., Tokita, K., Kumaki, K., 2008. Nerve fiber analysis of ansa cervicalis-vagus communications. Anat. Sci. Int. 83, 145–151.

Banneheka, S., 2008a. Anatomy of the ansa cervicalis: nerve fiber analysis. Anat. Sci. Int. 83, 61–67.

Benneheka, S., 2008b. Morphological study of the ansa cervicalis and the phrenic nerve. Anat. Sci. Int. 83, 31–44.

Blythe, J., Matharu, J., Reuther, W., Brennan, J., 2015. Innervation of the lower third of the sternocleidomastoid muscle by the ansa cervicalis through the C1 descendens hypoglossal branch: a previously unreported anatomical variant. Br. J. Oral Maxillofac. Surg. 53, 470–471.

Caliot, P., Dumont, D., Bousquet, V., Midy, D., 1986. A note on the anastomoses between the hypoglossal nerve and the cervical plexus. Surg. Radiol. Anat. 8, 75–79.

Chaurasia, B., 1980. Human Anatomy—Regional and Applied, Head and Neck and Brain. CBS Publishers, Delhi.

Chhetri, D., Berke, G., 1997. Ansa cervicalis nerve: review of the topographic anatomy and morphology. Laryngoscope 107, 1366–1372.

Chhetri, D., Blumin, J., 2012. Laryngeal reinnervation for unilateral vocal fold paralysis using ansa cervicalis nerve to recurrent laryngeal nerve anastomosis. Oper. Tech. Otolaryngol. Head Neck Surg. 23, 173–177.

Clemente, C., 1986. International Dictionary of Medicine and Biology: Neuroanatomy and Neurophysiology. John Wiley, New York.

Crumley, R., 1994. Unilateral recurrent laryngeal nerve paralysis. J. Voice 8, 79–83.

D'Souza, A., Biswabina, R., 2010. Study of the formation and distribution of the ansa cervicalis and its clinical significance. Eur. J. Anat. 14, 143–148.

Deganello, A., Bree, R De, Dolivet, G., Leemans, C., 2005. Infrahyoid myocutaneous flap reconstruction after wide local excision of a merkel cell carcinoma ricostruzione con lembo miocutaneo infraioideo dopo ampia escissione locale di un merkel cell carcinoma. Acta Otorhinolaryngol. Ital. 00, 50–54.

Diego Sastre, JI de, Melcon Diez, E., Prim Espada, M.P., 1996. Neurilemmoma of the ansa cervicalis: a case report. Acta Otorrinolaringol. Esp. 47, 83–84.

Frazier, C., 1924. Anastomosis of the recurrent laryngeal nerve with the descendens noni: in cases of recurrent laryngeal paralysis. J. Am. Med. Assoc. 83, 1637–1641.

Hirabayashi, S., Sakurai, A., Fukuda, O., 1987. Neurilemoma of the ansa cervicalis. Plast. Reconstr. Surg. 79, 809–811.

Indrasingh, I., Vettivel, S., 2000. A rare pseudo ansa cervicalis: a case report. J. Anat. Soc. India 49, 178–179.

Isshiki, N., Okamura, H., Ishikawa, T., 1975. Thyroplasty type I (lateral compression) for dysphonia due to vocal cord paralysis or atrophy. Acta Otolaryngol. 80, 465–473.

Isshiki, N., Tanabe, M., Sawada, M., 1978. Arytenoid adduction for unilateral vocal cord paralysis. Arch. Otolaryngol. 104, 555–558.

Jelev, L., 2013. Some unusual types of formation of the ansa cervicalis in humans and proposal of a new morphological classification. Clin. Anat. 26, 961–965.

Kamal, A., Abd El-Fattah, A., Tawfik, A., Abdel Razek, A., 2007. Cervical sympathetic schwannoma with postoperative first bite syndrome. Eur. Arch. Otorhinolaryngol. 264, 1109–1111.

Kang, G., Soo, K.-C., Lim, D., 2007. Extracranial non-vestibular head and neck schwannomas: a ten-year experience. Ann. Acad. Med. Singapore 36, 233–238.

Khaki, A.A., Shokouhi, G., Shoja, M.M., Farahani, R.M., Zarrintan, S., Khaki, A., Montazam, H., Tanoomand, A., Tubbs, R.S., 2006. Ansa cervicalis as a variant of spinal accessory nerve plexus: a case report. Clin. Anat. 19, 540–543.

Kikuchi, T., 1970. A contribution to the morphology of the ansa cervicalis and the phrenic nerve. J. Anat. 45, 242–281.

Kim, S., Kim, N., Kim, K., Lee, J., Choi, H., 2010. Schwannoma in head and neck: preoperative imaging study and intracapsular enucleation for functional nerve preservation. Yonsei Med. J. 51, 938–942.

Kumar, N., Patil, J., Rkg, M., Sirasanagandla, S., Sb, N., Guru, A., 2014. Rare case of double looped ansa cervicalis associated with its deep position in the carotid triangle of the neck. Ann. Med. Health Sci. Res. 4, 29–31.

Lippmann, R., 1910. Abnormer ursprung des ramus descendens N. Anat. Anz. 37, 1–4.

Loukas, M., Thorsell, A., Tubbs, R.S., Kapos, T., Louis, R.G., Vulis, M., Hage, R., Jordan, R., 2007. The ansa cervicalis revisited. Folia Morphol. (Warsz) 66, 120–125.

Machalek, L., Charamza, J., Kikalova, K., Bezdekova, M., 2009. A variant case of ansa cervicalis. Int. J. Anat. Var. 2, 150–152.

Manjunath, K.Y., 2000. Vagal origin of the ANSA cervicalis nerve - report of two cases. Indian J. Otolaryngol. Head Neck Surg. 52, 257–258.

Nayak, A.B., Shetty, P., Reghunathan, D., Aithal, A.P., Kumar, N., 2017. Descendens vagohypoglossi: rare variant of the superior root of ansa cervicalis. Br. J. Oral Maxillofac. Surg. 55, 834–835.

Okonkwo, O., Doshi, J., Minhas, S., 2011. Schwannoma of the ansa cervicalis. J. Surg. Case Rep. 3.

Olry, R., Haines, D.E., 2002. Ansa hypoglossi or ansa cervicalis? That is the question. J. Hist. Neurosci. 11, 302–304.

Paniello, R.C., 2004. Laryngeal reinnervation. Otolaryngol. Clin. North Am. 37, 161–181 (vii-viii).

Park, J.H., Ahn, D., Hwang, K.H., Jeong, J.Y., 2014. Schwannoma of ansa cervicalis in the submandibular space. Korean J. Otorhinolaryngol. Head Neck Surg. 57, 616–619.

Prades, J.M., Gavid, M., Dubois, M.D., Dumollard, J.M., Timoshenko, A.T., Peoc'h, M., 2015. Surgical anatomy of the ansa cervicalis nerve: which branch to use for laryngeal reinnervation in humans? Surg. Radiol. Anat. 37, 139–145.

Quadros, L., Prasanna, L., D'Souza, A., Singh, A., Kalthur, S., 2015. Unilateral anatomical variation of the ansa cervicalis. Australas. Med. J. 8, 170–173.

Rao, T.R., Shetty, P., Rao, S.R., 2007. A rare case of formation of double ansa cervicalis. Neuroanatomy 6, 26–27.

Rath, G., Anand, C., 1994. Vagocervical complex replacing an absent ansa cervicalis. Surg. Radiol. Anat. 16, 441–443.

Rath, S., Sasmal, P.K., Saha, K., Deep, N., Mishra, P., Mishra, T.S., Sharma, R., 2015. Ancient schwannoma of ansa cervicalis: arare clinical entity and review of the literature. Case Rep. Surg. 578467.

Righini, C.A., Motto, E., Faure, C., Karkas, A., Lefournier, V., Reyt, E., 2007. Schwannomas of the neck. About 3 cases, and literature review. Rev. Laryngol. Otol. Rhinol. (Bord) 128, 109–115.

Rodrigues, A., 1930a. Communicating branches between the cervical sympathetic and the descendens cervicalis. J. Anat. 64, 308–318.

Rodrigues, A., 1930b. Le descendens cervicalis chez l'homme et chez le mammifères (quelques notes sur son évolution phylogénique). Assoc. Anatomistes C. R. 25, 267–282.

Sangvichien, S., Putsom, O., Chuncharunee, A., 2017. Anatomical variations of the ansa cervicalis in Thais. Siriraj Med. J. 55, 91–99.

Schaefer, E., Symington, J., Bryce, T., 1915. Quain's Elements of Anatomy, eleventh ed. Longmans, Green, and Co, London.

Shoja, M.M., Griessenauer, C.J., Apaydin, N., Rizk, E., Tubbs, R.S., 2015. An ansa cervicalis with vagohypoglossal anastamosis, absent inferior root and unusual C1 contribution. J. Exp. Clin. Neurosci. 2, 1–5.1.

Standring, S., 2016. Gray's Anatomy, 41st Edition. Elsevier, Canada.

Tubbs, R.S., Salter, E.G., Oakes, W.J., 2005. Anatomic landmarks for nerves of the neck: a vade mecum for neurosurgeons. Neurosurgery 56, 256–260.

Tucker, H.M., Rusnov, M., 1981. Laryngeal reinnervation for unilateral vocal cord paralysis: long-term results. Ann. Otol. Rhinol. Laryngol. 90, 457–459.

Tunner, W., 1893. A phrenic nerve receiving a root of origin from the descendens hypoglossi. J. Anat. Physiol. 27, 427.

Venugopal, S., Mallula, S., 2010. Ansa cervicalis—without loop. Int. J. Anat. Var. 3, 153–155.

Verma, R., Das, S., Suri, R., 2005. Unusual organization of the ansa Cervicalis: a case report. Braz. J. Morphol. Sci. 22, 175–177.

Vollala, V.R., Bhat, S.M., Nayak, S., Raghunathan, D., Samuel, V.P., Rodrigues, V., Mathew, J.G., 2005. A rare origin of upper root of ansa cervicalis from vagus nerve: a case report. Neuroanatomy 4, 8–9.

Winckler, G., 1955. A propros des relations que relations que existent entre le plexus cervical et le nerf grand hypoglosse. Assoc. Anatomistes C. R. 42, 1415–1419.

Wischnewsky, A., 1930. Die aufbautypes des ramus descendens nervi hypoglossi. Z. Anat. Entwicklungsgeschichte 92, 551–564.

Yoleri, L., Songur, E., Yoleri, O., Vural, T., Cagdas, A., 2000. Reanimation of early facial paralysis with hypoglossal/facial end-to-side neurorrhaphy: a new approach. J. Reconstr. Microsurg. 16, 346–347.

Zapata, P., Torrealba, G., 1988. Reflex effects evoked by stimulation of hypoglossal afferent fibers. Brain Res. 445, 19–29.

Zhang, H., Cai, C., Wang, S., Liu, H., Ye, Y., Chen, X., 2007. Extracranial head and neck schwannomas: a clinical analysis of 33 patients. Laryngoscope 117, 278–281.

CHAPTER 8

The Spinal Accessory Nerve

R. SHANE TUBBS

INTRODUCTION

The spinal accessory nerve (Fig. 8.1), named by Thomas Willis (Willis, 1965) cranial nerve XI, innervates the sternocleidomastoid (SCM) and trapezius muscles. It has a complex anatomy and shares a unique relationship with the cervical plexus. From a clinical perspective, this nerve is significant because it can be injured during surgical interventions involving the neck, namely in the posterior cervical triangle, potentially resulting in loss of movement of the aforementioned muscles (Inoue et al., 2006; Durazzo et al., 2009; Benninger, 2015). The nerve consists almost entirely of motor fibers, but recent studies have suggested that it might transmit sensory/nociceptive signals as well (Bremner-Smith et al., 1999; Tubbs et al., 2014a,b; Restrepo et al., 2015; Overland et al., 2016). The number of myelinated fibers contained in the spinal accessory nerve can range from 1700 to 2000 and its diameter is close to 2 mm (Saxod et al., 1985; Alnot and Narakas, 1996).

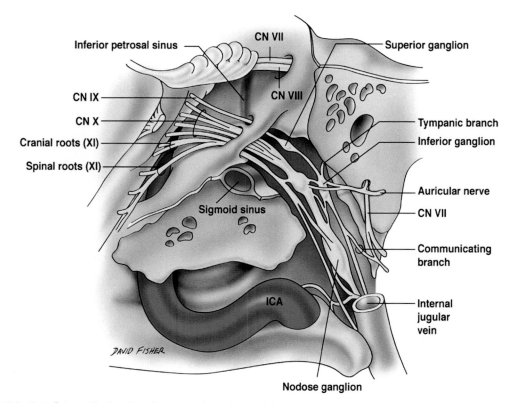

FIG. 8.1 Schematic drawing of a posterolateral view of the opened jugular foramen noting the course of the proximal components of the spinal accessory nerve.

Surgical Anatomy of the Cervical Plexus and its Branches. https://doi.org/10.1016/B978-0-323-83132-1.00004-4

Historically, the terms "accessory nerve" and "spinal accessory nerve" have been used interchangeably (Benninger, 2015). More recent anatomical texts differentiate between the two and describe the spinal accessory nerve as comprising two distinct portions (Alnot and Narakas, 1996; Benninger, 2015; Watkinson and Gleeson, 2016). One portion is the spinal root (Figs. 8.2 and 8.3), which is derived from the spinal cord. The other, the cranial root(s), arises from the brain stem (Fig. 8.4) (Alnot and Narakas, 1996; Linn et al., 2009; Benninger, 2015) (Fig. 8.2). The accessory branch leaves the skull as the external ramus or branch, which innervates the SCM and trapezius muscles (DeToledo and Dow, 1998; DeToledo and David, 2001; Falla et al., 2002; Benninger, 2015) (Fig. 8.5). The cranial portions join the vagus nerve as the internal branch or ramus (Linn et al., 2009; Benninger, 2015) (Fig. 8.5). Together with the vagus nerve, these latter parts of the spinal accessory nerve are thought to innervate the palatal, pharyngeal, and laryngeal muscles.

Some authors have proposed that the true spinal accessory nerve consists only of the spinal root, and that the cranial root is independent of it (Wiles et al., 2007; Kappers et al., 1967). Instead, the cranial root should be classified as a caudal portion of the vagus nerve, and this view has been supported by research on various species (Kappers et al., 1967; Barbas-Henry and Lohman, 1984; de Oliveria et al., 1985; Oka et al., 1987; Kitamura et al., 1989). However, human cadaveric studies have confirmed the existence of a cranial root contributing to the spinal accessory nerve and it can be considered as one of the two roots contributing to the spinal accessory nerve proper (Ryan et al., 2007; Wiles et al., 2007; Tubbs et al., 2014a) (Fig. 8.2).

ANATOMY

The spinal accessory nerve is derived from a nucleus of motor neurons located laterally in the ventral horn. The contributing rootlets take a variable course in their route to the nerve, some emerging directly and others joining after a more circuitous, irregular path. The rootlets themselves have various origins and are classified on the basis of their point of genesis as contributing to either the cranial or the spinal root (Watkinson and Gleeson, 2016). The spinal portion arises from the upper five or six rootlets originating from the spinal nucleus of the lateral gray matter of cervical spinal levels C1–C5, and the cranial portion arises from four or five rootlets originating from the dorsolateral surface of the medulla oblongata (Salgarelli et al., 2009; Ryan

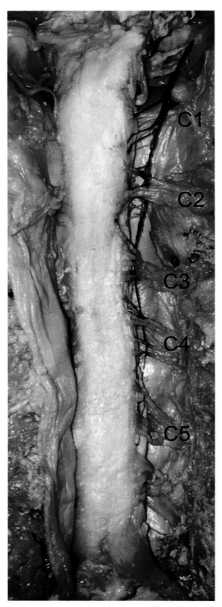

FIG. 8.2 Posterior cadaveric dissection of the entire spinal part of the spinal accessory nerve (here colored in purple). The cervical spinal dorsal rootlets are labeled. Also observe that the posterior rootlets of C1 are absent in this case.

et al., 2007; Overland et al., 2016). The spinal rootlets ascend through the spinal canal and enter the posterior cranial fossa via the foramen magnum, traveling behind the vertebral artery and dorsal to the denticulate ligaments.

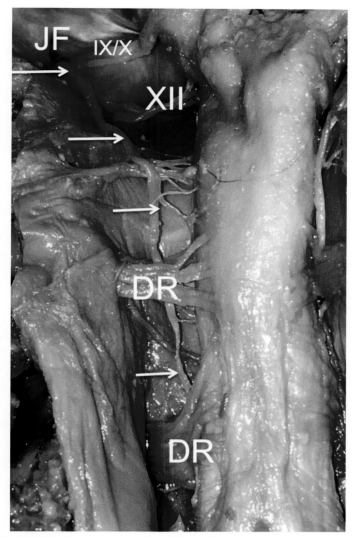

FIG. 8.3 Posterior cadaveric dissection following removal of the vertebral artery. Note the relationship of the spinal accessory nerve (arrows) anteriorly with the hypoglossal nerve (XII). Also note the relationship between the spinal accessory nerve and the dorsal rootlets (DR). The jugular foramen (JF) and cranial nerves IX and X are also shown. Also observe that the posterior rootlets of C1 are absent in this case.

These rootlets then connect with the cranial root to constitute a common trunk of the spinal accessory nerve (Alnot and Narakas, 1996).

The trunk then turns upwards and travels laterally to pass through the jugular foramen. During this passage through the jugular foramen, it runs through a dural sheath while traveling lateral to the vagus nerve and anterior to the internal jugular vein (IJV) (Watkinson and Gleeson, 2016). While passing or transiting the IJV, the spinal accessory nerve forms connections with the vagus nerve via its internal ramus or pars vagalis with the superior ganglion of the vagus nerve (Fig. 8.5) (Lang, 1989; Katsuta et al., 1997). These connections are believed to allow the cranial part of the spinal accessory nerve to be distributed via the recurrent laryngeal nerve branch of the vagus (Ling and Smoll, 2016; Polednak, 2017). These crosslinks can be considered as more proximal interconnections between the accessory and vagus nerves, and are sometimes termed Lobstein's anastomoses (Olry, 1995).

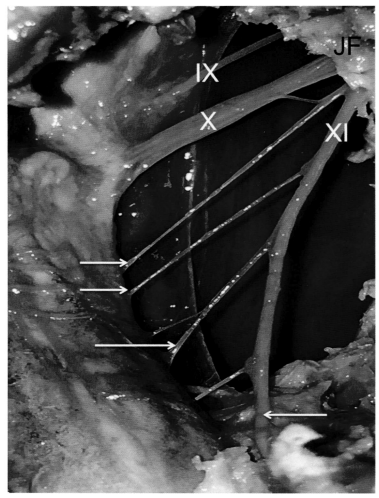

FIG. 8.4 Anterior dissection of the skull base emphasizing the anatomy of the right sided CNs IX-XII as they arise from the brain stem and spinal cord and exit via the jugular foramen (JF). The upper three arrows mark the cranial roots of the spinal accessory nerve and the lower arrow marks the spinal part.

After passing through the jugular foramen, the spinal accessory nerve trunk enters the neck and lies snugly between the internal carotid artery and the IJV. The common trunk enters the retrostyloid space and then separates once again into fibers derived from spinal and cranial roots (Salgarelli et al., 2009; Iwanaga et al., 2017). The cranial roots (internal branches) join the vagus nerve and the spinal roots (external branch) then progresses onward and travels past the IJV laterally, although there is a degree of variation in this part of its route (Overland et al., 2016). The spinal accessory nerve then travels past the transverse process of the atlas,

anteriorly in most cases, although there is some variation; less commonly, it lies lateral or medial to the transverse process of the atlas (Durazzo et al., 2009). It then descends medially to the styloid process and travels past the stylohyoid and digastric muscles (Overland et al., 2016). It runs alongside the superior SCM branch of the occipital artery and enters the deep surface of the upper portion of the SCM muscle. Once within the muscle, it forms a connection with fibers from C2 alone, C3 alone, or both C2 and C3 (Watkinson and Gleeson, 2016). The spinal accessory nerve is the only nerve that transmits motor signals to the SCM. C2

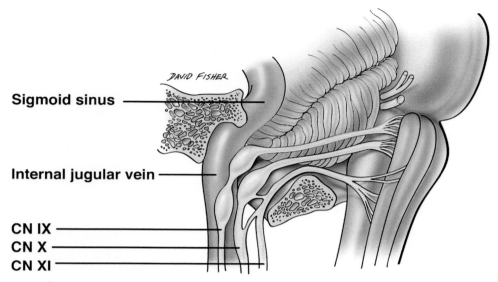

FIG. 8.5 Schematic drawing through the jugular foramen in coronal section illustrating the anatomy of the spinal accessory nerve.

and C3 cervical nerve fibers are said to carry prioprioceptive fibers (DeToledo and David, 2001; Fitzgerald et al., 1982; Watkinson and Gleeson, 2016).

The spinal accessory nerve exits from along the posterior border of the SCM muscle, at which point it often receives a communicating branch from the great auricular nerve (Brown et al., 2000). During its passage through the posterior cervical triangle, the nerve is relatively superficial is separated from the overlying skin by a thin sheet of deep cervical fascia and adipose tissue. It then travels to the anterior border of the trapezius muscle and forms a plexus at its surface about 3—5 cm superior to the clavicle. This plexus also receives branches from C2—C4 ventral rami and then enters the deep surface of the trapezius muscle (Fig. 8.6) or some of these cervical nerve fibers may join the spinal accessory nerve more proximally (Watkinson and Gleeson, 2016) (Fig. 8.7). Most of the motor supply to the trapezius muscle is derived from the spinal accessory nerve, with some contribution from the cervical plexus. This latter contribution is variable, but C2, C3, and C4 are believed to contribute to the cervical motor supply to the trapezius (Tubbs et al., 2011b; Kim et al., 2014; Watkinson and Gleeson, 2016). Pu et al. (2008) showed that the C2 nerve mostly innervates the trapezius muscle via communication with the spinal accessory nerve, whereas the C3 and C4 nerves innervate the muscle independently. The extension to the trapezius muscle serves

as the terminal trunk of the spinal accessory nerve (Figs. 8.7—8.9) (Alnot and Narakas, 1996).

Recently, Brinzeu and Sindou (2017) intraoperatively mapped contributions to the spinal accessory nerve using electromyography. The authors performed 262 stimulation sites on 49 patients. A vocal cord response was obtained by stimulation of the cranial root in 84.2% of stimulations. No stimulation of spinal roots resulted in vocal cord responses. Stimulation at C-1 resulted in a 95.8% response of the sternal head of the sternocleidomastoid muscle. Stimulation of C-2 resulted in a 90.0% response of the clavicular head of the sternocleidomastoid muscle. C-3 stimulation resulted in responses in the superior part of the trapezius muscle 66.6% of the time. Inferior to C3, stimulation resulted in only middle part of the trapezius being activated.

VARIATIONS

Some degree of anatomical variation in the course taken by the spinal accessory nerve has been reported in the literature. The spinal contribution is located close to the anterior and posterior rootlets of the upper five cervical nerves (Kumaki, 1970; Moriishi et al., 1989). Four different patterns of intradural communication between the spinal accessory nerve and the first cervical nerve rootlets have been described (Ouaknine and

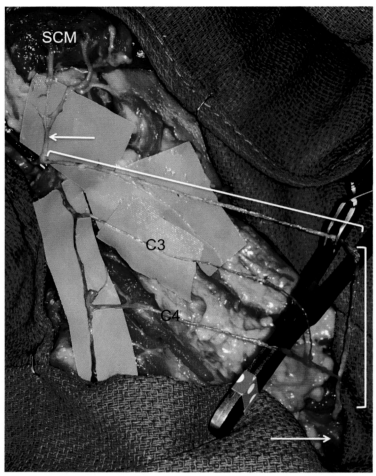

FIG. 8.6 Right neck dissection illustrating the proximal spinal accessory nerve branches (upper arrow) to the sternocleidomastoid muscle (SCM) and continuation (brackets) to the trapezius muscle (lower arrow). Also, note the contributions from C3 and C4 spinal nerves to the distal spinal accessory nerve en route to the trapezius muscle.

Nathan, 1973; Hagenah et al., 1983). In the type I variant, the posterior C1 root is absent and the spinal accessory nerve occasionally connects to the anterior C1 rootlets. In the type II variant, there is no communication with the posterior C1 nerve rootlets. The type III variant features a connection between the spinal accessory nerve and the posterior C1 rootlets either at their crossing point or through a posterior C1 rootlet anastomotic branch (Fig. 8.8). Finally, the type IV variant presents with a spinal accessory nerve forming a connection with the posterior C1 root that is not connected to the spinal cord (Ouaknine and Nathan, 1973; Hagenah et al., 1983).

As previously described, the spinal accessory nerve most commonly traverses lateral to the IJV. However, it can less commonly travel medial to the IJV, through the IJV, or even divide and come back together to travel both medial and lateral to the IJV (Saman et al., 2011; Hashimoto et al., 2012; Taylor et al., 2013). In rare cases, the SCM muscle can serve as the nerve's terminus with the trapezius being exclusively innervated by cervical nerve fibers. However, the spinal accessory nerve more often exits from along the midpoint of the posterior border of the SCM muscle (Watkinson and Gleeson, 2016). A recent cadaveric study by Tubbs et al. (2016) revealed that there can be multiple anatomical variations along its length. One area of variability reported in this study was the course taken by the spinal accessory nerve through the jugular foramen, as in one

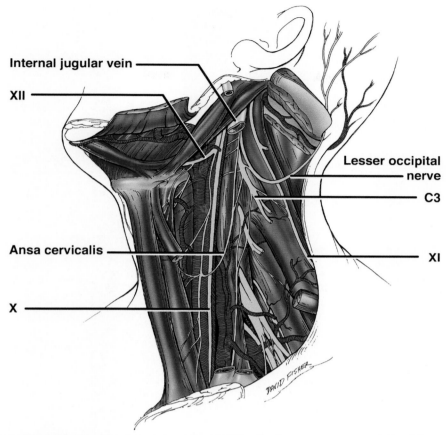

FIG. 8.7 Schematic drawing of the left neck and illustrating the course of the spinal accessory nerve superficial to the levator scapulae and to the trapezius muscle.

specimen the spinal accessory nerve lay within its own dural compartment and formed a plexus of nerves with the vagus. Other variations reported included intracranial duplication of the spinal accessory nerve and a direct connection with the facial nerve, with both nerves commonly innervating the SCM muscle (Tubbs et al., 2016).

LANDMARKS

Awareness of the anatomical landmarks associated with the spinal accessory nerve is important for any surgeon operating within its vicinity, given the clinical consequences of injuring it intraoperatively. This sensitivity to operative injury is most prominent when procedures of the posterior triangle of the neck are involved, and multiple landmarks have been identified to help orient surgeons in this area (Overland et al., 2016). Within the posterior cervical triangle, this nerve lies between the superficial and prevertebral layers of the cervical fascia and is just lateral to the levator scapulae muscle. The spinal accessory nerve crosses the anterior surface of the transverse process of the atlas. At a point midway between the mastoid process and angle of the mandible, it inclines posteriorly deep to the occipital artery and enters the sternocleidomastoid muscle at the junction of its upper and second quarters and leaves at the junction of the upper and second thirds (Brash and Jamieson, 1942). This emergence from the sternocleidomastoid is approximated by the superior border of the thyroid cartilage (Schaeffer, 1953). The fibers to the trapezius enter this muscle anteriorly approximately 5 cm superior to the muscle's attachment to the lateral one-third of the clavicle (Grant, 1940). The spinal accessory nerve travels anterior to the internal jugular vein in approximately 70%−80% of cases (Agur and Lee, 1991).

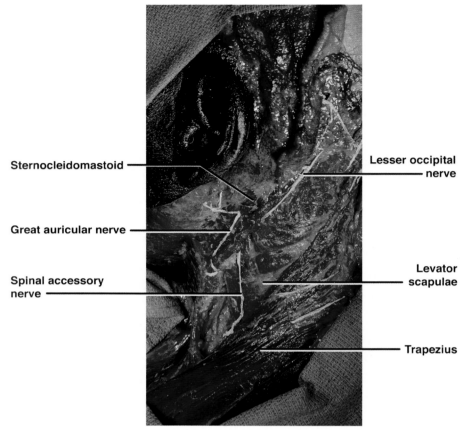

Sternocleidomastoid

Great auricular nerve

Spinal accessory nerve

Lesser occipital nerve

Levator scapulae

Trapezius

FIG. 8.8 Posterolateral view of the left posterior cervical triangle. Note the spinal accessory nerve leaving the posterior border of the sternocleidomastoid and traveling distally to the trapezius.

In approximately 20%–30% of individuals, it may pass posterior to this vessel and in approximately 3%, this nerve will pierce the internal jugular vein in route to the sternocleidomastoid muscle (Williams and Warwick, 1975). The spinal accessory nerve enters the deep surface of the sternocleidomastoid muscle approximately 5 cm (2–3 finger breadths) inferior to the apex of the mastoid process (Grant 1940). Treves (1907) note that this distance is 2.5 cm inferior to the tip of the mastoid process. Branches of cervical nerves 3 and 4 travel approximately a finger's breadth inferior and parallel to the spinal accessory nerve in route to the trapezius muscle. The approximate path of the spinal accessory nerve can also be represented by a line drawn inferiorly from the lower and anterior part of the tragus to the tip of the transverse process of the atlas, and then inferiorly and posteriorly, across the elevation produced by the sternocleidomastoid and the depression corresponding to the posterior triangle of the neck, to a point on the anterior border of the trapezius at the approximate 5 cm superior to the clavicle mentioned earlier (Williams and Warwick, 1975).

In a cadaveric study, Tubbs et al. (2005a,b) found that the distance between the midpoint of the clavicle to the entrance of the spinal accessory nerve into the trapezius ranged from 5 to 7.5 cm (mean 6 cm; SD 1.9). The distance from the inferior aspect of the mastoid process to the spinal accessory nerve's entrance into the trapezius ranged from 6.5 to 8.5 cm (mean 7 cm; SD 1.7). The distance from the acromion process of the scapula to the spinal accessory nerve's entrance into the trapezius ranged from 5 to 7 cm (mean 5.5 cm; SD 3.1). The distance from the posterior border of the sternocleidomastoid muscle to the entrance site

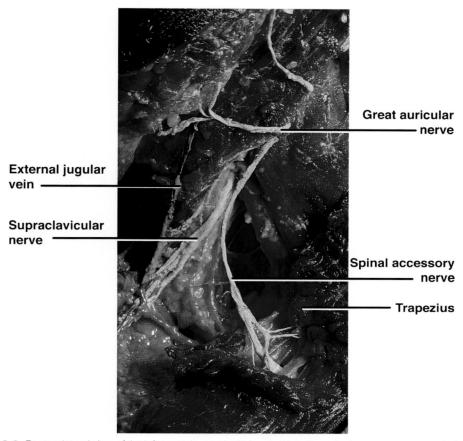

External jugular vein

Supraclavicular nerve

Great auricular nerve

Spinal accessory nerve

Trapezius

FIG. 8.9 Posterolateral view of the left posterior cervical triangle. Note the spinal accessory nerve entering the deep surface of the trapezius, which has been dissected.

of the spinal accessory nerve into the trapezius (i.e., the entire course of the spinal accessory nerve in the posterior cervical triangle) ranged from 2.5 to 4 cm (3.5 cm; SD 2.2). The distance from the angle of the mandible to the exit site of the spinal accessory nerve from the posterior border of the sternocleidomastoid muscle ranged from 4.5 to 7 cm (mean 6 cm; SD 1.5). The distance from the inferior aspect of the mastoid process to the exit site of the spinal accessory nerve from the posterior border of the sternocleidomastoid muscle ranged from 4.5 to 6.5 cm (mean 5 cm; SD 1.3). The width of the spinal accessory nerve while in the posterior cervical triangle ranged from 2 to 5 mm (mean 3 mm) and the length of the spinal accessory nerve while in the posterior cervical triangle ranged from 2 to 5 cm (mean 3.5 cm).

Kim et al. (2003) have said that the course of the spinal accessory nerve can be found by palpating the transverse process of C2 and then projecting a line from this point to the tip of the shoulder although the latter point was not defined. Treves et al. (1907) has noted that the spinal accessory nerve often exits the posterior border of the sternocleidomastoid muscle at the junction of the upper and second thirds of this muscle. However, Brown (2002) states that this point is at the midpoint of the muscle or at the junction of its upper and middle third. Lu et al. (2002) found that the spinal accessory nerve exited the posterior border of the sternocleidomastoid muscle 50.7 ± 12.9 mm superior to the clavicle. Kierner et al. (2000) have reported that the spinal accessory nerve exited the posterior border of the sternocleidomastoid muscle 8.2 ± 1.01 cm superior to the clavicle. The exit of the great auricular nerve posterior to the sternocleidomastoid may also serve as a landmark for the spinal accessory nerve with the spinal accessory nerve being superior to and within 2 cm from the great auricular nerve at its exit from the posterior border of the sternocleidomastoid muscle. The spinal accessory nerve has been noted to enter the trapezius from 2 to 10 cm superior to the clavicle. We found that this distance had a mean of 6 cm. The discrepancy in distances may simply be the varied concavity of the clavicle or the differences in muscle bulk of the trapezius. Bonnard and Narakas (1996) have mentioned that the transverse cervical vessels pass superficial to the spinal accessory nerve 4 cm superior to the clavicle.

At a point around midway between the mastoid process and angle of the mandible, it enters the SCM muscle at the junction between its upper and second quarters. It emerges from the SCM muscle at a point landmarked by the superior border of the thyroid cartilage (Schaeffer, 1953).

The nerve then traverses through the posterior cervical triangle on its approach to the trapezius. Its point of entry to the trapezius muscle is around 5 cm medial to the attachment of trapezius to the lateral one-third of the clavicle (Peck and Luce, 1988; Aramrattana et al., 2005; Tatla et al., 2005). Another point that helps orient surgeons within the posterior triangle is the nerve point or punctum nervosum, which is located around the midpoint of the posterior border of the SCM muscle (Frank et al., 1997; Tubbs et al., 2007). This point is mistakenly referred to as Erb's point by many anatomists and clinicians, as demonstrated by Tubbs et al. (2007). The nerve point serves as a landmark to approximate the location at which the bundle of sensory nerves from the cervical plexus emerges from the posterior border of the SCM muscle (Salagrelli et al., 2009; Durazzo et al., 2009; Overland et al., 2016). The spinal accessory nerve is usually found just proximal to the nerve point as it enters the posterior cervical triangle from the posterior border of the sternocleidomastoid muscle.

EMBRYOLOGY

For much of its embryological development, the spinal accessory nerve exists as a common structure that also gives rise to the vagus nerve. This structure comprises both sensory and motor roots with ganglia derived from the same ganglionic crest. As development proceeds, its cranial end becomes more sensory while the caudal end is predominantly motor in nature (Streeter, 1905). The series of structures that eventually give rise to the spinal accessory nerve is not defined until around the third week of development. Around day 20, the ganglion crest has lateralized into left and right halves and the part of the crest giving rise to the spinal cord arranges

itself into a flattened compact structure, the dorsal bridge (Streeter, 1905).

A series of rounded segmental clusters of cells project ventrally from this structure and eventually form the primitive spinal ganglia. The ganglionic crest of the vagus exists as a spindle-shaped structure that proceeds caudally, ending just beyond the fourth brachial arch. At the caudal end of this ganglion crest, there is a well-defined bundle of fibers that represents the future spinal accessory nerve. This bundle lies enclosed within a sleeve of cells, distinguishing it from the vagal ganglionic crest. It is located at the fourth, fifth, and sixth cervical vertebral segments. At irregular intervals, fibers connect to this bundle from the dorsolateral border of the neural tube. During the fourth week of development, the spinal accessory nerve remains enclosed within the sleeve of cells, but it extends forward and turns the curve on the back of the trunk of the vagus nerve. As it frees itself from the vagus nerve, it proceeds a short distance laterally and then ends in a mass of condensed mesoderm, which is a precursor to the SCM muscle (Streeter, 1905).

By day 30 of development, the cellular and fibrous elements have increased considerably. A chain of ganglia is observed among the rootlets of the spinal accessory nerve as the cell masses become segmented into ganglionic clumps. At the end of the fifth week, the developing spinal accessory nerve lies medial to the dorsal rootlets and is connected at irregular intervals to the spinal cord. It usually adheres to the first spinal ganglion, and at this point cell masses are attached to the trunk of the nerve itself. Toward the cranial end of the spinal accessory nerve is a row of ganglia that eventually gives rise to the accessory root ganglia. These ganglia become successively larger throughout development and eventually form a connection with the jugular ganglion of the vagus nerve. Initially, the accessory root ganglia comprise three or four principal masses with several smaller clumps scattered among the rootlets (Streeter, 1905).

During the second and third months of development, the spinal accessory nerve elongates and becomes more sharply defined. The continuous growth of the fiber elements separates the ganglionic masses more widely from one another. Two root ganglia appear along the trunk of the spinal accessory nerve between the first cervical ganglion and the jugular ganglion. A third ganglionic mass is also observed partially attached to the jugular ganglion. This complex eventually rearranges itself such that the cranial end is predominantly sensory and the caudal or accessory division is predominantly motor (Streeter, 1905). As development proceeds, the spinal accessory nerve eventually adapts a form similar to the anatomy previously described for adults.

MOLECULAR DEVELOPMENT

The molecular development of the spinal accessory nerve has been a more recent area of study, and a few molecular pathways have been implicated (Tada and Kuratano, 2015). A homeodomain-containing transcription factor, *Nkx2.9*, has been proposed to play some role in regulating the development of the spinal accessory nerve. *Nkx2.9*-null mutant mice consistently developed shorter and thinner spinal accessory nerve axons than wild type mice. In 50% of *Nkx2.9* mutant mice, the vagus and glossopharyngeal nerves were also malformed (Pabst et al., 2003; Tada and Kuratano, 2015). The *Gli2* gene regulates the initial extension of axons from spinal accessory nerve cell bodies, and the receptor-encoding gene *Dcc* functions alongside netrin-1 to allow for the dorsal migration of the nerve (Dillon et al., 2005). The development of spinal accessory nerve axons is also regulated in part by *UNC5C*, a gene that encodes the UNC5 receptor. This receptor facilitates migration of the spinal accessory nerve away from the ventral midline, and *UNC5C* mutant mice have inappropriately clustered spinal accessory nerve cell bodies within the ventrolateral spinal cord (Dillon et al., 2007; Tada and Kuratano, 2015).

HISTOLOGY

The categorization of the spinal accessory nerve as a purely motor nerve has been challenged by more recent studies, which have revealed the potential of the spinal accessory nerve to carry sensory fibers as well (Tubbs et al., 2014b). The earliest evidence for the potential of the spinal accessory nerve to carry sensory signals came from experiments highlighting the presence of sensory fibers in the spinal accessory nerves of monkeys and cats (Windle, 1931) and anecdotal pain syndromes following spinal accessory nerve injury. These findings were supplemented by subsequent simulation experiments in cats, which showed that the spinal accessory nerve can carry sensory fibers that are proprioceptive rather than nocioceptive in function (Windle and DeLozier, 1932). It has also been proposed that this nerve holds the requisite apparatus to carry sensory fibers; there is evidence of connections with C2 and C3 fibers, and a dorsal root ganglion is shared between the first cervical nerve and the spinal accessory nerve (Pearson, 1937; Tubbs et al., 2011b, 2014b).

A recent histological investigation by Tubbs et al. (2014b) revealed occasional microganglia cells along the periphery of spinal accessory nerve fibers. These microganglia cells were always on the nerve's periphery and were most abundant within its intracranial segment. They were shown to be neuronal in composition by reacting positively to synaptophysin. In other animals, similar cells carry nociceptive signals (Tubbs et al., 2014b). A study of rats highlighted clusters of pseudounipolar sensory neurons associated with the spinal accessory nerve. It was concluded that these fibers serve a nociceptive function for the muscles innervated by the spinal accessory nerve (Wetmore and Elde, 1991). In humans, the spinal accessory nerve contains a bundle of unmyelinated fibers that can be classified as dorsal C root fibers, which are known to transmit sensory modalities such as pain, temperature, mechanoreception, and reflex responses (Bremner-Smith et al., 1999). One symptom associated with spinal accessory nerve injury is pain within its area of distribution, and injury to nociceptive fibers within the spinal accessory nerve could produce such outcomes (Tubbs et al., 2014b).

PATHOLOGY

The spinal accessory nerve holds important clinical significance for surgeons who operate in and around the posterior triangle of the neck, as injury to it at this point can cause severe shoulder disability. The nerve itself follows a long and superficial course through the posterior triangle and is at risk of iatrogenic injury during surgical procedures (Mirjalili et al., 2012). Isolated palsy of the spinal accessory nerve can also be produced iatrogenically during IJV cannulation in the posterior triangle of the neck, during carotid endarterectomy, coronary bypass surgery, and radiation therapy (Brazis et al., 2011). Aside from iatrogenic injury, palsy of the spinal accessory nerve can result secondary to blunt or penetrating trauma to the lateral neck, and as a result of cervical stretch injury. Injury to the spinal accessory nerve produces a cluster of signs and symptoms characterized by scapular, shoulder and neck pain, weakness and drooping of the shoulder, trapezius atrophy, and limited active coronal plane abduction (Kelley et al., 2008). In chronic cases, compensatory hypertrophy of the levator scapulae muscle can also occur (Ong and Chong, 2010).

Most cases involving iatrogenic injury to the spinal accessory nerve are thought to occur during lymph node biopsies performed by general surgeons and otolaryngologists in the posterior triangle of the neck (Kretschmer et al., 2001; Kim et al., 2003; Mirjalili et al., 2012). Roughly 3—8% of posterior cervical triangle lymph node biopsy procedures result in such injury (Kim et al., 2003; Morris et al., 2008). Ewing and Martin

(1952) were the first to present a comprehensive review of the cluster of symptoms following radical neck dissection. They described a significant incidence of disfigurement of the shoulder with drooping or undue prominence on one side, a vaguely defined pain within the shoulder region, and some weakness within the arm (Ewing and Martin, 1952). This clinical presentation was described by Nahum et al. (1961) as "shoulder syndrome," comprising pain within and drooping of the shoulder, impaired abduction of the shoulder, and atrophy of the SCM and trapezius muscles coupled with compensatory hypertrophy of the other shoulder muscles (Nahum et al., 1961; Overland et al., 2016). More recent surgical advances have led to the development of procedures that attempt to spare injury to the spinal accessory nerve, but even these produce shoulder complaints in up to a third of all patients (van Wilgen et al., 2004).

Rarely, clinical pathologies such as schwannoma of the spinal accessory nerve are also observed. Reporting on a case of schwannoma within the cervical portion of the nerve, Kohli et al. (2013) noted that only 28 cases of schwannomas along the spinal accessory nerve had previously been reported. These tumors most commonly present as a gradually enlarging, painless lump causing no neurological signs or symptoms. Intracranial schwannomas of the spinal accessory nerve can be classified as cervical, intracisternal, or occurring within the jugular foramen. Tumors within the jugular foramen occur at the complex formed by the accessory, vagus, and glossopharyngeal nerves and are defined without identification of any individual cranial nerve (Kohli et al., 2013). These tumors are most commonly the result of paragangliono-mas, which result from paraganglionic tissue located in the adventitia of the jugular vein (glomus jugulare), or in and around the vagus nerve (glomus vagale) (Ramina et al., 2004).

SURGERY

As mentioned previously, iatrogenic injury to the spinal accessory nerve following its manipulation during procedures at the posterior triangle of the neck is a common cause of morbidity (Cesmebasi and Spinner, 2015). This nerve is particularly vulnerable to iatrogenic injury owing to its relatively superficial location within the posterior cervical triangle (Matz and Barbaro, 1996). Contributing to the intraoperative difficulty of avoiding injury to the spinal accessory nerve is the tortuous, coiled route it takes through the posterior cervical triangle while it has a straight gross configuration proximal to the posterior triangle (Tubbs et al., 2010).

This coiling could be attributed to biomechanical functional necessity, given the stretch experienced by structures within the posterior triangle during movements of the shoulder. The alteration in shape and pattern of the spinal accessory nerve during its descent through the posterior triangle does not appear to result from histological or structural differences (Tubbs et al., 2010).

Modified surgical techniques have been developed to avoid injury to the spinal accessory nerve during surgical interventions in and around the posterior cervical triangle, the original having been proposed by Bocca and Pignataro (1967). These authors showed that during its course through the posterior triangle, the spinal accessory nerve is located within an aponeurotic compartment separated from the cervical nodes and this is probably the same as the classically described thin sheet of deep cervical fascia in this area. They used this finding to develop a surgical technique that allows the nerve to be preserved (Bocca and Pignataro, 1967; Chaukar et al., 2006). A more recent paper by Chaukar et al. (2006) proposes using a small but constant vein that runs anterior to the spinal accessory nerve during its course through the posterior cervical triangle as a landmark to identify the nerve and prevent iatrogenic injury. This vein drains the SCM muscle into the pharyngeal plexus, and it emerges from the junction of the upper and middle thirds of the muscle. The spinal accessory nerve runs approximately 2 mm deep to this vein, so it could serve as a useful identifying landmark for surgical procedures involving the posterior triangle (Chaukar et al., 2006).

The spinal accessory nerve can be used as a transferable nerve in neurotization and reinnervation procedures. These procedures are performed to manage suprascapular and musculocutaneous nerve lesions (Tubbs et al., 2011a). The concept of using the spinal accessory nerve as a transferable nerve was pioneered by Kotani et al. (1971), who used it for reinnervation of the upper trunk and the radial and musculocutaneous nerves. Allieu et al. (1984) successfully transferred long cutaneous grafts from the spinal accessory nerve to the musculocutaneous and axillary nerves. If the spinal accessory nerve is approached anteriorly, the length available for transfer can be limited (Vathana et al., 2007; Tubbs et al., 2011a). More recent studies have suggested that a posterior approach could allow it to be harvested for ipsilateral neurotization procedures (Schaakxs et al., 2009). The posterior approach could even allow the spinal accessory nerve to be harvested for use in neurotization procedures involving the radial nerve branches to the triceps brachii muscle, and the axillary nerve at its exit from the quadrangular space (Vathana et al., 2007; Tubbs et al., 2011a). A recent cadaveric feasibility study by Tubbs et al. (2008) showed that the spinal accessory nerve would be feasible for use in neurotization of the phrenic nerve in patients with high cervical quadriplegia (Tubbs et al., 2008). Additionally, Tubbs et al. (2017) have shown that the spinal accessory nerve in the posterior cervical triangle can be lengthening in order to use it for neurotization procedures more distally. For example, in their cadaveric study, the nerve, following disconnection from its tetherings to cervical nerves, could be grafted to the musculocutaneous nerve via a subclavicular tunneling procedure.

IMAGING

The use of imaging techniques for investigating the spinal accessory nerve and its associated clinical pathologies has not been well researched. A recent study by Li et al. (2016) investigated the utility of MRI in assessing patients with suspected neuropathies of the spinal accessory nerve. They found that MRI evaluation of the SCM and trapezius muscles can identify areas of denervation and atrophy secondary to spinal accessory nerve neuropathy. These MRI findings can be used alongside EMG studies and clinical assessment to verify a diagnosis of spinal accessory nerve neuropathy (Li et al., 2016). Imaging can also be used to assess a patient for tumors along the length of the spinal accessory nerve. Paraganglionomas, which have been known to cause spinal accessory nerve neuropathy at the jugular foramen, appear on MRI as isointense lesions that are heavily enhanced after gadolinium administration. Larger tumors can have a characteristic salt-and-pepper appearance, with T-weighted hyperintense foci representative of subacute hemorrhage, and associated T2-weighted hypointense foci (Vogl and Bisdas, 2009).

CONCLUSIONS

Our knowledge of the spinal accessory nerve has increased and changed over the decades. Although we have learned more about this nerve's neuroanatomy, much is still to be learned about this enigmatic cranial nerve.

REFERENCES

Agur, M.R., Lee, M.J., 1991. Grant's Atlas of Anatomy, tenth ed. Lippincott Williams & Wilkins, Philadelphia. 760 pp.

Allieu, Y., Privat, J.M., Bonnel, F., 1984. Paralysis in root avulsion of the brachial plexus: neurotization by the spinal accessory nerve. Clin. Plast. Surg. 11, 133–136.

Alnot, J.Y., Narakas, A., 1996. Traumatic Brachial Plexus Injuries. Expansion Scientifique Française, Paris, pp. 33–35.

Aramrattana, A., Sittitrai, P., Harnsiriwattanagit, K., 2005. Surgical anatomy of the spinal accessory nerve in the posterior triangle of the neck. Asian J. Surg. 28, 171–173.

Barbas-Henry, H.A., Lohman, A.H., 1984. The motor nuclei and primary projections of the IXth, Xth, XIth, and XIIth cranial nerves in the monitor lizard, Varanusexanthematicus. J. Comp. Neurol. 226, 565–579.

Benninger, B., 2015. The accessory nerve (CN XI). In: Tubbs, R.S., Rizk, E., Shoja, M.M., Loukas, M., Barbaro, N., Spinner, R.J. (Eds.), Nerve and Nerve Injuries Volume 1: History, Embryology, Anatomy, Imaging, and Diagnostics. Academic Press, London, pp. 399–415.

Bocca, E., Pignataro, O., 1967. A conservation technique in radical neck dissection. Ann. Otol. Rhinol. Laryngol. 76, 975–987.

Bonnard, C., Narakas, A., 1996. Neurotization using the spinal accessory nerve in the brachial plexus lesions. In: Alnot, J.Y., Narakas, A. (Eds.), Traumatic Brachial Plexus Injuries. Expansion Scientifique Française, Paris, pp. 156–166.

Brash, J.C., Jamieson, E.B., 1942. Cunningham's Manual of Practical Anatomy, tenth ed. Oxford University Press, New York, p. 190.

Brazis, P.W., Masdeu, J.C., Biller, J., 2011. Localization in Clinical Neurology. Lippincott Williams & Wilkins, Philadelphia, pp. 369–376.

Bremner-Smith, A.T., Unwin, A.J., Williams, W.W., 1999. Sensory pathways in the spinal accessory nerve. J. Bone Jt. Surg. Br. 81, 226–228.

Brînzeu, A., Sindou, M., 2017. Functional anatomy of the accessory nerve studied through intraoperative electrophysiological mapping. J. Neurosurg. 126, 913–921.

Brown, H., 2002. Anatomy of the spinal accessory nerve plexus: relevance to head and neck cancer and atherosclerosis. Exp. Biol. Med. 227, 570–578.

Brown, H., Hidden, G., Ledroux, M., Poitevan, L., 2000. Anatomy and blood supply of the lower four cranial and cervical nerves: relevance to surgical neck dissection. Proc. Soc. Exp. Biol. Med. 223, 352–361.

Cesmebasi, A., Spinner, R.J., 2015. An anatomic-based approach to the iatrogenic spinal accessory nerve injury in the posterior cervical triangle: how to avoid and treat it. Clin. Anat. 28, 761–766.

Chaukar, D.A., Pai, A., D'Cruz, A.K., 2006. A technique to identify and preserve the spinal accessory nerve during neck dissection. J. Laryngol. Otol. 120, 494–496.

de Oliviera, E., Rhoton Jr., A.L., Pearce, D., 1985. Microsurgical anatomy of the region of the foramen magnum. Surg. Neurol. 24, 293–352.

DeToledo, J.C., David, N.J., 2001. Innervation of the sternocleidomastoid and trapezius muscles by the accessory nucleus. J. Neuro Ophthalmol. 21, 214–216.

DeToledo, J.C., Dow, R., 1998. Sternomastoid function during hemispheric suppression by amytal: insights into the inputs to the spinal accessory nucleus. Mov. Disord. 13, 809–812.

Dillon, A.K., Fujita, S.C., Matise, M.P., Jarjour, A.A., Kennedy, T.E., Kollmus, H., Arnold, H.H., Weiner, J.A.,

Sanes, J.R., Kaprielian, Z., 2005. Molecular control of spinal accessory motor neuron/axon development in the mouse spinal cord. J. Neurosci. 25, 10119–10130.

Dillon, A.K., Jevince, A.R., Hinck, L., Ackerman, S.L., Lu, X., Tessier-Lavigne, M., Kaprielian, Z., 2007. UNC5C is required for spinal accessory motor neuron development. Mol. Cell. Neurosci. 35, 482–489.

Durazzo, M.D., Furlan, J.C., Teixeira, G.V., Friguglietti, C.U., Kulcsar, M.A., Magalhães, R.P., Ferraz, A.R., Brandão, L.G., 2009. Anatomic landmarks for localization of the spinal accessory nerve. Clin. Anat. 22, 471–475.

Ewing, M.R., Martin, H., 1952. Disability following radical neck dissection: an assessment based on the postoperative evaluation of 100 patients. Cancer 5, 873–883.

Falla, D., Dall'Alba, P., Rainoldi, A., Merletti, R., Jull, G., 2002. Repeatability of surface EMG variables in the sternocleidomastoid and anterior scalene muscles. Eur. J. Appl. Physiol. 87, 542–549.

Fitzgerald, M.J.T., Comerford, P.T., Tuffery, A.R., 1982. Sources of innervation of the neuromuscular spindles in sternomastoid and trapezius. J. Anat. 134, 471–490.

Frank, D.K., Wenk, E., Stern, J.C., Gottlieb, R.D., Moscatello, A.L., 1997. A cadaveric study of the motor nerves to the levator scapulae muscle. Otolaryngol. Head Neck Surg. 117, 671–680.

Grant, J.C.B., 1940. A Method of Anatomy Descriptive and Deductive, second ed. Williams and Wilkins, Baltimore. 794 pp.

Hagenah, R., Kosak, M., Freckmann, N., 1983. Anatomic topographic relationship of the intraspinal accessory root to the upper cervical roots and to the vessels of the cranical cervical region. Acta Anat. 115, 158–167.

Hashimoto, Y., Otsuki, M., Morimoto, K., Saito, M., Nibu, K., 2012. Four cases of spinal accessory nerve passing through the fenestrated internal jugular vein. Surg. Radiol. Anat. 34, 373–375.

Inoue, H., Nibu, K., Saito, M., Otsuki, N., Ishida, H., Onitsuka, T., Fujii, T., Kawabata, K., Saikawa, M., 2006. Quality of life after neck dissection. Arch. Otolaryngol. Head Neck Surg. 132, 662–666.

Iwanaga, J., Fisahn, C., Alonso, F., DiLorenzo, D., Grunert, P., Kline, M.T., Watanabe, K., Oskouian, R.J., Spinner, R.J., Tubbs, R.S., 2017. Microsurgical anatomy of the hypoglossal and C1 nerves: description of a previously undescribed branch to the atlanto-occipital joint. World Neurosurg. 100, 590–593.

Kappers, A., Huber, G., Crosby, E., 1967. The Comparative Anatomy of the Nervous System of Vertebrates, Including Man, vol. II. Hafner Publishing Company, New York.

Katsuta, T., Rhoton Jr., A.L., Matsushima, T., 1997. The jugular foramen: microsurgical anatomy and operative approaches. Neurosurgery 41, 149–201.

Kelley, M.J., Kane, T.E., Leggin, B.G., 2008. Spinal accessory nerve palsy: associated signs and symptoms. J. Orthop. Sports Phys. Ther. 38, 78–86.

Kierner, A.C., Zelenka, I., Heler, S., Burian, M., 2000. Surgical anatomy of the spinal accessory nerve and the trapezius branches of the cervical plexus. Arch. Surg. 135, 1428–1431.

Kim, D.H., Cho, Y.J., Tiel, R.L., Kline, D.G., 2003. Surgical outcomes of 111 spinal accessory nerve injuries. Neurosurgery 53, 1106–1113.

Kim, J.H., Choi, K.Y., Lee, K.H., Lee, D.J., Park, B.J., Rho, Y.S., 2014. Motor innervation of the trapezius muscle: intraoperative motor conduction study during neck dissection. J. Otorhinolaryngol. Relat. Spec. 76, 8–12.

Kitamura, S., Nishiguchi, T., Ogata, K., Sakai, A., 1989. Neurons of origin of the internal ramus of the rabbit accessory nerve: localization in the dorsal nucleus of the vagus nerve and the nucleus retroambigualis. Anat. Rec. 224, 541–549.

Kohli, R., Singh, S., Gupta, S.K., Matreja, P.S., 2013. Schwannoma the spinal accessory nerve: a case report. J. Clin. Diagn. Res. 7, 1732–1734.

Kotani, T., Toshima, Y., Matsuda, H., Suzuki, T., Ishizaki, Y., 1971. Postoperative results of nerve transposition in brachial plexus injury. Seikei Geka 22, 963–966.

Kretschmer, T., Antoniadis, G., Braun, V., Rath, S.A., Richter, H.P., 2001. Evaluation of iatrogenic lesions in 722 surgically treated cases of peripheral nerve trauma. J. Neurosurg. 94, 905–912.

Kumaki, K., 1970. The cervical and the spinal accessory nerves: an account by means of fiber analysis. Acta Anat. Nippon. 45, 311–344.

Lang, J., 1989. Clinical Anatomy of the Nose, Nasal Cavity and Paranasal Sinuses. Georg ThiemeVerlag, Stuttgart.

Li, A.E., Greditzer 4th, H.G., Melisaratos, D.P., Wolfe, S.W., Feinberg, J.H., Sneag, D.B., 2016. MRI findings of spinal accessory neuropathy. Clin. Radiol. 71, 316–320.

Ling, X.Y., Smoll, N.R., 2016. A systematic review of variations of the recurrent laryngeal nerve. Clin. Anat. 29, 104–110.

Linn, J., Moriggl, B., Schwarz, F., Naidich, T.P., Schmid, U.D., Wiesmann, M., Bruckmann, H., Yousry, I., 2009. Cisternal segments of the glossopharyngeal, vagus, and accessory nerves: detailed magnetic resonance imaging — demonstrated anatomy and neurovascular relationships. J. Neurosurg. 110, 1026–1041.

Lu, L., Haman, S.P., Ebraheim, N.A., 2002. Vulnerability of the spinal accessory nerve in the posterior triangle of the neck: a cadaveric study. Orthopedics 25, 71–74.

Matz, P.G., Barbaro, N.M., 1996. Diagnosis and treatment of iatrogenic spinal accessory nerve injury. Am. Surg. 62, 682–685.

Mirjalili, S.A., Muirhead, J.C., Stringer, M.D., 2012. Ultrasound visualization of the spinal accessory nerve in vivo. J. Surg. Res. 175, e11–e16.

Moriishi, J., Otani, K., Tanaka, K., Inoue, S.I., 1989. The intersegmental anastomoses between spinal nerve roots. Anat. Rec. 224, 110–116.

Morris, L.G., Ziff, D.J., DeLacure, M.D., 2008. Malpractice litigation after surgical injury of the spinal accessory nerve: an evidence-based analysis. Arch. Otolaryngol. Head Neck Surg. 134, 102–107.

Nahum, A.M., Mullally, W., Marmor, L., 1961. A syndrome resulting from radical neck dissection. Arch. Otolaryngol. 74, 424–428.

Oka, Y., Satou, M., Ueda, K., 1987. Morphology and distribution of the motor neurons of the accessory nerve (nXI) in the Japanese toad: a cobaltic lysine study. Brain Res. 400, 383—388.

Olry, R., 1995. Dictionary of Anatomical Eponyms. Verlag, New York, p. 99.

Ong, C.K., Chong, V.F., 2010. The glossopharyngeal, vagus and spinal accessory nerves. Eur. J. Radiol. 74, 359—367.

Ouaknine, G., Nathan, H., 1973. Anastomotic connections between the eleventh nerve and the posterior root of the first cervical nerve in humans. J. Neurosurg. 38, 189—197.

Overland, J., Hodge, J.C., Breik, O., Krishnan, S., 2016. Surgical anatomy of the spinal accessory nerve: review of the literature and case report of a rare anatomical variant. J. Laryngol. Otol. 130 (10), 969—972.

Pabst, O., Rummelies, J., Winter, B., Arnold, H.H., 2003. Targeted disruption of the homeobox gene Nkx2.9 reveals a role in development of the spinal accessory nerve. Development 130, 1193—1202.

Pearson, A.A., 1937. The spinal accessory nerve in human embryos. J. Comp. Neurol. 68, 243—266.

Peck, D., Luce, E.A., 1988. A method for locating the external ramus of the accessory nerve in the posterior cervical triangle. Clin. Anat. 1, 53—58.

Polednak, A.P., 2017. Relationship of the recurrent laryngeal nerve to the inferior thyroid artery: a comparison of findings from two systematic reviews. Clin. Anat. 30, 318—321.

Pu, Y.M., Tang, E.Y., Yang, X.D., 2008. Trapezius muscle innervation from the spinal accessory nerve and branches of the cervical plexus. Int. J. Oral Maxillofac. Surg. 37 (6), 567—572.

Ramina, R., Maniglia, J.J., Fernandes, Y.B., Paschoal, J.R., Pfeilsticker, L.N., Neto, M.C., Borges, G., 2004. Jugular foramen tumors: diagnosis and treatment. Neurosurg. Focus 17, e5.

Restrepo, C.E., Tubbs, R.S., Spinner, R.J., 2015. Expanding what is known of the anatomy of the spinal accessory nerve. Clin. Anat. 28, 467—471.

Ryan, S., Blyth, P., Duggan, N., Wild, M., Al-Ali, S., 2007. Is the cranial accessory nerve really a portion of the accessory nerve? Anatomy of the cranial nerves in the jugular foramen. Anat. Sci. Int. 82, 1—7.

Salgarelli, A.C., Landini, B., Bellini, P., Multinu, A., Consolo, U., Collini, M., 2009. A simple method of identifying the spinal accessory in modified radical neck dissection: anatomic study and clinical implications for resident training. Oral Maxillofac. Surg. 13, 69—72.

Saman, M., Etebari, P., Pakdaman, M.N., Urken, M.L., 2011. Anatomic relationship between the spinal accessory nerve and the jugular vein: a cadaveric study. Surg. Radiol. Anat. 33, 175—179.

Saxod, R., Torch, S., Vila, A., Laurent, A., Stoebner, P., 1985. The density of myelinated fibres is related to the fascicle diameter in human superficial peroneal nerve: statistical study of 41 normal samples. J. Neurol. Sci. 71, 49—64.

Schaakxs, D., Bahm, J., Sellhaus, B., Weis, J., 2009. Clinical and neuropathological study about the neurotization of the suprascapular nerve in obstetric brachial plexus lesions. J. Brachial Plexus Peripher. Nerve Inj. 11 (4), 15.

Schaeffer, J.P., 1953. Morris' Human Anatomy: A Complete Systematic Treatise, eleventh ed. Blakiston Company, New York.

Streeter, G.L., 1905. The development of the cranial and spinal nerves in the occipital region of the human embryo. Am. J. Anat. 4, 83—116.

Tada, M.N., Kuratani, S., 2015. Evolutionary and developmental understanding of the spinal accessory nerve. Zool. Lett. 1, 4.

Tatla, T., Kanagalingam, J., Majithia, A., Clarke, P.M., 2005. Upper neck spinal accessory nerve identification during neck dissection. J. Laryngol. Otol. 119, 906—908.

Taylor, C.B., Boone, J.L., Schmalbach, C.E., Miller, F.R., 2013. Intraoperative relationship of the spinal accessory nerve to the internal jugular vein: variation from cadaver studies. Am. J. Otolaryngol. 34, 527—529.

Treves, F., 1907. Surgical Applied Anatomy, fifth ed. Lea Brothers, Philadelphia. 640 pp.

Tubbs, R.S., Pearson, B., Loukas, M., Shokouhi, G., Shoja, M.M., Oakes, W.J., 2008. Phrenic nerve neurotization utilizing the spinal accessory nerve: technical note with potential application in patients with high cervical quadriplegia. Childs Nerv. Syst. 24 (11), 1341—1344.

Tubbs, R.S., Salter, E.G., Oakes, W.J., 2005a. Anatomic landmarks for nerves of the neck: a vade mecum for neurosurgeons. Neurosurgery 56, 256—260.

Tubbs, R.S., Salter, E.G., Wellons 3rd, J.C., Blount, J.P., Oakes, W.J., 2005b. Superficial landmarks for the spinal accessory nerve within the posterior cervical triangle. J. Neurosurg. Spine 3, 375—378.

Tubbs, R.S., Loukas, M., Salter, E.G., Oakes, W.J., 2007. William Erb and Erb's point. Clin. Anat. 20, 486—488.

Tubbs, R.S., Stetler, W., Louis Jr., R.G., Gupta, A.A., Loukas, M., Kelly, D.R., Shoja, M.M., Cohen-Gadol, A.A., 2010. Surgical challenges associated with the morphology of the spinal accessory nerve in the posterior cervical triangle: functional or structural? J. Neurosurg. Spine 12, 22—24.

Tubbs, R.S., Mortazavi, M.M., Shoja, M.M., Loukas, M., Cohen-Gadol, A.A., 2011a. Contralateral spinal accessory nerve for ipsilateral neurotization of branches of the brachial plexus: a cadaveric feasibility study. J. Neurosurg. 114, 1538—1540.

Tubbs, R.S., Shoja, M.M., Loukas, M., Lancaster, J., Mortazavi, M.M., Hattab, E.M., Cohen-Gadol, A.A., 2011b. Study of the cervical plexus innervation of the trapezius muscle. J. Neurosurg. Spine 14, 626—629.

Tubbs, R.S., Ajayi, O.O., Fries, F.N., Spinner, R.J., Oskouian, R.J., 2016. Variations of the accessory nerve: anatomical study including previously undocumented findings — expanding our misunderstanding of this nerve. Br. J. Neurosurg. 31 (1), 113—115 (Epub ahead of print).

Tubbs, R.S., Benninger, B., Loukas, M., Cohen-Gadol, A.A., 2014a. Cranial roots of the accessory nerve exist in the majority of adult humans. Clin. Anat. 27, 102—107.

Tubbs, R.S., Sorenson, E.P., Watanabe, K., Loukas, M., Hattab, E., Cohen-Gadol, A.A., 2014b. Histologic confirmation of neuronal cell bodies along the spinal accessory nerve. Br. J. Neurosurg. 28, 746—749.

Tubbs, R.S., Maldonado, A.A., Stoves, Y., Fries, F.N., Li, R., Loukas, M., Oskouian, R.J., Spinner, R.J., 2017. A novel method of lengthening the accessory nerve for direct coaptation during nerve repair and nerve transfer procedures. J. Neurosurg. 3, 1—5.

van Wilgen, C.P., Dijkstra, P.U., van der Laan, B.F., Plukker, J.T., Roodenburg, J.L., 2004. Shoulder complaints after nerve sparing neck dissections. Int. J. Oral Maxillofac. Surg. 33, 253—257.

Vathana, T., Larsen, M., de Ruiter, G.C., Bishop, A.T., Spinner, R.J., Shin, A.Y., 2007. An anatomic study of the spinal accessory nerve: extended harvest permits direct nerve transfer to distal plexus targets. Clin. Anat. 20, 899—904.

Vogl, T.J., Bisdas, S., 2009. Differential diagnosis of jugular foramen lesions. Skull Base 19, 3—16.

Watkinson, J.C., Gleeson, M., 2016. Neck: the accessory nerve. In: Standring, S. (Ed.), Gray's Anatomy: The Anatomical Basis of Clinical Practice, forty oneth ed. Elsevier Limited, London, pp. 467—468.

Wetmore, C., Elde, R., 1991. Detection and characterization of a sensory microganglion associated with the spinal accessory nerve: a scanning laser confocal microscopic study of the neurons and their processes. J. Comp. Neurol. 305, 148—163.

Wiles, C.C., Wrigley, B., Greene, J.R., 2007. Re-examination of the medullary rootlets of the accessory and vagus nerves. Clin. Anat. 20, 19—22.

Williams, P.L., Warwick, R., 1975. Functional Neuroanatomy of Man. W.B. Saunders, Philadelphia, 460 pp.

Willis, T., 1965. The Anatomy of the Brain and Nerves. McGill University press, Montreal, pp. 137—144.

Windle, W.F., 1931. The sensory components of the spinal accessory nerve. J. Comp. Neurol. 53, 115—127.

Windle, W.F., DeLozier, L.C., 1932. The absence of painful sensation in the cat during stimulation of the spinal accessory nerve. J. Comp. Neurol. 54, 97—101.

FURTHER READING

Lang, J., 1993. Clinical Anatomy of the Cervical Spine. Thieme, New York, 192 pp.

CHAPTER 9

The Sympathetics and Cervical Nerves

TYLER WARNER • R. SHANE TUBBS

ANATOMY

The first-order neurons of the sympathetic tract descend from the hypothalamus to the spinal cord to synapse with second-order neurons in the lateral horns at the thoracic and lumbar levels. These second-order sympathetic nerves leave the spinal cord through the anterior horn and reach the paravertebral sympathetic trunk via the white rami, which are bilateral and receive fibers from the cell bodies of nerves in the lateral horns. After entering the sympathetic trunk, these sympathetic nerves can move superiorly or inferiorly depending on the target organ. The sympathetic nerves associated with the cervical ganglia course superiorly into the head and neck giving rise to three separate ganglia bilaterally. At these cervical ganglia, second-order preganglionic sympathetic fibers arising from the lateral horns of the spinal cord synapse with postganglionic sympathetic fibers as they ascend superiorly. The superior cervical ganglion usually appears at the C2 and C3 levels lateral to the longus colli muscle. This ganglion is used as a surgical landmark and is located anteromedial or medial to the internal carotid (Mitsuoka et al., 2017; Yokota et al., 2018). It is important to note that the preganglionic fibers do not supply the dermatome associated with the radicular nerve with which they leave the spinal cord. Each preganglionic nerve supplies several postganglionic sympathetic nerves, which join with sensory cerebrospinal nerve fibers and travel toward the skin to supply the dermatome associated with the accompanying nerve.

The postganglionic sympathetic fibers from the superior cervical ganglion travel as gray rami communicantes to innervate structures including the eye, face, pharynx, lacrimal glands, salivary glands, pineal gland, glands of the palate and nasal cavity, sweat glands, dilator pupillae, superior tarsal muscle, carotid body, heart, and arterial smooth muscle. There are four other ganglia in the head: the ciliary, sphenopalatine, otic, and submaxillary ganglia. Although they comprise parasympathetic interactions, it is important to note that postganglionic sympathetic fibers arising from the gray rami communicantes pass through them without synapsing to reach their targets of innervation (Collins, 1991). The middle cervical ganglion typically lies at C6 and is closely associated with the inferior thyroid artery. The postganglionic sympathetic fibers from this ganglion innervate the larynx, trachea, pharynx, upper esophagus, heart, and arterial smooth muscle. The inferior cervical ganglion frequently gives rise to the stellate ganglion as it merges with the first thoracic ganglion, but several variations of the associations between these ganglia have been reported (Jamieson et al., 1952). The postganglionic sympathetic nerves from this ganglion typically innervate the heart and arterial smooth muscle.

VARIANTS

The gray rami communicantes were shown by Langley (1896) to contain sympathetic fibers that join spinal nerves in the same segment. Variations in the distribution of gray rami comminicantes have been observed among the superior cevical, middle, and inferior cervical ganglia. Early studies identified little variation in the distribution of gray rami communicantes to spinal nerves. Each postganglionic sympathetic fiber joined C1, C2, or C3 with almost no overlap between the innervations (Fig. 9.1). Sheehan found several specimens in which it was difficult to separate the vagus nerve from the superior cervical, but there were few such cases among the specimens observed (Sheehan and Pick, 1943). Although human studies have revealed variation, Sheehan found consistency across the middle cervical ganglion of most specimens. This ganglion was identified between the seventh vertebral disc and the first thoracic vertebra.

No rami communicantes were identified between the middle cervical ganglion and any of the cervical nerves, in contrast to specimens examined in human

Surgical Anatomy of the Cervical Plexus and its Branches. https://doi.org/10.1016/B978-0-323-83132-1.00016-0

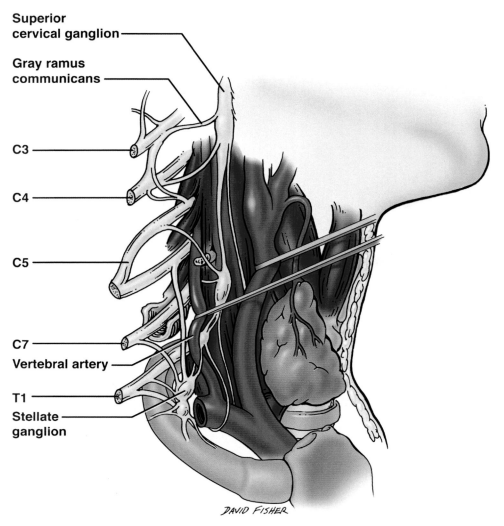

Superior cervical ganglion

Gray ramus communicans

C3

C4

C5

C7

Vertebral artery

T1

Stellate ganglion

DAVID FISHER

FIG. 9.1 Schematic drawing of the sympathetic trunk of the right neck. Note the gray rami communicantes joining it to the upper cervical nerves.

studies, but there was a significant interaction with the recurrent laryngeal nerve. The stellate ganglion contained the inferior cervical, first and second thoracic ganglia in most specimens, but lacked the second thoracic ganglion in 12. The stellate ganglion distributed fibers to the brachial plexus and consistently supplied sympathetics to C4, C5, and C6. However, there was a great deal of variation in the rami supplying C7, C8, T1, and T2. Among the 40 specimens studied, the seventh cervical nerve had no rami in 20, one ramus

in 17, and two rami in three. The eighth cervical nerve had no rami in 15, one ramus in 20, two rami in three, three in one, and four in one. The first thoracic nerve had one ramus in 10, two rami in 20, and three in 10. The second thoracic nerve had no rami in one, one ramus in 30, two rami in seven, and three in two (Sheehan and Pick, 1943).

Axford also explored variations in the anatomy of the sympathetics, emphasizing the anatomy of the middle cervical ganglion. As described by Potts (1925), most specimens studied fell into one of two categories. In the first type, referred to as the high type, the middle cervical ganglion was closely associated with the inferior thyroid artery around the sixth vertebra. It was closely related to the carotid tubercle of Chassaignac. This ganglion was typically flat, oval, and lying on the longus colli muscle. In the second type, referred to as the low type, the middle cervical ganglion lay at the ventral aspect of the vertebral artery around the seventh vertebra. This ganglion was pyramidal in shape and the rami communicantes derived from it provided sympathetics to the fifth, sixth, and seventh cervical nerves, among which there was a great deal of variation. In cases without a clear middle ganglion, thickenings in the cervical sympathetic trunk were hypothesized to act as ganglia, though others have questioned whether such thickenings truly serve as sympathetic ganglia (Jonnesco, 1923). Examination of the gray rami communicantes from the superior cervical ganglion revealed that they typically supplied the first three cervical nerves and occasionally the fourth. The rami themselves had several variations, the uppermost ramus being doubled in some specimens and the lowest absent in several. The author also reported cases in which a ramus derived directly from the sympathetic trunk, below the superior cervical ganglion, joined with the fourth or fifth cervical nerve. Some of the rami supplied by the inferior cervical ganglion were consistent. The first constant ramus was a thick branch of nerves that joined the eighth cervical nerve posterior to the scalene muscle close to the first rib. It was typically doubled and gave three different branches in several cases. The second constant ramus coursed caudally along the posteromedial aspect of the vertebral artery and typically joined the eighth cervical nerve on its anterior portion. The third constant ramus traveled vertically and crossed the eighth cranial nerve to join the seventh. The gray ramus communicans to the first thoracic nerve was typically single, but also presented as a double ramus with variable thickness across the two types (Axford, 1928).

Jamieson also studied anatomical variations associated with the sympathetic nervous system, observing the positions of the cervical ganglia in 100 cervicothoracic dissections to identify their relationships to anatomical landmarks. The superior cervical ganglion spanned the transverse processes of C1–C3 in 61% of the specimens observed; in 29%, the superior cervical ganglion lay opposite the transverse processes of C1 and C2. In the remaining specimens, one lay opposite the C1 vertebra and the other opposite the transverse process of C2. The average length of this ganglion was 18 mm and its average width was 8 mm. In this study, the position of the middle ganglion was as previously described by Axford—high type or low type—which also described the different types of relationship of the middle cervical ganglion to the vertebral artery. Some specimens had no perceptible middle cervical ganglion, but the sympathetic chain was thickened and fibers branched off the thickened portions, which served as gray rami communicantes. Fibers were mentioned running anterior to the subclavian artery to connect the middle and inferior cervical ganglia, which the author referred to as the ansa.

These fibers also ran along the subclavian artery to innervate this plexus and course toward the mammary artery. The middle ganglion was identified in 53 of the 100 specimens studied and was the smallest of the cervical ganglia, measuring an average of 14 mm in length and 4 mm in width. The inferior cervical ganglion was identified in only 18 of the 100 specimens; it was 15 mm long and just under 6 mm wide on average. The stellate ganglion was the last sympathetic ganglion and often contained the inferior cervical ganglion. It was present in 82 of the 100 specimens and was 22 mm long and 8 mm wide on average (Jamieson et al., 1952). Kiray later performed a similar cadaveric study with a smaller sample size, about 12 formalin-fixed cadavers and 24 specimens. This study, along with Saylam's dissections of 20 formalin-fixed cadavers, found similarities in the average relative sizes of the cervical and stellate ganglia, and in the frequency with which the ganglia occurred (Kiray et al., 2005; Saylam et al., 2009).

Recent studies have shown that about 80% of the population has an inferior cervical ganglion fused with the first thoracic ganglion, giving rise to the stellate ganglion. Song studied the variations of the gray rami communicantes distributed from the stellate ganglion to the brachial plexus in 33 formalin-fixed cadavers, 27 males and six females. These rami communicantes could be divided into medial and lateral groups. The lateral group coursed to join C8 and T1, with variable interaction with each of those spinal nerves. The T1 spinal nerve interacted with as few as one ramus and as many as four rami in particular specimens. The C8 spinal nerve joined between zero and three rami in particular specimens. The medial group interacted with cervical nerves C6, C7, and C8. The study identified several different patterns taken by the gray rami communicantes from the stellate ganglion to C8. In 45 specimens, the branches traveled through the traverse foramina, and in the remaining six they passed anterior to the transverse processes. Branches that joined C7 showed a similar pattern. In 41 specimens, they traveled through the foramen transversarium at the C6 level, close to the vertebral artery, to join C7. Six branches joined the C6 spinal nerve that ascended posteromedially with the vertebral artery (Song et al., 2010).

APPLICATIONS

Horner's syndrome is a common result of iatrogenic injuries around the neck. Typically, it can result from any disruption of the sympathetic system, occurring anywhere along the tract between the hypothalamus and the target organ. Tumors located around the neck often require surgical intervention, which can inadvertently cause classic signs associated with Horner's syndrome such as miosis, ptosis, and anhidrosis. Such symptoms result from the unopposed parasympathetic input to the eye and face on the ipsilateral side of the sympathetic chain injury. Lyons observed some of these radical head and neck dissections resulting from a variety of tumors including squamous cell carcinoma and medullary thyroid carcinomas. The injury could occur at any point along the sympathetic trunk, but several specimens had injuries at the superior cervical ganglion (Lyons and Mills, 1998). Surgical procedures for cervical spondylotic myelopathy, cervical disc herniation, or diseased vertebral bodies can also lead to a Horner's syndrome presentation.

Civelek studied the benefits of an anterolateral approach for a cervicothoracic procedure. The sympathetic chain lies posteromedial to the carotid sheath and the approach is less likely to cause iatrogenic injuries, except for extensive procedures that result in the dissection of the longus colli muscle. Thorough knowledge of sympathetic chain anatomy and ganglia is imperative for reducing the risk of iatrogenic injury significantly (Civelek et al., 2008). Anatomical knowledge is also vital for performing anesthetic nerve blocks. Usui conducted an ultrasound study to improve accuracy and reduce the risk of injury, particularly to the sympathetic trunk, when these nerve blocks are performed (Usui et al., 2010).

REFERENCES

Axford, M., 1928. Some observations on the cervical sympathetic in man. J. Anat. 62, 301–318.

Civelek, E., Karasu, A., Cansever, T., Hepgul, K., Kiris, T., Sabancı, A., Canbolat, A., 2008. Surgical anatomy of the cervical sympathetic trunk during anterolateral approach to cervical spine. Eur. Spine J. 17 (8), 991–995. https://doi.org/10.1007/s00586-008-0696-8.

Collins, S.L., 1991. The cervical sympathetic nerves in surgery of the neck. Otolaryngol. Head Neck Surg. (Tokyo) 105 (4), 544–555. https://doi.org/10.1177/019459989110500406.

Jamieson, R.W., Smith, D.B., Anson, B.J., 1952. The cervical sympathetic ganglia: an anatomical study of 100 cervicothoracic dissections. Q. Bull. Northwest Univ. Med. Sch. 26 (3), 219–227.

Jonnesco, T., 1923. Le Sympathetique Cervico-Thoracique. Paris.

Kiray, A., Arman, C., Naderi, S., Güvencer, M., Korman, E., 2005. Surgical anatomy of the cervical sympathetic trunk. Clin. Anat. 18 (3), 179–185. https://doi.org/10.1002/ca.20055.

Langley, J.N., 1896. J. Physiol. 20, 55–76.

Lyons, A., Mills, C., 1998. Anatomical variants of the cervical sympathetic chain to be considered during neck dissection. Br. J. Oral Maxillofac. Surg. 36 (3), 180–182. https://doi.org/10.1016/s0266-4356(98)90493-4.

Mitsuoka, K., Kikutani, T., Sato, I., 2017. Morphological relationship between the superior cervical ganglion and cervical nerves in Japanese cadaver donors. Brain Behav. 7 (2), e00619. Feb.

Potts, T.K., 1925. The main peripheral connections of the human sympathetic nervous system. J. Anat. LIX, 129 (January).

Saylam, C.Y., Ozgiray, E., Orhan, M., Cagli, S., Zileli, M., 2009. Neuroanatomy of cervical sympathetic trunk: a cadaveric study. Clin. Anat. 22 (3), 324–330. https://doi.org/10.1002/ca.20764.

Sheehan, D., Pick, J., 1943. The rami communicantes in the rhesus monkey. J. Anat. 77 (Pt 2), 125–139. Jan.

Song, Z.-F., Sun, M.-M., Wu, Z.-Y., Xia, C.-L., 2010. Anatomical study and clinical significance of the rami communicantes between cervicothoracic ganglion and brachial plexus. Clin. Anat. 23 (7), 811–814. https://doi.org/10.1002/ca.21008.

Usui, Y., Kobayashi, T., Kakinuma, H., Watanabe, K., Kitajima, T., Matsuno, K., 2010. An anatomical basis for blocking of the deep cervical plexus and cervical sympathetic tract using an ultrasound-guided technique. Anesth. Analg. 110 (3), 964–968. https://doi.org/10.1213/ane.0b013e3181c91ea0.

Yokota, H., Mukai, H., Hattori, S., Yamada, K., Anzai, Y., Uno, T., 2018. MR imaging of the superior cervical ganglion and inferior ganglion of the vagus nerve: structures that can mimic pathologic retropharyngeal lymph nodes. AJNR Am. J. Neuroradiol. 39 (1), 170–176. Jan.

CHAPTER 10

Comparative Anatomy of the Cervical Plexus

MALCON ANDREI MARTINEZ-PEREIRA, SR.

Peripheral nerve lesions and plexopathies are common in routine clinical practice and surgery. In the cervical region, cervicalgia can compromise quality of life and incapacitate the individual; it is associated with many professions and bad postural activities (Fonseca et al., 2001; Valachi and Valachi, 2003; Melo and Pereira, 2011; Sobral et al., 2013). Cervicobrachialgia differs; here, the pain is associated with the shoulder and arm, being caused by (among other things) clamping of or injury to the nerve responsible (Hurwitz et al., 2002; Sepúlveda, 2004; Melo and Pereira, 2011; Sobral et al., 2013). Knowledge of the origin, route, and destination of cervical plexus components is needed to diminish the risk of iatrogenic injury during locoregional anesthesia and surgical interventions and to help in the examination and diagnosis of injuries (Hurwitz et al., 2002). Various authors have described the relationship between cervical and mandibular innervation in odontological interventions. The mapping provided can correlate each nerve to the target organ, allowing the neurological injury to be identified and treatment and rehabilitation managed.

This chapter presents a comparative review of the topography, origin, and distribution of the nerves that constitute the cervical plexus. Unfortunately, in contrast to the brachial and lumbosacral plexuses, cervical innervation has been little studied and described in species used as experimental models for plexopathies and peripheral nerve injuries, such as the rat (*Rattus norvegicus*), guinea pig (*Cavia porcellus*), and rabbit (*Oryctolagus cuniculus*), or in lower tetrapods. For this reason, the topography, origin, and distribution of the nerves of the cervical plexus are compared among dogs, cats, pigs, and some nonhuman primates. Despite this limitation, the comparative approach to neuroanatomy of the peripheral nervous system can help us to understand the functional aspects of neural structure design.

The cervical spinal cord begins at the level of the foramen magnum of the occipital bone in a not-well-defined margin rostral to the origin of the first cervical nerve (Dyce et al., 2009; Getty, 1975). In contrast to other spinal regions, the segments and nerves of the cervical cord are constant throughout mammal species (Table 10.1, Hepburn, 1892a,b; Hill, 1955, 1957, 1960, 1966, 1972; Dyce et al., 2009; Getty, 1975). The first pair of spinal nerves emerges from the spinal cord between the base of the skull and the first cervical vertebra. The other cervical nerves are located cranially to their corresponding vertebrae, except for the eighth pair, which emerge cranially to the first thoracic vertebra (Dyce et al., 2009; Getty, 1975). The diameter in this region is not uniform because the caudal portion of the cervical spine is enlarged (*intumescentia cervicalis, cervical enlargement*) owing to the greater numbers of cells and nerve fibers involved in thoracic limb innervation via the *brachial plexus* (Dyce et al., 2009; Getty, 1975).

The spinal cord in birds extends along the whole of the vertebral canal. In contrast to the spinal cord in mammals, the cervical region is longer and differs among avian species, although it always shows the *intumescentia cervicalis* (Baumel, 1975; Nickel et al., 1977; Dubbeldam, 1993; Orosz and Bradshaw, 2007). The reptilian spinal cord has a segmented organization as in other vertebrates; however, it lacks some of the functional regionalization seen in mammals. The cervical region has a larger cross-section near the brainstem, filling 50% of the lumen in alligators and 29%–34% in several lizard species, while snakes and limbless lizards lack the *intumescentia cervicalis* (Ashley, 1962; Kusuma et al., 1979; Wyneken, 2003, 2007; Arantes, 2016). In amphibians, there is no cervical region in the spine, although an *intumescentia cervicalis* can be observed (Underhill, 1987).

Surgical Anatomy of the Cervical Plexus and its Branches. https://doi.org/10.1016/B978-0-323-83132-1.00014-7

TABLE 10.1
Number of Vertebrae, Medullary Segments in the Cervical Spinal Cord, and Level of Intumescentia Cervicalis in Different Species.

Specie	Vertebrae	Spine Segments	Intumescentia Cervicalis
HUMAN	7	8	C4-T1
NONHUMAN PRIMATES			
Ateles	7	8	C4-T2
Cebus	7	8	C4-T2
Chimpanzee	7	8	C4-T1
Cynomolgus	7	8	C4-T2
Gibbon	7	8	C4-T1
Gorilla	7	8	C4-T1
Lagothrix	7	8	C4-T1
Orangutans	7	8	C4-T1
Rhesus macaque	7	8	C4-T2
OTHER MAMMALS			
Cat	7	8	C3-T1
Chinchilla	7	8	C5-T2
Dog	7	8	C4-T1
Guinea pig	7	8	C4-T1
Swine	7	8	C4-T1
Rabbit	7	8	C5-T2
Rat	7	8	C5-T1
OTHER TETRAPODS			
Birds	Variable	Variable	C11-T2
Crocodilians	8	8–9	PSSN6-11
Iguana	8	8	C8-PSV3
Varanus	8	9	C9-PSV2
Tortoise	8	8–9	C5-T1
Anurans	Absent	Absent	SN1-3

PSS, presacral medullary segments; *PSSN*, presacral spinal nerve; *PSV*, presacral vertebrae; *SN*, spinal nerve.

GENERAL ASPECTS

In humans, the cervical plexus is formed by anastomosis of the ventral rami of the first four cervical nerves (C1-C4). Each nerve, except for C1, divides into ascending and descending branches, which unite with branches of contiguous nerves to form the loops and branches that constitute the plexus (Di Dio, 2002; Standring, 2009). These ventral rami receive one or more gray *rami communicantes* from the superior cervical ganglion of the sympathetic trunk. The plexus comprises three major divisions:

posterior, ventral, and deep. There are four major nerves in the posterior division: the lesser occipital nerve, *great auricular nerve* and *transverse cervical, nerve* all originating from the C2-3 loop, and the *supraclavicular nerve* from the C3-4 loop. The ventral division has two branches (the *phrenic* from (C3-5) and the *ansa cervicalis* or *ansa hypoglossi* divided into superior (C1-2) and inferior (C2-3) roots (Di Dio, 2002; Standring, 2009). However, Loukas and Colleagues (2007) observed that the *ansa cervicalis* fibers could come from C3 alone (40%), C2-3 (38%), or in few cases C2 or C2-4. The branches of the deep division are divided into lateral (sternocleidomastoid muscle from C2-4, trapezius from C3-4, *levator scapulae* from C3-4, scalenus medius from C3-4, and communicating branches to the spinal accessory nerve from C2-4) and medial (to prevertebral muscles from C1-4 and communicating branches to the vagus from C1-2, to the hypoglossal nerve from C1-2, and to the superior cervical ganglion from C1-4) (Di Dio, 2002; Standring, 2009). This brief contextualization is necessary for a better understanding of comparative anatomy. A more accurate description of the cervical nerves and plexus can be found in other chapters of this book.

Nonhuman Primates

The study of nonhuman primates is important because the anatomical, physiological and ethological similarities between these animals and humans can help to elucidate evolutionary aspects of human development. The description of the cervical plexus is based on three genera of Hominidae (*Gorilla*, *Pan* or chimpanzee, and *Pongo* or orangutans), on the genus *Hylobates* (gibbon; superfamily Hominoidea), and some primate species of experimental interest such as *Cebus apella*, *Macaca mulatta*, *Lagothrix lagothrica*, and *Ateles*. For example, studies of nerve segmentations in the rhesus macaque (*Macaca mulatta*, Hartmann and Straus, 1932; Pietrzk et al., 1964) provided major information on the functions of the spinal reflexes and their territories of innervation, helping to elucidate human neurophysiology. As described elsewhere (Martinez-Pereira and Zancan, 2015, 2018; Martinez-Pereira, 2021), when the plexuses of humans and other primates (mostly the rhesus macaque) are compared, the points of similarity in the basic plane are more striking than the slight differences. Plexus branches in the posterior, ventral and *deep* divisions are very similar to those in humans, especially when the individual distribution of each nerve is considered.

Other Mammals

In contrast to the *brachial* and *lumbosacral* plexuses, there have been few comparisons among experimental models of the cervical plexus. Only general descriptions are available for dogs, cats, and swine, for example, Getty (1975), while for rodents and rabbits the descriptions are based on drawings by Hunt (1924), Greene (1968), Chiasson (1980), and Cooper and Schiller (1975), or by Bensley and Craigie (1938), Barone and Colleagues (1973), and Mclaughlin and Chiasson (1987), respectively.

Before the cervical nerve and plexus are described anatomically, some characteristics of the experimental models, particularly in the quadrupedal position,

must be considered; the researcher needs to apply the correct anatomical terms when studying experimental species. Most anatomical structures in animals have the same names as in humans, but some names differ because of the standing positions of the animals. Fig. 10.1 briefly reviews the orientation planes and axes of the head and neck in vertebrate quadrupeds, and the terms for position, situation, and location. However, when an animal is observed in an anatomical position, it can be imagined within a parallelepiped. Each face of the parallelepiped constitutes a delimitation plane: the face adjacent to the head is the cranial plane, while the face tangent to the tail is the caudal plane; a plane tangential to the vertebral column corresponds to the dorsal plane, and the base of the parallelepiped is the ventral plane; the remaining sides delimit the right and left planes. By demarcating the midpoints of each pair of opposite planes and tracing straight lines between them, three axes are defined: craniocaudal, dorsal-ventral, and latero-lateral. The section planes of the body are: (1) the craniocaudal axis divides the body into right and left antimers by the longitudinal median plane; (2) the sagittal or paramedian planes are parallel to the longitudinal plane; (3) the transverse planes are vertical sections on the craniocaudal axis; (4) the horizontal plane is parallel to the dorsoventral axis and divides the body into dorsal and ventral halves. These planes and axes guide the application of the following terms to localize structures: (1) cranial and caudal (structures nearest to or toward the head or tail, respectively; head structures can be also referred to as oral); (2) dorsal and ventral refer to back side and belly side, respectively, as opposed to anterior and posterior in humans; (3) medial and lateral (close or distant to the median plane, respectively) and intermediate (between lateral and medial structures) (Dyce et al., 2009; Nomina Anatomica Veterinaria, 2017).

According to Getty (1975), the cervical nerves generally comprise eight pairs, the first emerging from the *foramen alare* of the atlas and the last from the *intervertebral foramen* between the C7 and Th1 vertebrae. The dorsal rami innervate the skin and dorsolateral muscles of the neck, and those from C3 to C6 anastomose to produce a dorsal cervical plexus. Medial rami run over the *multifidus* to supply the lateral deep muscles and the skin of the neck, while the lateral branch is essentially muscular. The C1-8 ventral cervical branches innervate areas of skin on the head, neck, and thorax, some cervical muscles, the diaphragm, and muscles of the thoracic limb. The ventral branches of C1-C4(5) are minor compared to the dorsal ones, and the last three cervical nerves contribute to forming the *brachial plexus*. The ventral C1-4(5) branches form three anastomotic loops

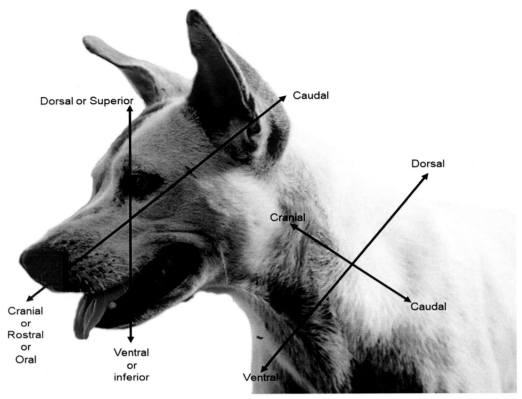

FIG. 10.1 Direction planes and terms for situation and location in the head and neck.

constituting the ventral cervical plexus, divided into superficial (sensory fibers to the skin in the surrounding region of the neck and pinna) and deep (essentially motor fibers to the ventrolateral muscles of the neck and diaphragm) (Dyce et al., 2009; Getty, 1975). On the other hand, according to the Nomina Anatomica Veterinaria (2017), the cervical nerves comprise the *suboccipital* and *greater occipital* (*dorsal rami*), the *great auricular, transverse cervical* and the *supraclavicular* (*ventral rami*) nerves, while the *plexus cervicalis* is constituted only by the *ansa cervicalis* and the *phrenic nerve*.

CERVICAL NERVES AND PLEXUS

In this section, the nerves will be described in accordance with the perspective of the Nomina Anatomica Veterinaria (2017), considering the distinction between nerves and cervical plexus, and indicating differences in the segmental participation of certain nerves and their participation in tissue innervation, as with other peripheral plexuses.

Suboccipital Nerve

The *suboccipital nerve* (C1) is the first dorsal cervical dorsal. It emerges superior to the posterior arch of the atlas and inferior to the vertebral artery and contains a few sensory fibers. It is located in the suboccipital triangle and supplies the muscles that bound this (*rectus capitis posterior* (*dorsalis*) *major* and *minor*, *obliqui superior* (*cranialis*) and *inferior* (*caudalis*) and *semispinalis capitis*). Occasionally, it gives off a cutaneous branch, which accompanies the occipital artery to the scalp and communicates with the *greater occipital* and *lesser occipital* nerves (observed in nonhuman primates: Champneys, 1871; Hartmann and Straus, 1932; Hill, 1955, 1957, 1960, 1972; Pietrzk et al., 1964; absent in dog, cat, and other mammals: Getty, 1975; Hunt, 1924; Cooper and Schiller, 1975; Chiasson, 1980).

Nevertheless, in dogs and cats, the *suboccipital nerve* does not emit dorsal and medial branches (Getty, 1975), but presents cutaneous rami that join the *auricularis caudalis, facial* and *great auricular nerves* (C2: Ellenberger and Baun, 1891). Nevertheless, this nerve is connected to the *vagus* and the *sympathetic trunk* in these species (Ellenberger and Baun, 1891; Bradley and Grahame, 1959), while it also communicates with the *distal ganglion* of the *vagus nerve* only in the cat (Taylor and Weber, 1951). The *suboccipital* nerve also joins the *hypoglossal nerve* to form the *ansa cervicalis* in cats, dogs, and swine (Ellenberger and Baun, 1891; Bradley and Grahame, 1959; Ghoshal, 1975). In those animals, this nerve supplies the *sternothyroid* and *sternohyoid* muscles (Getty, 1975).

Greater occipital nerve
In nonhuman primates, especially anthropoid apes, this nerve is very similar to that in humans (Hepburn, 1892a,b; Bolk, 1932). Originating from the dorsal branch of C2-3 it is the main sensory nerve of the occipital region, ascending obliquely between the *obliquus inferior* and the *semispinalis capitis* muscles, piercing the latter and the *trapezius* (Eisler, 1890; Hepburn, 1892a,b; Hartmann and Straus, 1932; Hill, 1960, 1972; El Assy, 1966). The C2 medial posterior branch joins the C3 posterior division near the occipital artery, innervating the skin of the scalp as far the skull. This nerve emits branches communicating with the *lesser occipital nerve* (Eisler, 1890; Hepburn, 1892a,b; Hartmann and Straus, 1932; Hill, 1960, 1972; El Assy, 1966).

In dogs (Miller et al., 1964; Getty, 1975; Dyce et al., 2009), swine (Ghoshal, 1975), rabbit (Bensley and Craigie, 1938; Barone et al., 1973; Mclaughlin and Chiasson, 1987), and rodents (Hunt, 1924; Greene, 1968; Cooper and Schiller, 1975; Chiasson, 1980), the *greater occipital nerve* originates exclusively from the C2 ventral branch. However, in cats, the medial branch of this nerve anastomoses with C3 (Getty, 1975; Crouch, 1985); this is infrequent in dogs (Ellenberger and Baun, 1891; Bradley and Grahame, 1959). The *greater occipital nerve* emerges cranially to the *spinous process* of the axis, passing caudodorsally between this and the *obliquus capitis caudalis* muscle (Getty, 1975).

Great auricular nerve
The *great auricular nerve* is the largest of the cervical ventral branches, formed by anastomosis of the C2-3 nerves. However, in *Macaca fascicularis*, this nerve arises from C2 (C3-4) (Kato et al., 1990). In anthropoid apes (Hepburn, 1892a,b), it winds around the posterior border of the *sternocleidomastoid*, and, after perforating the deep fascia, ascends upon the platysma to the *parotid gland*, where it divides into anterior and a posterior branches. The *facial* or anterior branch is scattered in the skin of the face over the *parotid gland*, where it emits communicating rami to the *facial nerve* in the gland

(Eisler, 1890; El Assy, 1966; Raven and Hill, 1950). The *mastoid* or posterior branch innervates the skin over the *mastoid process* and on the inferior back of the auricula, and a small ramus pierces the auricle to reach its lateral surface, where it is distributed to the lobule and lower part of the concha. The *mastoid branch* emits communicating rami to the *lesser occipital nerve*, *auricular branch* of the *vagus*, and *ramus auricularis* posterior to the *facial nerve* (Eisler, 1890; El Assy, 1966; Raven and Hill, 1950). Other species are described similarly (Hartmann and Straus, 1932; Hill, 1957, 1960, 1972; El Assy, 1966).

Among the cervical ventral branches, the *great auricular nerve* is more important in dogs and cats because of their topography; this has clinical and surgical significance in these animals. In general, this nerve originates from the C2 ventral branch, which crosses the *sternocephalicus* and *cleidocephalicus* of the *brachiocephalicus* muscles superficially and dorsocranially, emerging near the *parotid gland* and parallel to the caudal margin of the *parotidoauricularis* muscle (Miller et al., 1964; Getty, 1975; Crouch, 1985; Dyce et al., 2009). This nerve supplies the *parotid* region and the *cartilago scutiformis* and part of *external acoustic meatus* of the *external ear*. However, in cats, the C2 ventral ramus anastomoses with C1 and C3 nerves and emits a branch to the *accessory* nerve (Getty, 1975; Crouch, 1985), while in swine it arises from the C2-3 nerves (Getty, 1975; Ghoshal, 1975). Drawings of rabbits (Bensley and Craigie, 1938; Barone et al., 1973; Mclaughlin and Chiasson, 1987) and rats (Hunt, 1924; Greene, 1968; Chiasson, 1980) show similar origin and topography. In all species, it contributes with the *trigeminal* and *vagus* nerves to forming the *internal auricular nerve*.

Transverse cervical nerve
Originating from the (C2)C3(4) ventral rami in a common trunk with the *great auricular nerve*, the *transverse cervical nerve* is also called the cutaneous cervical or *cutaneous colli*, or the superficial or transverse cervical nerve (Bolk, 1932; Hartmann and Straus, 1932; Kato et al., 1990). After emerging around the posterior border of the *sternocleidomastoid* at about its middle, it passes anterior obliquely to the margin of this muscle, beneath the *external jugular vein*. It then perforates the *lamina prevertebralis* or the profunda of the *cervical fascia* and divides beneath the *platysma* into ascending (superior) and descending (inferior) branches, which are distributed anterolaterally in the neck. This description is the same as for anthropoid apes (Eisler, 1890; El Assy, 1966; Raven and Hill, 1950) and other families and genera of nonhuman primates (Hartmann and Straus, 1932;

Hill, 1957, 1960, 1972; El Assy, 1966). Despite some peculiarities in *Ateles* (Hill, 1957; El Assy, 1966), *Cebus* (Hill, 1960), and *rhesus macaque* (Hartmann and Straus, 1932), the ascending branches or *rami superiores* generally run upwards to the submaxillary region and, beneath the *platysma*, join the cervical ramus of the *facialis*. Some perforating fibers cross the *platysma*, innervating the anterior and frontal face of the neck. Like the ascending branches, the descending or *rami inferiores* pierce the *platysma*, and are distributed to the skin of the lateral and frontal faces of the neck as low as the sternum (Eisler, 1890; Hartmann and Straus, 1932; Raven and Hill, 1950; Hill, 1957, 1960, 1972; El Assy, 1966).

In other mammals, the *transverse cervical nerve* also originates from the C2 ventral branch of a common trunk with the *great auricular nerve* (Getty, 1975), though in cats and swine it receives a branch of the C3 nerve (Reignhard and Jennings, 1935; Taylor and Weber, 1951). This nerve crosses the *cleidocephalicus* of the *brachiocephalicus*, in parallel with the vena jugularis externa, and passes the *platysma* cranioventrally upwards in the mandibular space (Getty, 1975). However, in dogs, Bradley and Grahame (1959) describe branches from this nerve to the laryngeal region and the cervical branch of the *facial*, as also to the *accessory* nerve. Drawings of the cervical region in rabbits (Bensley and Craigie, 1938; Barone et al., 1973; Mclaughlin and Chiasson, 1987) and rats (Hunt, 1924; Greene, 1968; Chiasson, 1980) revealed the same pattern. This nerve supplies the *cutaneous colli* muscle and the skin over the parotid and laryngeal regions.

Supraclavicular nerves

As in humans, there are three *supraclavicular nerves* in nonhuman primates (medial, intermediate, and lateral) originating from C3-4 (Eisler, 1890; Hepburn, 1892a,b; Hartmann and Straus, 1932; Raven and Hill, 1950; Hill, 1957, 1960, 1972; El Assy, 1966). However, according to Kato et al. (1990), these nerves originate only from C4 in *Macaca fascicularis*. They all emerge beneath the posterior border of the *sternocleidomastoid* and run to the neck posteriorly to the *platysma* and the *lamina prevertebralis* of the *cervical fascia*. Near the *clavicle*, they pierce the fascia and the *platysma* where they divide to become cutaneous (Hepburn, 1892a,b; Hartmann and Straus, 1932; Raven and Hill, 1950; Hill, 1957, 1960, 1972; El Assy, 1966). The *anterior supraclavicular*, or medial or suprasternal nerves, cross the *external jugular vein* and the *clavicular* and *sternal* heads of the *sternocleidomastoid* obliquely, innervating the sternoclavicular joint and skin as far as the midline. The *middle*

supraclavicular or intermediate group runs on the *clavicle* and innervates the skin over the *pectoralis major* and *deltoid* muscles, communicating with the cutaneous branches of the upper intercostal nerves. The *posterior supraclavicular nerves* or lateral or supraacromial nerves pass obliquely across the surface of the *trapezius* and *acromion* to supply the skin of the *articulatio humeri* dorsoposteriorly (Hepburn, 1892a,b; Hartmann and Straus, 1932; Raven and Hill, 1950; Hill, 1957, 1960, 1972; El Assy, 1966).

The cutaneous ventral rami of C4-5 join to form the three *supraclavicular* (*ventralis*, *intermedii*, and *dorsalis*) nerves in dogs, cats, and swine (Miller et al., 1964; Getty, 1975; Ghoshal, 1975; Crouch, 1985). They are observed along the deep face of the *omotransversarius* muscle. However, Taylor and Weber (1951) observed a ventral ramus of C5 that anastomosed with the *accessory nerve* near the aponeurosis between the *cervical and thoracic parts* of the *trapezius* in the cat. These rami innervate the skin surrounding and over the *articulatio humeri*. Similar patterns are observed in drawings of rabbits (Bensley and Craigie, 1938; Barone et al., 1973; Mclaughlin and Chiasson, 1987) and some rodents (Hunt, 1924; Greene, 1968; Chiasson, 1980).

Cervical Plexus

As mentioned previously, the cervical plexus is formed from the anterior primary rami of C1-4, and sometimes C5, deep to the *sternocleidomastoid*, in the anterior position of the scalenus medius and *levator scapulae* muscles and deep to the *internal jugular vein*. The C2-4 nerves divide into ascending and descending branches, which join the rami of contiguous nerves to form loops. These loops constitute ventral motor branches, the *ansa cervicalis* and *phrenic nerves* being most important (Hepburn, 1892a,b). However, the lateral ventral branches innervate the muscles of the cervical region: from C2-4 to the *sternocleidomastoid*, from C3-4 to the *trapezius*, *levator scapulae*, and *scalenus medius*, and C2-C4 communicating branches to the *accessory nerve*. In anthropoid apes, as in humans, there are additional connections of C2-5 to the *levator scapulae* and from C3-6 to the *rhomboids* (Hepburn, 1892a,b). However, fibers of C3-4 carry additional motor innervation to the *trapezius*, independently of the *accessory nerve*.

Following the Nomina Anatomica Veterinaria (2017), the cervical plexus is composed of the *ansa cervicalis* and *phrenic* nerves. However, Getty (1975) states that in dogs, cats, and swine, this plexus forms a dorsal cervical plexus (C3-6) to the superficial and deep muscles of the neck. In other experimental models, the architecture is similar to that of the first-mentioned species (Hunt, 1924; Bensley and Craigie, 1938; Greene, 1968; Barone et al., 1973; Chiasson, 1980; Mclaughlin and Chiasson, 1987). In general, the dorsal cervical plexus innervates the *splenius cervicis, scalenus, transverso-spinalis* muscles, and by joining the *accessory nerve*, the *trapezius, sternocephalicus, longus colli* muscles, and the *cleidocephalicus* of the *brachiocephalicus* (Dyce et al., 2009; Getty, 1975).

Ansa cervicalis

The *ansa cervicalis*, also called *ansa hypoglossi*, is formed by the union of the ventral rami of C1-3 after interjoining through two main roots (superior and inferior). Its main role is to supply the infrahyoid muscles (*sternohyoid, sternothyroid,* and *omohyoid*); it is then joined by the inferior root. The superior root is represented by C1 fibers that join the *hypoglossal* nerve and descend the neck to form the descending ramus of that nerve (Hepburn, 1892a,b). It lies superficial to the *internal jugular vein* in the carotid triangle and supplies the superior parts of the *sternohyoid* and *sternothyroid*, and the *superior belly* of the *omohyoid*. C2-3 fibers form the inferior root, also known as *descendens cervicalis*, innervating the inferior parts of the *sternohyoid* and *sternothyroid* and the *superior belly* of the *omohyoid*. The *descendens cervicalis* also innervates the inferior parts of the *vagina carotica* on the surface of the internal jugular vein and bends anteroinferiorly to join the superior root (Champneys, 1871; Hepburn, 1892a,b; Hartmann and Straus, 1932; Pietrzk et al., 1964; Hill, 1960, 1972).

As in humans and nonhuman primates, there are two roots of the *ansa cervicalis* in other mammals. However, these are called *radixes cranialis* and *caudalis* owing to their anatomical positions in the experimental models (Nomina Anatomica Veterinaria, 2017). Nevertheless, considering the descriptions in anatomical textbooks, this can be compared to the ventral cervical plexus (Dyce et al., 2009; Getty, 1975).

Phrenic *nerve*

The *phrenic nerve* receives its fibers from (C3)C4(5) and emerges near the *thyroid cartilage* of the larynx, extending along the *scalenus anterior* muscle with the *internal jugular vein*. As in humans, its trajectory differs between the left and right antimeres. In anthropoid apes, the *phrenic* nerve crosses the *scalenus anterior* anteriorly to the first parts of the *subclavian artery and vein* in the left antimere, while in the right this crossing occurs anterior to the second parts of the vessels (Hepburn, 1892a,b). However, in other genera, the trajectory is the same in the left

and right antimeres: both nerves cross over the anterior part of the *subclavian artery and vein* in the *mediastinum* (Hartmann and Straus, 1932; Hill, 1957, 1960, 1972; Pietrzk et al., 1964; El Assy, 1966). In all species, there is a *rami pericardiaci* innervating the *mediastinal pleura*. This nerve supplies the *mediastinal pleura* with sensory fibers and the *diaphragma* with motor innervation. The *accessory phrenic* nerve, originating from (C4)C5(6) or from the *ansa cervicalis*, is infrequent in *Cebus* (Hill, 1960), *Plathyrrhinos, Alouattinae* (Hill, 1960, 1972), and the rhesus macaque (Hartmann and Straus, 1932; Pietrzk et al., 1964). However, when present, it runs in the neck and goes on to join the *phrenic nerve* near the *clavicle* or in the entrance of the *cavum thoracis*.

Ellenberger and Baum (1891), Zimmerl (1909, 1930), Lesbre (1923), and Dyce et al. (2009) describe the *phrenic nerve* as emerging from the C5-7 nerves, and its roots run along the *scalenus* muscle toward the *thoracis*, joining in a single structure that goes to the *diaphragm* to form its motor innervation. Similar patterns are observed in dogs (Miller et al., 1964; Getty, 1975) and swine (Getty, 1975; Ghoshal, 1975), while in cats this nerve arises from C5-6 (Getty, 1975; Crouch, 1985). In contrast, the *phrenic* nerve in rats (Hunt, 1924; Greene, 1968; Scheidegger and Van der Zypen, 1974; Chiasson, 1980) and rabbits (Barone et al., 1973; Marie et al., 1999) arises from C4-5, while in guinea pigs it originates from C4-7 (Cooper and Schiller, 1975; Salgado et al., 1983). In these rodents, there is lateral asymmetry, the left nerve usually being smaller than the right, particularly in the distal segment (Scheidegger and Van der Zypen, 1974; Cooper and Schiller, 1975; Chiasson, 1980; Salgado et al., 1983). However, in rabbits, the C4 root is either short or long (Barone et al., 1973; Marie et al., 1999). Although not described in dogs, cats, and pigs (Miller et al., 1964; Getty, 1975; Ghoshal, 1975; Crouch, 1985), an *accessory phrenic* nerve emerges from C6 in rats (Gottschall and Gruber, 1977), while in rabbits it arises from C5 or C6 owing to the inconstancy of the C6 root, which is at times absent or sometimes double (Marie et al., 1999).

REFERENCES

Arantes, R.C., 2016. Ossos da coluna vertebral e origens dos plexos braquial e lombossacral da iguana *Iguana iguana*. Tese (doutorado). Universidade Federal de Uberlândia, Programa de Pós-Graduação em Ciências Veterinárias, p. 47.

Ashley, L.M., 1962. Laboratory Anatomy of the Turtle. WM C. Brown Company Publishers, Iowa.

Barone, R., Pavaux, C., Blin, P.C., Cuq, P., 1973. Atlas of Rabbit Anatomy. Masson & Cie, Paris.

Baumel, J.J., 1975. Aves nervous system. In: Getty, R. (Ed.), Sisson and Grossman's. The Anatomy of the Domestic Animals, fifth ed., vol. 2. W.B. Saunders Company, Philadelphia, PA, USA, pp. 2044—2052.

Bensley, B.A., Craigie, E.H., 1938. Practical Anatomy of the Rabbit an Elementary Text-Book in Mammalian Anatomy, sixth ed. The University of Toronto Press, Toronto.

Bolk, L., 1932. Beitrdge zur Affenanatomie. III. Der Cervicobrachialis der Primaten. Petrus Camper I, 371—567.

Bradley, O.C., Grahame, T., 1959. Topographical Anatomy of the Dog, 6th. Ed. The Macmillan Co, New York.

Champneys, F., 1871. The muscles and nerves of a chimpanzee (*Troglodytes niger*) and a *Cynocephalus anubis*. J. Anat. Physiol. 6, 176—211.

Chiasson, R.B., 1980. Laboratory Anatomy of the White Rat. Brown Company Publisher, Iowa.

Cooper, G., Schiller, A.L., 1975. Anatomy of the Guinea Pig. Harvard University Press, Cambridge, Massachusetts.

Crouch, J.E., 1985. Text-atlas of Cat Anatomy. Lea & Febiger, Philadelphia.

Di Dio, L.J.A., 2002. Tratado de anatomia aplicada, second ed, 2 v. Póluss Editorial, São Paulo.

Dubbeldam, J.L., 1993. Systema nervosum periphericum. In: Baumel, J.J. (Ed.), Handbook of Avian Anatomy: Nomina Anatomica Avium, second ed. Nuttall Ornithological Club, Cambridge, pp. 555—584.

Dyce, K.M., Sack, W.O., Wensing, C.J.G., 2009. Textbook of Veterinary Anatomy, fourth ed. Elsevier.

Eisler, P., 1890. Das Gefass- und Periphere Nervensystem des Gorilla. Tausch & Grosse, Halle.

El Assy, Y.S., 1966. Beitrage zur morphologie des peripheren nervensystems der primaten, vol. 27. Gegenbaurs Morphologisches Jahrbuch, Frankfurt, pp. 476—567.

Ellenberger, W., Baun, H., 1891. Systematische und topographische Anatomie des Hundes. Paul Parey, Berlin.

Fonseca, K.G., Duarte, H.E., Rosário, A.R.V., 2001. Chronic cervicalgy main causes and preventions. ACM Arq. Catarin. Med. 30 (3/4), 10—14.

Getty, R., 1975. Sisson and Grossman's the Anatomy of the Domestic Animals, fifth ed. W. B. Saunders Company, Philadelphia.

Ghoshal, N.G., 1975. Spinal nerves of the swine, 1975. In: Getty, R. (Ed.), Sisson and Grossman's the Anatomy of the Domestic Animals, fifth ed. Saunders Company, Philadelphia: WB.

Gottschall, J., Gruber, H., 1977. The accessory phrenic nerve in the rat. Anat. Embryol. 151, 63—69.

Greene, E.C., 1968. Anatomy of the Rat. Hafner Publishing Company, New York and London.

Hartmann, C.G., Straus Junior, W.L., 1932. Anatomy of the Rhesus Monkey. Press, New York.

Hepburn, D., 1892a. The comparative anatomy of the muscles and nerves of the superior and inferior extremities of the anthropoid apes. Part I. J. Anat. Physiol. 26, 149—186.

Hepburn, D., 1892b. The comparative anatomy of the muscles and nerves of the superior and inferior extremities of the anthropoid apes Part II. J. Anat. Pshysol. 26, 324—356.

Hill, W.C.O., 1955. Primates: Comparative Anatomy and Taxonomy II — Haplorrini - Tarsoidea. Edinburgh University Press, Edinburgh.

Hill, W.C.O., 1957. Primates: Comparative Anatomy and Taxonomy III Pithecoidea — Platyrrhini - Hapalidae. Edinburgh University Press, Edinburgh.

Hill, W.C.O., 1960. Primates: Comparative Anatomy and Taxonomy IV Cebidae: Part A. Edinburgh University Press, Edinburgh.

Hill, W.C.O., 1966. Primates: Comparative Anatomy and Taxonomy VI Catarrhini — Cercopithecoidea - Cercopithecinae. Edinburgh University Press, Edinburgh.

Hill, W.C.O., 1972. Primates: Comparative Anatomy and Taxonomy V Cebidae: Part B. Edinburgh University Press, Edinburgh.

Hunt, H.R.A., 1924. Laboratory Manual of the Anatomy of the Rat. Macmillan Company, New York.

Hurwitz, E.L., Morgenstern, H., Harber, P., Kominski, G.F., Yu, F., Adams, A.H., 2002. A randomized trial of chiropractic manipulation and mobilization for patients with neck pain: clinical outcomes from the UCLA neck-pain study. Am. J. Publ. Health 92 (10), 1634—1641.

Kato, K., Hopwood, P., SATO, T., 1990. The cutaneous cervical plexus nerves of the crab-eating macaque (Macaca fascicularis), eastern grey Kangaroo (Macropus giganteus), and Koala (Phascolarctos cinereus). Okajimas Folia Anat. Jpn. 67 (5), 315—324.

Kusuma, A., ten Donkelaar, H.J., Nieuwenhuvs, R., 1979. Intrinsic organization of the spinal cord. In: Gans, C., Northcutt, R.G., Ulinski, P. (Eds.), Biology of the Reptila, vol. 10. Academic, New York, pp. 59—109.

Lesbre, F.X., 1923. Appareil de innervation. In: Lesbre, F.X. (Ed.), Précis d' Anatomie Comparée de Animaux Domestiques, vol. 2. J.B. Bailliére, Paris, pp. 668—669.

Loukas, M., Thorsell, A., Tubbs, R.S., Kapos, T., Louis, R.G., Jr Vulis, M., Hage, R., Jordan, R., 2007. The ansa cervicalis revisited. Folia Morphol. (Warsz) 66, 120—125.

Marie, J.P., Lerosey, Y., Dehesdin, D., Tadié, M., Andrieu-Guitrancourt, J., 1999. Cervical anatomy of phrenic nerve roots in the rabbit. European Group for Research on the Larynx. Ann. Otol. Rhinol. Laryngol. 108 (5), 516—521.

Martinez-Pereira, M.A., 2021. Chapter 19 comparative anatomy of the lumbosacral plexus. In: Tubbs, R.S., Iwanaga, J., Loukas, M., Dumont, A.S., Reina, M.A. (Eds.), Surgical Anatomy of the Sacral Plexus and its Branches. Academic Press Elsevier, London, pp. 189—204.

Martinez-Pereira, M.A., Zancan, D.M., 2015. Comparative anatomy of the peripheral nerves. In: Tubbs, R.S., Rizk, E., Shoja, M., Loukas, M., Spinner, R.J. (Eds.), Nerves and Nerves Injuries. Academic Press Elsevier, London, pp. 55—77.

Martinez-Pereira, M.A., Zancan, D.M., 2018. Comparative anatomy of the lumbar plexus. In: Tubbs, R.S., Loukas, M., Hanna, A.S., Oskouian, R.J. (Eds.), Surgical Anatomy of the Lumbar Plexus. Thieme Publishers, New York.

Mclaughlin, C.A., Chiasson, R.B., 1987. Laboratory Anatomy of the Rabbit. W. C. Brown Company, Iowa.

Melo, R.S., Pereira, T.R., 2011. Prevalência de algias vertebrais em cirurgiões dentistas. Lecturas EFDeportes.com Available from: http://www.efdeportes.com/efd157/algiasvertebrais-em-cirurgioes-dentistas.htm.

Miller, M., Christensen, G., Evans, H., 1964. Anatomy of the Dog. W. B. Saunders Company, Philadelphia.

Nickel, R., Schummer, A., Seiferle, E., 1977. Peripheral nervous system. In: Nickel, R., Schummer, A., Seiferle, E. (Eds.), Anatomy of the Domestic Birds. Parey, Berlin, pp. 131–139.

Nomina Anatomica Veterinaria, 2017. Copyright by the Word Association of Veterinary Anatomists, sixth ed. (revised version). Editorial Committee, Hanover, Germany.

Orosz, S.E., Bradshaw, G.A., 2007. Avian neuroanatomy revisited: from clinical principles to avian cognition. Vet. Clin. North Am. Exot. Anim. Pract. 10, 775–802.

Pietrzk, K., Urbanowick, Z., Zaluska, S., 1964. Nerwy pachowy I promieniowy. U Macacus rhesus. Folia Morphol. 15, 425–436.

Raven, H.C., Hill, J.E., 1950. Regional anatomy of the Gorilla. In: Gregory, W.K. (Ed.), The Anatomy of the Gorilla. Columbia University Press, New York.

Reignhard, J., Jennings, H.S., 1935. Anatomy of the Cat, third ed. Henry Holt & Co. Inc, New York.

Salgado, M.C., Orsi, A.M., Vicentini, C.A., Mello Dias, S., 1983. The phrenic nerve in the Guinea pig (*Cavia porcellus* L. 1756). Anat. Anz. 154 (3), 217–220.

Scheidegger, D., Van der Zypen, E., 1974. Über das Verhalten der motorischen Endplatten des Diaphragma der Ratte nach proximaler und distaler Durchtrennung des Nervus phrenic. Acta Anat 88, 580–599.

Sepúlveda, T.A., 2004. Cervicalgia y cervicobraquialgia en el adulto mayor. Rev. Chil. Reumatol. 20 (2), 81–83.

Sobral, L.P., Badessa, M.P.S.G., Sobral, M.L., Oliveira Júnior, J.B., 2013. Study of the prevalence of the spine pains in residents of cardiovascular surgery: initial study Marcelo. Rev. Bras. Med. Trab. 11 (2), 82–89.

Standring, S., 2009. Gray's Anatomy: The Anatomical Basis of Clinical Practice, Expert Consult, 40th Ed. Elsevier.

Taylor, W.T., Weber, R.J., 1951. Functional Mammalian Anatomy, with Special Reference to the Cat. N. J. D. Van Nostrand Company Inc, Princeton.

Underhill, R.A., 1987. Laboratory Anatomy of the Frog, fifth ed. WM C. Brown Company Publishers, Iowa.

Valachi, B., Valachi, K., 2003. Mechanisms leading to musculoskeletal disorders in dentistry. J. Am. Dent. Assoc. 134 (10), 1344–1350.

Wyneken, J., 2003. The external morphology, musculoskeletal system, and neuroanatomy of sea turtles. In: Lutz, P.L., et al. (Eds.), The Biology of Sea Turtles, Volume 2. CRC Marine Biology Series, vol. 4, pp. 39–77.

Wyneken, J., 2007. Reptilian neurology: anatomy and function. Vet. Clin. Exot. Anim. 10, 837–853.

Zimmerl, U., 1909. Sistema nervoso. In: Bossi, V., Caradonna, G.B., Spampani, G., Varaldi, L., Zimmerl, U. (Eds.), Trattato di Anatomia Veterinária, vol. 3. Francesco Vallardi, Milano, pp. 228–229.

Zimmerl, U., 1930. Apparecchio nervoso. In: Bruni, A.C., Caradonna, G.B., Mannu, A., Preziuso, L., Zimmerl, U. (Eds.), Trattato di Anatomia Veterinaria, vol. 3. Francesco Vallardi, Milano, p. 476.

CHAPTER 11

Anatomical Variations of the Cervical Plexus

TYLER WARNER • R. SHANE TUBBS

Three loops usually form the cervical plexus. The anterior primary division of the first cervical nerve gives off a large branch that merges with the hypoglossal or cervical loop. The first loop of the cervical plexus receives the remaining branches that arise from the first cervical nerve. From this plexus, two of the branches emerging from the first cervical root will typically pass into the sheath of the hypoglossal nerve and course inferiorly where they enter the hypoglossal or cervical loop. The descendens cervicalis or descendens hypoglossi will form after the first cervical nerve departs from the hypoglossal (or vagus). The descendens cervicalis will supply the communicans cervicalis, which receives innervation from the second and third cervical nerves. The communication between these nerves forms the remaining parts of the hypoglossal or cervical loop, which often varies in its location. The cervical loop typically courses superficially to the internal jugular vein between the carotid artery and the sheath of the sternocleidomastoid. The cervical loop may also be seen between the jugular vein and the carotid artery, or posterior to the artery and vein, but these findings rarely occur (Fig. 11.1). The loop may descend below the levels of the thyroid cartilage, or at the level of the hyoid bone, and variations within this range have been reported. The descendens hypoglossi (or cervicalis) may lie within the sheath or just superior to the great vessels as it continues to course inferiorly. The second cervical nerve will provide fibers in the first and second loops of the cervical plexus. The third cervical nerve concludes the lower loops of the plexus after it fuses with the second and fourth cervical nerve (Henle, 1868; Schaefer et al., 1915; Jackson, 1933; Cordier and Devos, 1936; Latarjet, 1948).

ANSA CERVICALIS
Branches of the second cervical ramus and the third cervical ramus will converge and form the inferior root of the ansa cervicalis, also referred to as the ramus descendens cervicalis. It will course inferiorly along the lateral side of the internal jugular vein. The descendens cervicalis then crosses the internal jugular vein below the middle of the neck, and anterior to the common carotid artery, where it will combine with the superior root, or the ramus descendens hypoglossi. This forms the ansa cervicalis, or ansa hypoglossi, which will innervate all of the infrahyoid, with the exception of the thyrohyoid. The inferior root originates from the second and third cervical ventral rami in 75% of cases, second to fourth cervical rami in 15% of cases, and from the third cervical ramus alone in 5% of cases. Reports have shown origins from the second cervical ramus alone or combinations of the first to third cervical rami (Standring, 2008). The variation among the cervical roots that form the anatomy of the ansa cervicalis causes asymmetry across the inferior roots of the specimens observed (Khaki et al., 2006). One study found the variation in 75% of the inferior roots among the 80 cadaver dissections performed. Aside from cadavers with absent inferior roots (3%), they described seven different classifications of the root including a simple classic form (27%), short single form (1.2%), double classic form (40%), double form with two separate roots (11%), double short form (7.5%), triple form (8.7%), and quadruple form (1.2%) (Caliot et al., 1986; Kikuta et al., 2019). Jelev (2013) also proposed a classification system that consisted of five types. The first has no ansa cervicalis formation, which means the hypoglossal and cervical nerves are present, but there is no communication between them. The second type would be considered "typical" where the inferior loop connects to the superior loop. The third type consists of double loops that comprise the hypoglossal, vagal, and cervical nerves. The fourth type has a vagocervical ansa that will form a loop with the hypoglossal nerve. The fifth type does not form an ansa cervicalis, but has a hypoglossal and

Surgical Anatomy of the Cervical Plexus and its Branches. https://doi.org/10.1016/B978-0-323-83132-1.00015-9

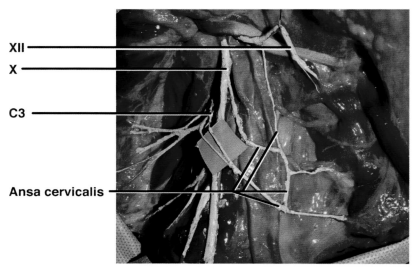

XII

X

C3

Ansa cervicalis

FIG. 11.1 Right cadaveric dissection noting an ansa cervicalis partially contributed to by the vagus nerve (X). The hypoglossal nerve (XII) and C3 spinal nerve are also seen contributing to the ansa.

vagal component present. These variations seldom occur with the exception of type two (Kikuta et al., 2019). These groups could also be subclassified based on the interaction between the cervical roots and vagal, or hypoglossal nerves (Jelev, 2013).

Rao et al. (2007) reported a case with a duplicated ansa cervicalis. The ramus descendens hypoglossi may also be substituted by the vagus (CN X). Banneheka et al. (2008) noticed that the interactions between the ansa cervicalis and vagus nerve can broadly be classified as either false (pseudo) communications, bound together exclusively by connective tissue, or true communications, which involve neuronal interaction. This true communication typically occurred at the base of the skull and knowledge of these variants may prove useful during surgical intervention (Banneheka et al., 2008). When there is no ansa cervicalis present, branches from the second and third cervical roots will directly innervate the infrahyoid muscles. The descendens hypoglossi may give off a branch to provide supply the thyrohyoid and may even contribute to the phrenic nerve. There have also been reports of interactions between the sympathetic trunk and a communicating branch from the fourth cervical nerve, which will merge with the descending cervical nerve in the ansa cervicalis (Turner, 1893; Lippmann, 1910; Schaefer et al., 1915; Rodrigues, 1930; Wischnewsky, 1930; Langsam, 1941; Winckler, 1955). In 18% of subjects, Lang found that the most inferior part of the ansa cervicalis would not pass the lowest point of the cervical part

of the hypoglossal nerve. It would also interact with the intermediate tendon of the omohyoid muscle in 6.5% of subjects (Lang, 1993).

Some studies have found variations in the superior roots of the ansa cervicalis as well. Rare variants include specimens where the vagus and hypoglossal nerves were fused proximally, superior roots branching off of hypoglossal, or vague nerves (Fig. 11.2), even the absence of the ansa cervicalis. In its absence, a vagocervical complex was identified, which originated from the C1 root, C2 root, and the vagus nerve (Nayak et al., 2017; Rath and Anand, 1994; Verma et al., 2009).

PHRENIC NERVE

Studies have been performed to investigate and identify variations in the origin, course, and distribution of the phrenic nerve. Roots from one or more of the following nerves may supply the phrenic nerve: nerve to subclavius; nerve to sternohyoid; second, or rarely sixth, cervical nerve; descendens cervicalis; ansa cervicalis; and brachial plexus. Branches from CN XII (hypoglossal) can communicate with CN XI (spinal accessory) and may supply the phrenic nerve as well. It can also arise exclusively from the nerve to the subclavius; this nerve may innervate the subclavius muscle. The phrenic nerve can travel along the lateral border of the anterior scalene muscle and may run through the muscle as well. The nerve consolidates to a single branch when it enters the thorax, and the size of the nerve may have variability

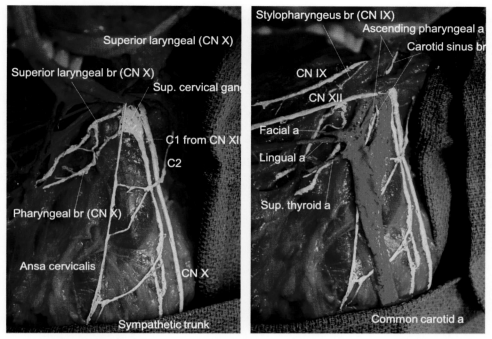

FIG. 11.2 Left neck dissection showing an ansa contributed to by the sympathetic trunk and traveling posterior to the carotid sheath.

bilaterally. The phrenic nerve can pass anterior to subclavian vein or even through a ring or annulus formed by the vein, rather than descending behind it. The fifth or fifth and sixth cervical nerves can give rise to an accessory phrenic nerve. The accessory phrenic will merge with the phrenic nerve at the root of the neck or within the thorax after it travels in front or behind the subclavian vein. Yano (1925) identified an accessory phrenic nerve in 75% of 309 cases studied. The scalenus anterior muscle is supplied by a branch from the phrenic nerve and can course inferiorly along the posterior surface of the sternocleidomastoid. It will then cross anterior to the right brachiocephalic vein and subclavian, and lie about 1.5 cm in front of the subclavian artery and scalenus anterior muscle. Yano (1925) found a case where the right phrenic nerve traveled through an annulus of the subclavian vein (Vieussens, 1664; Wrisberg, 1780; Ziemessen, 1882; Larkin, 1889; Turner, 1893; Wernicke, 1897; Haro, 1907; Sauerbruch, 1913; Schaefer et al., 1915; Felix, 1922a,b; Kiss and Ballon, 1925; Oliver and Minne, 1926; Ruhemann, 1926; Yano, 1928; Bertelli, 1933–34; Ono, 1934–35; Greenfield and Curtis, 1942; Kelley, 1950; Van der Stricht, 1950; Fontes, 1955; Prioton and Thevenet, 1957; Jaya, 1960; Minne et al., 1949).

Loukas et al. (2006) identified the accessory phrenic nerve to have variability in its origin. Fibers from the fifth cervical ventral ramus ran within a branch of the nerve to the subclavius and formed the accessory phrenic nerve. This nerve was just lateral to the phrenic nerve and descended posteriorly, or anteriorly to the subclavian vein. The accessory phrenic nerve typically merges with the phrenic nerve near the first rib and occasionally converges near the pulmonary hilum or distal to the hilum. There are several nerves that can provide it with branches, including the fourth cervical ventral rami, sixth cervical ventral rami, or ansa cervicalis (Standring, 2008).

The full length of the phrenic nerve was observed to be 24.6 cm ± 1.7 cm on the right and 30.6 cm ± 1.8 cm on the left (Jiang et al., 2011). While dissecting a 30-year-old male cadaver, Prakash et al. (2007) observed variations on the right side only. Early in its course, near the origin, the phrenic nerve gives off a communicating branch to the C5 root of the brachial plexus. This branch was located anterior to the subclavian vein. It is typically located posteriorly, between the subclavian vein and artery at the level of the root of the neck, just before entering the thorax. After identifying the variations of the phrenic nerve, the authors recognized that phrenic nerve variations may leave patients susceptible to injury during subclavian catheterization for vascular access (Prakash et al., 2007).

Loukas et al. (2006) reported phrenic nerve injury in 10%—85% of patients after cardiac operations, while discussing the necessity for accurate anatomical description of the innervation of the diaphragm to minimize iatrogenic injury, associated costs, and length of hospitalization. This study looked at 160 nerve specimens taken from 80 adult formalin-fixed cadavers. After crossing the anterior scalene, nerves branching to the phrenic nerve were identified as accessory phrenic nerves. 61.8% had an accessory phrenic nerve and a phrenic nerve present. The accessory phrenic nerve arose from the nerve to the subclavius in 60.6%, ansa cervicalis in 12.1%, and nerve to the sternohyoid in 7%. It merged with the phrenic nerve in the thorax anterior to the subclavian vein in 45.5% specimens and posterior to it in 22.2%. A phrenic nerve loop, also referred to as a phrenic accessory, was observed around the subclavian vein in 45 specimens and around the internal thoracic artery in 38 specimens. Loukas et al. (2006) mentioned that the presence of an accessory phrenic nerve should be considered before mobilization and skeletonization of the internal thoracic artery above the second rib.

Williams et al. (1995) identified that the phrenic nerve came from the fourth cervical nerve root. It originates from the fourth cervical nerve that also had several filaments from a communicating branch from the fifth and third cervical nerve. Codesido and Guerri-Guttenberg (2008) observed a case where the right accessory phrenic nerve went through a division of the subclavian vein before merging with the phrenic nerve. In this case, they noticed that the fifth cervical nerve gave rise to the accessory phrenic nerve, which was an unlikely origin for that nerve. On the anterior surface of the subclavian vein, the nerve ran through an opening located 1 cm away from the jugulo-subclavian junction. After traveling through this annulus, it emerged from the posterior surface of the vein to converge with the phrenic nerve in the thorax, which was the first reported case in the literature. The study suggested that these variations may leave patients susceptible to complications during subclavian venous catheterization because the lumen of the subclavian vein was transiently divided by the accessory phrenic nerve (Codesido and Guerri-Guttenberg, 2008).

Canella et al. (2010) demonstrated that an ultrasonography could show the cervical course of the phrenic nerve. The anterior scalene muscle, transverse cervical nerve, and cervical ascending arteries were landmarks that could easily be identified for ultrasound.

During an interscalene block, the phrenic nerve is frequently anesthetized, usually as a result of the roots of the cervical plexus getting blocked (Bigeleisen, 2003). It was typically anesthetized (36%—67%) when a supraclavicular block was performed as well (Knoblanche, 1979; Farrar et al., 1981; Lanz et al., 1983). Lanz et al. (1983) was surprised because the cervical roots are not blocked very often with this technique. Urmey et al. (1991) noticed the supraclavicular and interscalene approaches were used for blocks, but each approach had a different effect on the quality of the phrenic nerve block. With an interscalene block, there was a 100% incidence of paralysis in the diaphragm that resulted in a 25% reduction in forced vital capacity, but the supraclavicular block caused diaphragmatic paresis in only 50% of patients, which resulted in no loss of forced vital capacity (Neal et al., 1998). Clemente (1985) identified the phrenic nerve to typically originate from the root of the fourth cervical nerve with contributing branches from the third and fifth cervical nerves, previously considered part of the cervical plexus. Another study discussing variants of the phrenic nerve assumed the phrenic nerve would take its typical course (Bergman et al., 1988). They were able to determine that the phrenic nerve may also pass anterior to the subclavian vein instead of posterior to it. They noticed the fifth and sixth cervical nerve could supply the accessory phrenic nerve. The accessory phrenic nerve could also arise from the nerve to the subclavius muscle, which was found in as many as 75% of cadavers. Neal et al. (1998) found that branches from the cervical or brachial plexus supply the phrenic nerve. The 11th and 12th cranial nerves can contribute branches that have close proximity to the location where supraclavicular blocks are performed. The authors felt that the accessory phrenic nerve would lead to diminished ability to block the entire nerve, and should be considered because of the high frequency of accessory phrenic nerves. These situations could cause partial blockage of the ipsilateral hemidiaphragm, which aligned with the results from the study by Neal and colleagues (Bigeleisen, 2003). The clinical relevance is associated with the forced vital capacity in a supraclavicular block, particularly in patients with evidence of hemiparesis. The needle tip may be placed near one of the posterior divisions of the plexus giving rise to the radial nerve and parts of the phrenic nerve. Stimulation in this location would lead to contraction of the supinator and brachioradialis muscles, paresthesia in the thumb, and a diaphragmatic response based on the particular variation (Bigeleisen, 2003).

Bigeleisen (2003) assumed that distal blocks could cause partial phrenic nerve block regardless of the phrenic nerve anatomy, similar to interscalene or supraclavicular blocks. The local anesthetics may interact at the roots of the phrenic nerve causing this partial block, which is supported by the work of Neal and colleagues. Bigeleisen (2003) reported a case where there was a successful block in the diaphragmatic and brachial plexus. There were differences across the interscalene and supraclavicular blocks, which are believed to be the result of anatomical variations. This supports the need to further explore and evaluate the anatomical variants to successfully and safely administer anesthesia.

Rao et al. (2007) observed a subject with a left-sided phrenic nerve. This nerve formed a loop that traveled around the common arterial trunk from the subclavian artery, the source of the inferior thyroid, suprascapular and internal thoracic arteries. The nerve then traveled all along its typical course.

Golarz and White (2019) looked at 100 patients that fell within their inclusion criteria to observe the variants of the phrenic nerve. Of those 100, 28% of patients had some type of variation of the nerve, which included nine duplicated nerves, six lateral accessory nerves, eight medially displaced nerves, and five laterally displaced nerves. The study also looked at the variability of the brachial plexus, and observed these variations occurring simultaneously in patients with variable phrenic nerve anatomy 15% of the time. The phrenic nerve has also been seen giving communicating branches to the brachial plexus, usually in the upper trunk (Goyal and Jain, 2018). The phrenic nerve has variability, but no trends have been identified among sex, body height, body weight, or side on which the specimen was observed (Fazan et al., 2003; Mendelsohn et al., 2011).

LESSER OCCIPITAL NERVE

The lesser occipital nerve occasionally pierces through the sternocleidomastoid muscle. It is usually very small with a diameter of 1.2 mm ± 1.6 mm (Ducic et al., 2009) and distributed only to the skin of the neck, often interacting with branches of the occipital arteries along its course (Lee et al., 2013). This branch also communicates with the posterior branch of the great auricular nerve and is occasionally derived from the great occipital nerve. The greater occipital nerve may also provide innervation to areas usually supplied by the lesser occipital nerve.

Instead of its usual dorsal and upward course beneath the deep fascia along the posterior border of the sternocleidomastoid muscle, the lesser occipital nerve passes directly posteriorly, piercing the trapezius

muscle near its upper border before reaching the scalp in some cases. Its auricular branch can derive from the greater occipital. It usually arises from the second and third cervical nerves or the loop between them (Henle, 1868; Schaefer et al., 1915; Jackson, 1933; Cordier and Devos, 1936; Latarjet, 1948). Duplication (Fig. 11.3) and triplication of the lesser occipital nerves have been noted in the literature as well. These variations may have clinical significance when performing a neurectomy, or oblation to relieve pain in patients with compressions or cervicogenic headaches (Dash et al., 2005; Madhavi and Holla, 2004; Lee et al., 2009). We have dissected a specimen with communication between the lesser occipital nerve and auriculotemporal nerve (Fig. 11.4).

TRANSVERSE CERVICAL NERVE

The superficial cervical nerve can have two or more branches arising from the cervical plexus, instead of a single nerve. The third or both the third and fourth cervical nerves can converge to form this nerve. It sometimes passes through an annulus in the external jugular as it courses through the neck (Henle, 1868; Schaefer et al., 1915; Bautzmann, 1930; Jackson, 1933; Cordier and Devos, 1936; Latarjet, 1948). One study identified a communication between the ascending branch and the marginal mandibular branch of the facial nerve instead of the cervical branch (Salinas et al., 2009).

There have been several reports of unique variants of the transverse cervical nerve. As a result of the high incidence of failure with inferior alveolar nerve blocks, Lin studied cadavers to determine the underlying cause and noticed accessory nerve innervations originating from the cervical plexus. One of the supplemental nerve supplies originated from the transverse cervical nerve, which innervated the inferior border of the posterior mandible (Lin et al., 2013). Another study identified branches of the transverse cervical nerve supplying the middle portion of the sternocleidomastoid. These fibers were determined to mainly provide proprioception, but the report speculated about possible motor innervation, which may have implications with the facial nerve (Paraskevas, 2015).

GREAT AURICULAR NERVE

The posterior or mastoid branch of the great auricular nerve may arise without branches originating from the cervical plexus. In this circumstance, the cervical plexus passes upward between the lesser occipital and the great auricular nerves on its course. The great auricular nerve will form from the third cervical nerve or both the third

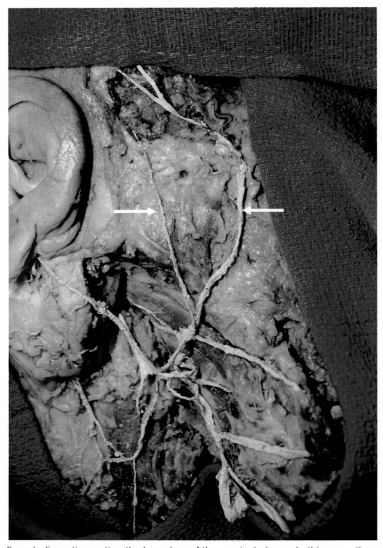

FIG. 11.3 Left neck dissection noting the branches of the cervical plexus. In this case, there are two lesser occipital nerves (arrows). In the older literature, some have termed the more anterior branch as the "mastoid branch" but earlier authors were not clear if this is a branch of the lesser occipital nerve or a separate and independent branch of the cervical plexus.

and fourth cervical nerves (Henle, 1868; Schaefer et al., 1915; Jackson, 1933; Cordier and Devos, 1936; Latarjet, 1948). It typically arises from the posterior border of the sternocleidomastoid at one-third the distance of the muscle from the mastoid process to the origin at the clavicle (Lefkowitz et al., 2013). It might be duplicated (Fig. 11.5).

There are conflicting opinions about the exact anatomical course of the great auricular nerve. Zohar

et al. (2002) observed the pathway of the anterior branch and endings of this nerve in relation to the parotid gland. The study used 19 fresh adult cadavers with causes of death that were not due to pathology in the parotid region. The study observed the parotid gland near the site of termination at the anterior branch of the nerve using these cadavers. In the majority of cases, there was no evidence of well-organized fibers

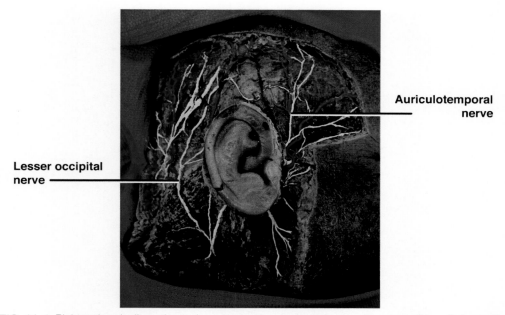

Auriculotemporal nerve

Lesser occipital nerve

FIG. 11.4 Right cadaveric dissection noting a more or less horizontal connection above the ear between the lesser occipital and auriculotemporal nerves.

of the great auricular nerve inside the parotid gland (21/37 = 57%). In several cadavers (5/37 = 13%), the nerve fibers were reported as penetrating the interlobular septa, and in others (11/37 = 30%), nerve bundles were found deep within the gland alongside small ducts, which ran within close proximity of thin-walled blood vessels. These findings further prove the existence of anatomical variations in the endings of the anterior branch of the great auricular nerve. Zohar et al. (2002) suggested that these nerve bundles deep in the gland along ducts and near vessels may have many clinical applications.

Another report noticed that an anterior branch of the great auricular nerve passed into the submandibular triangle. The nerve then coursed anterior to the facial vein where it converged with the deep surface of the marginal mandibular branch of the facial nerve (Brennan et al., 2008). Brennan conducted an anatomical study with 25 cadavers in search of variations of the great auricular nerve. Of the 25 cadavers, 2 had variations that interacted with the mandibular branch of the facial nerve (Brennan et al., 2010). Although there are few reported interacting with the facial nerve, these variations may prompt the need for further study because of their surgical implications, especially in maxillofacial surgery.

SUPRACLAVICULAR NERVES

Reports of several different variations have been identified in these nerves. A branch from the supraclavicular nerves will pass into the thorax and merge with the phrenic nerve once it has passed the subclavian artery or vein. This branch may also receive innervation from a bundle on nerves originating from the fifth cervical nerve. The rhomboids typically receive innervation from these nerves and will pass through the trapezius muscle until it reaches the skin near the midline. This will usually occur at the level of the fifth and sixth vertebrae. One study using 14 necks (8 embalmed cadavers) found that the average distance between the two farthest supraclavicular nerves was 98 mm (85–125) and the most distal from the clavicle was 46 mm (30–63). The study further analyzed the intermediate and lateral branches, and noticed they typically had two or three secondary rami, but the lateral branch did not divide in six of those cases. The lateral branches ended either lateral to or at the level of the acromion process with a mean distance of 10.4 mm (0–24) from the acromion (Havet et al., 2007). Another study reported 10 of 254 cases where the middle branch of the supraclavicular nerves would travel through the clavicle (Papadatos, 1980). They traversed the bone within intraclavicular canals, which could be visualized

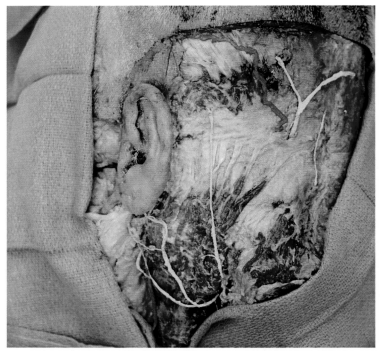

FIG. 11.5 Left cadaveric dissection noting duplicated great auricular nerves traveling with the external jugular vein. Posterior to this is the lesser occipital, greater occipital, and lesser occipital nerves. The occipital artery is seen between the lesser and greater occipital nerves.

with radiography (Henle, 1868; Kopsch, 1908; Schaefer et al., 1915; Oliver and Minne, 1926; Latarjet, 1948; Anson, 1966).

Tubbs et al. (2006) identified the right intermediate branch of the supraclavicular nerve to pierce the clavicle in a male cadaver. This variation was the only anomaly reported in this specimen. The intermediate branch of the supraclavicular nerve leads to the manifestation of several symptoms, but a review of the literature indicated that these were relatively rare. To alleviate the associated symptoms, a surgical decompression of the entrapped nerve would be necessary. Clinicians should consider an entrapment of the supraclavicular nerve within the clavicle as a differential diagnosis for shoulder pain even though this variation is not commonly found (Tubbs et al., 2006).

As a result of the proximity of the supraclavicular nerve to the clavicle, any fractures, or surgical innervation to repair fractures of the clavicle, may cause damage to the supraclavicular nerves and its branches. The literature has described the development of painful neuromas after iatrogenic transection and symptomatic nerve entrapment in fracture callus after healing.

Fracture fixation and nerve decompression are essential in a cases of acute supraclavicular nerve entrapment and tension to significantly reduce the pain in the patients (O'Neill et al., 2012). Rao et al. (2009) also reported a supraclavicular nerve that looped around the external jugular vein and the transverse cervical artery.

A number of clinical cases of this specific neuropathy have been reported after Gelberman et al. (1975) had defined the supraclavicular nerve entrapment syndrome. The supraclavicular nerve branch was found within a narrow canal in the clavicle that leads to nerve injuries in all these cases. However, reports in the anatomical literature have mentioned variants of the courses of the supraclavicular nerves. Reports of these nerves have identified branches to abnormal fibrous and muscular structures, not just bony canals. For the entrapment neuropathy to develop, the nerve must become compressed as a result of a narrow site with a rigid wall. The study by Jelev and Surchev (2007) examined all the possible variant anatomical structures that could lead to the development of a supraclavicular nerve entrapment. They categorized these variants using three groups of structures closely related to the course of the supraclavicular nerve: transclavicular canals, fibrous bands, and unusual muscular structures (supraclavicularis proprius muscle, cleidooccipitalis muscle, etc.). As a result of the characteristics of the variations identified, they implied that for the first time that certain fibrous, muscular structures may also have an anatomical basis for supraclavicular nerve entrapment syndrome, in addition to the bony canals through the clavicle.

Despite the rarity of this syndrome, it should be considered as a differential for causes of anterior shoulder girdle pain. It is usually related to anatomical variants (involving the bone structures, fibrous bands, or muscles and tendons), and computed tomography is the most useful investigation to observe these variations. Medications used to treat neuropathic pain can provide relief, but clinicians may resort to more invasive procedures if unsuccessful. A local glucocorticoid injection or even surgical decompression may be considered (Douchamps et al., 2012).

REFERENCES

Anson, B.J. (Ed.), 1966. Morris' Human Anatomy, twelfth ed. McGraw-Hill Book Company, New York.

Banneheka, S., Tokita, K., Kumaki, K., 2008. Nerve fiber analysis of ansa cervicalis-vagus communications. Anat. Sci. Int. 83, 145–151.

Bautzmann, H., 1930. Verlauf des Nervus cutaneous colli durch eine Insel der Vena jugularis externa. Anat. Anz. 70, 516–519.

Bergman, R.A., Thompson, S.A., Afifi, A.K., Saddeh, F.A., 1988. Compendium of Human Anatomical Variation. Urban and Schwarzenburg, Baltimore.

Bertelli, D., 1933-34. Distribuzione dei nervi frenici nel diaframma dei Mammiferi. Ital. J. Anat Embryol. 32, 110–148.

Bigeleisen, P.E., 2003. Anatomical variations of the phrenic nerve and its clinical implication for supraclavicular block. Br. J. Anaesth. 91, 916–917.

Brennan, P.A., Webb, R., Kemidi, F., Spratt, J., Standring, S., 2008. Great auricular communication with the marginal mandibular nerve—a previously unreported anatomical variant. Br. J. Oral Maxillofac. Surg. 46, 492–493.

Brennan, P., Gholmy, M., Ounnas, H., Zaki, G., Puxeddu, R., Standring, S., 2010. Communication of the anterior branch of the great auricular nerve with the marginal mandibular nerve: a prospective study of 25 neck dissections. Br. J. Oral Maxillofac. Surg. 48, 431–433.

Caliot, P., Dumont, D., Bousquet, V., Midy, D., 1986. A note on the anastomoses between the hypoglossal nerve and the cervical plexus. Surg. Radiol. Anat. 8, 75–79.

Canella, C., Demondion, X., Delebarre, A., Moraux, A., Cotten, H., Cotten, A., 2010. Anatomical study of phrenic nerve using ultrasound. Eur. J. Radiol. 20, 659–665.

Clemente, C.D. (Ed.), 1985. Anatomy of the Human Body. Lea & Febiger, Philadelphia, pp. 1203–1205.

Codesido, M., Guerri-Guttenberg, R.A., 2008. Right accessory phrenic nerve passing through an annulus of the subclavian vein. Clin. Anat. 21, 779–780.

Cordier, C., Devos, D., 1936. Contribution a l'étude de la constitution du plexus cervical chez l'homme et quelques primates. Assoc. Anat. C. R. 31, 114–123.

Dash, K., Janis, J., Guyuron, B., 2005. The lesser and third occipital nerves and migraine headaches. Plast. Reconstr. Surg. 115, 1752–1758.

Douchamps, F., Courtois, A.C., Bruyère, P.J., Crielaard, J.M., 2012. Supraclavicular nerve entrapment syndrome. Joint Bone Spine 79, 88–89.

Ducic, I., Moriarty, M., Al-Attar, A., 2009. Anatomical variations of the occipital nerves: implications for the treatment of chronic headaches. Plast. Reconstr. Surg. 123, 859–863.

Farrar, M.D., Scheybani, M., Nolte, H., 1981. Upper extremity block, effectiveness and complications. Reg. Anesth. Pain Med. 6, 133–134.

Fazan, V., Amadeu, A., Caleffi, A., Rodrigues Filho, O., 2003. Brachial plexus variations in its formation and main branches. Acta Cir. Bras. 18, 14–18.

Felix, W., 1922a. Anatomische, experimentelle und klinische Untersuchungen über den N. phrenicus und über die Zwerchfellinnervation. Deutsche Z Chir. 171, 283–397.

Felix, W., 1922b. Über den Nervus phrenicus und die Zwerchfellinnervation. Zentralbl Chir. 49, 1832.

Fontes, V., 1955. Les origines du nerf phrénique. Assoc. Anat. C. R. 42, 518–526.

Gelberman, R.H., Verdeck, W.N., Brodhea, d WT., 1975. Supraclavicular nerve-entrapment syndrome. J. Bone Joint Surg. 57, 119.

Golarz, S., White, J., 2019. Anatomic variation of the phrenic nerve and brachial plexus encountered during 100 supraclavicular decompressions for neurogenic thoracic outlet syndrome with associated post-operative neurologic complications. Ann. Vasc. Surg. 55, 13.

Goyal, N., Jain, A., 2018. Variant communication of phrenic nerve in neck. Surg. Radiol. Anat. 41, 151–152.

Greenfield, J., Curtis, G.M., 1942. The "sniff test" in thoracic surgery. With a review of 119 phrenic nerve interruptions. J. Thorac. Surg. 12, 79–85.

Haro, S., 1907. Ueber einige klinisch sehr wichtige Verlaufsanomalien des N. phrenicus. Tokyo J. Med. Sci. 21, 21–29.

Havet, E., Duparc, F., Tobenas-Dujardin, A., Muller, J., Fréger, P., 2007. Morphometric study of the shoulder and subclavicular innervation by the intermediate and lateral branches of supraclavicular nerves. Surg. Radiol. Anat. 29, 605–610.

Henle, J., 1868. Handbuch der Systematischen Anatomie des Menschen. von Friedrich Vieweg und Sohn, Braunschweig.

Jackson, C.M. (Ed.), 1933. Morris' Human Anatomy, ninth ed. P. Blakiston's Son & Co., Inc., Philadelphia. 1481 p.

Jaya, Y., 1960. Liver as a content of the right sided diaphragmatic hernia - a case report. J. Anat. Soc. India 9, 37–38.

Jelev, L., 2013. Some unusual types of formation of the ansa cervicalis in humans and proposal of a new morphological classification. Clin. Anat. 26, 961–965.

Jelev, L., Surchev, L., 2007. Study of variant anatomical structures (bony canals, fibrous bands, and muscles) in relation to potential supraclavicular nerve entrapment. Clin. Anat. 20, 278–285.

Jiang, S., Xu, W.D., Shen, Y.D., Xu, J.G., Gu, Y.D., 2011. An anatomical study of the full-length phrenic nerve and its blood supply: clinical implications for endoscopic dissection. Anat. Sci. Int. 86, 225–231.

Kelley, W.O., 1950. Phrenic nerve paralysis. Special considerations of the accessory phrenic nerve. J. Thorac. Surg. 19, 923–928.

Khaki, A., Shokouhi, G., Shoja, M., Farahani, R., Zarrintan, S., Khaki, A., Montazam, H., Tanoomand, A., Tubbs, R., 2006. Ansa cervicalis as a variant of spinal accessory nerve plexus: a case report. Clin. Anat. 19, 540–543.

Kikuta, S., Jenkins, S., Kusukawa, J., Iwanaga, J., Loukas, M., Tubbs, R., 2019. Ansa cervicalis: a comprehensive review of its anatomy, variations, pathology, and surgical applications. Anat. Cell. Biol. 52, 221.

Kiss, F., Ballon, H.C., 1925. Contribution to the nerve supply of the diaphragm. Anat. Rec. 41, 285–298.

Knoblanche, G.E., 1979. The incidence and aetiology of phrenic nerve blockade association with supraclavicular brachial plexus block. Anaesth. Intens. Care. 7, 346.

Kopsch, F., 1908. Rauber's Lehrbuch der Anatomie des Menschen. Georg Thieme, Leipzig.

Lang, J., 1993. Clinical Anatomy of the Cervical Spine. Thieme, New York.

Langsam, C.L.M., 1941. Omohyoideus in American whites and negroes. Am. J. Phys. Anthropol. 28, 249–259.

Lanz, E., Theiss, D., Jankovic, D., 1983. The extent of blockade following various techniques of brachial plexus block. Anesth. Analg. 62, 55–58.

Larkin, F.C., 1889. Accessory phrenic nerve. J. Anat. Physiol. 23, 340.

Latarjet, A., 1948. Testut's Traité d'Anatomie Humaine, ninth ed. G. Doin & Co, Paris.

Lee, S.H., Lee, J.K., Jin, S.M., Kim, J.H., Park, I.S., Chu, H.R., Ahn, H.Y., Rho, Y.S., 2009. Anatomical variations of the spinal accessory nerve and its relevance to level IIb lymph nodes. J. Otolaryngol. Head Neck Surg. 141, 639–644.

Lee, M., Brown, M., Chepla, K., Okada, H., Gatherwright, J., Totonchi, A., Alleyne, B., Zwiebel, S., Kurlander, D., Guyuron, B., 2013. An anatomic study of the lesser occipital nerve and its potential compression points. Plast. Reconstr. Surg. 1.

Lefkowitz, T., Hazani, R., Chowdhry, S., Elston, J., Yaremchuk, M., Wilhelmi, B., 2013. Anatomical landmarks to avoid injury to the great auricular nerve during rhytidectomy. Aesthet. Surg. J. 33, 19–23.

Lin, K., Uzbelger Feldman, D., Barbe, M., 2013. Transverse cervical nerve: implications for dental anesthesia. Clin. Anat. 26, 688–692.

Lippmann, R.V., 1910. Abnormer Ursprung des Ramus descendens N. hypoglossi aus dem N. vagus. Anat. Anz. 37, 1–4.

Loukas, M., Kinsella Jr., C.R., Louis Jr., R.G., Gandhi, S., Curry, B., 2006. Surgical anatomy of the accessory phrenic nerve. Ann. Thorac. Surg. 82, 1870–1875.

Madhavi, C., Holla, S., 2004. Triplication of the lesser occipital nerve. Clin. Anat. 17, 667–671.

Mendelsohn, A., DeConde, A., Lambert, H., Dodson, S., Daney, B., Stark, M., Berke, G., Wisco, J., 2011. Cervical variations of the phrenic nerve. Laryngoscope 121, 1920–1923.

Minne, J., Senneville, A., Guyot, A., 1949. Remarques sur la division et les branches terminales du nerf phrenique droit. Assoc. Anat. C. R. 36, 484–491.

Nayak, S., Shetty, P., Reghunathan, D., Aithal, A., Kumar, N., 2017. Erratum to "Descendens vagohypoglossi: rare variant of the superior root of ansa cervicalis" [Br J Oral Maxillofac Surg 55 (2017) 834–5]. Br. J. Oral Maxillofac. Surg. 55, 1049.

Neal, J.M., Moore, J.M., Kopacz, D.J., Liu, S.S., Kramer, D.J., Plorde, J.J., 1998. Quantitative analysis of respiratory, motor, and sensory function after supraclavicular block. Anesth. Analg. 86, 1239–1244.

Oliver, E., Minne, R., 1926. La traversée diaphragmatique du nerf phrénique droit et ses variations. Assoc. Anat. C. R. 21, 441–444.

Ono, N., 1934-35. Untersuchungen und Studien über die Ursprungszellen des N. phrenicus. Jpn J. Med. Sci. 5, 1–34.

O'Neill, K., Stutz, C., Duvernay, M., Schoenecker, J., 2012. Supraclavicular nerve entrapment and clavicular fracture. J. Orthop. Trauma 26, e63–65.

Papadatos, D., 1980. Supraclavicular nerves piercing the clavicle: a study of 10 cases. Anat. Anz. 147, 371–381.

Paraskevas, G., 2015. Aberrant innervation of the sternocleidomastoid muscle by the transverse cervical nerve: a case report. J. Clin. Diagn. Res. 9, AD01–AD02.

Prakash, P.,L.V., Madhyastha, S., Singh, G., 2007. A variation of the phrenic nerve: case report and review. Singap. Med. J. 48, 1156–1157.

Prioton, J.B., Thevenet, A., 1957. La distribution intra-diaphragmatique des nerfs phréniques. Assoc. Anat. C. R. 44, 635–645.

Rao, T.R., Kumar, B., Shetty, P., Rao, S.R., 2007. Variaiton in the course of the left phrenic nerve: a case report. Neuroanatomy 6, 24–25.

Rao, T.R., Shetty, P., Rao, S., 2009. A rare case of looping of supraclavicular nerve branches around external jugular vein and transverse cervical artery. Int. J. Anat. Var. 2, 48–50.

Rath, G., Anand, C., 1994. Vagocervical complex replacing an absent ansa cervicalis. Surg. Radiol. Anat. 16, 441–443.

Rodrigues, A., 1930. Le descendens cervicalis chez l'homme et chez le mammifères (quelques notes sur son évolution phylogénique). Assoc. Anat. C. R. 25, 267–282.

Ruhemann, E., 1926. Die Topographie des Nervus phrenicus unter abnormen Verhältnissen. Arch. Klin. Chirurgie 139, 557–562.

Salinas, N.L., Jackson, O., Dunham, B., Bartlett, S.P., 2009. Anatomical dissection and modified Sihler stain of the lower branches of the facial nerve. Plast. Reconstr. Surg. 124, 1905–1915.

Sauerbruch, F., 1913. Die Beeinflussung von Lungenerkrankungen durch künstliche Lähmung des Zwerchfells (phrenikotomie). Munch Med. Wochenschr. 60, 625–626.

Schaefer, E.A., Symington, J., Bryce, T.H. (Eds.), 1915. Quain's Anatomy, eleventh ed. Longmans, Green, and Co, London.

Standring, S., 2008. Gray's Anatomy, 40th ed. Churchill Livingstone, Edinburgh, pp. 456–460.

Tubbs, R.S., Salter, E.G., Oakes, W.J., 2006. Anomaly of the supraclavicular nerve: case report and review of the literature. Clin. Anat. 19, 599–601.

Turner, W., 1893. A phrenic nerve receiving a root of origin from the descendens hypoglossi. J. Anat. Physiol. 27, 427.

Urmey, W.F., Talts, K.H., Sharrock, N.E., 1991. One hundred percent incidence of hemidiaphragmatic paresis associated with interscalene brachial plexus anesthesia as diagnosed by ultrasonography. Anesth. Analg. 72, 498–503.

Van der Stricht, J., 1950. A propos d'une anomalie du nerf phrénique. Assoc. Anat. C. R. 37, 478–484.

Verma, R., Das, S., Suri, R., 2009. Unusual organization of the ansa cervicalis : a case report. Braz. J. Morphol. Sci. 22, 175–177.

Vieussens, R., 1664. Neurographia Universalis. Lugduni.

Wernicke, 1897. Insuffizienz der Nervi phrenici. Monatsschar. f. Psych. Neurol. 2, 200.

Williams, P.L., Bannister, L.H., Berry, M.M., Collins, P., Dyson, M., Dussek, J.E., Ferguson, M.W.J., 1995. Anatomı'a de Gray, 38th Ed. Hart-court, Madrid.

Winckler, G., 1955. A propros des relations que relations que existent entre le plexus cervical et le nerf grand hypoglosse. Assoc. Anat. C. R. 42, 1415–1419.

Wischnewsky, A.S., 1930. Die Aufbautypen des Ramus descendens nervi hypoglossi. Z. Anat. Entwicklungsgeschichte 92, 551–564.

Wrisberg, L., 1780. De Nervis Viscerum Abdominalium. Secto. I. De nervo Diaphragmatico, Gottingae.

Yano, K., 1925. Zur Anatomie des Nervus pherincus und Nebenphrenicus. Folia Anat. Jpn. 3, 95–106.

Yano, K., 1928. Zur Anatomie und Histologie des Nervus phrenicus und sogenannten Nebenphrenicus, nebst Bemerkungen uber ihre Verbindung mit Sympathicus. Folia Anat. Jpn. 6, 247–290.

Ziemessen, H., 1882. Erregbarkeit des N. phrenicus. Arch. Klin. Med. 30, 270.

Zohar, Y., Siegal, A., Siegal, G., Halpern, M., Levy, B., Gal, R., 2002. The great auricular nerve; does it penetrate the parotid gland? An anatomical and microscopical study. J Craniomaxillofac. Surg. 30, 318–321.

CHAPTER 12

Microanatomy of the Origin of the Cervical Plexus at the Spinal Cord, Nerve Root Cuffs, and Dorsal Root Ganglia Levels

IRENE RIQUELME • MIGUEL ANGEL REINA • ANDRÉ P. BOEZAART •
FRANCISCO REINA • VIRGINIA GARCÍA-GARCÍA • PALOMA FERNÁNDEZ •
ANNA CARRERA

In this chapter, we address the microanatomy of the structures that are enclosed within the cervical spine that give rise to the anterior branches of the cervical spinal nerves. The sequential images allow visualization of all the structures and their microscopic details from the spinal cord at C1—C4 levels. This includes the anterior and posterior roots that are separated by the denticulate ligaments within the subarachnoid space, the anterior and posterior roots within the nerve root cuffs, dorsal root ganglia, and the distal peripheral nerve formed by (motor and sensory axons). The spinal nerves give rise to the anterior rami, the origin of the cervical plexus. The sympathetic trunk and its ganglia located within the cervical region are also included in the images.

The figures show a sequence of successive and complete cross-sections of the cervical spine from C1 to C4. After each complete cross-section, further images with the details at higher magnification are also included.

Each image has a measurement bar for exact measurements of each of the structures included in the image. These bars are from slide-printed bars captured at the same magnification as the images by the same scanner. These bars are 1 cm (10 mm) with divisions at 1, 0.1, and 0.01 mm; 1 mm with 0.1 mm divisions, and 0.1 mm with 0.01 mm divisions.

$$0.1mm = 100\mu m; 0.01mm = 10\mu m$$

Note: The axons enter and leave the spinal cord through the rootlets. Grouped rootlets form the anterior and posterior spinal nerve roots within the spinal subarachnoid space. These grouped nerve roots exit from the spinal dural sac through the nerve root cuffs as anterior and posterior nerve roots of the spinal nerves.

The subdural space is not a natural anatomical space at this level. The spaces seen between arachnoid and dura mater layers are artifacts created during dedissection—thus they is an acquired subdural space (Figs. 12.1—12.58).

Surgical Anatomy of the Cervical Plexus and its Branches. https://doi.org/10.1016/B978-0-323-83132-1.00007-X

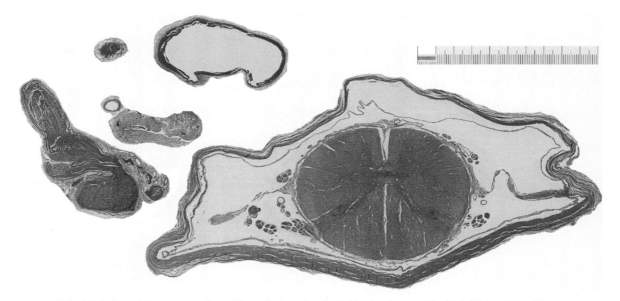

FIG. 12.1 Complete cross-section of the spinal cord and neighboring tissue at the high C1 level. Bar: 10 mm including divisions.

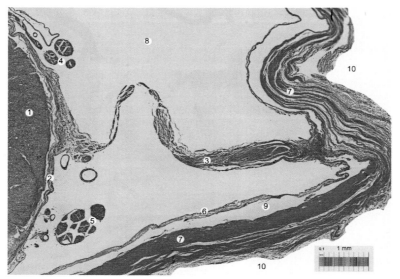

FIG. 12.2 Details of Fig. 12.1. 1: spinal cord, 2: pia mater, 3: denticulate ligament, 4: anterior spinal nerve roots within subarachnoid space, 5: posterior spinal nerve roots within subarachnoid space, 6: arachnoid layer, 7: dura mater, 8: subarachnoid space, 9: acquired subdural space, 10: epidural space. Bar: 1 mm including divisions.

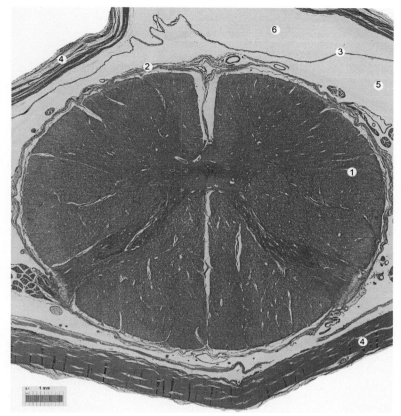

FIG. 12.3 Details of Fig. 12.1. 1: spinal cord, 2: pia mater, 3: arachnoid mater, 4: dura mater, 5: subarachnoid space, 6: acquired subdural space, 7: epidural space. Bar: 1 mm including divisions.

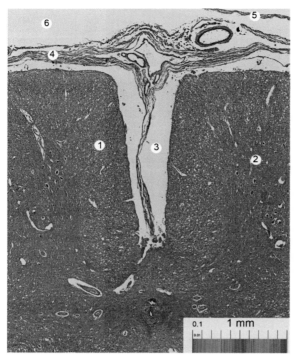

FIG. 12.4 Details of Fig. 12.1. 1: spinal cord, 2: anterior horn, 3: anterior median fissure 4: pia mater, 5: arachnoid layer, 6: subarachnoid space. Bar: 1 mm including divisions.

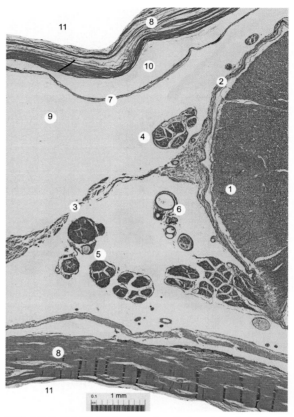

FIG. 12.5 Details of Fig. 12.1. 1: spinal cord, 2: pia mater, 3: denticulate ligament, 4: anterior spinal nerve roots within subarachnoid space, 5: posterior spinal nerve roots within subarachnoid space, 6: subarachnoid free vessels, 7: arachnoid layer, 8: dura mater, 9: subarachnoid space, 10: acquired subdural space, 11: epidural space. Bar: 1 mm including divisions.

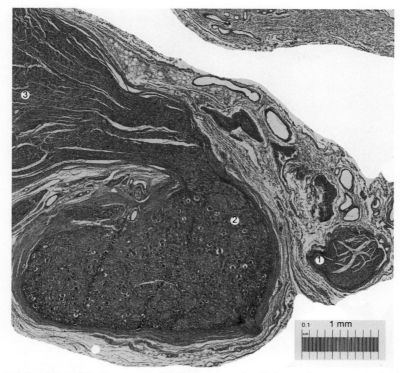

FIG. 12.6 Details of Fig. 12.1. Structures within the nerve root cuff. 1: anterior nerve root of spinal nerve, 2: dorsal root ganglion, 3: transitional area distal to dorsal root ganglion where axon from anterior and posterior nerve roots form the origin of peripheral nerve. Bar: 1 mm including divisions.

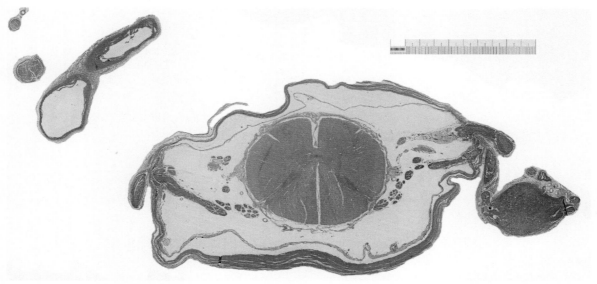

FIG. 12.7 Complete cross-section through the spinal cord and neighboring tissue at the inferior C1 level. Bar: 10 mm including divisions.

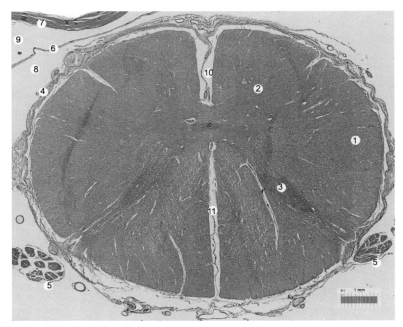

FIG. 12.8 Details of Fig. 12.7. 1: spinal cord, 2: anterior horn, 3: posterior horn, 4: pia mater, 5: posterior spinal nerve roots within subarachnoid space, 6: arachnoid layer, 7: dura mater, 8: subarachnoid space, 9: acquired subdural space, 10: anterior median fissure, 11: posterior median sulcus. Bar: 1 mm including divisions.

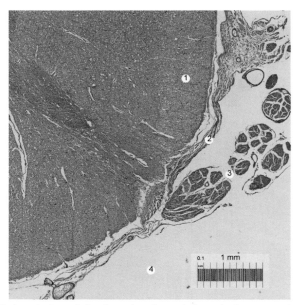

FIG. 12.9 Details of Fig. 12.7. 1: spinal cord, 2: pia mater, 3: posterior spinal nerve roots within subarachnoid space, 4: subarachnoid space. Bar: 1 mm including divisions.

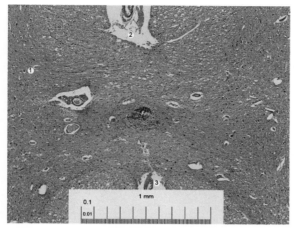

FIG. 12.10 Details of Fig. 12.7. 1: spinal cord. 2: anterior median fissure, 3: posterior median sulcus. Bar: 1 mm including divisions.

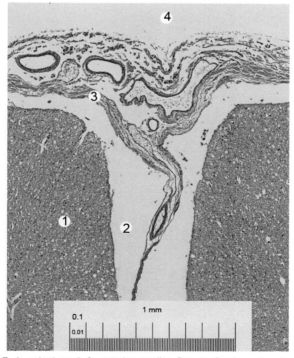

FIG. 12.11 Details of Fig. 12.7. 1: spinal cord, 2: anterior median fissure, 3: pia mater, 4: subarachnoid space. Bar: 1 mm including divisions.

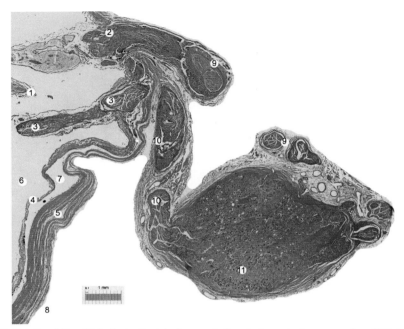

FIG. 12.12 Details of Fig. 12.7. 1: denticulate ligament, 2: anterior spinal nerve roots within subarachnoid space, 3: posterior spinal nerve roots within subarachnoid space, 4: arachnoid layer, 5: dura mater, 6: subarachnoid space, 7: acquired subdural space, 8: epidural space. Structures within nerve root cuff, 9: anterior root of spinal nerve, 10: posterior root of spinal nerve, 11: dorsal root ganglion. Bar: 1 mm including divisions.

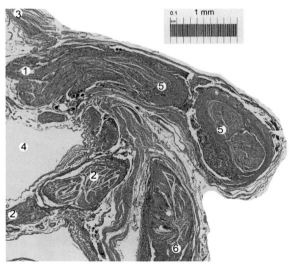

FIG. 12.13 Details of Fig. 12.7. 1: anterior spinal nerve roots within subarachnoid space, 2: posterior spinal nerve roots within subarachnoid space, 3: dura mater, 4: subarachnoid space 3. Structures within nerve root cuff, 5: anterior root of spinal nerve, 6: posterior root of spinal nerve. Bar: 1 mm including divisions.

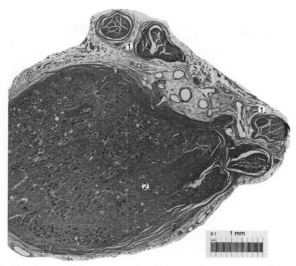

FIG. 12.14 Details of Fig. 12.7. Structures within nerve root cuff, 1: anterior nerve root of spinal nerve, 2: dorsal root ganglion. Bar: 1 mm including divisions.

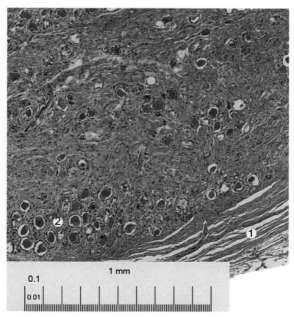

FIG. 12.15 Details of Fig. 12.7. Dorsal root ganglion. 1: transitional tissue dura mater-epineurium, 2: soma of sensory axons. Bar: 1 mm including divisions.

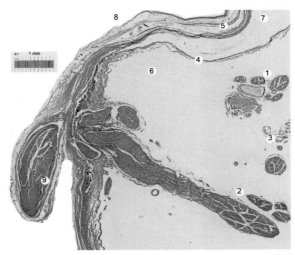

FIG. 12.16 Details of Fig. 12.7. 1: anterior spinal nerve roots within subarachnoid space, 2: posterior spinal nerve roots within subarachnoid space, 3: denticulate ligament, 4: arachnoid layer, 5: dura mater, 6: subarachnoid space, 7: acquired subdural space, 8: epidural space. Structures within nerve root cuff, 9: posterior root of spinal nerve. Bar: 1 mm including divisions.

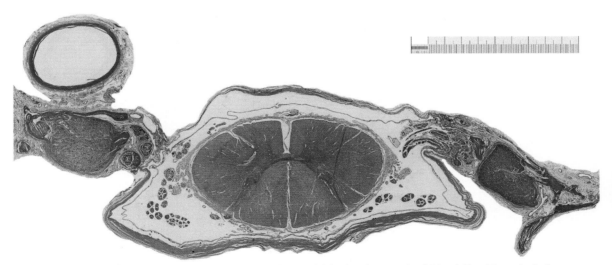

FIG. 12.17 Complete cross-section spinal cord and neighboring tissue at the C2 level. Bar: 10 mm including divisions.

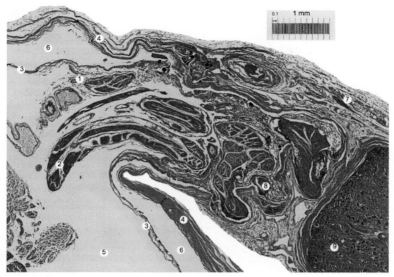

FIG. 12.18 Details of Fig. 12.17. 1: anterior spinal nerve roots within subarachnoid space, 2: posterior spinal nerve roots within subarachnoid space, 3: arachnoid layer, 4: dura mater, 5: subarachnoid space, 6: acquired subdural space. Structures within the nerve root cuff, 7: anterior nerve root of spinal nerve, 8: posterior nerve root of spinal nerve, 9: dorsal root ganglion. Bar: 1 mm including divisions.

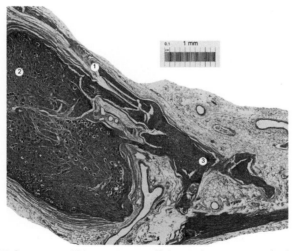

FIG. 12.19 Details of Fig. 12.17. Structures within nerve root cuff, 1: anterior nerve root of spinal nerve, 2: dorsal root ganglion, 3: origin of peripheral nerves including sensory and motor axons. Bar: 1 mm including divisions.

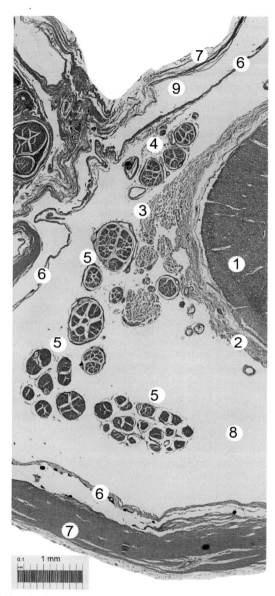

FIG. 12.20 Details of Fig. 12.17. 1: spinal cord, 2: pia mater, 3: denticulate ligament (reflected), 4: anterior spinal nerve roots within subarachnoid space, 5: posterior spinal nerve roots within subarachnoid space, 6: arachnoid layer, 7: dura mater, 8: subarachnoid space, 9: acquired subdural space. Bar: 1 mm including divisions.

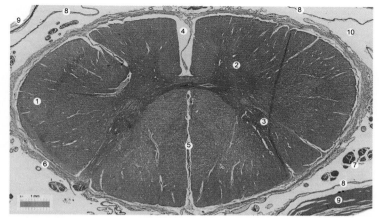

FIG. 12.21 Details of Fig. 12.17. 1: spinal cord, 2: anterior horn, 3: posterior horn, 4: anterior median fissure, 5: posterior median sulcus. 6: pia mater, 7: posterior spinal nerve roots within subarachnoid space, 8: arachnoid layer, 9: dura mater, 10: subarachnoid space. Bar: 1 mm including divisions.

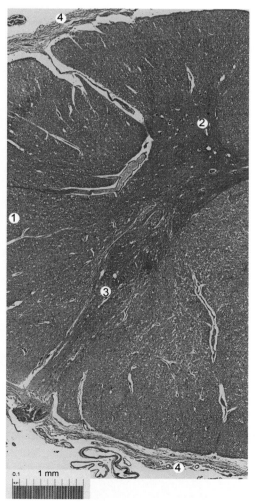

FIG. 12.22 Details of Fig. 12.17. 1: spinal cord, 2: anterior horn, 3: posterior horn, 4: pia mater. Bar: 1 mm including divisions.

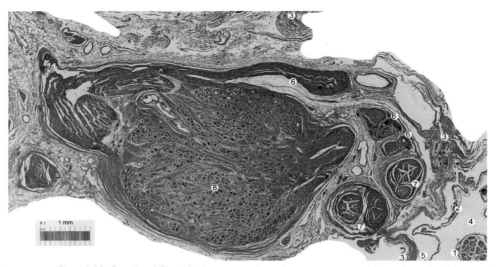

FIG. 12.23 Fig. 12.20. Details of Fig. 12.17. 1: posterior spinal nerve roots within subarachnoid space, 2: arachnoid layer, 3: dura mater, 4: subarachnoid space, 5: acquired subdural space. Structures within nerve root cuff, 6: anterior nerve root of spinal nerve, 7: posterior nerve root of spinal nerve, 8: dorsal root ganglion. Bar: 1 mm including divisions.

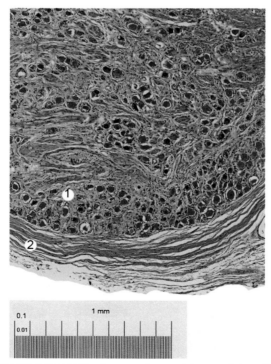

FIG. 12.24 Details of Fig. 12.17. Dorsal root ganglion, 1: soma of sensorial axons, 2: transitional tissue dura mater-epineurium. Bar: 1 mm including divisions.

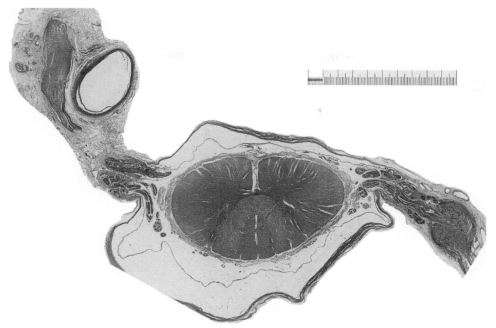

FIG. 12.25 Complete cross-section spinal cord and neighboring tissue at the C3 level. Bar: 10 mm including divisions.

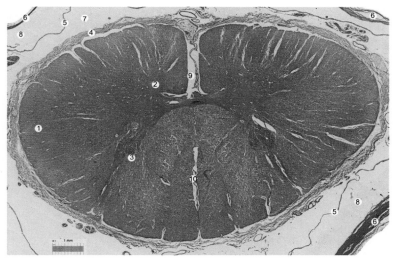

FIG. 12.26 Details of Fig. 12.25. 1: spinal cord, 2: anterior horn, 3: posterior horn, 4: pia mater, 5: arachnoid layer, 6: dura mater, 7: subarachnoid space, 8: acquired subdural space, 9: anterior median fissure, 10: posterior median sulcus. Bar: 1 mm including divisions.

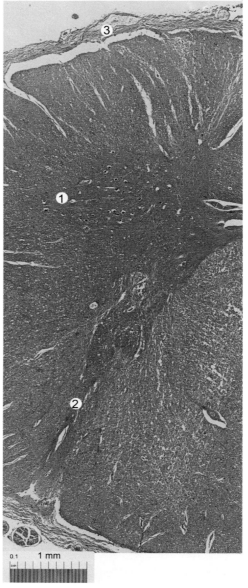

FIG. 12.27 Details of Fig. 12.25. Spinal cord, 1: anterior horn, 2: posterior horn, 3: pia mater. Bar: 1 mm including divisions.

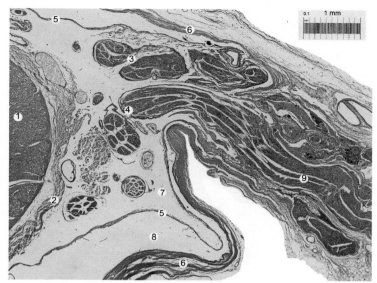

FIG. 12.28 Details of Fig. 12.25. 1: spinal cord, 2: pia mater, 3: anterior spinal nerve roots within the subarachnoid space, 4: posterior spinal nerve roots within the subarachnoid space, 5: arachnoid layer, 6: dura mater, 7: subarachnoid space, 8: acquired subdural space. Structures within nerve root cuff, 9: posterior nerve root of spinal nerve. Bar: 1 mm including divisions.

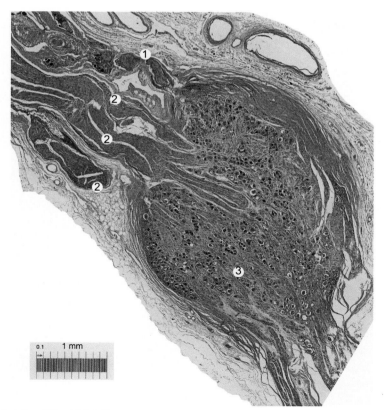

FIG. 12.29 Details of Fig. 12.25. Structures within nerve root cuff, 1: anterior nerve root of spinal nerve, 2: posterior nerve root of spinal nerve, 3: dorsal root ganglion. Bar: 1 mm including divisions.

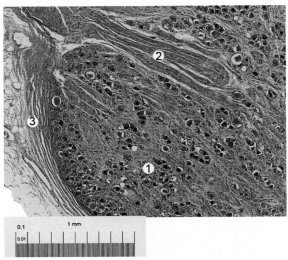

FIG. 12.30 Details of Fig. 12.25. Dorsal root ganglion, 1: somas of sensorial axons, 2: posterior root, 3: dura mater-epineurium transitional tissue. Bar: 1 mm including divisions.

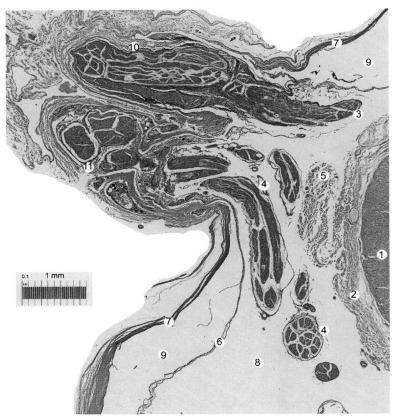

FIG. 12.31 Details of Fig. 12.25. 1: spinal cord, 2: pia mater, 3: anterior spinal nerve roots within subarachnoid space, 4: posterior spinal nerve roots within subarachnoid space, 5: denticulate ligament (reflected), 6: arachnoid layer, 7: dura mater, 8: subarachnoid space, 9: acquired subdural space. Structures within nerve root cuff, 10: anterior nerve root of spinal nerve, 11: posterior nerve root of spinal nerve. Bar: 1 mm including divisions.

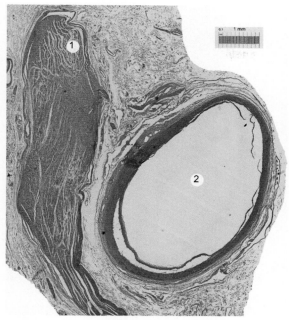

FIG. 12.32 Details of Fig. 12.25. 1: Anterior branch spinal nerve, 2: vertebral artery. Bar: 1 mm including divisions.

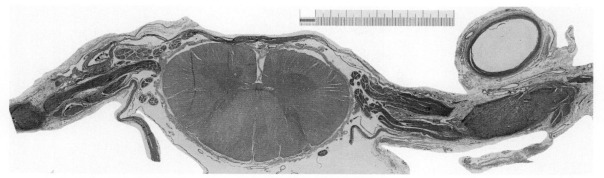

FIG. 12.33 Complete cross-section spinal cord and neighboring tissue at the C4 level. Bar: 10 mm including divisions.

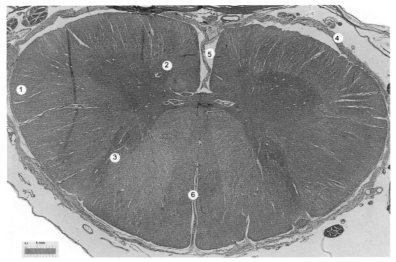

FIG. 12.34 Details of Fig. 12.33. 1: spinal cord, 2: anterior horn, 3: posterior horn, 4: pia mater, 5: anterior median fissure, 6: posterior median sulcus Bar: 1 mm including divisions.

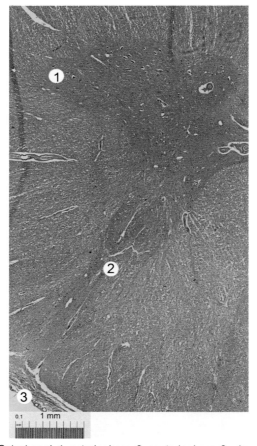

FIG. 12.35 Details of Fig. 12.33. Spinal cord, 1: anterior horn, 2: posterior horn, 3: pia mater. Bar: 1 mm including divisions.

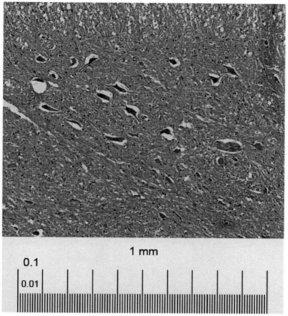

FIG. 12.36 Details of Fig. 12.33. Spinal cord, anterior horn, somas of motor neuron Bar: 1 mm including divisions.

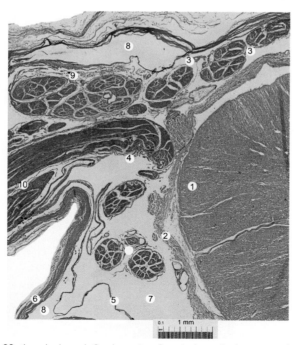

FIG. 12.37 Details of Fig. 12.33. 1: spinal cord, 2: pia mater, 3: anterior spinal nerve roots within subarachnoid space, 4: posterior spinal nerve roots within the subarachnoid space, 5: arachnoid layer, 6: dura mater, 7: subarachnoid space, 8: acquired subdural space. Structures within nerve root cuff, 9: anterior nerve root of spinal nerve, 10: posterior nerve root of spinal nerve. Bar: 1 mm including divisions.

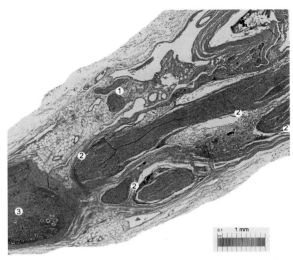

FIG. 12.38 Details of Fig. 12.33. Structures within nerve root cuff, 1: anterior nerve root of spinal nerve, 2: posterior nerve root of spinal nerve, 3: dorsal root ganglion. Bar: 1 mm including divisions.

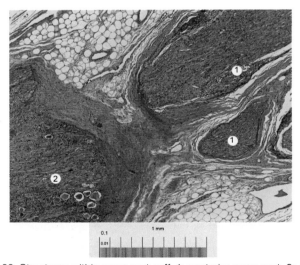

FIG. 12.39 Details of Fig. 12.33. Structures within nerve root cuff, 1: posterior nerve root, 2: dorsal root ganglion. Bar: 1 mm including divisions.

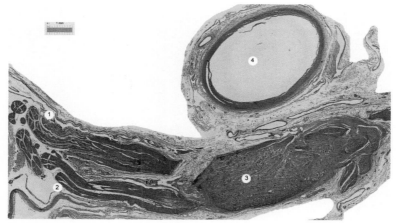

FIG. 12.40 Details of Fig. 12.33. Structures within nerve root cuff, 1: anterior nerve root of spinal nerve, 2: posterior nerve root of spinal nerve, 3: dorsal root ganglion, 4: vertebral artery. Bar: 1 mm including divisions.

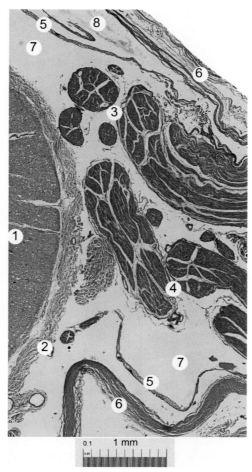

FIG. 12.41 Details of Fig. 12.33. 1: spinal cord, 2: pia mater, 3: anterior spinal nerve roots within subarachnoid space, 4: posterior spinal nerve roots within subarachnoid space, 5: arachnoid layer, 6: dura mater, 7: subarachnoid space, 8: acquired subdural space. Bar: 1 mm including divisions.

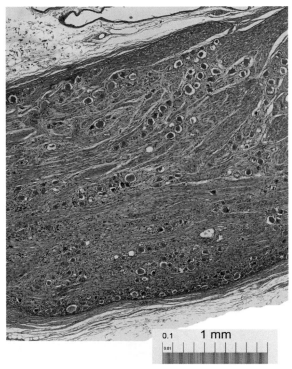

FIG. 12.42 Details of Fig. 12.33. Dorsal root ganglion, bodies of sensory axons. Bar: 1 mm including divisions.

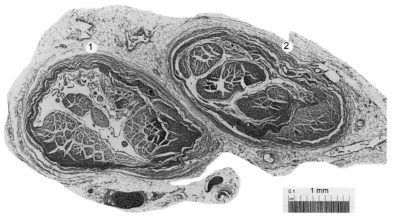

FIG. 12.43 Transverse cross-section of nerve root cuff at the C4 level. 1: anterior nerve root, 2: posterior nerve root. Bar: 1 mm including divisions.

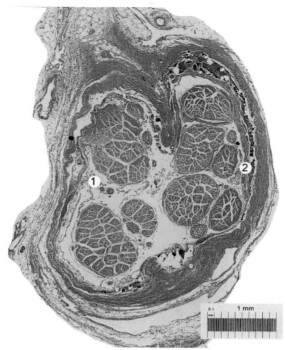

FIG. 12.44 Transverse cross-section of nerve root cuff at the C4 level. Following cross-section distal to Fig. 12.43. 1: anterior nerve root of spinal nerve, 2: posterior nerve root of spinal nerve. Bar: 1 mm including divisions.

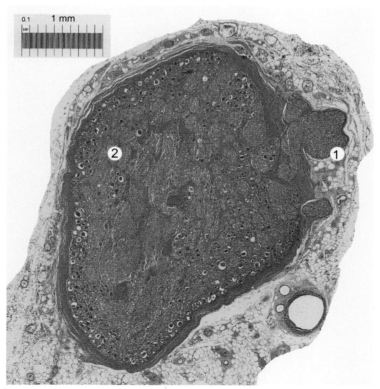

FIG. 12.45 Transverse cross-section of nerve root cuff at the C4 level. Following cross-section distal to Fig. 12.44. 1: anterior nerve root of spinal nerve, 2: dorsal root ganglion. Bar: 1 mm including divisions.

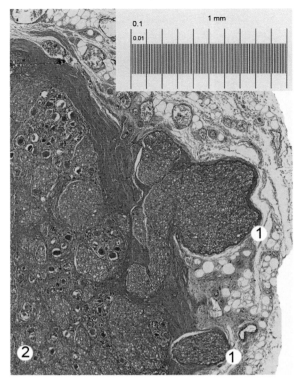

FIG. 12.46 Transverse cross-section of nerve root cuff at the C4 level. Following cross-section distal to Fig. 12.44. Detail of Fig. 12.45. 1: anterior nerve root of spinal nerve, 2: dorsal root ganglion. Bar: 1 mm including divisions.

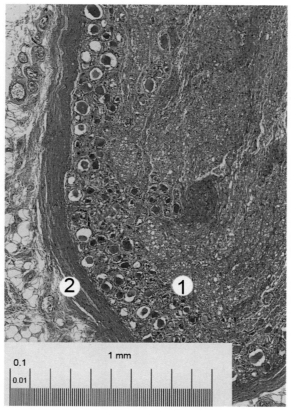

FIG. 12.47 Transverse cross-section of nerve root cuff at C4 level. Following cross-section distal to Fig. 12.44. Detail of Fig. 12.45. 1: dorsal root ganglion, 2: transitional dura mater-epineurium tissue. Bar: 1 mm including divisions.

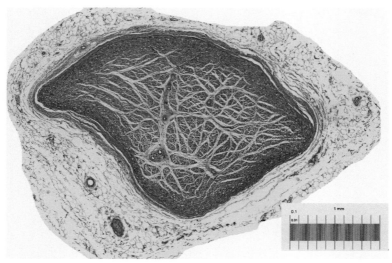

FIG. 12.48 Transverse cross-section of nerve root cuff at C4 level. Following cross-section distal to Fig. 12.45. Anterior branch of spinal nerve. Bar: 1 mm including divisions.

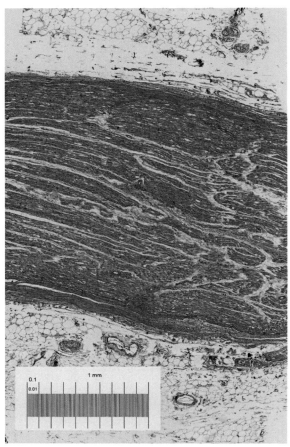

FIG. 12.49 Longitudinal section of nerve root cuff at C4 level. Following cross-section distal to Fig. 12.45. 1: anterior branch of spinal nerve. Bar: 1 mm including.

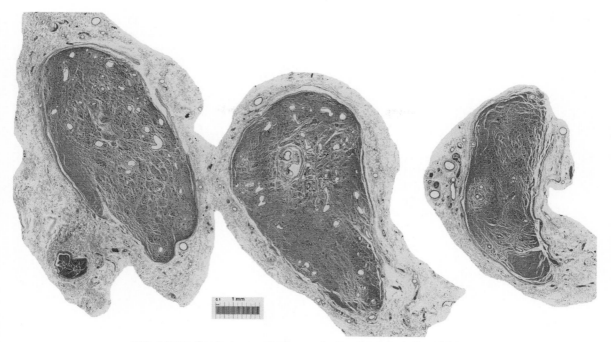

FIG. 12.50 Cervical sympathetic ganglia. Bar: 1 mm including divisions.

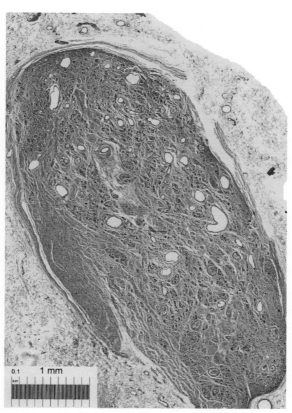

FIG. 12.51 Cervical sympathetic ganglia. Detail of Fig. 12.50. Bar: 1 mm including divisions.

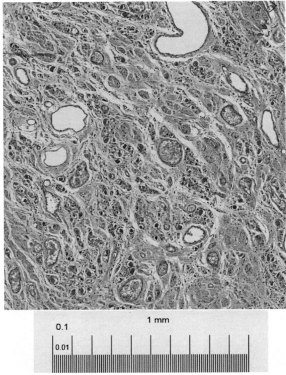

FIG. 12.52 Cervical sympathetic ganglia. Detail of Fig. 12.50. Bar: 1 mm including divisions.

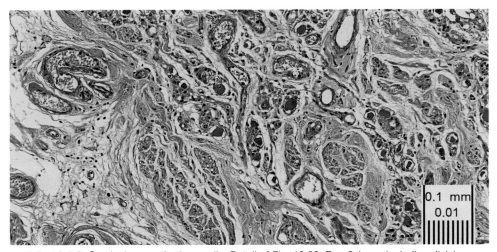

FIG. 12.53 Cervical sympathetic ganglia. Detail of Fig. 12.50. Bar: 0.1 mm including divisions.

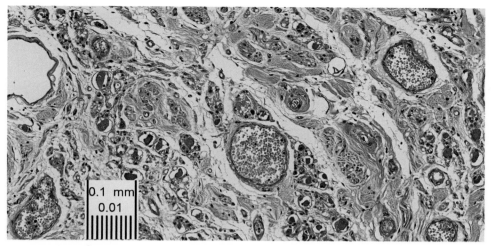

FIG. 12.54 Cervical sympathetic ganglia. Detail of Fig. 12.50. Bar: 0.1 mm including divisions.

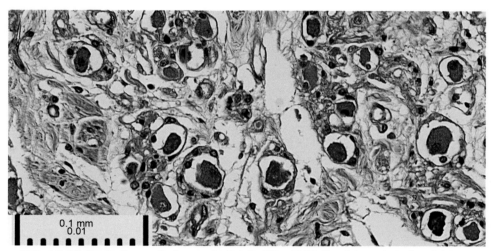

FIG. 12.55 Cervical sympathetic ganglia. Detail of Fig. 12.50. Bar: 0.1 mm including divisions.

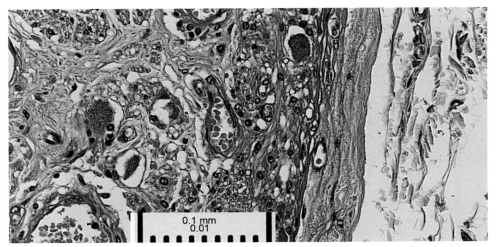

FIG. 12.56 Cervical sympathetic ganglia. Detail of Fig. 12.50. Bar: 0.1 mm including divisions.

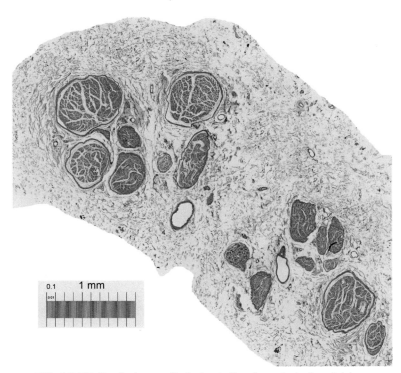

FIG. 12.57 Cervical sympathetic trunk. Bar: 1 mm including divisions.

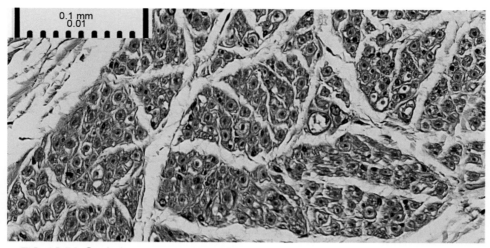

FIG. 12.58 Cervical sympathetic ganglia. Detail of Fig. 12.57. Bar: 0.1 mm including divisions.

Cross-Sectional Anatomy of the Cervical Plexus

FRANCISCO REINA • MIGUEL ANGEL REINA • ENRIQUE VERDÚ •
ANDRÉ P. BOEZAART • JAVIER MORATINOS-DELGADO • ANNA CARRERA

The images in this chapter are serial axial slices of the cervical region from the base of the posterior cranial fossa to the C5 vertebral body. The slices are 3 mm in thickness and are those of a 75-year-old at death male voluntary body donor. The cadaver was sectioned serially after freezing it at $-80°$C using a band saw with a blade thickness of 0.7 mm.

We performed a total of 16 sections (Figs. 13.1−13.16). The images correspond to the inferior face of the cross-section. The head of the cadaver was in approximately 30 degrees of extension and 2 mm of lateral flexion toward its right side. This caused the images not to be completely symmetrical. The image corresponding to the left side of the cadaver was thus, somewhat more cephalad. For orientation, the right and left sides of the cadaver have been marked R and L, respectively.

In each photograph, we used the following color code:

Osteoligamentous structures: gray
Musculature: white
Blood vessels: blue
Nerves: yellow

Surgical Anatomy of the Cervical Plexus and its Branches. https://doi.org/10.1016/B978-0-323-83132-1.00012-3

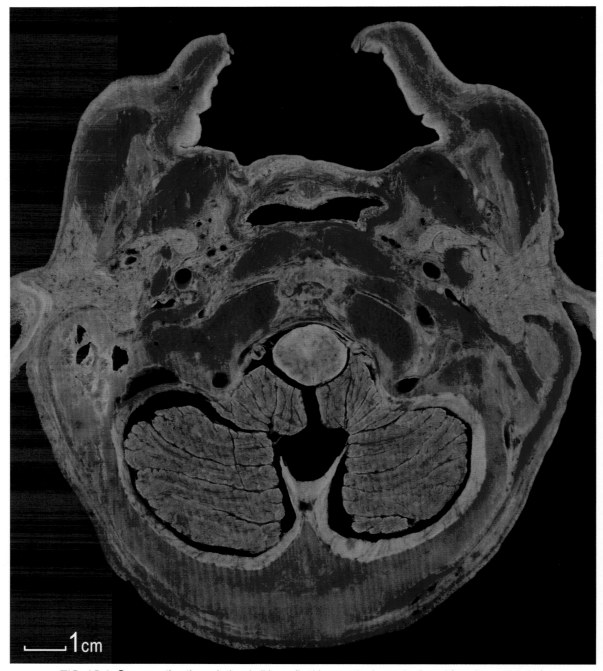

FIG. 13.1 Cross-section through the skull base (*in this case the image is viewed from its cranial side*).

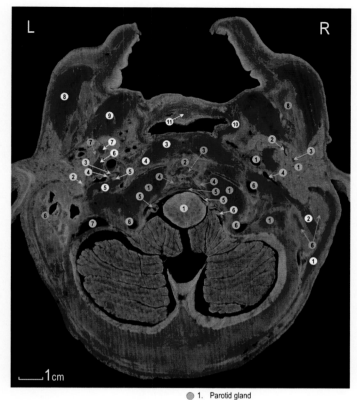

1cm

1. Parotid gland

BONES & LIGAMENTS
1. Occipital bone – lateral part
2. Atlas
3. Apex dentis and apical ligament of dens
4. Alar ligament
5. Tectorial membrane
6. Mastoid process and mastoid cells
7. Styloid process
8. Ramus of mandible

MUSCLES
1. Sternocleidomastoid muscle
2. Digastric muscle – posterior belly
3. Longus capitis muscle
4. Rectus capitis anterior muscle
5. Rectus capitis lateralis muscle
6. Stylopharyngeus and Stylohyoid muscles
7. Styloglossus muslce
8. Masseter muscle
9. Medial pterygoid muscle
10. Superior constrictor of the pharynx muscle
11. Musculus uvulae

VESSELS
1. Internal carotid artery
2. External carotid artery
3. Retromandibular vein
4. Internal jugular vein
5. Vertebral artery
6. Condylar emissary vein
7. Sigmoid sinus

NERVES
1. Medulla oblongata
2. 7th cranial; facial nerve
3. 9th cranial; Glossopharyngeal nerve
4. 10th cranial; Vagus nerve
5. 11th cranial; Accessory nerve
6. 12th cranial; Hypoglossal nerve

FIG. 13.1 cont'd.

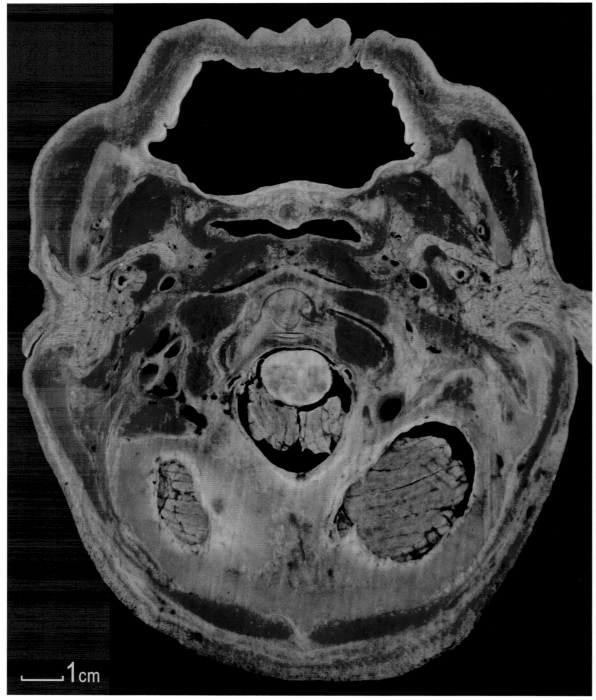

FIG. 13.2 Cross-section through the atlanto-occipital joint.

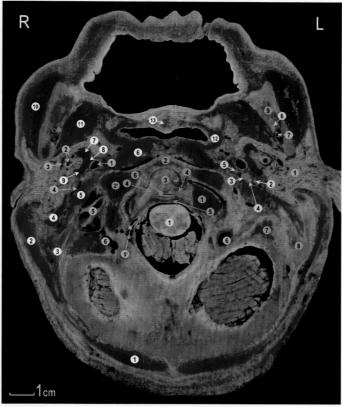

1cm

FIG. 13.2 cont'd.

1. Parotid gland

BONES & LIGAMENTS
1. Occipital condyle
2. Atlas - anterior arch - anterior tubercle
2'. Atlas - lateral mass
3. Axis - dens
4. Alar ligament
5. Tectorial membrane
6. Cruciate ligament of atlas – superior longitudinal band
7. Occipital bone – lateral part
8. Mastoid process
9. Ramus of mandible

MUSCLES
1. Semispinalis capitis muscle
2. Sternocleidomastoid muscle
3. Splenius capitis muscle
4. Digastric muscle – posterior belly
5. Rectus capitis lateralis muscle
6. Longus capitis muscle
7. Styloglossus muscle
8. Stylopharyngeus muscle
9. Stylohyoid muscle
10. Masseter muscle
11. Medial pterygoid muscle
12. Superior constrictor of the pharynx muscle
13. Musculus uvulae

VESSELS
1. Internal carotid artery
2. External carotid artery
3. Retromandibular vein
4. Internal jugular vein
5. Vertebral artery
5'. Vertebral artery (intracranial part)
6. Condylar emissary vein
7. Inferior alveolar artery

NERVES
1. Medulla oblongata
2. 9th cranial; Glossopharyngeal nerve
3. 10th cranial; Vagus nerve
4. 11th cranial; Accessory nerve
5. 12th cranial; Hypoglossal nerve
6. Inferior alveolar nerve

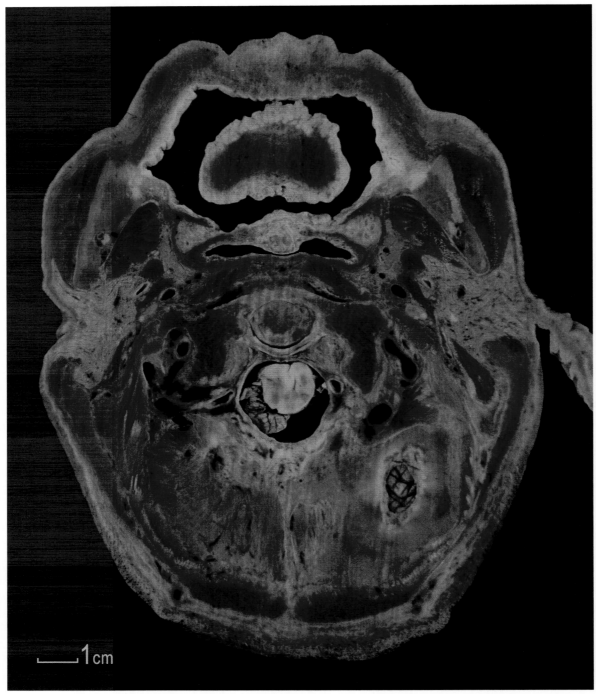

FIG. 13.3 Cross-section through the anterior arch of atlas and C_1 spinal nerve.

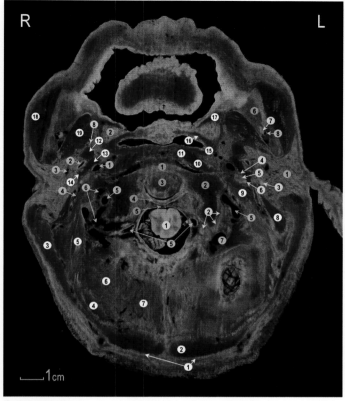

BONES & LIGAMENTS
1. Atlas - anterior arch
2. Atlas - lateral mass
3. Axis – dens
4. Cruciate ligament of atlas -Transverse ligament of atlas
5. Tectorial membrane
6. Ramus of mandible

MUSCLES
1. Trapezius muscle
2. Semispinalis capitis muscle
3. Sternocleidomastoid muscle
4. Splenius capitis muscle
5. Longissimus capitis muscle
6. Rectus capitis posterior major muscle
7. Rectus capitis posterior minor muscle
8. Digastric muscle – posterior belly
9. Rectus capitis lateralis muscle
10. Rectus capitis anterior muscle
11. Longus capitis muscle
12. Styloglossus muscle
13. Stylopharyngeus muslce
14. Stylohyoid muscle
15. Superior constrictor of the pharynx muscle
16. Palatopharingeus muscle
17. Palatoglossus muscle
18. Masseter muscle
19. Medial pterygoid muscle

1. Parotid gland
2. Palatine tonsil

VESSELS
1. Internal carotid artery
2. External carotid artery
3. Retromandibular vein
4. Internal jugular vein
5. Vertebral artery
6. Vertebral vein
7. Condylar emissary vein
8. Inferior alveolar artery

NERVES
1. Medulla oblongata
2. C_1 spinal nerve and anterior ramus
3. 7th cranial; Facial nerve
4. 9th cranial; Glossopharyngeal nerve
5. 10th cranial – 12th cranial
   Vagus nerve - Hypoglossal nerve
6. 11th cranial; Accessory nerve
7. Inferior alveolar nerve
8. Lingual nerve

FIG. 13.3 cont'd.

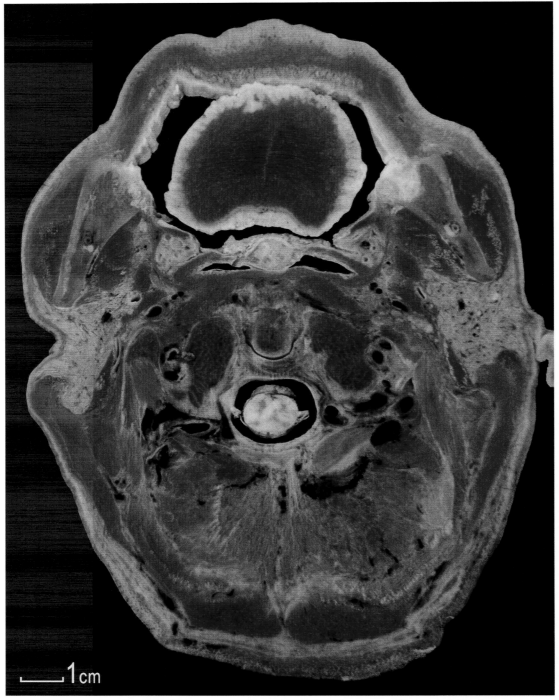

FIG. 13.4 Cross-section through the dens of the axis and transverse ligament of the atlas.

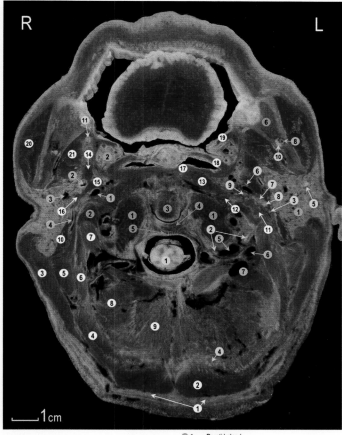

FIG. 13.4 cont'd.

BONES & LIGAMENTS
1. Atlas – lateral mass
2. Atlas – transverse process
3. Axis – dens
4. Cruciate ligament of atlas -Transverse ligament of atlas
5. Tectorial membrane
6. Ramus of mandible

MUSCLES
1. Trapezius muslce
2. Semispinalis capitis muscle
3. Sternocleidomastoid muscle
4. Splenius capitis muscle
5. Levator scapulae muscle
6. Longissimus capitis muscle
7. Obliquus capitis inferior muscle
8. Rectus capitis posterior major muscle
9. Rectus capitis posterior minor muscle
10. Digastric muscle – posterior belly
11. Rectus capitis lateralis muscle
12. Rectus capitis anterior muscle
13. Longus capitis muscle
14. Styloglossus muscle
15. Stylopharyngeus muscle
16. Stylohyoid muscle
17. Superior constrictor of the pharynx muscle
18. Palatopharingeus muscle
19. Palatoglossus muscle
20. Masseter muscle
21. Medial pterygoid muscle

1. Parotid gland
2. Palatine tonsil

VESSELS
1. Internal carotid artery
2. External carotid artery
3. Retromandibular vein
4. Internal jugular vein
5. Vertebral artery
6. Vertebral vein
7. Condylar emissary vein
8. Inferior alveolar artery

NERVES
1. Spinal cord
2. C_1 spinal nerve and anterior ramus
3. C_1-C_2 loop
4. Greater occipital nerve (C_2 posterior ramus)
5. 7th cranial; Facial nerve
6. 9th cranial; Glossopharyngeal nerve
7. 10th cranial; Vagus nerve
8. 11th cranial; Accessory nerve
9. 12th cranial; Hypoglossal nerve
10. Inferior alveolar nerve
11. Lingual nerve

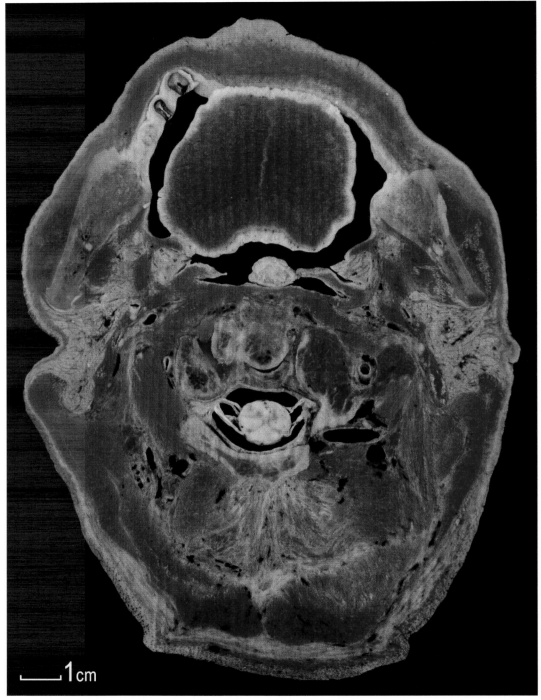

FIG. 13.5 Cross-section through the lateral atlanto-axial joint and the C$_2$ spinal nerve.

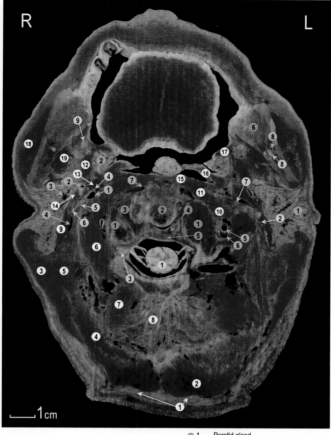

1. Parotid gland
2. Palatine tonsil

BONES & LIGAMENTS
1. Atlas
2. Axis – dens
3. Lateral atlanto-axial joint
4. Cruciate ligament of atlas- inferior longitudinal band
5. Tectorial membrane
6. Ramus of mandible

MUSCLES
1.   Trapezius muscle
2.   Semispinalis capitis muscle
3.   Sternocleidomastoid muscle
4.   Splenius capitis muscle
5.   Levator scapulae muscle
6.   Obliquus capitis inferior muscle
7.   Rectus capitis posterior major muscle
8.   Rectus capitis posterior minor muscle
9.   Digastric muscle – posterior belly
10. Rectus capitis anterior muscle
11. Longus capitis muscle
12. Styloglossus muscle
13. Stylopharyngeus muscle
14. Stylohyoid muscle
15. Superior constrictor of the pharynx muscle
16. Palatopharingeus muscle
17. Palatoglossus muscle
18. Masseter muscle
19. Medial pterygoid muscle

VESSELS
1. Internal carotid artery
2. External carotid artery
3. Retromandibular vein
4. Internal jugular vein
5. Vertebral artery
6. Vertebral vein
7. Ascending pharyngeal artery
8. Inferior alveolar artery

NERVES
1. Spinal cord
2. C_1-C_2 loop
3. C_2 spinal nerve
4. 9th cranial; Glossopharyngeal nerve
5. 10th cranial; Vagus nerve
6. 11th cranial; Accessory nerve
7. 12th cranial; Hypoglossal nerve
8. Inferior alveolar nerve
9. Lingual nerve

FIG. 13.5 cont'd.

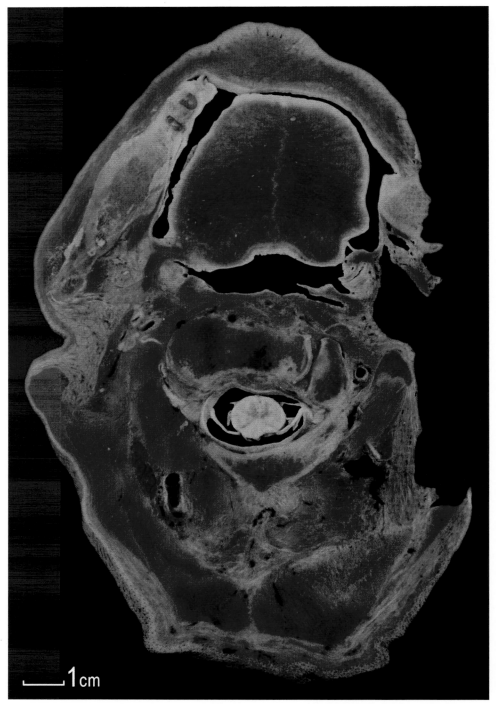

FIG. 13.6 Cross-section through the axis vertebral body and the C$_2$ spinal nerve.

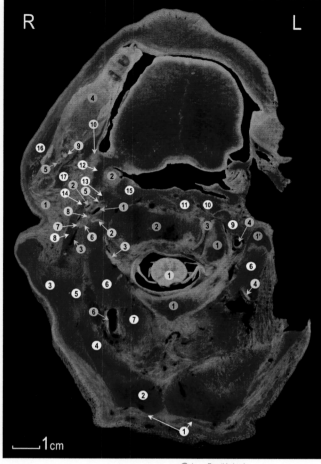

FIG. 13.6 cont'd.

BONES & LIGAMENTS
1. Atlas
2. Atlas – transverse process
3. Axis
4. Lateral atlanto-axial joint
5. Body of mandible

MUSCLES
1. Trapezius muscle
2. Semispinalis capitis muscle
3. Sternocleidomastoid muscle
4. Splenius capitis muscle
5. Levator scapulae muscle
6. Obliquus capitis inferior muscle
7. Rectus capitis posterior major muscle
8. Digastric muscle – posterior belly
9. Rectus capitis anterior muscle
10. Longus capitis muscle
11. Longus colli muscle
12. Styloglossus muscle
13. Stylopharyngeus muscle
14. Stylohyoid muscle
15. Middle constrictor of the pharynx muscle
16. Masseter muscle
17. Medial pterygoid muscle

1. Parotid gland
2. Palatine tonsil

VESSELS
1. Internal carotid artery
2. External carotid artery
3. Internal jugular vein
4. Vertebral artery
5. Inferior alveolar artery
6. Deep cervical artery and vein

NERVES
1. Spinal cord
2. Muscular branches from C_1
3. C_2 spinal nerve - anterior ramus
4. C_2 spinal nerve - posterior ramus
5. 9th cranial; Glossopharyngeal nerve
6. 10th cranial; Vagus nerve
7. 11th cranial; Accessory nerve
8. 12th cranial; Hypoglossal nerve
9. Inferior alveolar nerve
10. Lingual nerve

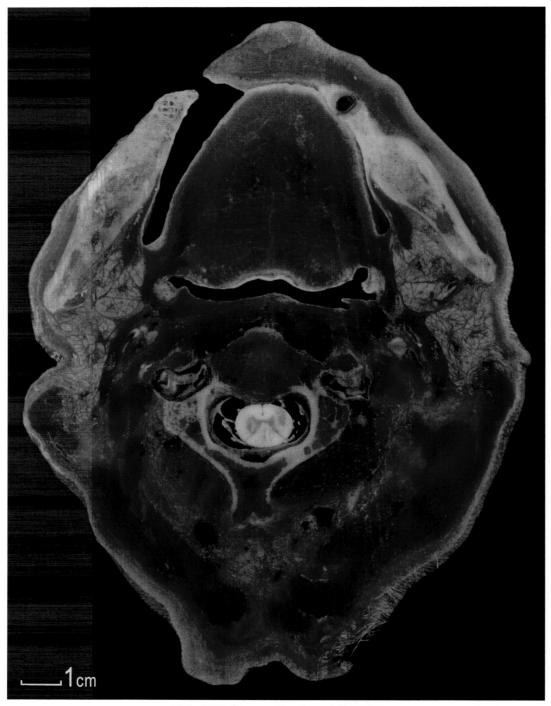

FIG. 13.7 Cross-section through the axis.

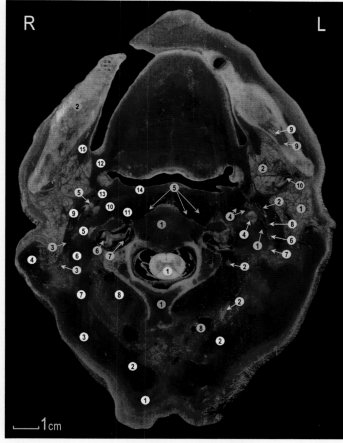

1. Parotid gland
2. Submandibular gland

VESSELS
1. Internal carotid artery
2. External carotid artery
3. Internal jugular vein
4. Ascendent pharyngeal artery and vein
5. Venous pharyngeal plexus
6. Vertebral artery
7. Vertebral vein
8. Deep cervical artery and vein
9. Inferior alveolar artery
10. Facial artery

NERVES
1. Spinal cord
2. C$_2$ spinal nerve - posterior ramus
3. Great auricular nerve
4. Superior cervical sympathetic ganglion
5. 9th cranial; Glossopharyngeal nerve
6. 10th cranial; Vagus nerve
7. 11th cranial; Accessory nerve
8. 12th cranial; Hypoglossal nerve
9. Inferior alveolar nerve

BONES & LIGAMENTS
2. Axis
3. Body of mandible

MUSCLES
1. Trapezius muscle
2. Semispinalis capitis muscle
3. Splenius muscles
4. Sternocleidomastoid muscle
5. Scalenus medius muscle
6. Levator scapulae muscle
7. Longissimus capitis muscle
8. Obliquus capitis inferior muscle
9. Digastric muscle – posterior belly muscle
10. Longus capitis muscle
11. Longus colli muscle
12. Styloglossus muscle
13. Stylopharyngeus muscle
14. Middle constrictor of the pharynx muscle
15. Mylohyoid muscle

FIG. 13.7 cont'd.

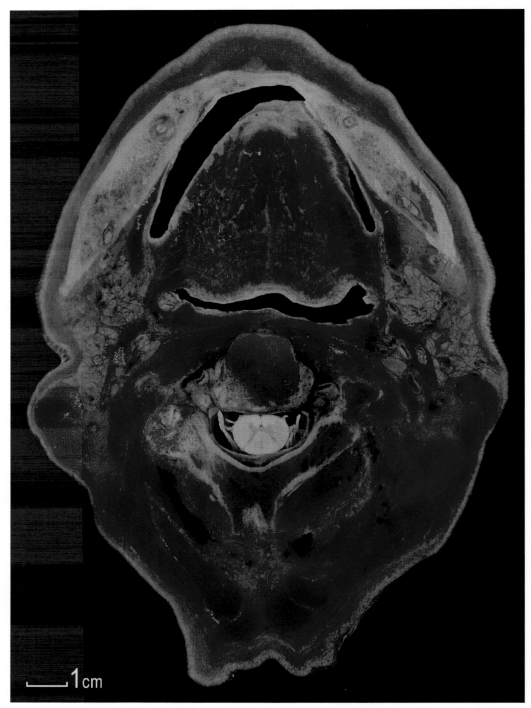

FIG. 13.8 Cross-section through the intervertebral foramen C2—C3.

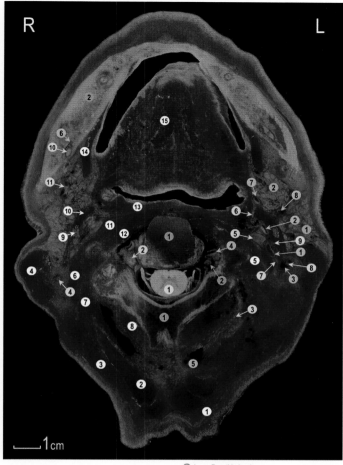

FIG. 13.8 cont'd.

1. Parotid gland
2. Submandibular gland

VESSELS
1. Internal carotid artery
2. External carotid artery
3. Internal jugular vein
4. Vertebral artery
5. Deep cervical artery and vein
6. Inferior alveolar artery
7. Facial artery
8. Facial vein

NERVES
1. Spinal cord
2. C₃ spinal nerve
3. Greater occipital nerve
4. Great auricular nerve
5. Superior cervical sympathetic ganglion
6. 9th cranial; Glossopharyngeal nerve
7. 10th cranial; Vagus nerve
8. 11th cranial; Accessory nerve
9. 12th cranial; Hypoglossal nerve
10. Inferior alveolar nerve
11. Lingual nerve

BONES & LIGAMENTS
1. Axis
2. C2-C3 intervertebral foramen
3. Body of mandible

MUSCLES
1. Trapezius muscle
2. Semispinalis capitis muscle
3. Splenius muscles
4. Sternocleidomastoid muscle
5. Scalenus medius muscle
6. Levator scapulae muscle
7. Longissimus cervicis muscle
8. Obliquus capitis inferior muscle
9. Digastric muscle - tendon and posterior belly
10. Stylohyoid muscle
11. Longus capitis muscle
12. Longus colli muscle
13. Middle constrictor of the pharynx muscle
14. Mylohyoid muscle
15. Genioglossus muscle

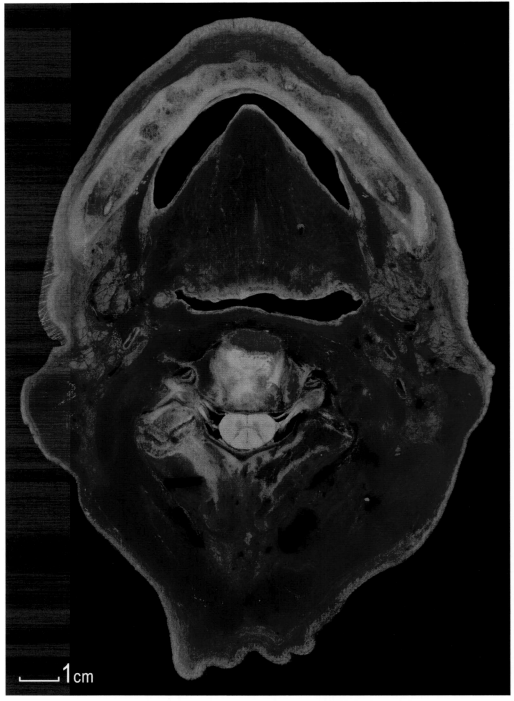

FIG. 13.9 Cross-section through the C2–C3 joint and the C$_3$ spinal nerve.

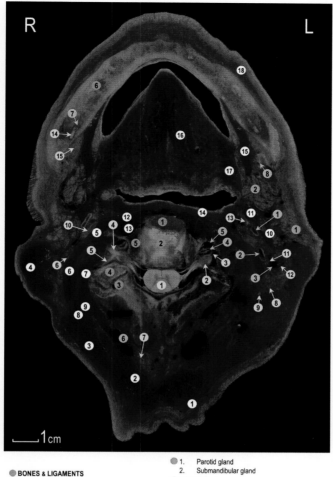

BONES & LIGAMENTS
1. Axis
2. C2-C3 intervertebral disc
3. C2 inferior articular process
4. C3 superior articular process
5. C3 uncinate process
6. Body of mandible

MUSCLES
1. Trapezius muscle
2. Semispinalis capitis muscle
3. Splenius muscles
4. Sternocleidomastoid muscle
5. Scalenus medius muscle
6. Levator scapulae muscle
7. Longissimus cervicis muscle
8. Longissimus capitis muscle
9. Iliocostalis cervicis muscle
10. Digastric muscle – tendon and posterior belly
11. Stylohyoid muscle
12. Longus capitis muscle
13. Longus colli muscle
14. Middle constrictor of the pharynx muscle
15. Mylohyoid muscle
16. Genioglossus muscle
17. Hyoglossus muscle
18. Platysma muscle

1. Parotid gland
2. Submandibular gland

VESSELS
1. Internal carotid artery
2. External carotid artery
3. Internal jugular vein
4. Vertebral artery
5. Vertebral vein
6. Deep cervical vein
7. Inferior alveolar artery
8. Facial artery

NERVES
1. Spinal cord
2. C_3 spinal sensory ganglion
3. C_3 spinal nerve
4. C_3 spinal nerve- anterior ramus
5. C_3 spinal nerve- posterior ramus
6. C_2-C_3 loop
7. C_2 spinal nerve -posterior ramus (medial branch)
8. Great auricular nerve
9. Lesser occipital nerve
10. Superior cervical sympathetic ganglion
11. 10th cranial; Vagus nerve
12. 11th cranial; Accessory nerve
13. 12th cranial; Hypoglossal nerve
14. Inferior alveolar nerve
15. Lingual nerve

FIG. 13.9 cont'd.

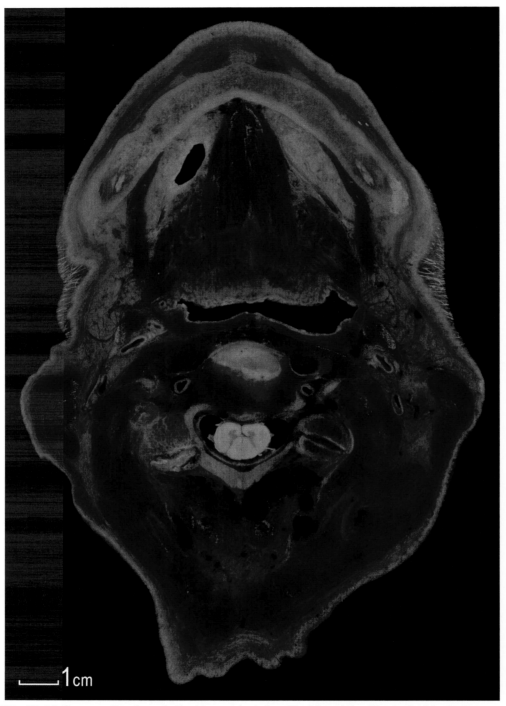

FIG. 13.10 Cross-section through the intervertebral disc C2–C3 and the C3 vertebral body. It passes through the C2–C3 zygapophysial joint.

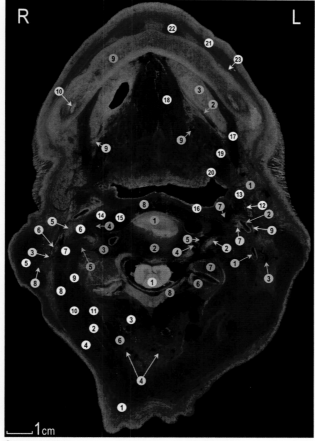

FIG. 13.10 cont'd.

● **BONES & LIGAMENTS**
1.   C2-C3 intervertebral disc
2.   C3 vertebral body
3.   C3 transverse process
4.   C3 anterior tubercle
5.   C3 posterior tubercle
6.   C2 inferior articular process
7.   C3 superior articular process
8.   C3 lamina
9.   Body of mandible

○ **MUSCLES**
1.   Trapezius muscle
2.   Semispinalis capitis muscle
3.   Semispinalis cervicis muscle
4.   Splenius muscles
5.   Sternocleidomastoid muscle
6.   Scalenus anterior muscle
7.   Scalenus medius muscle
8.   Levator scapulae muscle
9.   Longissimus cervicis muscle
10.   Longissimus capitis muscle
11.   Iliocostalis cervicis muscle
12.   Digastric muscle - tendon
13.   Stylohyoid muscle
14.   Longus capitis muscle
15.   Longus colli muscle
16.   Middle constrictor of the pharynx muscle
17.   Mylohyoid muscle
18.   Genioglossus muscle
19.   Hyoglossus muscle
20.   Styloglossus muscle
21.   Platysma muscle
22.   Mentalis muscle
23.   Depressor anguli oris muscle

● 1.   Submandibular gland
2.   Submandibular duct
3.   Sublingual gland

● **VESSELS**
1.   Internal carotid artery
2.   External carotid artery
3.   Internal jugular vein
4.   Vertebral artery
5.   Vertebral vein
6.   Deep cervical vein
7.   Ascendent pharyngeal artery
8.   Venous pharyngeal plexus
9.   Lingual artery and vein

○ **NERVES**
1.   Spinal cord
2. C_3 spinal nerve - anterior ramus
3.   Rami from C_7-C_3 loop
4. C_2 spinal nerve - posterior ramus (medial branch)
5.   Superior cervical sympathetic ganglion
6.   10th cranial; Vagus nerve
7.   Superior laryngeal nerve
8.   11th cranial; Accessory nerve
9.   12th cranial; Hypoglossal nerve
10.   Inferior alveolar nerve

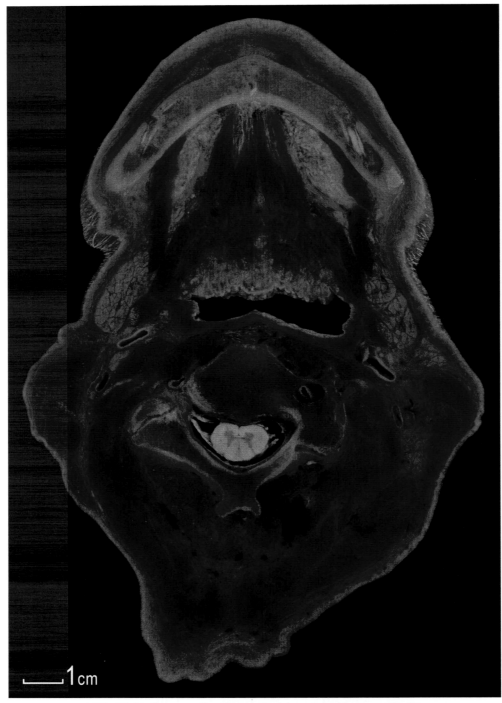

FIG. 13.11 Cross-section through the intervertebral foramen C3–C4.

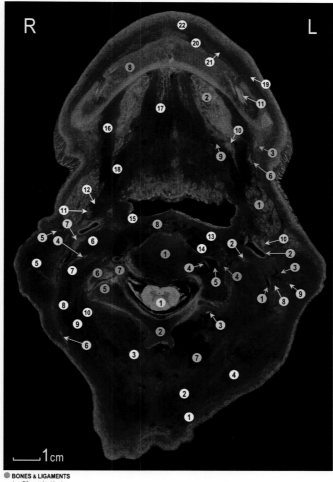

FIG. 13.11 cont'd.

BONES & LIGAMENTS
1. C3 vertebral body
2. C3 spinous process
3. C3 lamina
4. C3 transverse process
5. C3 inferior articular process
6. C4 superior articular process
7. Intervertebral foramen C3-C4
8. Body of mandible

MUSCLES
1. Trapezius muscle
2. Semispinalis capitis muscle
3. Semispinalis cervicis and multifidus muscles
4. Splenius muscles
5. Sternocleidomastoid muscle
6. Scalenus anterior muscle
7. Scalenus medius muscle
8. Levator scapulae muscle
9. Longissimus cervicis muscle
10. Iliocostalis cervicis muscle
11. Digastric muscle - tendon
12. Stylohyoid muscle
13. Longus capitis muscle
14. Longus colli muscle
15. Middle constrictor of the pharynx muscle
16. Mylohyoid muscle
17. Genioglossus muscle
18. Hyoglossus muscle
19. Platysma muscle
20. Mentalis muscle
21. Depressor anguli oris muscle
22. Depressor labii inferioris

1. Submandibular gland
2. Sublingual gland
3. Submandibular lymph node

VESSELS
1. Internal carotid artery
2. External carotid artery
3. Internal jugular vein
4. Vertebral artery
5. Vertebral vein
6. Mylohyoid artery and vein
7. Deep cervical vein
8. Venous pharyngeal plexus
9. Lingual artery and vein

NERVES
1. Spinal cord
2. C3 spinal nerve – anterior ramus
3. C3 spinal nerve – posterior ramus (medial branch)
4. C3-C4 loop
5. Transverse cervical nerve
6. Emergence of Lesser occipital and Great auricular nerves
7. Superior cervical sympathetic ganglion
8. 10th cranial; Vagus nerve
9. 11th cranial; Accessory nerve
10. 12th cranial; Hypoglossal nerve
11. Inferior alveolar nerve

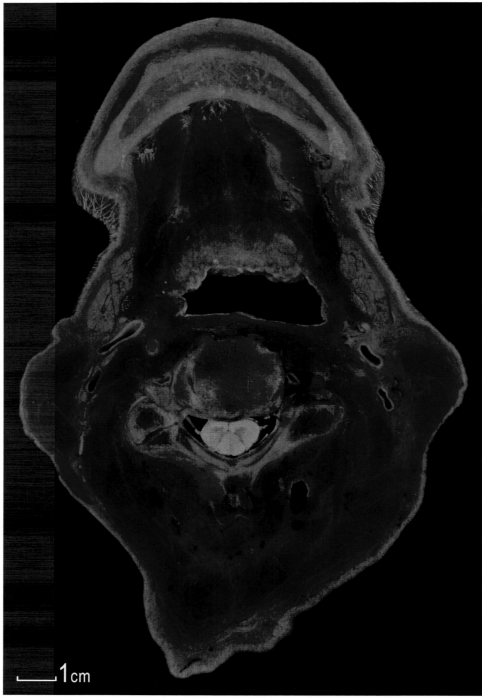

FIG. 13.12 Cross-section through the C3–C4 zygapophysial joint.

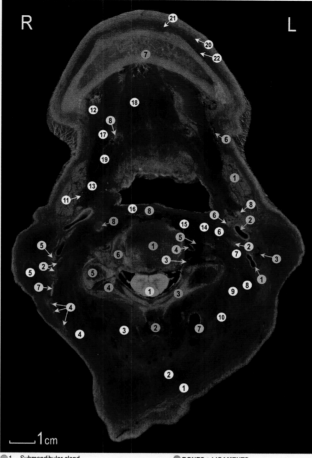

FIG. 13.12 cont'd.

1. Submandibular gland

○ **MUSCLES**
1. Trapezius muscle
2. Semispinalis capitis muscle
3. Semispinalis cervicis and multifidus muscles
4. Splenius muscles
5. Sternocleidomastoid muscle
6. Scalenus anterior muscle
7. Scalenus medius muscle
8. Levator scapulae muscle
9. Longissimus cervicis muscle
10. Iliocostalis cervicis muscle
11. Digastric muscle - tendon
12. Digastric muscle - anterior belly
13. Stylohyoid muscle
14. Longus capitis muscle
15. Longus colli muscle
16. Middle constrictor of the pharynx muscle
17. Mylohyoid muscle
18. Geniohyoid muscle
19. Hyoglossus muscle
20. Platysma muscle
21. Mentalis muscle
22. Depressor anguli oris muscle

● **BONES & LIGAMENTS**
1. C3 vertebral body
2. C3 spinous process
3. C3 lamina
4. C3 inferior articular process
5. C4 superior articular process
6. C4 uncinate process
7. Body of mandible
8. Hyoid bone

● **VESSELS**
1. Internal carotid artery
2. External carotid artery
3. Internal jugular vein
4. Vertebral artery
5. Vertebral vein
6. Mylohyoid artery and vein
7. Deep cervical vein
8. Venous pharyngeal plexus

○ **NERVES**
1. Spinal cord
2. C_3-C_4 loop
3. C_4 spinal nerve
4. Supraclavicular nerves
5. 10th cranial; Vagus nerve
6. Superior laryngeal nerve
7. 11th cranial; Accessory nerve
8. 12th cranial; Hypoglossal nerve

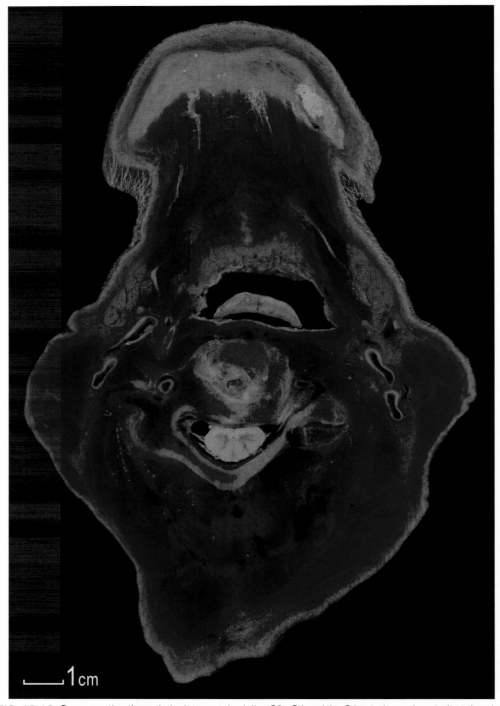

FIG. 13.13 Cross-section through the intervertebral disc C3—C4 and the C4 anterior and posterior tubercles.

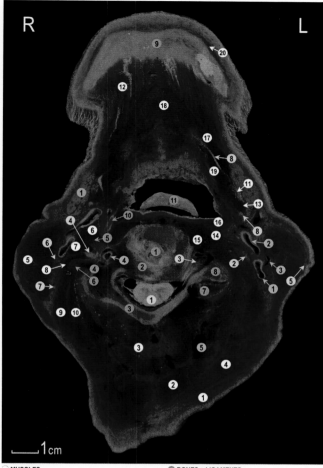

FIG. 13.13 cont'd.

○ **MUSCLES**
1. Trapezius muscle
2. Semispinalis capitis muscle
3. Semispinalis cervicis and multifidus muscles
4. Splenius muscles
5. Sternocleidomastoid muscle
6. Scalenus anterior muscle
7. Scalenus medius muscle
8. Scalenus posterior muscle
9. Levator scapulae muscle
10. Iliocostalis cervicis muscle
11. Digastric muscle - tendon
12. Digastric muscle – anterior belly
13. Stylohyoid muscle
14. Longus capitis muscle
15. Longus colli muscle
16. Middle constrictor of the pharynx muscle
17. Mylohyoid muscle
18. Geniohyoid muscle
19. Hyoglossus muscle
20. Platysma muscle

● **VESSELS**
1. Internal carotid artery
2. External carotid artery
3. Internal jugular vein
4. Vertebral artery
5. Deep cervical vein

● **BONES & LIGAMENTS**
1. C3-C4 intervertebral disc
2. C4 vertebral body
3. C4 lamina
4. C4 transverse process
5. C4 anterior tubercle
6. C4 posterior tubercle
7. C3 inferior articular process
8. C4 superior articular process
9. Body of mandible
10. Hyoid bone
11. Epiglottis

○ **NERVES**
1. Spinal cord
2. C_3-C_4 loop
3. C_4 spinal sensory ganglion
4. C_4 spinal nerve
5. Transverse cervical nerve
6. 10th cranial; Vagus nerve
7. 11th cranial; Accessory nerve
8. 12th cranial; Hypoglossal nerve

● 1. Submandibular gland

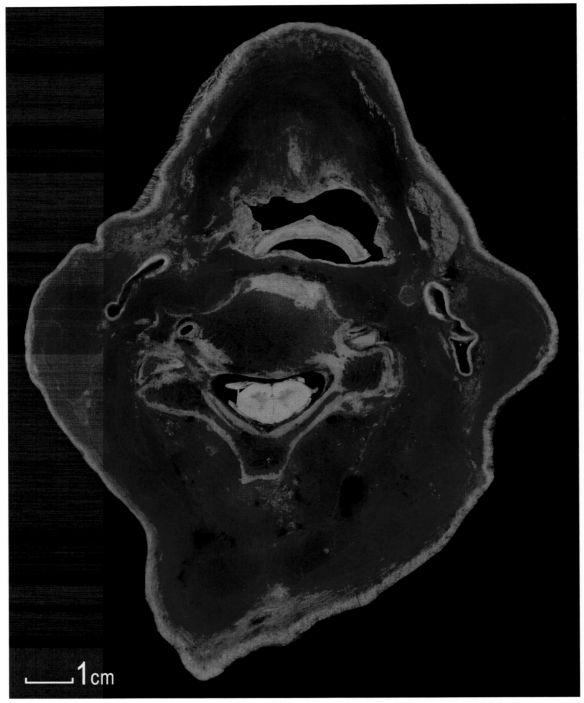

FIG. 13.14 Cross-section through the C_4 spinal nerve and C4–C5 zygapophysial joint.

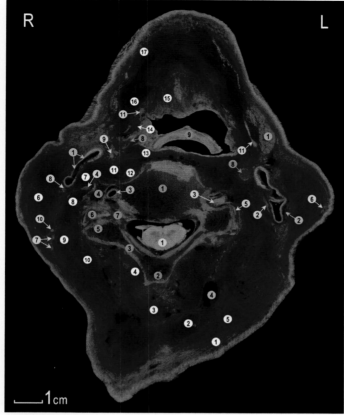

FIG. 13.14 cont'd.

BONES & LIGAMENTS
1. C4 vertebral body
2. C4 spinous process
3. C4 lamina
4. C4 transverse process
5. C4 inferior articular process
6. C5 superior articular process
7. C4-C5 intervertebral foramen
8. Hyoid bone
9. Epiglottis

MUSCLES
1. Trapezius muscle
2. Semispinalis capitis muscle
3. Semispinalis cervicis
4. Multifidus muscles
5. Splenius muscles
6. Sternocleidomastoid muscle
7. Scalenus anterior muscle
8. Scalenus medius and posterior muscles
9. Levator scapulae muscle
10. Iliocostalis cervicis muscle
11. Longus capitis muscle
12. Longus colli muscle
13. Inferior constrictor of the pharynx muscle
14. Stylohyoid muscle
15. Geniohyoid muscle
16. Hyoglossus muscle
17. Digastric muscle – anterior belly

1. Submandibular gland

VESSELS
1. Common carotid artery division
2. Internal jugular vein
3. Vertebral artery
4. Deep cervical vein

NERVES
1. Spinal cord
2. C_3-C_4 loop
3. C_4 spinal nerve
4. C_4 spinal nerve - anterior ramus
5. C_4 spinal nerve - posterior ramus
6. Transverse cervical nerve
7. Supraclavicular nerves
8. 10th cranial; Vagus nerve
9. Superior laryngeal nerve
10. 11th cranial; Accessory nerve
11. 12th cranial; Hypoglossal nerve

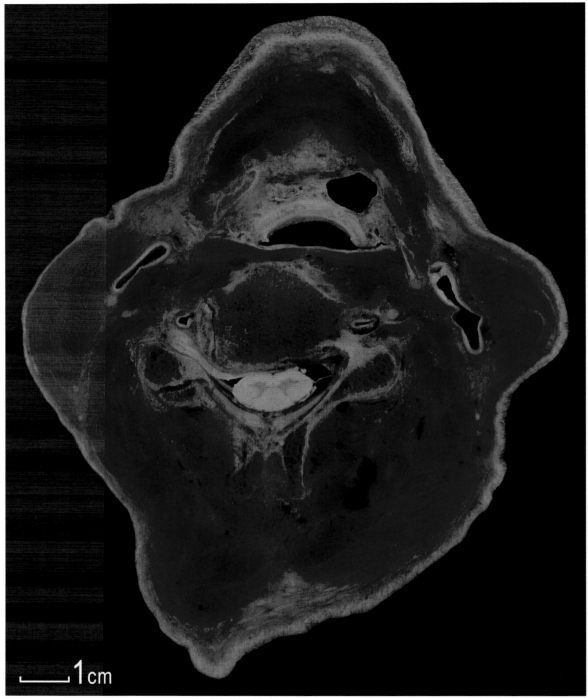

FIG. 13.15 Cross-section through the C4 vertebral body and the C5 spinal nerve passing in the intervertebral foramen C4–C5.

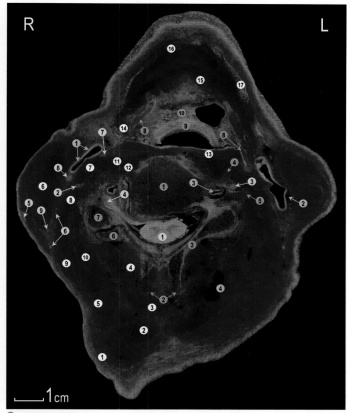

FIG. 13.15 cont'd.

● **BONES & LIGAMENTS**
1. C4 vertebral body
2. C4 spinous process
3. C4 lamina
4. C4 anterior tubercle
5. C4 posterior tubercle
6. C4 inferior articular process
7. C5 superior articular process
8. Hyoid bone
9. Epiglottis
10. Glosso-epiglottic folds

○ **MUSCLES**
1. Trapezius muscle
2. Semispinalis capitis muscle
3. Semispinalis cervicis muscle
4. Multifidus muscles
5. Splenius muscles
6. Sternocleidomastoid muscle
7. Scalenus anterior muscle
8. Scalenus medius and posterior muscles
9. Levator scapulae muscle
10. Iliocostalis cervicis muscle
11. Longus capitis muscle
12. Longus colli muscle
13. Inferior constrictor of the pharynx muscle
14. Stylohyoid muscle
15. Geniohyoid muscle
16. Mylohyoid muscle
17. Digastric muscle – anterior belly

● **VESSELS**
1. Common carotid artery division
2. Internal jugular vein
3. Vertebral artery
4. Deep cervical vein

○ **NERVES**
1. Spinal cord
2. C_3-C_4 loop and C_4 spinal nerve - anterior ramus
3. C_4 spinal nerve - anterior ramus
4. C_5 spinal nerve
5. Transverse cervical nerve
6. Supraclavicular nerves
7. Phrenic nerve
8. 10th cranial; Vagus nerve
9. 11th cranial; Accessory nerve

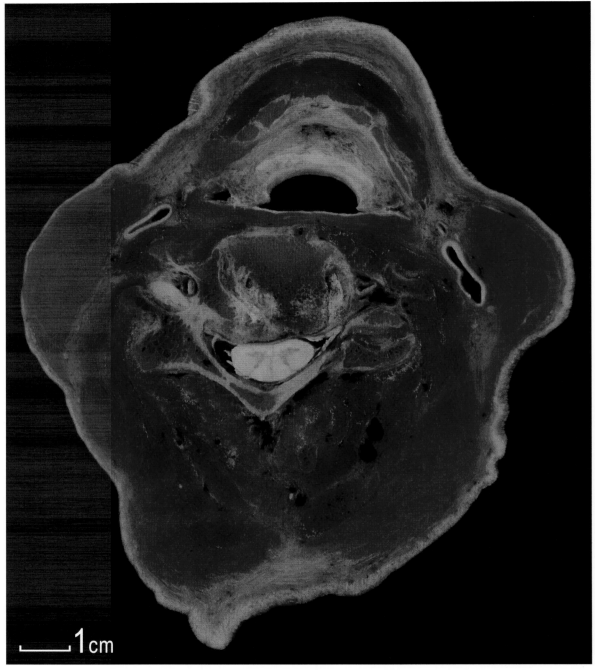

FIG. 13.16 Cross—section through the anterior and posterior C5 tubercles and the C$_5$ spinal nerve.

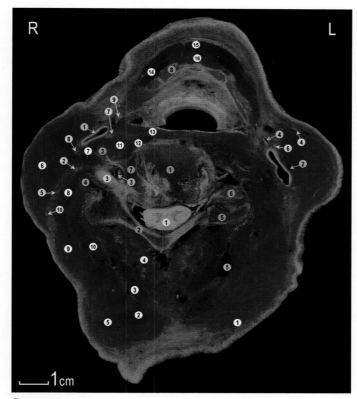

FIG. 13.16 cont'd.

BONES & LIGAMENTS
1. C4 vertebral body
2. C5 lamina
3. C5 anterior tubercle
4. C5 posterior tubercle
5. C4 inferior articular process
6. C5 superior articular process
7. C5 uncinate process
8. Hyoid bone

MUSCLES
1. Trapezius muscle
2. Semispinalis capitis muscle
3. Semispinalis cervicis muscle
4. Multifidus muscles
5. Splenius muscles
6. Sternocleidomastoid muscle
7. Scalenus anterior muscle
8. Scalenus medius and posterior muscles
9. Levator scapulae muscle
10. Iliocostalis cervicis muscle
11. Longus capitis muscle
12. Longus colli muscle
13. Inferior constrictor of the pharynx muscle
14. Omohyoid muscle
15. Mylohyoid muscle
16. Geniohyoid muscle

VESSELS
1. Common carotid artery
2. Internal jugular vein
3. Vertebral artery
4. Superior thyroid artery
5. Deep cervical vein

NERVES
1. Spinal cord
2. C_4 spinal nerve- anterior ramus
3. C_5 spinal nerve
4. Transverse cervical nerve
5. Supraclavicular nerves
6. Superior root of the ansa cervicalis
7. Phrenic nerve
8. 10th cranial; Vagus nerve
9. Superior laryngeal nerve
10. 11th cranial; Accessory nerve

ACKNOWLEDGMENTS

The authors sincerely thank those who donated their bodies to science so that anatomical research could be performed.

FURTHER READING

Clascá, F., Bover, R., Burón, J.A., Castro-Calvo, A., Díaz-Sastre, M.A., 2002. Anatomía seccional. Atlas de Esquemas axiales. Masson, SA, Barcelona.

Cunningham, D.J., 1972. The cervical plexus. In: Romanes, G. (Ed.), Cunningham's Text Book of Anatomy, eleventh ed. Oxford University Press, London, pp. 739—743.

FCAT, 2001. Terminologia Anatómica Internacional (FCAT). Editorial Médica Panamericana, Madrid.

Gardner, E.D., O'Rahilly, R., 1986. The head and the neck. In: Meier, A. (Ed.), Gardner-Gray-O'Rahilly Anatomy: A Regional Study of Human Structure, fifth ed. Saunders, Philadelphia, pp. 555—769.

Lazorthes, G., 1955. Le Système Nerveux Périphérique. Description, Systematisation, Exploration, Abord Chirurgical. Masson et Cie, Paris (editeurs).

Rouvière, H., Delmas, A., 2005. Anatomía Humana Descriptiva, Topográfica Y Funcional, 11a ed. Masson, Barcelona.

Schünke, M., Schulte, E., Schumacher, U., 2015. Prometheus. Texto y Atlas de Anatomía, 3a ed. Editorial Médica Panamericana, Madrid.

CHAPTER 14

Cervical Plexus Dissection

ANNA CARRERA • XAVIER SALA-BLANCH • ANA V. MONTAÑA •
ANDRÉ P. BOEZAART • MIGUEL ANGEL REINA • FRANCISCO REINA

The cervical plexus and its branches are situated in the lateral aspect of the neck between the sternocleidomastoid and trapezius muscles. The following images depict a step-by-step dissection of the cervical plexus and its branches.

After removing the skin and the subcutaneous tissue, including the platysma muscle, the different cutaneous nerves that form the **superficial cervical plexus** can be visualized (Fig. 14.1). For this Erb's point is key. It is where this bundle of nerves emerges from the deep plane. Here, a small area between 1 and 2 cm, situated at the posterior border of the sternocleidomastoid muscle, half-way between its clavicular and mastoid attachments course the **lesser occipital**, the **great auricular**, the **transverse cervical**, and the **supraclavicular nerves** from cranial to caudal. These nerves then extend radially, and each has a characteristic pathway. The **lesser occipital nerve** follows an ascending course along the posterior border of the sternocleidomastoid muscle, while the **great auricular nerve** ascends obliquely over this muscle toward the lower end of the pinna and parallel to and behind the external jugular vein (ressected in this dissection). The **transverse cervical nerve** crosses horizontally over the sternocleidomastoid muscle in the anterior direction. The **supraclavicular nerves**, which can be three individual branches or a single common trunk, follow a downward direction in the posterior triangle of the neck reaching the anterosuperior region of the thorax and shoulder, where they provide sensory innervation.

Advancing the dissection in the adipose tissue over the prevertebral layer of the cervical fascia, the inferolateral trajectory of the **11th cranial nerve (accessory nerve)** becomes visible. It is located in the posterior part of the posterior triangle of the neck, and follows a posteroinferior oblique course starting at a point between the mastoid process attachment and the midpoint of the sternocleidomastoid muscle at its posterior border, to the point of attachment of the middle and lower thirds of the anterior border of the trapezius muscle. When it reaches the trapezius muscle, it travels deep into this muscle. In this same plane of dissection, we can also identify the course of the transverse cervical artery and the anterior belly of the omohyoid muscle.

The objective of this dissection is to identify the **anterior rami of the cervical spinal nerves** from which the **cervical plexus** originates as well as the muscular nerves that emerge from it and form the **deep cervical plexus**(Fig. 14.2). To achieve this, we sectioned the distal end of the sternocleidomastoid muscle and reflected it medially to be able to perform removal of the prevertebral layer of the cervical fascia. By doing this we expose the neurovascular bundle of the neck and the deep muscular plane.

Focusing first on the lower portion of the plexus, between the longus capitis muscle anterior and the cervical insertion of the scalenus anterior muscles posterior, we visualize the anterior branches of the C_3 and C_4 cervical spinal nerves and the loop that is formed between them. From C_3, we find the branch that contributes to the formation of the **lower root of the ansa cervicalis**. This lower root passes behind the internal jugular vein (collapsed), joins the **upper root of the ansa cervicalis** on the common carotid artery, and forms the **ansa cervicalis**. From this nerve loop, we can further dissect the branches destined to innervate the infrahyoid muscles. Also, from C_3, we can locate the branch that contributes to the innervation of the trapezius muscle by the **cervical plexus** and other additional branches destined for the cutaneous territory of the **lesser occipital nerve**. From C_4, the course of the **phrenic nerve** can be followed on the anterior surface of the scalenus anterior muscle. The ascending cervical artery medially accompanies this nerve.

Surgical Anatomy of the Cervical Plexus and its Branches. https://doi.org/10.1016/B978-0-323-83132-1.00001-9

161

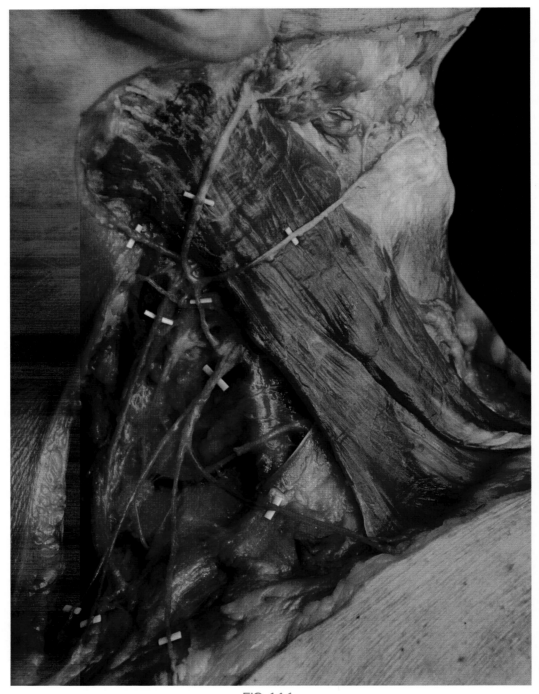

FIG. 14.1

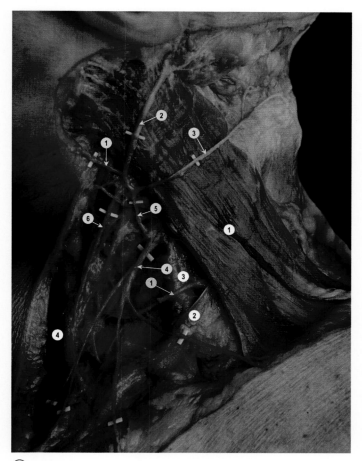

○ **MUSCLES**
  1. Sternocleidomastoid muscle
  2. Omohyoid (superior belly)
  3. Scalenus anterior
  4. Trapezius

● **VESSELS**
  1. Transverse cervical artery

○ **NERVES**
  1. Lesser occipital nerve
  2. Great auricular nerve
  3. Transverse cervical nerve
  4. Supraclavicular nerves
  5. C3-C4 loop
  6. 11th cranial; Accessory nerve

FIG. 14.1 cont'd.

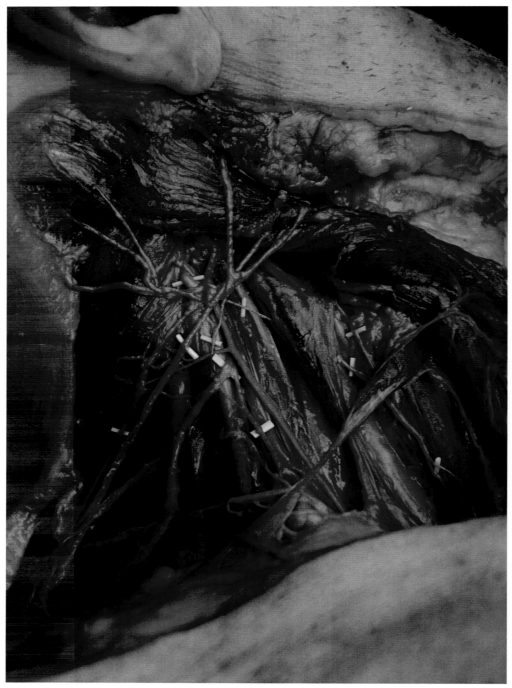

FIG. 14.2

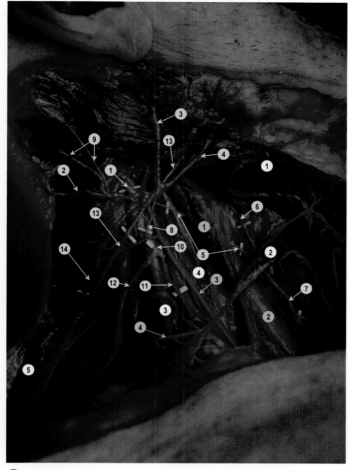

○ **MUSCLES**
   1. Sternocleidomastoid (reflected)
   2. Omohyoid (superior belly)
   3. Scalenus anterior
   4. Longus capitis
   5. Trapezius

● **VESSELS**
   1. Internal jugular vein
   2. Common carotid artery
   3. Ascending cervical artery
   4. Transverse cervical artery

○ **NERVES**
   1. C3
   2. Lesser occipital nerve
   3. Great auricular nerve
   4. Transverse cervical nerve
   5. Inferior root of the ansa cervicalis (C3 contribution)
   6. Superior root of the ansa cervicalis / descending branch of the hypoglossal nerve (C1 contribution trough hypoglossal nerve)
   7. Branches from cervicalis ansa to infrahioid muscles
   8. C3-C4 loop
   9. Complementary branches to lesser occipital nerve area
   10. C4
   11. Phrenic nerve
   12. Supraclavicular nerves
   13. 11th cranial; Accessory nerve
   14. C2-C3 propioceptive supply from cervical plexus to trapezius

FIG. 14.2 cont'd.

Continuing the dissection deeper in the upper region after medially reflecting the proximal part of the sternocleidomastoid muscle, the course of the **11th cranial nerve (accessory nerve)** can be observed (Fig. 14.3). It characteristically crosses through the muscle between its cleidomastoïd and cleidooccipital portions of the

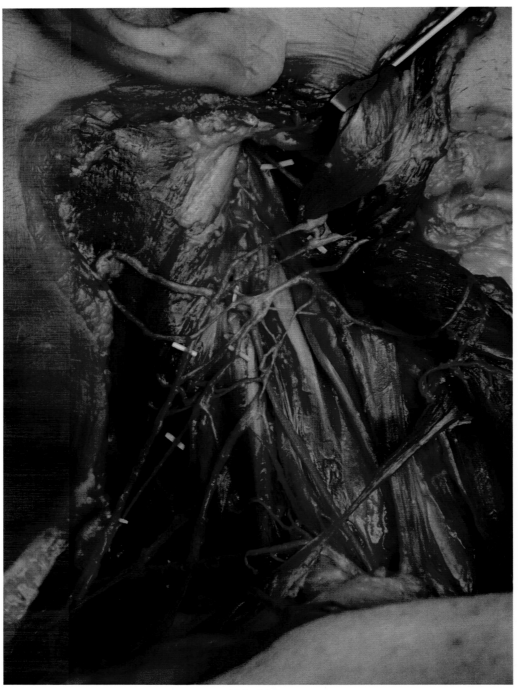

FIG. 14.3

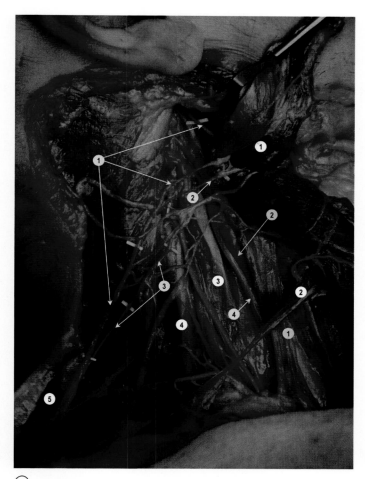

MUSCLES
1. Sternocleidomastoid (reflected)
2. Omohyoid (superior belly)
3. Longus capitits
4. Scalenus anterior
5. Trapezius

VESSELS
1. Internal jugular vein
2. Common carotid artery

NERVES
1. 11th cranial; Accessory nerve
2. C2-C3 propioceptive supply from cervical plexus to sternocleidomastoid
3. C2-C3 propioceptive supply from cervical plexus to trapezius
4. 10th cranial; Vagus nerve

FIG. 14.3 cont'd.

sternocleidomastoid muscle. The branch that innervates the sternocleidomastoid muscle originating from the **cervical plexus** can also be seen. Although the main motor innervation of the sternocleidomastoid and trapezius muscles comes from the **11th cranial nerve (accessory nerve)**, the **cervical plexus** also provides proprioceptive and possibly secondary motor innervation to these muscles.

Performing complete removal of the sternocleidomastoid muscle exposes the most cranial elements of the **cervical plexus**(Fig. 14.4). It is necessary to retract the internal jugular vein medially to uncover the C_1

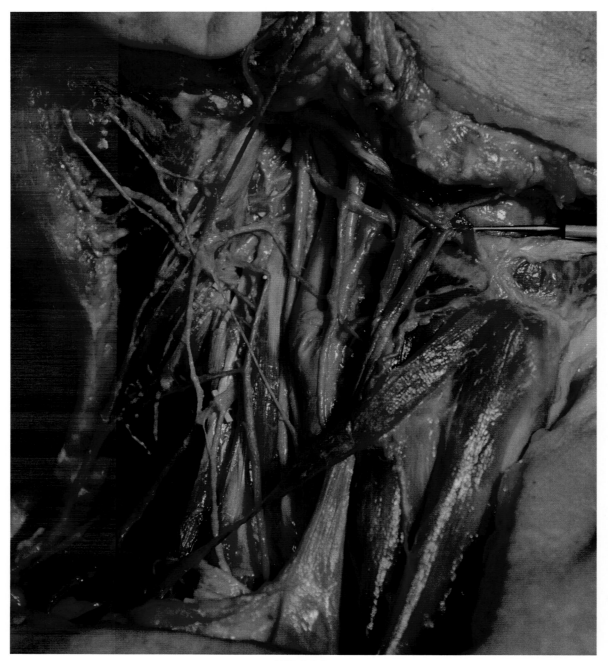

FIG. 14.4

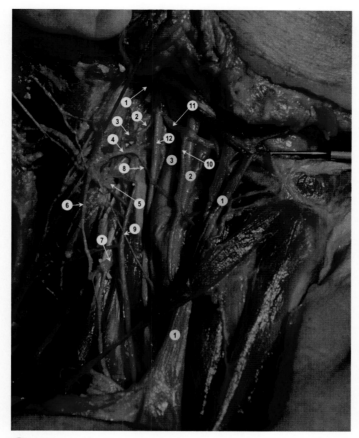

VESSELS
1. Internal jogular vein (reflected)
2. External carotid artery
3. Internal carotid artery

⬤ **NERVES**
1. C1
2. C1-C2 loop
3. C2
4. C2-C3 loop
5. C3
6. C3-C4 loop
7. C4
8. Inferior root of the ansa cervicalis (C2 contribution)
9. Inferior root of the ansa cervicalis (C3 contribution)
10. Superior root of the ansa cervicalis / descending branch of the hypoglossal nerve
        (C1 contribution trough hypoglossal nerve)
11. 12th cranial; Hypoglossal nerve
12. 10th cranial; Vagus nerve

FIG. 14.4 cont'd.

and C_2 **anterior rami of cervical spinal nerves** that emerge anterior to the cervical insertion of the splenius cervicis and levator scapulae muscles. Here, we can also visualize the C_1-C_2 and C_2-C_3 **loops**. From C_2, we can follow the branch which contributes to the formation of the **ansa cervicalis**. In this particular specimen, this contribution of C_2 to the loop was directly incorporated into the **superior root of the ansa cervicalis** (descending branch of the hypoglossal nerve). More distally, this superior root received input from C_3.

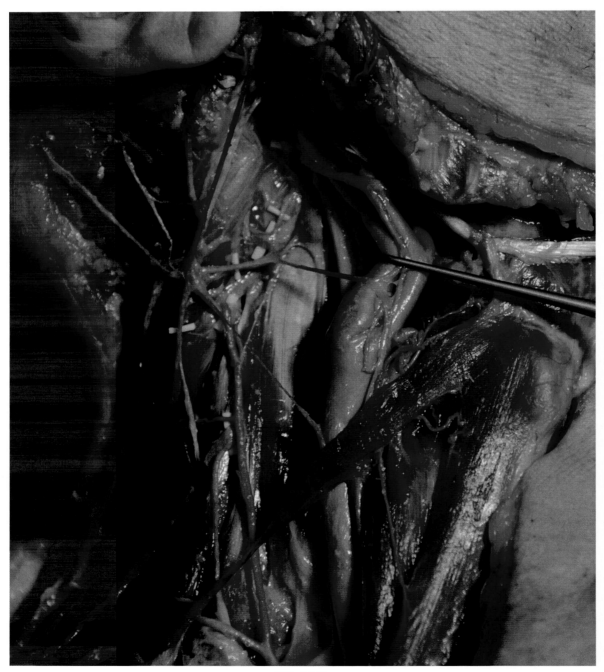

FIG. 14.5

In the deepest plane of dissection, after removing the internal jugular vein and retracting the external and internal carotid arteries medially, we can visualize the **sympathetic trunk** and the **superior cervical ganglion**, on the longus capitis muscle (Fig. 14.5). All the nerves of the origin of the cervical plexus are connected to this ganglion. The ramus communicans of C_2 is the thickest as seen in the image.

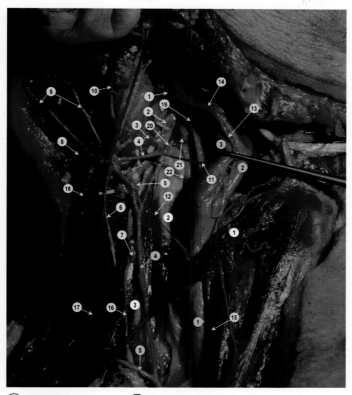

MUSCLES
1. Omohyoid (superior belly)
2. Longus capitis
3. Scalenus anterior

VESSELS
1. Common carotid artery
2. External carotid artery
3. Internal carotid artery
4. Ascendent cervical artery
5. Transverse cervical artery

NERVES
1. C1
2. C1-C2 loop
3. C2
4. C2-C3 loop
5. C3
6. C3-C4 loop
7. C4
8. Lesser occipital nerve
9. Complementary branches to lesser occipital nerve area
10. Great auricular nerve
11. Inferior root of the ansa cervicalis (C2 contribution)
12. Inferior root of the ansa cervicalis (C3 contribution)
13. Superior root of the ansa cervicalis / descending branch of the hypoglossal nerve
      (C1 contribution trough hypoglossal nerve)
14. 12th cranial; Hypoglossal nerve
15. Branches from ansa cervicalis to infrahyoid muscles
16. Phrenic nerve
17. Supraclavicular nerves
18. 11th cranial; Accessory nerve
19. 10th cranial; Vagus nerve
20. Simpathetic connection from superior cervical ganglion to C2 (grey ramus communicans)
21. Superior cervical ganglion
22. Simpathetic trunk

FIG. 14.5 cont'd.

ACKNOWLEDGMENTS

The authors sincerely thank those who donated their bodies to science so that anatomical research could be performed.

FURTHER READING

Cunningham, D.J., 1972. The cervical plexus. In: Romanes, G. (Ed.), Cunningham's Text Book of Anatomy, eleventh ed. Oxford University Press, London, pp. 739—743.

FCAT, 2001. In: FCAT (Ed.), Terminologia Anatómica Internacional. Editorial Médica Panamericana, Madrid.

Gardner, E.D., O'Rahilly, R., 1986. The head and the neck. In: Meier, A. (Ed.), Gardner-Gray-O'Rahilly Anatomy: A Regional Study of Human Structure, fifth ed. Saunders, Philadelphia, pp. 555—769.

Gray, H., Williams, P.L., 2001. Sistema nervioso periférico. In: Williams, P., Bannister, L., Berry, M., Collins, P., Dyson, M. (Eds.), Anatomía de Gray: bases anatómicas de la medicina y la cirugía, eleventh ed. Harcourt, Barcelona, pp. 1225—1291.

Lazorthes, G., 1955. Le système nerveux périphérique. Description, Systematisation, Exploration, Abord Chirurgical. Masson et Cie, Paris (editeurs).

Rouvière, H., Delmas, A., 2005. Anatomía humana descriptiva, topográfica y funcional, eleventh ed. Masson, Barcelona.

Schünke, M., Schulte, E., Schumacher, U., 2015. Prometheus. Texto y Atlas de Anatomía, third ed. Editorial Médica Panamericana, Madrid.

CHAPTER 15

High-Resolution Magnetic Resonance Neurography and Anatomy of the Cervical Plexus

CLAUDIA CEJAS • EMILIA OSA SANZ

INTRODUCTION

The cervical plexus (CP) is a complex network of nerves that gives rise to the innervation for some of the structures in the head, neck, and thorax (Slosar, 2016).

MR neurography (MRN) using a combination of two-dimensional and three-dimensional sequences is increasingly being used to diagnose a variety of peripheral nerve disorders (Fisher et al., 2016; Cejas, 2020).

Conventional MRI of the neck is limited for studying the CP owing to vascular signal artifacts, fat suppression, magnetic field inhomogeneity, and low resolution. Although the brachial plexus has been intensely investigated with MRI, there has been little research regarding the normal imaging appearance of the CP (Lee et al., 2017).

The purpose of this chapter is to reveal the anatomy of the CP through 3.0 T (3 T) high-resolution magnetic resonance neurography.

TECHNICAL ASPECTS OF MAGNETIC RESONANCE NEUROGRAPHY

Magnetic resonance neurography can be performed using both 1.5 and 3.0 T scanners, although 3.0 T is preferable when possible because of its higher signal-to-noise ratio and faster three-dimensional (3D) sequences. This is in part related to improved coil design, better gradient performance, and wider bandwidths (Chhabra et al., 2011). Also, fascicular detail is much more conspicuous on 3.0 T. However, 1.5 T imaging is preferred to 3.0 T in the presence of metallic implants to minimize artifacts (Chhabra et al., 2018).

An optimal MRN examination produces a multiplanar isotropic display of the nerve anatomy and neuronal lesions with a combination of high-resolution 2D and 3D spin-echo images. Sequences can be divided broadly into anatomical techniques (T1 and T2-weighted images (WI), fat-suppressed images) and functional techniques (diffusion-based images) (Chhabra, 2014).

The most important advantage of 3D acquisition is that it can be reformatted into any plane multiplanar recontruction (MPR) as required. It is also possible to make curved planar reformats and maximum intensity projections (MIP) to elucidate the paths of the nerves and their lesions (Schweitzer and Krol, 2016).

These isotropic (submillimeter) spin-echo techniques are referred to as 3D SPACE on Siemens MR Healthcare, VISTA on Philips Healthcare, and CUBE on General Electric (GE) Healthcare (Chhabra et al., 2011).

The 3D T2-WI sequence is useful for depicting variations in muscles and for spine imaging as part of plexus evaluation, because spine pathology is an important confounder in the diagnosis of regional peripheral neuropathy (Chhabra, 2013).

However, for homogeneous fat-water separation, multipoint Dixon protocols are used such as IDEAL (Iterative Decomposition of water and fat with Echo Asymmetry and Least-squares estimation) developed by GE Healthcare; Dixon TSE developed by Siemens Healthcare; or mDixon developed by Philips Healthcare. Fat suppression techniques such as short tau inversion recovery or spectral adiabatic inversion recovery are also used (Santini et al., 2014).

IDEAL-SPGR water—fat separation can be combined with T1 or T2-WI to provide high-quality images. Once water and fat have been separated, the IDEAL technique provides in-phase (water + fat) and opposed-phase (water—fat) images during each acquisition (Gerdes et al., 2007).

Surgical Anatomy of the Cervical Plexus and its Branches. https://doi.org/10.1016/B978-0-323-83132-1.00008-1

TABLE 15.1
Protocol of RMN to Evaluate the Cervical Plexus at 3.0

Sequences	TR/TE (ms)	GAP	FOV	Matrix (Ph/Fr)	NEX	Time (min)	Thick (mm)
CUBE DIR coronal[a]	6000/80	0	40	224/352	2	5:42	1,2 × 0
FIESTA coronal	4,4/Min	0	40	320/340	2	5:31	0,6 × 0
DWI axial	14555/1	4 × 1	30	128/80	-	7	2 × 9
SPGR 3D IDEAL[a]	6,4/Min	0	34	224/320	1	3:35	1 × 0
T2 HYPERCUBE	2000/90	0	38	384/384	1	3:42	1 × 0
T2 MERGE	499/5,8	4 × 1	16	224/228	2	2	4 × 1

[a] With and without contrast (Gadolinium). *DWI*, Diffusion-weighted images; *FOV*, Field of view; *Fr*, Frequency; *Min*, Minimum; *Ph*, Phase; *TE*, Echo time; *TR*, Repetition time.

Diffusion sequence imaging (DWI) enhances nerve visualization by suppressing the adjacent vascular, fat, and muscle signals, and also offers the potential to quantify the signal intensity of the nerve, ADC, and fractional anisotropy (Chhabra et al., 2011), although it is difficult to interpret in the CP owing to artifacts peculiar to the region.

A postcontrast T1-WI sequence (with or without fat suppression) should be obtained after intravenous administration of a gadolinium-based contrast agent (Schweitzer and Krol, 2016; Chhabra, 2014).

To study the CP in our radiology department, we add other sequences that should improve the visualization of the spinal nerves such as FIESTA. Also, CUBE DIR sequences with and without intravenous contrast (gadolinium) are better when pathology is suspected. In Table 15.1, we propose our imaging protocol for the CP.

ANATOMICAL IMAGING OF SPINAL NERVES

In humans, there are 31 pairs of spinal nerves: eight are cervical (C1—C8), the first seven of which emerge from the vertebral canal above their respective vertebrae.

The ventral roots predominantly consist of efferent somatic motor fibers (motor axons) derived from nerve cells of the ventral column. The spinal nerves are attached to the spinal cord by ventral (anterior) and dorsal (posterior) roots (Fig. 15.1). Each ventral root (also named the anterior root, radix anterior, radix ventralis, or radix motoria) is attached to the spinal cord by a series of rootlets that emerge from its ventrolateral sulcus. Each dorsal root (also named the posterior root, radix posterior, radix dorsalis, or radix sensoria) is attached to the dorsolateral sulcus of the spinal cord by a series of rootlets arranged in a line, the dorsal

root entry zone; they bear an ovoid swelling named the dorsal root (spinal) ganglion (DRG). The DRG is located close to the junction of the dorsal and ventral roots (Kayalioglu, 2009).

The spinal nerve runs from the lateral aspect of the dural sac, just posterolateral to the vertebral artery. It then runs to the intervertebral foramen in a tubular canal of variable length, a foramen distinct from other foramina because its boundaries consist of two movable joints, the ventral intervertebral joint and the dorsal zygapophysial joint (Gilchrist et al., 2002). Each nerve then divides into anterior (ventral) and posterior (dorsal) rami, which are found lateral to the vertebral artery (Tubbs et al., 2005) (Fig. 15.2).

ANATOMICAL IMAGING OF THE CERVICAL PLEXUS

The CP is formed from the anterior primary rami of the C1, C2, C3, and C4 spinal nerves (Fig. 15.3). The ventral ramus travels in a groove formed on the transverse process of the cervical vertebra. If present, the dorsal ramus of C1 is wedged between the posterior arch of the atlas and the vertebral artery as it courses in the groove for the latter. The first and second cervical nerves travel anterior to the vertebral artery, whereas the remaining cervical spinal nerves travel posterior to it (Tubbs et al., 2005).

The CP is located deep to the sternocleidomastoid muscle and the internal jugular vein and lies on the ventral surface of the medial scalene and levator scapulae muscles (Fig. 15.4) (Slosar, 2016).

Each ventral ramus, except C1, from the C2, C3, and C4 levels divides into two branches, superior and inferior, to form three communicating loops. These, in turn, unite in the following way: superior branch of C2 with C1, inferior branch of C2 with superior branch

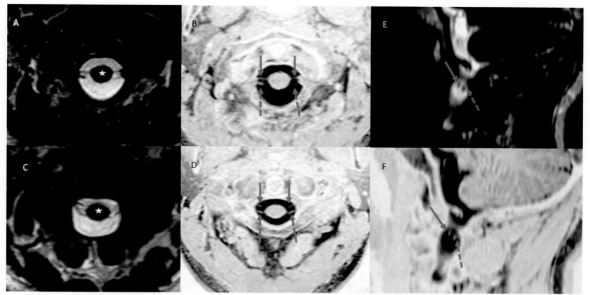

FIG. 15.1 Ventral and Posterior Roots: 3 D FIESTA sequence on axial plane **(A and C)**, and inverted images **(B and D)**, on parasagittal plane **(E)** on inverted image **(F)** of C2, shows the relationship between the spinal cord (asterisk in **A, C**) and, the ventral roots (arrows in **B, D–F**) and the posterior roots (*dotted arrows* in B, D, E, F).

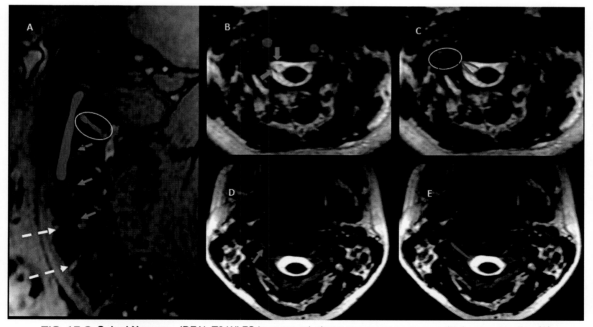

FIG. 15.2 Spinal Nerves: IDEAL T2 WI FS in opposed-phase sequence on parasagittal reconstruction **(A)** and, 3D FIESTA sequence on axial plane **(B–E)** observing the anterior and posterior rami of spinal nerves (arrows in **A, D** and orange in **E**) into the intervertebral foramina and, their relationship with the vertebral artery (red in **A** and **B**), the dorsal zygapophysial joint (circle in **A** and **C**) and the intervertebral joint (*dotted arrows* in **A**). Note: the ventral and posterior roots of the third rami (*thick arrow* in **B** and orange lines in **C**) and, the third spinal nerve (arrow in **D**, and orange line in **E**).

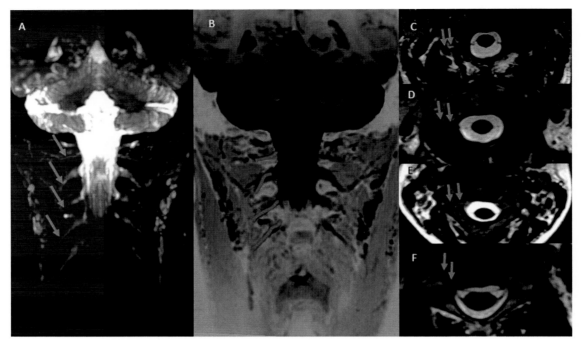

FIG. 15.3 **MR Neurography of the Normal Cervical Plexus:** 3D CUBE DIR sequence with contrast on coronal MIP reconstruction **(A)** inverted image **(B)**, shows the anterior primary from the first to the fourth rami (arrows in **A**, orange lines on **B**); 3D FIESTA sequence on axial reconstruction **(C–F)** demonstrate the anterior primary of the first (arrows on **C**), second (arrows on **D**), third (arrows on **E**) and, fourth (arrows on **F**) cervical spinal nerves.

of C3, inferior branch of C3 with superior branch of C4; and the inferior branch of C4 joins C5 to become part of the brachial plexus. These loops form the CP (Fig. 15.5) (Tubbs, 2011).

Terminal sensory, motor, and communicating branches supply skin and muscles in the occipital area, upper neck, supraclavicular region, upper pectoral region, and diaphragm (Schweitzer and Krol, 2016).

BRANCHES FROM THE CERVICAL PLEXUS

The CP can be divided into posterior and anterior branches.

SUPERFICIAL BRANCHES OF THE CERVICAL PLEXUS

The posterior branches of the CP supply sensory innervation to the lateral neck and upper thorax. Superficial (cutaneous) or sensory branches from the CP include the great auricular nerve (C2, 3), lesser occipital nerve (C2, 3), transverse cervical nerve (C2, 3), and supraclavicular nerve (C3, 4) (Tubbs, 2011).

The **great auricular nerve** (GAN) is a pure sensory nerve stemming from the second and third spinal nerves, emerging at the posterior border of the sternocleidomastoid muscle and ascending toward the angle of the mandible, parotid region, and auricle to provide cutaneous sensation. It is the largest branch of the CP and is frequently used as a jump graft in nerve repairs in the head and neck region. The GAN communicates with the facial and vagus nerves (Tayebi Meybodi et al., 2018; Ginsberg and Eicher, 2000) (Fig. 15.6).

The **lesser occipital nerve** arises from the second and third cervical nerves. It follows approximately the posterior border of the sternocleidomastoid muscle as it approaches the skin of the lateral occiput and ear (Tubbs et al., 2005) (Fig. 15.7).

The **transverse cervical nerve** arises from the second and third cervical anterior rami. It turns around the posterior edge of the sternocleidomastoid muscle, then divides into ascending and descending branches (Domet et al., 2005) (Fig. 15.8).

The **supraclavicular nerve** arises from a common trunk formed from the third and fourth cervical rami

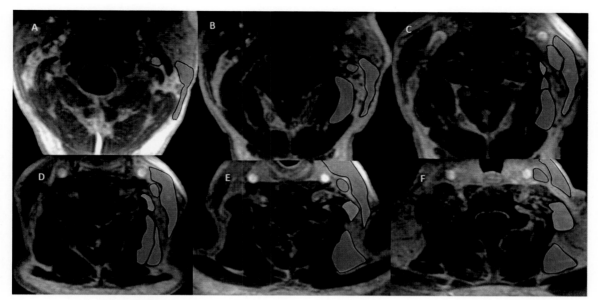

FIG. 15.4 Cervical Plexus Limits: IDEAL T2 WI FS in phase on axial reconstruction from C1–C2 to C6–C7 levels **(A–F)**, on coronal reconstruction **(G–I)** and, on sagittal reconstruction **(J–L)** shows the Cervical Plexus limits: deep to the sternocleidomastoid muscle (in green), the internal jugular vein (in blue) and, laying on the ventral surface of the medial scalene (in yellow) and levator scapulae (in brown) muscles. **Note:** the vertebral artery (red in **L**).

(Fig. 15.9). These emerge at the posterior border of the sternocleidomastoid muscle. The trunk descends under the platysma and the deep cervical fascia. It is divided into branches that diverge to pierce the deep fascia above the clavicle slightly (Fig. 15.10). It supplies the skin over the clavicle, upper chest, and part of the shoulder (Lee et al., 2017).

DEEP BRANCHES OF THE CERVICAL PLEXUS

The deep (muscular) or motor branches of the CP are divided into medial and lateral branches. The medial branches include the ansa cervicalis (C1–C3) to the infrahyoid muscles, branches to the prevertebral muscles (C1–C4), and the phrenic nerve (C3–C5) to the diaphragm. Communicating branches to the vagus nerve (C1–C2), hypoglossal nerve (C1–C2) (Fig. 15.11), and the superior cervical sympathetic ganglion (by gray rami communicants, C1–C4) also arise from the medial branches. The lateral branches are to the sternocleidomastoid (C2–C4) (Fig. 15.12), trapezius (C3–C4), levator scapulae (C3–C4), and scalenus medius (C3–C4) muscles, and communicating branches are to the accessory nerve (C2–C4) (Cesmebasi, 2015).

ANSA CERVICALIS

The ansa cervicalis is a neural complex formed by a combination of the ventral rami of three or four cervical spinal nerves. It comprises both superior and inferior roots. The superior root of the ansa cervicalis contains fibers from the first and second cervical spinal nerves. It travels with the hypoglossal nerve and descends along the anterior wall of the carotid sheath to run superficially lateral to and crossing the carotid internal artery, occipital artery, and external carotid artery in the carotid triangle (Fig. 15.13). It then joins the inferior root arising from fibers from the second and third spinal nerves to form the ansa cervicalis (Kikuta et al., 2019; Brandmeir, 2015). The morphology of the nerve is variable and many variations of it have been described; these are beyond the scope of this chapter (Khaki et al., 2006).

PHRENIC NERVE

The phrenic nerve comes from roots C3, C4, and C5 approximately at the midlevel of the thyroid cartilage. It runs downwards from lateral to medial on the surface of the scalenus anterior muscle behind the prevertebral fascia (Richards, 2015; Mancall and Brock, 2011) (Fig. 15.14).

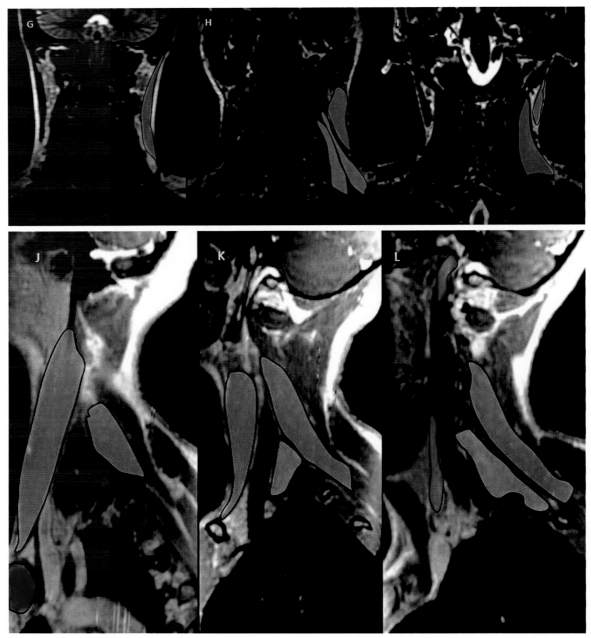

FIG. 15.4 Cont'd

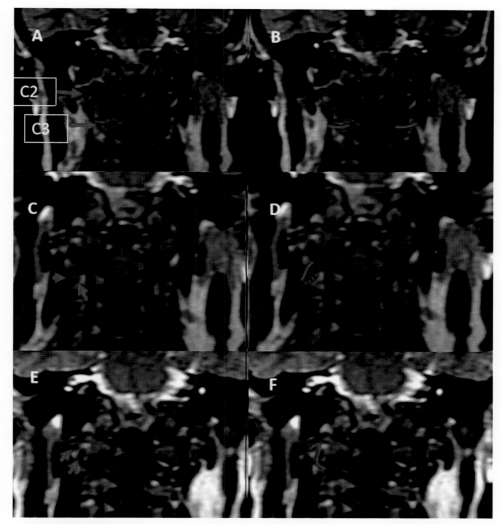

FIG. 15.5 **Neurography of the Ramus C2, C3 and the Communicating Loops of Cervical Plexus:**   CUBE T2-WI on coronal oblique reconstruction. Ramus from C2 and C3 levels (arrows in **A** and **C**, orange in **B** and **D**) and, communicating loops between C2–C3 (arrows in **E**, orange in **F**).

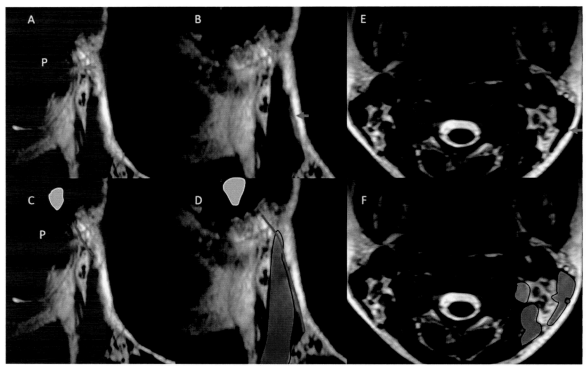

FIG. 15.6 **Greater Auricular Nerve:** CUBE T2-WI sequence on parasagittal-oblique reconstruction **(A—D)** and 3D FIESTA axial plane **(E and F)**, show the great auricular nerve (arrows in **A**, **B**, and **E**, orange in **C**, **D**, and **F**), behind the posterior border of sternocleidomastoid muscle (green in **D** and **F**) ascending toward the parotid region (P in **A** and **C**), and external auditory canal (white in **C** and **D**). Note: The medial scalene (yellow in **E**) and, levator scapulae (brown in **E**) muscles.

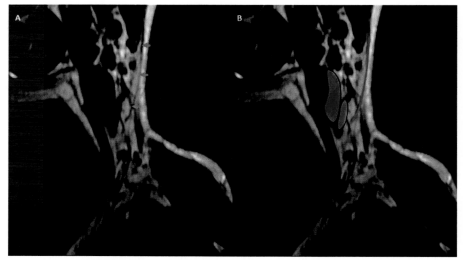

FIG. 15.7 **Lesser Occipital Nerve:** CUBE T2-WI sequence on parasagittal-oblique reconstruction shows the lesser occipital nerve (arrows in **A**, and orange in **B**), from the posterior edge of the sternocleidomastoid muscle (green in **B**) ascending to approach the superficial subcutaneous cell tissue of the lateral occiput and ear.

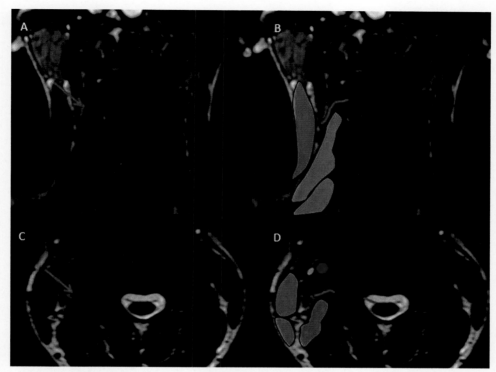

FIG. 15.8 Transverse Cervical Nerve: 3D FIESTA sequence, show the relationship of the transverse cervical nerve (arrow in **A** and **C**, and orange in **B** and **D**) when it pass to the anterior edge of sternocleidomastoid muscle (green in **B** and **D**) and, posterior to the internal jugular vein (blue in **D**). Note: the carotid artery (red in **D**), scalene muscle (yellow in **B**) and, levator scapulae (brown in **D**).

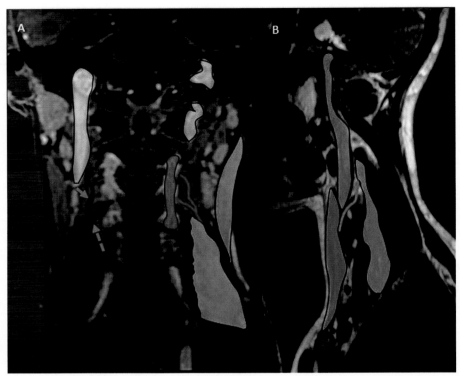

FIG. 15.9 **Third and Fourth Cervical Rami:** 3D IDEAL T1-WI in coronal reconstruction with contrast **(A)** and CUBE T2-WI parasagittal-oblique reconstruction **(B)**, show third (arrow in **A**) and fourth (*dotted-arrow* in **A**) cervical rami to form the trunk of the supraclavicular nerve (orange in **A** and **B**). Note: the relationship with jugular vein (blue), vertebral artery (red in **A**), scalene muscle (yellow in **A** and **B**), and sternocleidomastoid muscle (green in **A** and **B**).

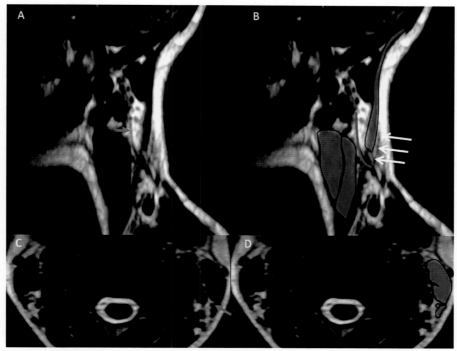

FIG. 15.10 **Supraclavicular Nerve:**   CUBE T2-WI sequence in parasagittal-oblique reconstruction **(A** and **B)**, 3D FIESTA axial reconstruction **(C** and **D)**, demonstrate the supraclavicular nerve (orange arrow in **A, C;** orange in **B** and **D)** behind the sternocleidomastoid muscle (green in **B** and **D)**. Note: the proximity with the lesser occipital nerve (*white arrows* in **B)**.

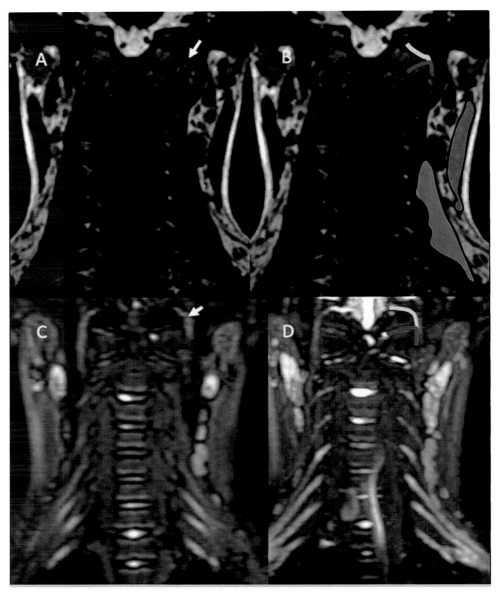

FIG. 15.11 **Medial Motor Branches of Cervical Plexus:** 3D FIESTA sequence **(A** and **B)**, CUBE DIR sequence with contrast **(C** and **D)** in coronal reconstruction, show the first cervical rami (orange in **B** and **D**) communicating with the hypoglossal nerve (*white arrow* in **A** and **C** and, yellow line in **B** and **D**). Note: sternocleidomastoid muscle in green, scalene muscle in brown.

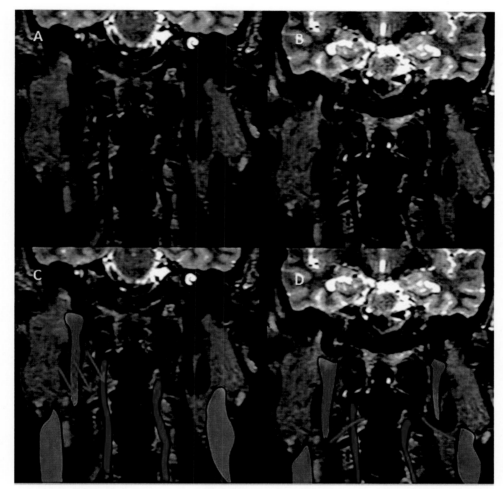

FIG. 15.12 **Lateral Motor Branches of Cervical Plexus: Sternocleidomastoid Nerve:** CUBE T2-WI sequence in corona-oblique reconstruction **(A–D)**, show the sternocleidomastoid nerve (arrows in **C**, orange line in **D**), one of the lateral branches from cervical plexus (C2–C4). Note: Sternocleidomastoid muscle in green, internal jugular vein in blue, vertebral arteries in red.

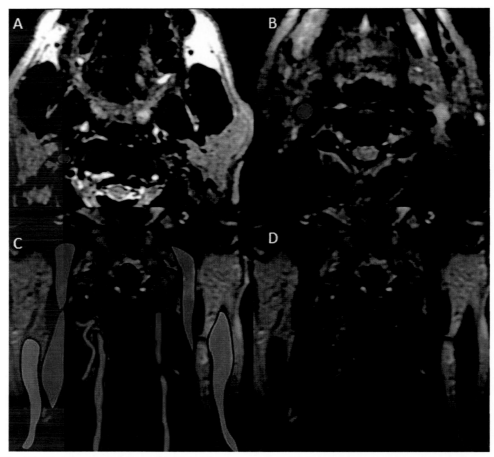

FIG. 15.13 **Ansa Cervicalis:** CUBE T2-WI sequence in axial (**A** and **B**) and coronal-oblique (**C** and **D**) reconstruction, demonstrate the superior root (arrow in **A**), and inferior root (arrow in **B**) of the ansa cervicalis (orange line in **C**). Note: internal jugular vein in blue, sternocleidomastoid muscle in green, vertebral artery in red.

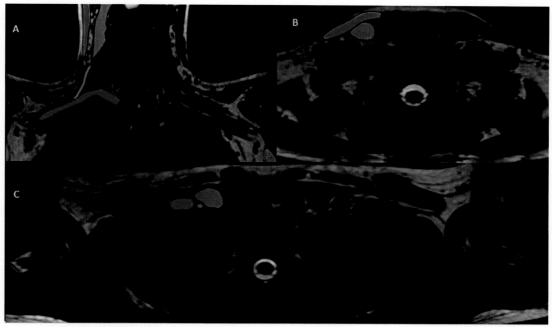

FIG. 15.14 **Phrenic Nerve:**   3D FIESTA sequence in coronal (**A**) and axial reconstruction (**B** and **C**), show the phrenic nerve (orange in **A**—**C**) running downward on the neck, on the anterior surface of the anterior scalenus muscle (violet in **A**, **B**) and, between the subclavian vessels in the upper thorax. Note: Subclavian vein in blue; subclavian artery in red.

REFERENCES

Brandmeir, N., 2015. Nerve Injuries of the Neck. In: Nerves and Nerve Injuries, vol. 2. Elsevier Ltd. https://doi.org/10.1016/B978-0-12-802653-3.00081-6, 493—504 pp. Available from:

Cejas, C., 2020. Neurografía por RM: Plexos y nervios periféricos. Ciudad Autonoma de Buenos Aires, first ed. 229 pp.

Cesmebasi, A., 2015. Anatomy of the Cervical Plexus and its Branches. In: Nerves and Nerve Injuries, vol. 1. Elsevier Ltd. https://doi.org/10.1016/B978-0-12-410390-0.00032-9, 441—449 pp. Available from:

Chhabra, A., Andreisek, G., Soldatos, T., Wang, K.C., Flammang, A.J., Belzberg, A.J., et al., 2011. MR neurography: past, present, and future. Am. J. Roentgenol. 197 (3), 583—591.

Chhabra, A., Madhuranthakam, A.J., Andreisek, G., 2018. Magnetic resonance neurography: current perspectives and literature review. Eur. Radiol. 28 (2), 698—707.

Chhabra, A., 2013. Magnetic resonance neurography-simple guide to performance and interpretation. Semin. Roentgenol. 48 (2), 111—125. https://doi.org/10.1053/j.ro.2012.11.004. Available from:

Chhabra, A., 2014. Peripheral MR neurography. Approach to interpretation. Neuroimaging Clin. N. Am. 24 (1), 79—89. https://doi.org/10.1016/j.nic.2013.03.033. Available from:

Domet, M.A., Connor, N.P., Heisey, D.M., Hartig, G.K., 2005. Anastomoses between the cervical branch of the facial nerve and the transverse cervical cutaneous nerve, 26, 168—171.

Fisher, S., Wadhwa, V., Manthuruthil, C., Cheng, J., Chhabra, A., 2016. Clinical impact of magnetic resonance neurography in patients with brachial plexus neuropathies. Br. J. Radiol. 89 (1067), 1—9.

Gerdes, C.M., Kijowski, R., Reeder, S.B., 2007. IDEAL imaging of the musculoskeletal system: robust water-fat separation for uniform fat suppression, marrow evaluation, and cartilage imaging. Am. J. Roentgenol. 189 (5), 1198.

Gilchrist, R.V., Slipman, C.W., Bhagia, S.M., 2002. Anatomy of the intervertebral foramen. Pain Physician 5 (4), 372—378.

Ginsberg, L.E., Eicher, S.A., 2000. Case report great auricular nerve : anatomy and imaging in a case of perineural tumor spread. Am. J. Neuroradiol. (March), 568—571.

Kayalioglu, G., 2009. The Spinal Nerves. The Spinal Cord. Elsevier Ltd. https://doi.org/10.1016/B978-0-12-374247-6.50008-0, 37—56 pp. Available from:

Khaki, A.A., Shokouhi, G., Shoja, M.M., 2006. Ansa cervicalis as a variant of spinal accessory nerve plexus: a case report. Clin. Anat. 543 (January 2005), 540—543.

Kikuta, S., Jenkins, S., Kusukawa, J., Iwanaga, J., Loukas, M., Tubbs, R.S., 2019. Ansa cervicalis: a comprehensive review of its anatomy, variations, pathology, and surgical applications. Anat. Cell Biol. 52 (3), 221–225.

Lee, J.H., Cheng, K.L., Choi, Y.J., Baek, J.H., 2017. High-resolution imaging of neural anatomy and pathology of the neck. Korean J. Radiol. 18 (1), 180–193.

Mancall, E.L., Brock, D.G., 2011. Cervical plexus. In: Mancall, E.L., Brock, D.G. (Eds.), Gray's Clinical Neuroanatomy: The Anatomic Basis for Clinical Neuroscience. Elsevier Health Sciences, Philadelphia, pp. 315–317.

Richards, A.T., 2015. Surgical Exposures for the Nerves of the Neck. In: Nerves and Nerve Injuries, vol. 2. Elsevier Ltd. https://doi.org/10.1016/B978-0-12-802653-3.00063-4, 201–213 pp. Available from:

Santini, F., Aro, M.R., Gold, G.E., Carrino, J.A., 2014. Fat-Suppression Techniques for 3-T MR Imaging of the Musculo.

Schweitzer, A.D., Krol, G., 2016. Imaging of plexopathy in oncologic patients. In: Handb Neuro-Oncology Neuroimaging, second ed., pp. 763–775.

Slosar, P., 2016. Cervical Spinal Nerves. Netter's Atlas Neurosci, pp. 153–231. Available from: https://linkinghub.elsevier.com/retrieve/pii/B9780323265119000096.

Tayebi Meybodi, A., Gandhi, S., Lawton, M.T., Preul, M.C., 2018. Anterior greater auricular point: novel anatomic landmark to facilitate harvesting of the greater auricular nerve. World Neurosurg. 119, e64–70. https://doi.org/10.1016/j.wneu.2018.07.001. Available from:

Tubbs, R.S., Salter, E.G., Oakes, W.J., 2005. Anatomic landmarks for nerves of the neck: a vade mecum for neurosurgeons. Neurosurgery 56 (4 Suppl.), 256–260.

Tubbs, S., 2011. Study of the cervical plexus innervation of the trapezius muscle, 14 (May), 626–629.

CHAPTER 16

Cervical Plexus Block

JIN-SOO KIM • HA YEON KIM

INTRODUCTION

The cervical plexus block (CPB) provides effective anesthesia and analgesia to the head and neck region (Kesisoglou et al., 2010; Perisanidis et al., 2013; Mariappan et al., 2015; Shin et al., 2014; Thawale et al., 2019; James and Niraj, 2020). Its most common clinical use has been in carotid endarterectomy (CEA) (Stoneham et al., 2015). Traditionally, CPB was classified into superficial and deep blocks (Winnie et al., 1975), but in 2004 Telford and Stoneham (2004), on the basis of a cadaveric study by Pandit et al. (2003), suggested an "intermediate" CPB of injection below the investing fascia in addition to superficial and deep CPBs. In 2010, Choquet et al. (2010) attempted to refine the intermediate CPB using ultrasound. Currently, it would be more acceptable to classify CPB techniques as superficial, intermediate, and deep (Kim et al., 2018a). Furthermore, as the use of ultrasound in the head and neck region has increased, CPB can be performed more safely and accurately under ultrasound guidance.

ANATOMY

Understanding the anatomy related to CPB is important, although the structural characteristics of the cervical fasciae and their permeabilities have not been fully investigated from the perspective of regional anesthesia. Moreover, there have been disagreements concerning the recognition of the deep cervical fascia especially in the lateral cervical region (Zhang et al., 2006; Natale et al., 2015), and there are anatomical variations (Shakespeare and Tsui, 2013; Lyons and Mills, 1998). Also, complications associated with CPB could result from the complex anatomical relationship between the cervical plexus and cranial nerves.

Cervical Fasciae

The cervical fasciae are clinically important in predicting the spread of disease (Levitt, 1970; Gidley et al., 1997; Granite, 1976), optimizing surgical management (Moncada et al., 1978), and performing regional anesthesia

in the neck area (Pandit et al., 2003; Shakespeare and Tsui, 2013; Guay and Grabs, 2011; Seidel et al., 2015); they are also related to chronic neck pain (Stecco et al., 2014; Tschopp and Gysin, 1996). However, descriptions of fascial arrangements and definitions of spaces in the neck area are inconsistent and unclear, and the terminology is variable. According to Gray's Anatomy (Standring, 2016a), the fascia is described as "sheaths, sheets or other masses of connective tissue large enough to be visible to the unaided eye," and the Fascia Nomenclature Committee of the Fascia Research Congress describes it as "a sheath, a sheet, or any other dissectible aggregation of connective tissue that forms beneath the skin to attach, enclose, and separate muscles and other internal organs." (Adstrum et al., 2017). Nonetheless, the cervical fasciae have been a subject of controversy despite the use of more recent techniques or materials for preserving and studying fascial structures. As Grodinsky and Holyoke (1938) described in their 1938 cadaver dissection study, the difficulties inherent in dissecting out cervical fascial spaces and the obvious artificiality of grouping them could lead to confusion in descriptions of cervical fasciae and to discrepancies among authors. According to recent work by Guidera et al. (2014), the cervical fasciae can be classified as superficial and deep; although the more specific term "subcutaneous tissue" instead of "superficial cervical fascia" has been suggested to reduce confusion with the "superficial layer" of the deep cervical fascia (Guidera et al., 2012). The deep cervical fascia can be divided into three layers (Guidera et al., 2014): (1) superficial layer, which was also called the investing fascia but its suggested synonyms are now masticator fascia, submandibular fascia, or sternocleidomastoid (SCM)-trapezius fascia; (2) middle layer, for which the names strap muscle fascia or visceral fascia are suggested; and (3) deep layer, for which perivertebral fascia is suggested instead of prevertebral fascia because "prevertebral fascia" should be used only for the anterior part. The carotid space containing major vessels, deep cervical lymph nodes, and nerves, usually referred

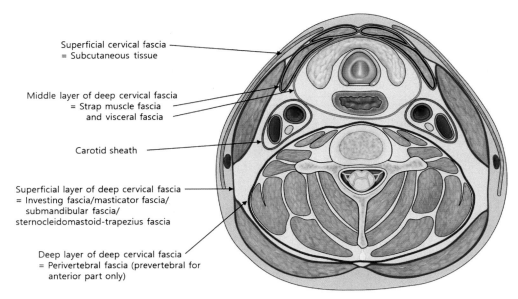

Superficial cervical fascia = Subcutaneous tissue

Middle layer of deep cervical fascia = Strap muscle fascia and visceral fascia

Carotid sheath

Superficial layer of deep cervical fascia = Investing fascia/masticator fascia/ submandibular fascia/ sternocleidomastoid-trapezius fascia

Deep layer of deep cervical fascia = Perivertebral fascia (prevertebral for anterior part only)

FIG. 16.1 The layers of cervical fascia (C6 transverse section) as suggested by Guidera et al. (2014). (The illustration is adapted from Smoker, W.R., Harnsberger, H.R., 1991. Differential diagnosis of head and neck lesions based on their space of origin. The infrahyoid portion of the neck. Am. J. Roentgenol. 157 (1), 155–159. doi:10.2214/ajr.157.1.2048511.)

to the "carotid sheath and its contents," is an important structure that can be affected during CPB (Guidera et al., 2012). Fig. 16.1 shows a schematic drawing of the cervical fasciae as Guidera et al. (2014) suggested.

Cervical Plexus

The cervical plexus is situated in a groove between the longus capitis and middle scalene muscles underneath the prevertebral fascia, but not in the interscalene groove because the anterior scalene muscle is almost absent cephalad to the C4 or C3 level (Usui et al., 2010). Two nerve loops formed by the union of the adjacent anterior spinal nerves from C2 to C4 give off four superficial sensory branches. In craniocaudal order, these are the following: the lesser occipital (C2,3), great auricular (C2,3), transverse cervical (C2,3), and supraclavicular (C3,4) nerves. Initially, they run posteriorly and soon pierce the prevertebral fascia. Afterward, they pass through the interfascial space between the SCM and the prevertebral muscles before radiating to the skin and superficial structures of the neck via the nerve point of the SCM muscle (Moore et al., 2014; Havet et al., 2007). Thus, superficial branches of the cervical plexus travel relatively long distances from the paravertebral space to their superficial endpoints: the skin and subcutaneous tissues of the neck and posterior aspect of the head and shoulders (de Arruda et al., 1974; Standring,

2016b). In contrast, fibers emanating anteromedially from the superior (C1–C2) and inferior (C2-3) roots unite at the level of the omohyoid central tendon to form a loop, the ansa cervicalis (Paraskevas et al., 2014). The ansa cervicalis supplies motor branches to the infrahyoid and SCM muscles (Brennan et al., 2016). Its origin and distribution are highly variable (Jelev, 2013); however, it has been suspected of having an afferent neuronal component (Khaki et al., 2006). Anterior rami of C3 and C4 form a loop, and branches of this loop join C5 to give rise to the phrenic nerve. The cervical plexus anastomoses with the spinal accessory, hypoglossal, facial, vagus, and glossopharyngeal nerves, and with the sympathetic trunk (Moore et al., 2014; Jelev, 2013; Shoja et al., 2014). Fig. 16.2 shows a schematic drawing of the deep and superficial cervical plexuses.

CERVICAL PLEXUS BLOCK METHODS

CPB has been performed at superficial, intermediate, or deep levels, although "deep," "superficial" and "intermediate" are poorly defined terms. Nonetheless, on the basis of anatomical studies of the cervical fasciae, nerve innervation, and relevant clinical reports, CPB techniques can be classified as superficial, intermediate, and deep (Fig. 16.3) (Kim et al., 2018a).

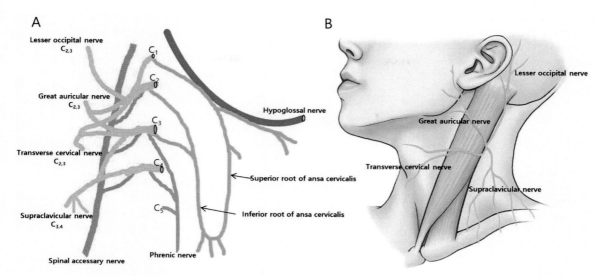

FIG. 16.2 Schematic drawing of deep and superficial cervical plexuses. **(A)** Four superficial branches of the cervical plexus are depicted in yellow, and deep branches (ansa cervicalis) are depicted in green. The cervical plexus is known to anastomose with several cranial nerves and the sympathetic trunk. **(B)** The superficial cervical plexus emerges behind the posterior border of the sternocleidomastoid muscle and innervates the head, neck, and shoulder areas. (The illustration is adapted from Restrepo, C.E., Tubbs, R.S., Spinner, R.J., 2015. Expanding what is known of the anatomy of the spinal accessory nerve. Clin. Anat. 28 (4), 467–471. doi: 10.1002/ca.22492.)

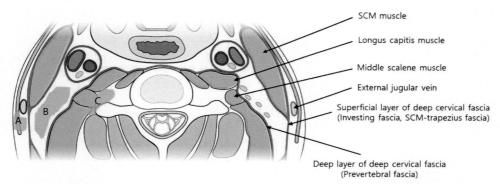

FIG. 16.3 Three different target areas of cervical plexus block (CPB) in the cervical fascial spaces are depicted schematically (C4 transverse section). **(A)** The target area for superficial CPB is subcutaneous tissue around the midportion of the posterior border of the sternocleidomastoid (SCM) muscle. **(B)** The target area for intermediate CPB is the space between the SCM muscle and the prevertebral fascia. **(C)** The target area for deep CPB is the space between the prevertebral fascia and the target transverse process.

Deep Cervical Plexus Block

Deep CPB is described as a paravertebral block targeting the C2–C4 spinal nerves (Winnie et al., 1975; Restrepo et al., 2015). It can be achieved by either a single injection or three separate injections (Winnie et al., 1975; Masters et al., 1995; Merle et al., 1999). Deep CPB performed at the paravertebral space can block not only superficial branches but also deep branches of the cervical plexus, resulting in relaxation of the neck muscles, though this has not been shown to be important clinically (Stoneham et al., 1998, 2015; Telford and Stoneham, 2004). On the other hand, if the ansa cervicalis also has an afferent neuronal component (Khaki et al., 2006), deep CPB would have more clinical significance in treating postoperative pain after neck surgeries involving the infrahyoid and/or SCM muscles, or pain originating in the neck. Wan et al. (2017) and Goldberg et al. (2008) reported that deep CPB in the C2 or C3 transverse process could treat cervicogenic headache effectively. Deep CPB has also been used in the thyroid or parathyroid surgery (Aunac et al., 2002; Pintaric et al., 2007), oral and maxillofacial surgery (Perisanidis et al., 2013), and CEA (Stoneham et al., 2015; Sait Kavakli et al., 2015) to obtain adequate anesthesia and/or analgesia. Owing to its deep endpoint, it can produce major complications such as intravascular injection, epidural or subarachnoid injection, and phrenic nerve palsy (Carling and Simmonds, 2000; Pandit et al., 2007). However, since the introduction of several different ultrasound techniques, deep CPB has become a relatively safe and simple procedure (Perisanidis et al., 2013; Sandeman et al., 2006; Saranteas et al., 2011). For ultrasound-guided (USG) deep CPB, Perisanidis et al. (2013) and Saranteas et al. (2011) simply injected local anesthetics into the space between the prevertebral fascia and the cervical transverse process under ultrasound guidance, but Wan et al. (2017) and Sandeman et al. (2006) injected local anesthetics after the needle touched the target cervical transverse process.

Superficial Cervical Plexus Block

Superficial CPB is conventionally described as subcutaneous injection in the midportion of the posterior border of the SCM muscle targeting superficial branches of the cervical plexus (Winnie et al., 1975; Pandit et al., 2007). This conventional subcutaneous infiltration of superficial CPB can be performed using ultrasound (Shin et al., 2014), and one or more superficial branches of the cervical plexus can be blocked selectively, depending on the type of surgery in the head and neck region, using landmarks (Kesisoglou et al., 2010; Suresh et al., 2002) or ultrasound (Maybin et al., 2011; Flores and Herring, 2016). Unlike deep CPB, superficial CPB carries a low risk of complications and is easy to master (Pintaric et al., 2007; Pandit et al., 2007; Guay, 2008). Nonetheless, it is important to make sure that the needle tip is positioned in the subcutaneous tissue during superficial CPB to avoid the adverse effects of the deep block (Broderick and Mannion, 2010; Cornish, 1999). Unilateral or bilateral superficial CPB can be used to produce postoperative analgesia after a variety of head and neck surgeries such as thyroidectomy (Kesisoglou et al., 2010; Kannan et al., 2018), minimally invasive parathyroidectomy (Pintaric et al., 2007), tympanomastoid surgery (Suresh et al., 2002), anterior cervical discectomy and fusion (Mariappan et al., 2015), and

infratentorial and occipital craniotomy (Girard et al., 2010). It can also be used as the sole anesthetic modality for external ear surgery (Ritchie et al., 2016). The present authors have applied landmark-based superficial CPB to various superficial head, neck, and upper chest wall surgeries to obtain anesthesia and/or analgesia in both pediatric and adult patients (Fig. 16.4). Superficial CPB also can be used as an adjuvant block for shoulder, clavicle, breast, and upper chest wall surgeries, particularly by blocking supraclavicular branches.

Intermediate Cervical Plexus Block

History: In 2002, Zhang and Lee (2002) reported that there is no investing fascia in the space between the SCM and trapezius muscles, which is called the posterior cervical triangle (Tubbs et al., 2006). They conducted a sectional anatomical investigation using epoxy sheet plastination of cadavers, but their results are still controversial (Natale et al., 2015; Guidera et al., 2012, 2014). Interestingly, in Gray's Anatomy (Standring, 2016c), the investing fascia between the SCM and trapezius muscles is said to be formed of areolar tissue, which is indistinguishable from that in the superficial cervical fascia. Nonetheless, in 2003, Pandit et al. (2003) introduced a new concept of subinvesting fascial injection (superficial to the prevertebral fascia but under the investing fascia) as one method for obtaining superficial CPB. These authors (Pandit et al., 2003) hypothesized that there is communication between the superficial and deep spaces through the prevertebral fascia, which could explain why superficial CPB is more effective than deep or combined-deep-and-superficial CPB during CEA (Stoneham et al., 1998; Pandit et al., 2000). In 2004, Telford and Stoneham (2004) suggested that Pandit's technique of subinvesting fascial injection could more correctly be termed "intermediate CPB," which could constitute a third type of CPB. They expected that this intermediate CPB could also produce the effects of deep CPB while avoiding some of its practical difficulties; however, this would be possible only if there really is a communication through the prevertebral fascia. In this context, the permeability of the prevertebral fascia must be important because it can eventually determine the characteristics of intermediate CPB. However, Kim et al. (2020) demonstrated for the first time that the prevertebral fascia has low permeability to the local anesthetic, and contended that intermediate CPB is not likely to produce deep cervical plexus block; although several articles (Martusevicius et al., 2012; Merdad et al., 2012; Kokofer et al., 2015; Barone et al., 2010) had already been published on the basis of Pandit's anatomical study (Pandit et al., 2003).

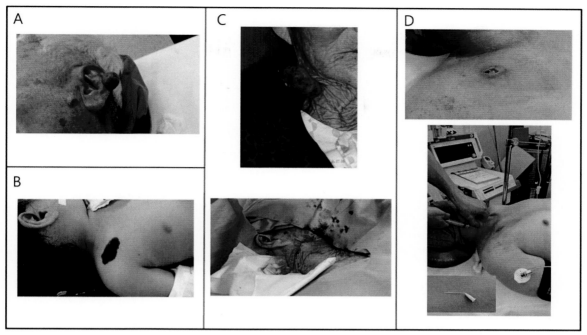

FIG. 16.4 Landmark-based superficial cervical plexus blocks have been performed in our institution for ear, neck, and upper chest wall surgeries to obtain adequate anesthesia and/or analgesia. **(A)** Great auricular and lesser occipital nerve blocks were performed on a 77-year-old male patient undergoing excision of an ear hemangioma. **(B)** Selective supraclavicular nerve block was performed on a four-year-old female patient undergoing excision of a congenital melanocytic nevus on the right upper chest wall. **(C)** Great auricular and transverse cervical nerve blocks were performed on a 94-year-old female patient undergoing excision of a squamous cell carcinoma on the right neck area. **(D)** Selective supraclavicular nerve block was performed on a 52-year-old male patient undergoing incision and drainage of an abscess on the right upper chest wall. To avoid deep injection, the needle was bent slightly.

Technique and nomenclature: Since Kefalianakis et al. (2005) published the first report of USG CPB targeting the space between the SCM and anterior scalene muscles for CEA in 2005, USG CPB has become more popular because it can be performed safely and accurately in the target space (Ciccozzi et al., 2014). In 2010, Choquet et al. advocated that intermediate CPB should target the posterior cervical space (PCS) at the C4 level. The PCS described by Choquet et al. (2010) is the interfascial space between the SCM and prevertebral muscles, which can be seen on cross-sectional imaging. They used the ultrasound technique and contended that the PCS corresponds to the subinvesting fascial space described by Pandit et al. (2003). The superficial branches of the cervical plexus arising from deep tissues pass through this space after piercing the prevertebral fascia and then radiate to the skin and superficial tissues via the posterior border of the SCM muscle (Choquet et al., 2010).

As Choquet et al. (2010) introduced intermediate CPB using ultrasonography, many studies have been published under the label "USG intermediate CPB." For the posterior approach to USG intermediate CPB, after the target cervical level is identified by moving upwards from C7 with ultrasound scanning, the SCM and middle scalene muscles are positioned in the middle of the screen. At this point, the needle is advanced into the PCS (between the SCM muscle and the prevertebral fascia) in a lateromedial direction (in-plane technique) using the anterior border of the middle scalene muscle as the landmark for placing the needle tip. Afterward, a local anesthetic is injected slowly and carefully while its spread in the PCS is observed (Kim et al., 2016, 2018b, 2020). The anterior approach to USG intermediate CPB could provide similar results to other regional techniques during CEA (Calderon et al., 2015). According to Leblanc et al. (2015), USG intermediate CPB is easy to perform, safe, and reliable.

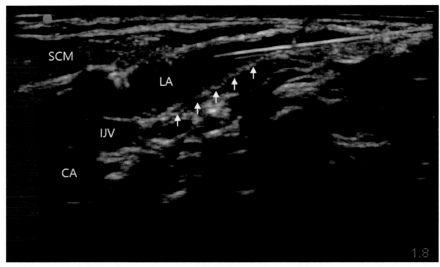

FIG. 16.5 Ultrasound image of posterior approach to intermediate cervical plexus block at C4-5 level in a 3-year-old torticollis patient undergoing unipolar SCM release with myectomy. Hydrodissection of the posterior cervical space between the sternocleidomastoid muscle and prevertebral fascia by local anesthetic is seen, and the local anesthetic spreads to the area near the carotid sheath. *CA*, carotid artery; *IJV*, internal jugular vein; *LA*, local anesthetic; *SCM*, sternocleidomastoid muscle. White arrow points: prevertebral fascia.

Effects of intermediate cervical plexus block: Importantly, intermediate CPB can provide different anesthetic and analgesic effects from superficial CPB. The cervical plexus (C2−C4) supplies sensation to the SCM muscle, including proprioception, with variable anastomosis with the spinal accessory nerve (Moore et al., 2014; Caliot et al., 1984; Koizumi et al., 1993; Cvetko, 2015; Paraskevas et al., 2015; Hayward, 1986). Therefore, the SCM muscle seems to have a complex innervation, but cervical branches of the nerve to this muscle, after piercing the prevertebral fascia, anastomose with the spinal accessory nerve at the posterior surface of or inside the SCM muscle (Caliot et al., 1984, 1989; Koizumi et al., 1993). While the spinal accessory nerve itself also has a sensory function (Restrepo et al., 2015; Tubbs et al., 2014; Bremner-Smith et al., 1999), the cervical plexus (ansa cervicalis) is believed to constitute another source of motor innervation to the SCM muscle in addition to the spinal accessory nerve (Brennan et al., 2016; Restrepo et al., 2015; Pu et al., 2008; Fitzgerald et al., 1982; Yoshizaki, 1961). Therefore, it is possible that USG intermediate CPB, performed accurately in the PCS at the proper cervical vertebral level, can block all four cutaneous branches of the cervical plexus and the sensory/motor branches of the cervical plexus supplying the SCM muscle simultaneously, thus providing good anesthesia and analgesia for neck surgeries manipulating (Kim et al., 2016) or resecting the SCM muscle (Fig. 16.5) (Kim et al., 2018b). Similarly, Yerzingatsian (1989) suggested that local anesthetic be deposited directly into the SCM muscle to block the sensory branches of the cervical plexus that innervate this muscle during local anesthesia for thyroidectomy. Also, the pain associated with the SCM muscle in SCM syndrome (Missaghi, 2004) or associated with trigger points in this muscle (Bodes-Pardo et al., 2013) can in principle be treated by this technique. Recently, intermediate CPB has become an effective modality for treating chronic neck pain (Thawale et al., 2019; James and Niraj, 2020).

CERVICAL PLEXUS BLOCK AND CAROTID ENDARTERECTOMY

The most common clinical use of CPB has been for CEA. CEA is a validated intervention for stroke prevention associated with symptomatic carotid stenosis (North American Symptomatic Carotid Endarterectomy Trial C, 1991; Bonati et al., 2015), which involves incisions in the skin, platysma muscle, carotid sheath, and carotid artery. Since the first report of CPB for CEA (Parrot et al., 1988) in 1988, various alternative techniques have been evaluated, but the ideal anesthetic technique for CEA remains a matter of debate (Merle et al., 1999;

Kfoury et al., 2015). Stoneham et al. (1998) in 1998 and Pandit et al. (2000) in 2000 reported that superficial CPB is as effective as deep or combined deep and superficial CPB in this context. However, during CEA under CPB, local anesthesia to subcutaneous or deep tissues is often supplemented by the surgeon regardless of the type of CPB method (Seidel et al., 2016), probably because in the neck structures including the carotid sheath there are areas innervated by cranial nerves that even deep CPB cannot reach (Shoja et al., 2014; Ramachandran et al., 2011; Einav et al., 1996), or there can be incisional pain near the midline, presumably mediated by contralateral fibers (Ramachandran et al., 2011; Capek et al., 2015). Seidel et al. (2015) demonstrated a constant anastomosis between the cervical branch of the facial nerve and the transverse cervical nerve of the cervical plexus. The pain associated with incision of the carotid sheath during CEA was completely relieved by a lidocaine spray (Einav et al., 1996), and involvement of cranial nerves (glossopharyngeal and vagus) and the sympathetic trunk in sensory innervation of the carotid artery and sheath was suggested (Shoja et al., 2014; Seidel et al., 2016; Einav et al., 1996); therefore, delivery of local anesthetic close to the carotid artery during CEA seems reasonable. Recently, single USG intermediate CPB (Kokofer et al., 2015; Calderon et al., 2015; Alilet et al., 2017) or USG intermediate CPB combined with USG infiltration of a local anesthetic to the perivascular area of the carotid artery (Seidel et al., 2016; Madro et al., 2016) has become an option for reducing the amount of intraoperative local anesthetic supplementation by the surgeon during CEA, while the use of deep CPB for CEA has been declined. However, direct infiltration of local anesthetic into the perivascular area of the carotid artery can produce adverse effects related to cranial nerve palsy (Seidel et al., 2016; Madro et al., 2016; Harris and Benveniste, 2000; Kwok et al., 2006).

SAFETY CONCERNS WITH CERVICAL PLEXUS BLOCK
Phrenic Nerve Palsy

The phrenic nerve is formed from the ventral rami of C3–C5. It runs from lateral to medial in a downwards oblique direction on the surface of the anterior scalene muscle, beneath the prevertebral fascia. According to Castresana et al. (1994), combined deep and superficial CPB produces acute abnormalities of diaphragmatic motion in 61% of patients. However, conventional superficial CPB seems unable to affect the phrenic nerve provide the injection is made accurately into the

subcutaneous tissue (Cornish, 1999). One reason why not all patients receiving deep CPB develop an abnormality of diaphragmatic motion could be anatomical variations, including the predominance of the fifth cervical nerve and presence or absence of an accessory phrenic nerve (Castresana et al., 1994).

The prevertebral fascia (deep layer of deep cervical fascia) forms a tubular sheath around the vertebral column and the muscles associated with it such as the longus colli and longus capitis anteriorly, the scalenes laterally, and the deep cervical muscles posteriorly (Winnie et al., 1975; Moore et al., 2014). Pandit et al. hypothesized that the prevertebral fascia is porous, but Seidel et al. (2015) investigated the dissemination of dye solution injected into the PCS using ultrasonography; they found that the dye remained in the PCS, implying that the prevertebral fascia is impermeable, contrary to Pandit's hypothesis (Pandit et al., 2003). Recently, Kim et al. (2020) demonstrated that the prevertebral fascia has low permeability to the local anesthetic, so phrenic nerve paralysis after intermediate CPB is very unlikely.

Airway Obstruction

Mechanical airway obstruction due to tissue edema or hematoma is a well-recognized surgical complication after various neck surgeries including thyroidectomy (Suzuki et al., 2016) and CEA (Carmichael et al., 1996; Kwok et al., 2004). Particularly during CEA, surgical procedures including dissection, traction, and retraction can injure the facial nerve, hypoglossal nerve, vagus nerve and its branches (recurrent and superior laryngeal nerves), or the glossopharyngeal nerve within the operative field (Fokkema et al., 2014). Among these, bilateral injury to the vagus, recurrent laryngeal, or hypoglossal nerve can result in fatal upper airway obstruction (Basile and Sadighi, 1989; Bageant et al., 1975). Although there are few data on cranial nerve blockades associated with single deep CPB, it is plausible that deep CPB can paralyze the glossopharyngeal, vagus, hypoglossal, and accessory nerves particularly when local anesthetic spreads cephalad, because there are extensive neural anastomoses between the lower and upper cervical nerves, although these vary widely among individuals (Shoja et al., 2014; Masters et al., 1995). Accordingly, we should bear in mind that bilateral deep CPB can cause not only bilateral phrenic nerve palsy but also fatal airway obstruction by paralyzing the vagus or hypoglossal nerve. More importantly, in patients with preexisting contralateral vagus (or recurrent laryngeal) or hypoglossal nerve injury, even unilateral deep CPB can lead to total airway obstruction;

therefore, although preexisting unilateral vocal cord paralysis is usually clinically asymptomatic (Harris and Benveniste, 2000; Weiss et al., 2005) and unilateral hypoglossal nerve palsy entails minimal disability (Bageant et al., 1975), preoperative routine history taking and physical examination of the tongue and vocal cord would be necessary for patients receiving deep CPB (Pintaric et al., 2007) or those undergoing CEA (Espinoza et al., 1999), regardless of anesthetic techniques.

As described earlier, direct infiltration of local anesthetic into the paracarotid area during CEA by either the surgeon or the anesthesiologist can be effective for blocking incisional pain from the carotid sheath or artery (Einav et al., 1996; Casutt et al., 2015), but it can also produce adverse effects related to blockade of the cranial nerves besides impairing the baroreceptor reflex (Seidel et al., 2016). Recently, USG infiltration of local anesthetic into the paracarotid area has been combined with subcutaneous infiltration or intermediate CPB to decrease intraoperative supplementation of local anesthetic during CEA. According to Casutt et al. (2015), USG carotid sheath block achieved by injecting a mixture of local anesthetic and contrast medium into the ventral side of the carotid artery leads to extensive spread of the drug, as confirmed by a postblock CT image. Martusevicius et al. (2012) reported that temporary hoarseness, facial palsy, and dysphagia occurred in 72%, 13%, and 12% of patients, respectively, who had received combined USG intermediate CPB and USG paracarotid infiltration of local anesthetics. Accordingly, bilateral infiltration of a local anesthetic to the paracarotid area can cause fatal airway obstruction.

The spread pattern of the local anesthetic in the PCS can be important in intermediate CPB. During the interfascial plane block, many factors can influence the spread of local anesthetic and the quality of block; precise needle placement and deep understanding of fascial tissue anatomy and structure are basic requirements (Elsharkawy et al., 2018). Therefore, it can be inferred that the incidence of hoarseness and dysphagia after a single USG intermediate CPB depends on the block technique and the volume of local anesthetic injected. On the other hand, when intermediate CPB was combined with the paracarotid infiltration of local anesthetic, a much higher incidence of hoarseness and dysphagia resulted (Martusevicius et al., 2012; Seidel et al., 2016; Madro et al., 2016).

Hoarseness (dysphonia), which is likely to be associated with blockades of the vagus nerve or its branches (recurrent and superior laryngeal nerves), difficulty in swallowing (dysphagia), which is likely to be associated with vagus, glossopharyngeal, or hypoglossal nerve blockade, and facial nerve blockade, can all result from the medial and upward spread of local anesthetic during USG intermediate CPB. Temporary dysphonia due to ipsilateral blockade of the vagus, recurrent laryngeal, or superior laryngeal nerve after USG intermediate CPB is not usually clinically significant. However, bilateral blockade of the vagus, recurrent laryngeal, or hypoglossal nerve can induce fatal airway obstruction. Therefore, bilateral intermediate CPB can be dangerous, and even unilateral CPB can lead to airway obstruction in patients with preexisting contralateral vagus or hypoglossal nerve injury, which can require routine preoperative examination. To avoid inadvertent cranial nerve blockades during USG intermediate CPB, the recommendations are to place the needle tip in the PCS well outside the carotid sheath, to use a small volume of local anesthetic, and to inject the anesthetic slowly while observing its spread and restricting medial spread toward the carotid sheath (Kim et al., 2016, 2018b), unless carotid sheath block is required.

Other Adverse Effects

Horner's syndrome has no clinical consequence in itself but it is an unpleasant side effect, although not necessarily described as a complication (Avidan, 2004). The occurrence of Horner's syndrome after intermediate CPB could be debatable because it could be affected by the location of the cervical sympathetic chains in relation to the prevertebral fascia, the permeability of the prevertebral fascia, and the extent of local anesthetic spread in the PCS toward the carotid sheath during intermediate CPB. Usui et al. (2010) and Civelek et al. (2008) showed that the cervical sympathetic chains are situated immediately beneath the prevertebral fascia covering the longus muscles. In contrast, the latest edition of Gray's Anatomy (Standring, 2017) states that the cervical sympathetic trunk lies on the prevertebral fascia behind the carotid sheath. Nonetheless, Horner's syndrome has been reported after superficial CPB (Pintaric et al., 2007), combined superficial and deep CPB (Pintaric et al., 2007; Sait Kavakli et al., 2015), single USG intermediate CPB (Leblanc et al., 2015), and combined USG intermediate CPB and paracarotid infiltration of local anesthetic (Martusevicius et al., 2012; Seidel et al., 2016; Rossel et al., 2013). On the other hand, according to Lyons and Mills (1998), the cervical sympathetic chain was found within the carotid sheath in two of 12 cadaveric neck dissections. This anatomical variation could facilitate sympathetic chain injury during neck dissection or simple catheterization of the internal jugular vein (Ahmad and Hayat, 2008) and also influence the occurrence of Horner's syndrome during CPB with/without paracarotid infiltration of local anesthetic.

The most common cause of spinal accessory nerve palsy is iatrogenic insult during neck surgeries, especially those located in the posterior cervical triangle (Tubbs et al., 2014; Nason et al., 2000). Anatomically, the spinal accessory nerve enters the posterior cervical triangle within 2 cm above Erb's point and then courses obliquely across the triangle to end in the anterior surface of the superior part of the trapezius muscle; but there are many variations (Symes and Ellis, 2005). In the posterior cervical triangle, the accessory nerve lies superficial to the prevertebral fascia (Tubbs et al., 2005), so it can be affected during superficial CPB (Masters et al., 1995). However, intermediate CPB targeting the PCS under the SCM muscle is not likely to affect the spinal accessory nerve (Townsley et al., 2011).

SUMMARY

As we learn more about CPB, its indications are gradually expanding. However, CPB is performed in the neck area, a highly complicated segment of the body with multiple fascial layers in a narrow space. Recently, a new and more specific terminology for cervical fasciae has been suggested, but there is still controversy over their recognition and description, including the investing and prevertebral fasciae, and the carotid sheath. Furthermore, anatomical variations in the cervical fascial layers can significantly influence the effects of each method of CPB. Currently, therefore, it seems difficult to describe the true effects of each CPB approach, although most CPB methods are now being performed accurately and safely under ultrasound guidance. In this chapter, we included a detailed discussion of intermediate CPB, a relatively new technique involving some controversies related to phrenic and cranial nerve palsies. Although unilateral USG intermediate CPB is safe, a bilateral block in a narrow neck area with complex fascial and neural structures should be performed with caution.

REFERENCES

Adstrum, S., Hedley, G., Schleip, R., Stecco, C., Yucesoy, C.A., 2017. Defining the fascial system. J. Bodyw. Mov. Ther. 21 (1), 173–177. https://doi.org/10.1016/j.jbmt.2016.11.003.

Ahmad, M., Hayat, A., 2008. Horner's syndrome following internal jugular vein dialysis catheter insertion. Saudi J. Kidney Dis. Transpl. 19 (1), 94–96.

Alilet, A., Petit, P., Devaux, B., et al., 2017. Ultrasound-guided intermediate cervical block versus superficial cervical block for carotid artery endarterectomy: the randomized-controlled CERVECHO trial. Anaesth. Crit. Care Pain Med. 36 (2), 91–95. https://doi.org/10.1016/j.accpm.2016.03.007.

Aunac, S., Carlier, M., Singelyn, F., De Kock, M., 2002. The analgesic efficacy of bilateral combined superficial and deep cervical plexus block administered before thyroid surgery under general anesthesia. Anesth. Analg. 95 (3), 746–750. https://doi.org/10.1097/00000539-200209000-00039.

Avidan, A., 2004. Horner's syndrome is not a complication of a brachial plexus block. RAPM 29 (4), 378. https://doi.org/10.1016/j.rapm.2004.02.006.

Bageant, T.E., Tondini, D., Lysons, D., 1975. Bilateral hypoglossal-nerve palsy following a second carotid endarterectomy. Anesthesiology 43 (5), 595–596. https://doi.org/10.1097/00000542-197511000-00026.

Barone, M., Diemunsch, P., Baldassarre, E., et al., 2010. Carotid endarterectomy with intermediate cervical plexus block. Tex. Heart Inst. J. 37 (3), 297–300.

Basile, R.M., Sadighi, P.J., 1989. Carotid endarterectomy: importance of cranial nerve anatomy. Clin. Anat. 2 (3), 147–155. https://doi.org/10.1002/ca.980020304.

Bodes-Pardo, G., Pecos-Martin, D., Gallego-Izquierdo, T., Salom-Moreno, J., Fernandez-de-Las-Penas, C., Ortega-Santiago, R., 2013. Manual treatment for cervicogenic headache and active trigger point in the sternocleidomastoid muscle: a pilot randomized clinical trial. J. Manip. Physiol. Ther. 36 (7), 403–411. https://doi.org/10.1016/j.jmpt.2013.05.022.

Bonati, L.H., Dobson, J., Featherstone, R.L., et al., 2015. Long-term outcomes after stenting versus endarterectomy for treatment of symptomatic carotid stenosis: the international carotid stenting study (ICSS) randomised trial. Lancet 385 (9967), 529–538. https://doi.org/10.1016/S0140-6736(14)61184-3.

Bremner-Smith, A.T., Unwin, A.J., Williams, W.W., 1999. Sensory pathways in the spinal accessory nerve. J. Bone Jt. Surg. Br. 81 (2), 226–228. https://doi.org/10.1302/0301-620x.81b2.9027.

Brennan, P.A., Alam, P., Ammar, M., Tsiroyannis, C., Zagkou, E., Standring, S., 2016. Sternocleidomastoid innervation from an aberrant nerve arising from the hypoglossal nerve: a prospective study of 160 neck dissections. Surg. Radiol. Anat. 39 (2), 205–209. https://doi.org/10.1007/s00276-016-1723-9.

Broderick, A.J., Mannion, S., 2010. Brachial plexus blockade as a result of aberrant anatomy after superficial cervical plexus block. RAPM 35 (5), 476–477. https://doi.org/10.1097/AAP.0b013e3181ef4b90.

Calderon, A.L., Zetlaoui, P., Benatir, F., et al., 2015. Ultrasound-guided intermediate cervical plexus block for carotid endarterectomy using a new anterior approach: a two-centre prospective observational study. Anaesthesia 70 (4), 445–451. https://doi.org/10.1111/anae.12960.

Caliot, P., Cabanie, P., Bousquet, V., Midy, D., 1984. A contribution to the study of the innervation of the sterno-cleidomastoid muscle. Anat. Clin. 6 (1), 21–28. https://doi.org/10.1007/BF01811210.

Caliot, P., Bousquet, V., Midy, D., Cabanie, P., 1989. A contribution to the study of the accessory nerve: surgical implications. Surg. Radiol. Anat. 11 (1), 11–15. https://doi.org/10.1007/BF02102238.

Capek, S., Tubbs, R.S., Spinner, R.J., 2015. Do cutaneous nerves cross the midline? Clin. Anat. 28 (1), 96–100. https://doi.org/10.1002/ca.22427.

Carling, A., Simmonds, M., 2000. Complications from regional anaesthesia for carotid endarterectomy. Br. J. Anaesth. 84 (6), 797–800. https://doi.org/10.1093/oxfordjournals.bja.a013595.

Carmichael, F.J., McGuire, G.P., Wong, D.T., Crofts, S., Sharma, S., Montanera, W., 1996. Computed tomographic analysis of airway dimensions after carotid endarterectomy. Anesth. Analg. 83 (1), 12–17. https://doi.org/10.1097/00000539-199607000-00004.

Castresana, M.R., Masters, R.D., Castresana, E.J., Stefansson, S., Shaker, I.J., Newman, W.H., 1994. Incidence and clinical significance of hemidiaphragmatic paresis in patients undergoing carotid endarterectomy during cervical plexus block anesthesia. J. Neurosurg. Anesthesiol. 6 (1), 21–23. https://doi.org/10.1097/00008506-199401000-00003.

Casutt, M., Breitenmoser, I., Werner, L., Seelos, R., Konrad, C., 2015. Ultrasound-guided carotid sheath block for carotid endarterectomy: a case series of the spread of injectate. Heart Lung Vessel 7 (2), 168–176.

Choquet, O., Dadure, C., Capdevila, X., 2010. Ultrasound-guided deep or intermediate cervical plexus block: the target should be the posterior cervical space. Anesth. Analg. 111 (6), 1563–1564. https://doi.org/10.1213/ANE.0-b013e3181f1d48f author reply 1564-1565.

Ciccozzi, A., Angeletti, C., Guetti, C., et al., 2014. Regional anaesthesia techniques for carotid surgery: the state of art. J. Ultrasound 17 (3), 175–183. https://doi.org/10.1007/s40477-014-0094-5.

Civelek, E., Karasu, A., Cansever, T., et al., 2008. Surgical anatomy of the cervical sympathetic trunk during anterolateral approach to cervical spine. Eur. Spine J. 17 (8), 991–995. https://doi.org/10.1007/s00586-008-0696-8.

Cornish, P.B., 1999. Applied anatomy of cervical plexus blockade. Anesthesiology 90 (6), 1790–1791.

Cvetko, E., 2015. Sternocleidomastoid muscle additionally innervated by the facial nerve: case report and review of the literature. Anat. Sci. Int. 90 (1), 54–56. https://doi.org/10.1007/s12565-013-0224-8.

de Arruda, J.V., Sartini Filho, R., Neder, A.C., Ranali, J., 1974. Intraoral anesthesia of the cervical plexus responsible for the sensory innervation of the platysma muscle or skin of the neck. Rev. Bras. Odontol. 31 (190), 229–231 (Anestesia intra-oral do plexo cervical responsavel pela inervacao sensitiva do musculo platisma ou cutaneo do pescoco).

Einav, S., Landesberg, G., Prus, D., Anner, H., Berlatzky, Y., 1996. A case of nerves. Reg. Anesth. 21 (2), 168–170.

Elsharkawy, H., Pawa, A., Mariano, E.R., 2018. Interfascial plane blocks: back to basics. RAPM 43 (4), 341–346. https://doi.org/10.1097/AAP.0000000000000750.

Espinoza, F.I., MacGregor, F.B., Doughty, J.C., Cooke, L.D., 1999. Vocal fold paralysis following carotid endarterectomy. J. Laryngol. Otol. 113 (5), 439–441. https://doi.org/10.1017/s002221510014416.

Fitzgerald, M.J., Comerford, P.T., Tuffery, A.R., 1982. Sources of innervation of the neuromuscular spindles in sternomastoid and trapezius. J. Anat. 134 (Pt 3), 471–490.

Flores, S., Herring, A.A., 2016. Ultrasound-guided greater auricular nerve block for emergency department ear laceration and ear abscess drainage. J. Emerg. Med. 50 (4), 651–655. https://doi.org/10.1016/j.jemermed.2015.10.003.

Fokkema, M., de Borst, G.J., Nolan, B.W., et al., 2014. Clinical relevance of cranial nerve injury following carotid endarterectomy. Eur. J. Vasc. Endovasc. Surg. 47 (1), 2–7. https://doi.org/10.1016/j.ejvs.2013.09.022.

Gidley, P.W., Ghorayeb, B.Y., Stiernberg, C.M., 1997. Contemporary management of deep neck space infections. Otolaryngol. Head Neck Surg. 116 (1), 16–22. https://doi.org/10.1016/s0194-5998(97)70345-0.

Girard, F., Quentin, C., Charbonneau, S., et al., 2010. Superficial cervical plexus block for transitional analgesia in infratentorial and occipital craniotomy: a randomized trial. Can. J. Anaesth. 57 (12), 1065–1070. https://doi.org/10.1007/s12630-010-9392-3.

Goldberg, M.E., Schwartzman, R.J., Domsky, R., Sabia, M., Torjman, M.C., 2008. Deep cervical plexus block for the treatment of cervicogenic headache. Pain Physician 11 (6), 849–854.

Granite, E.L., 1976. Anatomic considerations in infections of the face and neck: review of the literature. J. Oral Surg. 34 (1), 34–44.

Grodinsky, M., Holyoke, E.A., 1938. The fasciae and fascial spaces of the head, neck and adjacent regions. Am. J. Anat. 63, 367–393.

Guay, J., 2008. Regional anesthesia for carotid surgery. Curr. Opin. Anaesthesiol. 21 (5), 638–644. https://doi.org/10.1097/ACO.0b013e328308bb70.

Guay, J., Grabs, D., 2011. A cadaver study to determine the minimum volume of methylene blue or black naphthol required to completely color the nerves relevant for anesthesia during breast surgery. Clin. Anat. 24 (2), 202–208. https://doi.org/10.1002/ca.21085.

Guidera, A.K., Dawes, P.J., Stringer, M.D., 2012. Cervical fascia: a terminological pain in the neck. ANZ J. Surg. 82 (11), 786–791. https://doi.org/10.1111/j.1445-2197.2012.06231.x.

Guidera, A.K., Dawes, P.J., Fong, A., Stringer, M.D., 2014. Head and neck fascia and compartments: no space for spaces. Head Neck 36 (7), 1058–1068. https://doi.org/10.1002/hed.23442.

Harris, R.J., Benveniste, G., 2000. Recurrent laryngeal nerve blockade in patients undergoing carotid endarterectomy under cervical plexus block. Anaesth. Intensive Care 28 (4), 431–433. https://doi.org/10.1177/0310057X0002800413.

Havet, E., Duparc, F., Tobenas-Dujardin, A.C., Muller, J.M., Freger, P., 2007. Morphometric study of the shoulder and subclavicular innervation by the intermediate and lateral branches of supraclavicular nerves. Surg. Radiol. Anat. 29 (8), 605–610. https://doi.org/10.1007/s00276-007-0258-5.

Hayward, R., 1986. Observations on the innervation of the sternomastoid muscle. J. Neurol. Neurosurg. Psychiatry 49 (8), 951–953. https://doi.org/10.1136/jnnp.49.8.951.

James, A., Niraj, G., 2020. Intermediate cervical plexus block: a novel intervention in the management of refractory chronic neck and upper back pain following whiplash injury: a case report. AA Pract. 14 (6), e01197. https://doi.org/10.1213/XAA.0000000000001197.

Jelev, L., 2013. Some unusual types of formation of the ansa cervicalis in humans and proposal of a new morphological classification. Clin. Anat. 26 (8), 961–965. https://doi.org/10.1002/ca.22265.

Kannan, S., Surhonne, N.S., Chetan Kumar, R., Kavitha, B., Devika Rani, D., Raghavendra Rao, R.S., 2018. Effects of bilateral superficial cervical plexus block on sevoflurane consumption during thyroid surgery under entropy-guided general anesthesia: a prospective randomized study. Korean J. Anesthesiol. 71 (2), 141–148. https://doi.org/10.4097/kjae.2018.71.2.141.

Kefalianakis, F., Koeppel, T., Geldner, G., Gahlen, J., 2005. Carotid-surgery in ultrasound-guided anesthesia of the regio colli lateralis. Anasthesiol. Intensivmed. Notfallmed. Schmerzther. 40 (10), 576–581. https://doi.org/10.1055/s-2005-870377. Ultraschallgestutzte Blockade der Regio colli lateralis zur Karotis-Chirurgie – eine Fallserie.

Kesisoglou, I., Papavramidis, T.S., Michalopoulos, N., et al., 2010. Superficial selective cervical plexus block following total thyroidectomy: a randomized trial. Head Neck 32 (8), 984–988. https://doi.org/10.1002/hed.21286.

Kfoury, E., Dort, J., Trickey, A., et al., 2015. Carotid endarterectomy under local and/or regional anesthesia has less risk of myocardial infarction compared to general anesthesia: an analysis of national surgical quality improvement program database. Vascular 23 (2), 113–119. https://doi.org/10.1177/1708538114537489.

Khaki, A.A., Shokouhi, G., Shoja, M.M., et al., 2006. Ansa cervicalis as a variant of spinal accessory nerve plexus: a case report. Clin. Anat. 19 (6), 540–543. https://doi.org/10.1002/ca.20299.

Kim, J.S., Lee, J., Soh, E.Y., et al., 2016. Analgesic effects of ultrasound-guided serratus-intercostal plane block and ultrasound-guided intermediate cervical plexus block After single-incision transaxillary robotic thyroidectomy: a prospective, randomized, controlled trial. RAPM 41 (5), 584–588. https://doi.org/10.1097/AAP.0000000000000430.

Kim, J.S., Ko, J.S., Bang, S., Kim, H., Lee, S.Y., 2018. Cervical plexus block. Korean J. Anesthesiol. 71 (4), 274–288. https://doi.org/10.4097/kja.d.18.00143.

Kim, J., Joe, H.B., Park, M.C., Lee, S.Y., Chae, Y.J., 2018. Post-operative analgesic effect of ultrasound-guided intermediate cervical plexus block on unipolar sternocleidomastoid release with myectomy in pediatric patients with congenital muscular torticollis: a prospective, randomized, controlled trial. RAPM 43 (6), 534–640. https://doi.org/10.1097/AAP.0000000000000797.

Kim, H.Y., Soh, E.Y., Lee, J., et al., 2020. Incidence of hemi-diaphragmatic paresis after ultrasound-guided intermediate cervical plexus block: a prospective observational study. J. Anesth. 34 (4), 483–490. https://doi.org/10.1007/s00540-020-02770-2.

Koizumi, M., Horiguchi, M., Sekiya, S., Isogai, S., Nakano, M., 1993. A case of the human sternocleidomastoid muscle additionally innervated by the hypoglossal nerve. Okajimas Folia Anat. Jpn. 69 (6), 361–367. https://doi.org/10.2535/ofaj1936.69.6_361.

Kokofer, A., Nawratil, J., Felder, T.K., Stundner, O., Mader, N., Gerner, P., 2015. Ropivacaine 0.375% vs. 0.75% with prilocaine for intermediate cervical plexus block for carotid endarterectomy: a randomised trial. Eur. J. Anaesthesiol. 32 (11), 781–789. https://doi.org/10.1097/EJA.0000000000000243.

Kwok, O.K., Sun, K.O., Ahchong, A.K., Chan, C.K., 2004. Airway obstruction following carotid endarterectomy. Anaesth. Intensive Care 32 (6), 818–820. https://doi.org/10.1177/0310057X0403200615.

Kwok, A.O., Silbert, B.S., Allen, K.J., Bray, P.J., Vidovich, J., 2006. Bilateral vocal cord palsy during carotid endarterectomy under cervical plexus block. Anesth. Analg. 102 (2), 376–377. https://doi.org/10.1213/01.ane.0000189189.47768.42.

Leblanc, I., Chterev, V., Rekik, M., et al., 2015. Safety and efficiency of ultrasound-guided intermediate cervical plexus block for carotid surgery. Anaesth. Crit. Care Pain Med. 35 (2), 109–114. https://doi.org/10.1016/j.accpm.2015.08.004.

Levitt, G.W., 1970. Cervical fascia and deep neck infections. Laryngoscope 80 (3), 409–435. https://doi.org/10.1288/00005537-197003000-00004.

Lyons, A.J., Mills, C.C., 1998. Anatomical variants of the cervical sympathetic chain to be considered during neck dissection. Br. J. Oral Maxillofac. Surg. 36 (3), 180–182. https://doi.org/10.1016/s0266-4356(98)90493-4.

Madro, P., Dabrowska, A., Jarecki, J., Garba, P., 2016. Anaesthesia for carotid endarterectomy. Ultrasound-guided superficial/intermediate cervical plexus block combined with carotid sheath infiltration. Anaesthesiol. Intensive Ther. 48 (4), 234–238. https://doi.org/10.5603/AIT.2016.0043.

Mariappan, R., Mehta, J., Massicotte, E., Nagappa, M., Manninen, P., Venkatraghavan, L., 2015. Effect of superficial cervical plexus block on postoperative quality of recovery after anterior cervical discectomy and fusion: a randomized controlled trial. Can. J. Anaesth. 62 (8), 883–890. https://doi.org/10.1007/s12630-015-0382-3.

Martusevicius, R., Swiatek, F., Joergensen, L.G., Nielsen, H.B., 2012. Ultrasound-guided locoregional anaesthesia for carotid endarterectomy: a prospective observational study. Eur. J. Vasc. Endovasc. Surg. 44 (1), 27–30. https://doi.org/10.1016/j.ejvs.2012.04.008.

Masters, R.D., Castresana, E.J., Castresana, M.R., 1995. Superficial and deep cervical plexus block: technical considerations. Am. Assoc. Nurse Anesth. J. 63 (3), 235–243.

Maybin, J., Townsley, P., Bedforth, N., Allan, A., 2011. Ultrasound guided supraclavicular nerve blockade: first technical description and the relevance for shoulder surgery under regional anaesthesia. Anaesthesia 66 (11), 1053—1055. https://doi.org/10.1111/j.1365-2044.2011.06907.

Merdad, M., Crawford, M., Gordon, K., Papsin, B., 2012. Unexplained fever after bilateral superficial cervical block in children undergoing cochlear implantation: an observational study. Can. J. Anaesth. 59 (1), 28—33. https://doi.org/10.1007/s12630-011-9607-2.

Merle, J.C., Mazoit, J.X., Desgranges, P., et al., 1999. A comparison of two techniques for cervical plexus blockade: evaluation of efficacy and systemic toxicity. Anesth. Analg. 89 (6), 1366—1370. https://doi.org/10.1097/00000539-199912000-00006.

Missaghi, B., 2004. Sternocleidomastoid syndrome: a case study. J. Can. Chiropr. Assoc. 48 (3), 201—205.

Moncada, R., Warpeha, R., Pickleman, J., et al., 1978. Mediastinitis from odontogenic and deep cervical infection. Anatomic pathways of propagation. Chest 73 (4), 497—500. https://doi.org/10.1378/chest.73.4.497.

Moore, K., Dalley, A.F., Agur, A.M.R., 2014. Clinically Oriented Anatomy, seventh ed. Lippincott Williams & Wilkins, Wolters Kluwer business, p. 988.

Nason, R.W., Abdulrauf, B.M., Stranc, M.F., 2000. The anatomy of the accessory nerve and cervical lymph node biopsy. Am. J. Surg. 180 (3), 241—243. https://doi.org/10.1016/s0002-9610(00)00449-9.

Natale, G., Condino, S., Stecco, A., Soldani, P., Belmonte, M.M., Gesi, M., 2015. Is the cervical fascia an anatomical proteus? Surg. Radiol. Anat. 37 (9), 1119—1127. https://doi.org/10.1007/s00276-015-1480-1.

North American Symptomatic Carotid Endarterectomy Trial Collaborators, 1991. Beneficial effect of carotid endarterectomy in symptomatic patients with high-grade carotid stenosis. N. Engl. J. Med. 325 (7), 445—453. https://doi.org/10.1056/NEJM199108153250701.

Pandit, J.J., Bree, S., Dillon, P., Elcock, D., McLaren, I.D., Crider, B., 2000. A comparison of superficial versus combined (superficial and deep) cervical plexus block for carotid endarterectomy: a prospective, randomized study. Anesth. Analg. 91 (4), 781—786. https://doi.org/10.1097/00000539-200010000-00004.

Pandit, J.J., Dutta, D., Morris, J.F., 2003. Spread of injectate with superficial cervical plexus block in humans: an anatomical study. Br. J. Anaesth. 91 (5), 733—735. https://doi.org/10.1093/bja/aeg250.

Pandit, J.J., Satya-Krishna, R., Gration, P., 2007. Superficial or deep cervical plexus block for carotid endarterectomy: a systematic review of complications. Br. J. Anaesth. 99 (2), 159—169. https://doi.org/10.1093/bja/aem160.

Paraskevas, G.K., Natsis, K., Nitsa, Z., Mavrodi, A., Kitsoulis, P., 2014. Unusual morphological pattern and distribution of the ansa cervicalis: a case report. Rom. J. Morphol. Embryol. 55 (3), 993—996.

Paraskevas, G., Lazaridis, N., Spyridakis, I., Koutsouflianiotis, K., Kitsoulis, P., 2015. Aberrant innervation of the sternocleidomastoid muscle by the transverse cervical nerve: a case report. J. Clin. Diagn. Res. 9 (4), AD01—2. https://doi.org/10.7860/JCDR/2015/11787.5757.

Parrot, D., Fontaine, P., Coulon, C., Guyon, P., David, M., 1988. Carotid endarterectomy under cervical plexus block. Cahiers d'anesthesiologie. 36 (4), 255—259 (Endarterectomie carotidienne sous bloc plexique cervical).

Perisanidis, C., Saranteas, T., Kostopanagiotou, G., 2013. Ultrasound-guided combined intermediate and deep cervical plexus nerve block for regional anaesthesia in oral and maxillofacial surgery. Dentomaxillofac. Radiol. 42 (2), 29945724. https://doi.org/10.1259/dmfr/29945724.

Pintaric, T.S., Hocevar, M., Jereb, S., Casati, A., Novak Jankovic, V., 2007. A prospective, randomized comparison between combined (deep and superficial) and superficial cervical plexus block with levobupivacaine for minimally invasive parathyroidectomy. Anesth. Analg. 105 (4), 1160—1163. https://doi.org/10.1213/01.ane.0000280443.03867.12.

Pu, Y.M., Tang, E.Y., Yang, X.D., 2008. Trapezius muscle innervation from the spinal accessory nerve and branches of the cervical plexus. Int. J. Oral Maxillofac. Surg. 37 (6), 567—572. https://doi.org/10.1016/j.ijom.2008.02.002.

Ramachandran, S.K., Picton, P., Shanks, A., Dorje, P., Pandit, J.J., 2011. Comparison of intermediate vs subcutaneous cervical plexus block for carotid endarterectomy. Br. J. Anaesth. 107 (2), 157—163. https://doi.org/10.1093/bja/aer118.

Restrepo, C.E., Tubbs, R.S., Spinner, R.J., 2015. Expanding what is known of the anatomy of the spinal accessory nerve. Clin. Anat. 28 (4), 467—471. https://doi.org/10.1002/ca.22492.

Ritchie, M.K., Wilson, C.A., Grose, B.W., Ranganathan, P., Howell, S.M., Ellison, M.B., 2016. Ultrasound-guided greater auricular nerve block as sole anesthetic for ear surgery. Clin. Pract. 6 (2), 856. https://doi.org/10.4081/cp.2016.856.

Rossel, T., Kersting, S., Heller, A.R., Koch, T., 2013. Combination of high-resolution ultrasound-guided perivascular regional anesthesia of the internal carotid artery and intermediate cervical plexus block for carotid surgery. Ultrasound Med. Biol. 39 (6), 981—986. https://doi.org/10.1016/j.ultrasmedbio.2013.01.002.

Sait Kavakli, A., Kavrut Ozturk, N., Umut Ayoglu, R., et al., 2015. Comparison of combined (deep and superficial) and intermediate cervical plexus block by use of ultrasound guidance for carotid endarterectomy. J. Cardiothorac. Vasc. Anesth. 30 (2), 317—322. https://doi.org/10.1053/j.jvca.2015.07.032.

Sandeman, D.J., Griffiths, M.J., Lennox, A.F., 2006. Ultrasound guided deep cervical plexus block. Anaesth. Intensive Care 34 (2), 240—244. https://doi.org/10.1177/0310057X0603400201.

Saranteas, T., Kostopanagiotou, G.G., Anagnostopoulou, S., Mourouzis, K., Sidiropoulou, T., 2011. A simple method for blocking the deep cervical nerve plexus using an ultrasound-guided technique. Anaesth. Intensive Care 39 (5), 971—972.

Seidel, R., Schulze, M., Zukowski, K., Wree, A., 2015. Ultrasound-guided intermediate cervical plexus block. Anatomical study. Anaesthesist 64 (6), 446–450. Ultraschallgesteuerte intermediare zervikale Plexusanasthesie: Anatomische Untersuchung doi.org/10.1007/s00101-015-0018-6.

Seidel, R., Zukowski, K., Wree, A., Schulze, M., 2016. Ultrasound-guided intermediate cervical plexus block and perivascular local anesthetic infiltration for carotid endarterectomy : a randomized controlled trial. Anaesthesist. https://doi.org/10.1007/s00101-016-0230-z. Ultraschallgesteuerte intermediare Blockade des Plexus cervicalis und perivaskulare lokale Infiltrationsanasthesie vor Karotisendarteriektomie : Eine randomisierte, kontrollierte Studie.

Shakespeare, T.J., Tsui, B.C., 2013. Intermittent hoarseness with continuous interscalene brachial plexus catheter infusion due to deficient carotid sheath. Acta Anaesthesiol. Scand. 57 (8), 1085–1086. https://doi.org/10.1111/aas.12147.

Shin, H.J., Yu, H.N., Yoon, S.Z., 2014. Ultrasound-guided subcutaneous cervical plexus block for carotid endarterectomy in a patient with chronic obstructive pulmonary disease. J. Anesth. 28 (2), 304–305. https://doi.org/10.1007/s00540-013-1702-9.

Shoja, M.M., Oyesiku, N.M., Shokouhi, G., et al., 2014. A comprehensive review with potential significance during skull base and neck operations, part II: glossopharyngeal, vagus, accessory, and hypoglossal nerves and cervical spinal nerves 1-4. Clin. Anat. 27 (1), 131–144. https://doi.org/10.1002/ca.22342.

Smoker, W.R., Harnsberger, H.R., 1991. Differential diagnosis of head and neck lesions based on their space of origin. The infrahyoid portion of the neck. Am. J. Roentgenol. 157 (1), 155–159. https://doi.org/10.2214/ajr.157.1.2048511.

Standring, S., 2016. Gray's anatomy. In: The Anatomical Basis of Clincal Practice, forty oneth ed. Churchill Livingstone Elsevier, Edinburg, p. 41.

Standring, S., 2016. Gray's anatomy. In: The Anaotomical Basis of Clinical Practice, forty oneth ed. Churchill Livingstone Elsevier, Edinburg, pp. 463–464.

Standring, S., 2016. Gray's anatomy. In: The Anatomical Basis of Clinical Practice, forty oneth ed. Churchill Livingstone Elsevier, Edinburg, p. 445.

Standring, S., 2017. Gray's anatomy. In: The Anatomical Basis of Clinical Practice, forty oneth ed. Churchill Livingstone Elsevier, Edinburg, p. 468.

Stecco, A., Meneghini, A., Stern, R., Stecco, C., Imamura, M., 2014. Ultrasonography in myofascial neck pain: randomized clinical trial for diagnosis and follow-up. Surg. Radiol. Anat. 36 (3), 243–253. https://doi.org/10.1007/s00276-013-1185-2.

Stoneham, M.D., Doyle, A.R., Knighton, J.D., Dorje, P., Stanley, J.C., 1998. Prospective, randomized comparison of deep or superficial cervical plexus block for carotid endarterectomy surgery. Anesthesiology 89 (4), 907–912.

Stoneham, M.D., Stamou, D., Mason, J., 2015. Regional anaesthesia for carotid endarterectomy. Br. J. Anaesth. 114 (3), 372–383. https://doi.org/10.1093/bja/aeu304.

Suresh, S., Barcelona, S.L., Young, N.M., Seligman, I., Heffner, C.L., Cote, C.J., 2002. Postoperative pain relief in children undergoing tympanomastoid surgery: is a regional block better than opioids? Anesth. Analg. 94 (4), 859–862. https://doi.org/10.1097/00000539-200204000-00015.

Suzuki, S., Yasunaga, H., Matsui, H., Fushimi, K., Saito, Y., Yamasoba, T., 2016. Factors associated with neck hematoma after thyroidectomy: a retrospective analysis using a Japanese inpatient database. Medicine 95 (7), e2812. https://doi.org/10.1097/MD.0000000000002812.

Symes, A., Ellis, H., 2005. Variations in the surface anatomy of the spinal accessory nerve in the posterior triangle. Surg. Radiol. Anat. 27 (5), 404–408. https://doi.org/10.1007/s00276-005-0004-9.

Telford, R.J., Stoneham, M.D., 2004. Correct nomenclature of superficial cervical plexus blocks. Br. J. Anaesth. 92 (5), 775. https://doi.org/10.1093/bja/aeh550 author reply 775-6.

Thawale, R., Alva, S., Niraj, G., 2019. Ultrasound-guided intermediate cervical plexus block with depot steroids in the management of refractory neck pain secondary to cervicothoracic myofascial pain syndrome: a case series. AA Pract. 13 (12), 446–449. https://doi.org/10.1213/XAA.0000000000001102.

Townsley, P., Ravenscroft, A., Bedforth, N., 2011. Ultrasound-guided spinal accessory nerve blockade in the diagnosis and management of trapezius muscle-related myofascial pain. Anaesthesia 66 (5), 386–389. https://doi.org/10.1111/j.1365-2044.2011.06691.x.

Tschopp, K.P., Gysin, C., 1996. Local injection therapy in 107 patients with myofascial pain syndrome of the head and neck. ORL J. Otorhinolaryngol. Relat. Spec. 58 (6), 306–310. https://doi.org/10.1159/000276860.

Tubbs, R.S., Salter, E.G., Wellons 3rd, J.C., Blount, J.P., Oakes, W.J., 2005. Superficial landmarks for the spinal accessory nerve within the posterior cervical triangle. J. Neurosurg. Spine 3 (5), 375–378. https://doi.org/10.3171/spi.2005.3.5.0375.

Tubbs, R.S., Loukas, M., Shoja, M.M., Salter, E.G., Oakes, W.J., Blount, J.P., 2006. Approach to the cervical portion of the vagus nerve via the posterior cervical triangle: a cadaveric feasibility study with potential use in vagus nerve stimulation procedures. J. Neurosurg. Spine 5 (6), 540–542. https://doi.org/10.3171/spi.2006.5.6.540.

Tubbs, R.S., Sorenson, E.P., Watanabe, K., Loukas, M., Hattab, E., Cohen-Gadol, A.A., 2014. Histologic confirmation of neuronal cell bodies along the spinal accessory nerve. Br. J. Neurosurg. 28 (6), 746–749. https://doi.org/10.3109/02688697.2014.920485.

Usui, Y., Kobayashi, T., Kakinuma, H., Watanabe, K., Kitajima, T., Matsuno, K., 2010. An anatomical basis for blocking of the deep cervical plexus and cervical sympathetic tract using an ultrasound-guided technique. Anesth. Analg. 110 (3), 964–968. https://doi.org/10.1213/ANE.0b013e3181c91ea0.

Wan, Q., Yang, H., Li, X., et al., 2017. Ultrasound-guided versus fluoroscopy-guided deep cervical plexus block for the treatment of cervicogenic headache. Biomed Res. Int. 2017, 4654803. https://doi.org/10.1155/2017/4654803.

Weiss, A., Isselhorst, C., Gahlen, J., et al., 2005. Acute respiratory failure after deep cervical plexus block for carotid endarterectomy as a result of bilateral recurrent laryngeal nerve paralysis. Acta Anaesthesiol. Scand. 49 (5), 715−719. https://doi.org/10.1111/j.1399-6576.2005.00694.x.

Winnie, A.P., Ramamurthy, S., Durrani, Z., Radonjic, R., 1975. Interscalene cervical plexus block: a single-injection technic. Anesth. Analg. 54 (3), 370−375. https://doi.org/10.1213/00000539-197505000-00030.

Yerzingatsian, K.L., 1989. Thyroidectomy under local analgesia: the anatomical basis of cervical blocks. Ann. R. Coll. Surg. Engl. 71 (4), 207−210.

Yoshizaki, F., 1961. Innervation of sternocleidomastoid muscle of man and the rabbit. Okayama Igakkai Zasshi 73 (1), 159−171.

Zhang, M., Lee, A.S., 2002. The investing layer of the deep cervical fascia does not exist between the sternocleidomastoid and trapezius muscles. Otolaryngol. Head Neck Surg. 127 (5), 452−454. https://doi.org/10.1067/mhn.2002.129823.

Zhang, M., Nicholson, H.D., Nash, L., 2006. Investing layer of the cervical fascia of the neck may not exit. Anesthesiology 104, 1344. https://doi.org/10.1097/00000542-200606000-00038 author reply 1344-1345.

CHAPTER 17

Surgery of the Cervical Plexus

MITCHELL D. KILGORE • CASSIDY WERNER • MANSOUR MATHKOUR • C.J. BUI •
R. SHANE TUBBS

ANSA CERVICALIS

Anatomy and Clinical Significance

The ansa cervicalis is a complex of nerves that receives contributions from C1 through C3 and provides efferent innervation to the infrahyoid muscles of the anterior neck (Kikuta et al., 2019). While it commonly exhibits variable anatomy, the nerve typically consists of a superior root that arises from C1 and C2 and descends alongside the hypoglossal nerve inferiorly where it then meets the inferior root that arises from C2 and C3 and forms a loop, of which several branches are projected to innervate individual infrahyoid muscles (Kikuta et al., 2019). Given its large anatomic distribution, the ansa cervicalis is understandably vulnerable to iatrogenic damage during many anterior neck procedures (Kikuta et al., 2019).

Use in Neurotization Procedures

The ansa cervicalis is a particularly useful candidate in the setting of unilateral vocal fold paralysis (UVFP), where it may be used to reinnervate intrinsic muscles of the larynx (Paniello, 2004). Neuropathic loss of these muscles in UVFP results in several significant adverse manifestations including impaired deglutition and phonation, and in severe instances, aspiration that may become life-threatening (Hartl and Brasnu, 2000). UVFP may arise from several etiologies and, interestingly, the choice of surgical reinnervation technique is largely etiology-specific (Aynehchi et al., 2010). Accordingly, an ansa cervicalis to recurrent laryngeal nerve anastomosis (ansa-RLN) has been most frequently studied for use in patients with UVFP caused by mediastinal tumors or prior spine surgery (Aynehchi et al., 2010). The most effective branch for use in ansa-RLN, however, depends on the goal of reinnervation (Paniello, 2004). Due to differences in normal physiologic function, the branch of the ansa cervicalis that innervates the sternohyoid may be best for adductor reinnervation, whereas abductor reinnervation may be best achieved by the branches to the sternothyroid and omohyoid (Paniello, 2004). In any case, it has been shown that early ansa-RLN is associated with significantly better functional outcomes compared to longer durations of denervation and, in instances of UVFP of iatrogenic etiology, this makes a strong case for pursuing immediate neurotization whenever possible (Li et al., 2014).

LESSER OCCIPITAL NERVE

Anatomy and Clinical Significance

Predominantly arising from the ventral ramus of C2 with contributions from C3, the lesser occipital nerve is responsible for supplying sensation to portions of the occipital and postauricular scalp (Cesmebasi et al., 2015). Due to its anatomical course, the lesser occipital nerve may be stretched, compressed, or otherwise damaged while traversing several structures including the inferior oblique muscle, the atlantoaxial junction, or the vertebral artery en route to its distal regions of innervation (Cesmebasi et al., 2015). The resultant local perineural irritation may be implicated in occipital neuralgias and other head and neck pain syndromes and, as such, the nerve is occasionally targeted for therapeutic surgical decompression in pathologies that are refractory to medical management (Blake and Burstein, 2019; Lee et al., 2013).

The lesser occipital nerve remains indirectly implicated in many head and neck procedures due to its close proximity to the surgical field. For instance, during retrosigmoid craniotomy, the traditional approach involves a linear incision that begins just posterior to the mastoid groove and transverses laterally toward the external occipital protuberance (Tubbs et al., 2016). Such an incision is likely to transect the lesser occipital nerve proximal to its trunk, which may cause chronic postoperative neuralgia and discomfort for the patient (Tubbs et al., 2016). Accordingly, a modified

Surgical Anatomy of the Cervical Plexus and its Branches. https://doi.org/10.1016/B978-0-323-83132-1.00010-X

curvilinear "U" incision, which is designed to circum-navigate the more common lesser occipital nerve courses, is a useful alternative approach for sparing the nerve to prevent these postoperative deficits in this setting (Tubbs et al., 2016). Similar modified, sensory-sparing surgical approaches have been described in other related settings, all of which have been designed with the vulnerable superficial anatomy of this nerve in mind (Pantaloni and Sullivan, 2000; Lee et al., 2017; Chen et al., 2018; Zeng et al., 2020).

Surgical Decompression and Neurectomy

Several superficial surgical approaches may be utilized successfully in this context. In focal neuralgias, one such approach is to instruct the patient to accurately define the region of the occiput associated with maximal pain and discomfort and to subsequently incise and explore the region locally to isolate involved segments of the lesser occipital nerve, at which time targeted neurolysis or neurectomy may be performed (Lee et al., 2013). Using this same technique, branches of the occipital artery that are found to cross or intertwine with the involved portions of the lesser occipital nerve may concurrently be isolated or considered for ligation (Lee et al., 2013). An alternative approach targeted for total lesser occipital neuralgia release may be performed via a small incision along the middle third of the posterior border of the sternocleidomastoid, at which point the proximal trunk of the lesser occipital nerve is identifiable just deep to the deep fascia and may be decompressed or resected entirely (Ducic et al., 2009; Afifi et al., 2019). In any case, decompression and neurolysis without neurectomy have been shown to be highly successful and preserve lesser occipital nerve distribution sensation, which suggests these approaches should be used as first-line surgical treatments followed by neurectomy in instances where they are unsuccessful (Peled et al., 2016).

To a lesser extent, lesser occipital neuralgias may be associated with C2 or C3 root entrapment, which most often occurs secondary to cervical spondylosis (Poletti, 1983). In this setting, fascial and foraminal decompression may result in favorable regression of lesser occipital nerve-related pathologies (Ducic et al., 2009). Other, more aggressive denervating procedures including gangliotomy or rhizotomy of the involved cervical rootlets may also provide some therapeutic relief, though these procedures are associated with significant adverse outcomes including severe postoperative vertigo and nausea, scalp anesthesia, and, in rare instances, cerebrospinal fluid leak (Ducic et al., 2009; Dubuisson, 1995). It is also important to consider that neuralgias due to C2 root entrapment may involve distributions of several additional nerves including the greater occipital, great auricular, and transverse cervical nerves due to their receiving shared input from this spinal level, and all may benefit from cervical decompression when implicated. However, these procedures should not be performed in instances of isolated lesser occipital neuralgias due to the unavoidable and unnecessary sacrifice of these other sensory innervations.

GREAT AURICULAR NERVE
Anatomy and Clinical Significance

The great auricular nerve (GAN) is a cutaneous branch of the cervical plexus that arises from spinal nerves C2 and C3 (Humphrey and Kriet, 2008). It ascends superiorly along the posterior border of the sternocleidomastoid (SCM) muscle before coursing obliquely toward the ear, where it most commonly bifurcates into anterior and posterior branches (Werner et al., 2020). The areas supplied by the GAN include the skin over the mandible, parotid gland, mastoid process, external acoustic meatus, and parts of the auricle (Alberti, 1962; Som et al., 2011; Sharma et al., 2017). Clinical significance of the GAN is primarily related to its incidental resection during parotidectomy to increase exposure (Fiacchini et al., 2018) or inadvertent neurapraxia during rhytidectomy secondary to manipulation of the SCM in the proximity of the posterior branch of the GAN (Lefkowitz et al., 2013). In the case of resection, symptoms include chronic hypoesthesia and dysesthesia along its cutaneous distribution (Werner et al., 2020; Altafulla et al., 2019). Sensory changes after rhytidectomy are typically transient (Lefkowitz et al., 2013).

Facial Nerve Reconstruction

Nerve grafting for facial nerve reconstruction was historically conducted using sural nerve grafts until the late 20th century when surgeons began using the GAN (Werner et al., 2020). Major benefits, when compared to the sural nerve, include closer proximity to the facial nerve (Alberti, 1962) and numerous surgical landmarks owing to the GAN's consistent anatomical position (McKinney and Katrana, 1980). The major disadvantage is that GAN nerve resection confers more noticeable sensory deficits (Wolford and Rodrigues, 2011). Classically, the anatomical landmark for identifying the GAN is McKinney's point (6.5 cm below the inferior wall of the external acoustic meatus and 0.5 cm posterior to the external jugular vein) (McKinney and Katrana, 1980); however various authors have described additional landmarks (Altafulla et al., 2019; Raikos et al., 2017; Tubbs et al., 2007a,b). Many surgeons have reported successful repair of facial nerve function using the GAN as the donor (Werner et al., 2020). Koshima et al. described a one-stage pedicle graft technique and postulated that a vascularized nerve graft is more suitable for elderly patients with diminished revascularization ability or patients undergoing radiation therapy (Koshima et al., 2004).

Additionally, GAN grafts have been used to repair the inferior alveolar nerve (Taraquois et al., 2016) and spinal accessory nerve (Weisberger et al., 1998).

Use in Neurotization Procedures

The GAN has recently been employed for corneal neurotization in patients with neurotrophic keratopathy secondary to trigeminal nerve insult (Benkhatar et al., 2018; Jowett and Pineda Ii, 2019). An ipsilateral GAN interposition graft has been used to bridge the gap between the supratrochlear and supraorbital nerves and the anesthetic cornea (Jowett and Pineda Ii, 2019). Scleral-corneal tunnel incisions were used to facilitate neurotization. As compared to direct use of the contralateral supratrochlear nerve, neurotization with the GAN provides a larger nerve with a higher axon count and can lead to restored ipsilateral referred sensation. Moreover, the diameter of the sural nerve is significantly larger than that of the supratrochlear nerve, and thus the smaller GAN is a more suitable donor (Benkhatar et al., 2018).

Local Anesthetic Blockade

Trigeminal (Rowland, 1955), glossopharyngeal (Aoki and Tokunaga, 1965), and great auricular (Duvall et al., 2020) neuralgias have all been temporarily treated with GAN blocks. Although there are currently many available preferred treatments for trigeminal neuralgia (Jones et al., 2019), in 1955 Rowland described his technique of procaine injection of the GAN on the deep cervical fascia at the posterior border of the SCM one-third of its length from the inferior border (Rowland, 1955).

In one case report, lidocaine was into the layer between the platysma and SCM to treat glossopharyngeal neuralgia. In a second case, the same authors performed a great auricular neurotomy that showed a reduction in neuralgia symptoms. A cadaveric study with dogs revealed overlap between sensory nerves from the upper cervical segment (e.g., the GAN) and the glossopharyngeal nerves in the pharynx, which provided an anatomical explanation for the treatment's success. In contrast to direct glossopharyngeal nerve blocks, the GAN method avoided incidental weakness of the facial, vagus, and hypoglossal nerves (Aoki and Tokunaga, 1965).

TRANSVERSE CERVICAL NERVE
Anatomy and Clinical Significance

The transverse cervical nerve receives contributions from the ventral rami of C2 and C3 to provide sensation to the skin of the anterolateral neck (Brennan et al., 2017). The nerve is grossly identifiable on cervical dissection where it traverses the posterior border of the midpoint of the sternocleidomastoid and courses anteriorly before dividing into ascending and descending cutaneous branches (Brennan et al., 2017).

Intraoperative transverse cervical nerve injury may be a result of direct neurectomy during dissection of the anterolateral neck but may also be caused by stretching, clamping, or retraction of proximal tissues containing minor branches of the nerve (Schauber et al., 1997). Historically, the risk of nerve damage of this etiology has remained high in all anterior neck procedures, as postoperative transverse cervical nerve injury has been demonstrated to occur in more than two-thirds of patients in certain surgical contexts, where only mild function recovery is reported by a small proportion of patients at long-term follow-up (Dehn and Taylor, 1983; Aldoori and Baird, 1988). However, recent advances in high-resolution ultrasound have allowed for the direct visualization of the transverse cervical nerve in real-time, which may aid in preoperative diagnosis as well as intraoperative navigation to decrease the risk of these possible adverse outcomes (Drlicek et al., 2020). It is also important to note that, in instances where other nearby critical nerves are acutely injured during anterolateral neck surgery, the transverse cervical nerve may be a suitable candidate to sacrifice for use in immediate intraoperative grafting to reanneal the damaged nerve and preserve function (Simó et al., 2020).

Maxillofacial Implications

Surgical implications of the transverse cervical nerve may concern its superficial anesthetization before head and neck procedures as well as its potential to sustain intraoperative damage therein. The former may especially relate to maxillofacial procedures, as nervous anastomoses may occasionally be encountered between the transverse cranial nerve and the lower branches of the facial nerve (Domet et al., 2005; Brennan et al., 2019; Marcuzzo et al., 2020). Interestingly, in patients with these anatomical variations, intraoperative stimulation of the transverse cervical nerve may deceitfully cause contractions of muscles innervated by the facial nerve despite its physiologic role as a sensory tract, which may confuse the surgeon and highlights the need to remain vigilant when identifying and operating around nerves in this region (Brennan et al., 2017, 2019). The transverse cervical nerve has also been shown to occasionally enter the lingual foramina, which may necessitate the administration of extraalveolar anesthesia in procedures involving the mandible (Bitner et al., 2015; Kim et al., 2016).

SUPRACLAVICULAR NERVE
Anatomy and Clinical Significance
The supraclavicular nerve receives contributions from C3 and C4 before dividing into the medial, intermediate, and lateral branches (Tubbs et al., 2006). Respectively, these provide sensation to the skin from the midclavicle inferiorly to the sternal angle, the anterior axial line, and the pectoralis major and anterolateral deltoid (Tubbs et al., 2006). Given its expansive sensory distribution, the nerve is frequently implicated in pathologies and surgeries that involve the superior thorax, shoulder, and upper extremity.

Injury to the supraclavicular nerve is frequently due to either clavicular fracture or subsequent surgical repair. The nerve's branches are particularly susceptible to damage during diaphyseal clavicle fracture given their anatomical course directly superior to this region (Labronici et al., 2013). At the time of fracture, patients may sustain damage that presents with neuropathic symptoms in the distributions of the nerve, though in some instances, these may resolve spontaneously (Labronici et al., 2013). However, persistent symptomatology may indicate that the supraclavicular nerve has become encased in the healing bone callus or proximal fibrous scar tissue, which may necessitate surgical exploration and subsequent neurolysis to resolve (Mehta and Birch, 1997; Jupiter and Leibman, 2007). Furthermore, severe open or comminuted clavicular fractures require open reduction and internal fixation (ORIF) to accommodate healing, which is associated with iatrogenic supraclavicular neuropathy in as many as one out of every two cases (Wang et al., 2010). To minimize this risk, vertical incisions that parallel the course of the supraclavicular nerve may be used in conjunction with intentional suprascapular nerve-sparing dissection techniques, although the effectiveness of these measures is limited by the moderately variable course of the nerve's branches (Wang et al., 2010; Huang et al., 2020; Nathe et al., 2011). However, recently developed alternatives to conventional clavicular ORIF including minimally invasive plate osteosynthesis have also shown promise for further reducing iatrogenic supraclavicular neuropathy rates in this setting (You et al., 2018).

Use in Neurotization Procedures
The supraclavicular nerve has also been used as a donor sensory tract in several novel neurotization procedures. One such application was demonstrated in sternoclavicular joint reconstruction using an autografted metatarsophalangeal joint, in which the supraclavicular nerve was coapted to the grafted tissue's deep fibular nerve trunk to provide restored sensation to the joint (Bendon and Giele, 2014). Another involved superior reflection of the supraclavicular nerve with subsequent coaptation to the mental nerve of the trigeminal distribution to restore lower lip sensation in a patient suffering palsy following cerebrovascular accident (Mucci and Dellon, 1997). However, perhaps the most common neurotization application of the supraclavicular nerve is in sensory reinnervation following upper brachial plexus injury. In these patients, damage to the plexus's upper cervical contributions results in an array of neuropathies that include loss of sensation to portions of the hand. With this in mind, the supraclavicular nerve has several advantages as a sensory donor in this setting, considering its anatomic location, size, and identifiability (Seruya et al., 2013). Thus, attempts have been successfully made to coapt the nerve to several regions of the brachial plexus including the roots of C5 and C6, the lateral cord, and the median nerve directly, with the goal of restoring some degree of sensate prehensile function to the hand (Seruya et al., 2013; Doi et al., 1991, 1995; Ihara et al., 1996). Notably, the utility of this methodology extends to the setting of pediatric brachial plexus injury, which may otherwise be a devastating pathology with life-long consequences (Seruya et al., 2013). However, given the supraclavicular nerve's exclusive role as a cutaneous nerve, it is important to recognize that its use in brachial plexus reinnervation will not address the motor deficits associated with the pathology and must be used in tandem with other motor reinnervation procedures if these are to be addressed.

PHRENIC NERVE
Anatomy and Clinical Significance
Arising from the ventral rami of C3 through C5, the phrenic nerve courses inferiorly through the superior thoracic aperture and the mediastinum, where it ultimately provides motor innervation to the diaphragm, allowing for respiration and sensory innervation of the central diaphragm (Ricoy et al., 2019). It also provides afferent visceral sensation to the diaphragmatic and mediastinal parts of the parietal pleura as well as the fibrous pericardium. Lesions to the phrenic nerve may cause hemidiaphragm paralysis, which results in

significant respiratory dysfunction. Accordingly, it is one of the most important nerves of the body.

Unsurprisingly, cardiothoracic surgery is a major cause of iatrogenic injury to the phrenic nerve (Ostrowska and de Carvalho, 2012). Its intricate anatomical relationship with the compact contents of the mediastinum makes unintentional contact inevitable during many surgical procedures (Aguirre et al., 2013). Additionally, phrenic nerve sacrifice may be necessary for many mediastinal neoplastic processes where nerve infiltration occurs (Kawashima et al., 2015).

Nerve Reconstruction

Surgical reconstruction of this vital nerve remains a highly relevant area of study. In instances where sufficient viable phrenic nerve trunk is available on either side of the lesion such that anastomotic tension can be prevented, the direct end-to-end anastomosis may be performed (Kawashima et al., 2015; Shinohara et al., 2017). If there is not sufficient phrenic trunk for direct coaptation, portions of the intercostal nerve may be harvested for grafting between proximal and distal ends of the phrenic nerve (Kawashima et al., 2015). However, in either case, treatment should ideally be pursued immediately upon recognition of the phrenic nerve deficit.

Phrenic Nerve Stimulation

Phrenic nerve palsy may also be caused by high cervical spinal cord injury if it occurs at or above the level of the phrenic motor neurons, which leads to diaphragmatic paralysis necessitating long-term mechanical ventilation unless innervation can be restored (Sieg et al., 2016). The outlook is poor in these patients and, unfortunately, surgical intervention in this setting currently remains limited. Phrenic nerve stimulation is a potentially safe and effective surgical option for decreasing ventilator dependence, although many critical questions regarding periprocedural variables including optimal surgical approach and intervention timing following injury, long-term efficacy, and impact on the quality of life have yet to be answered (Sieg et al., 2016). Notably, this technique requires an intact phrenic nerve to be successful, so in cases where phrenic integrity is known to be impaired, intercostal to phrenic nerve neurotization may be performed and subsequently followed by implantation of a diaphragmatic pacer to achieve successful reinnervation (Nandra et al., 2017). Aside from nerve stimulation, a cadaveric study has demonstrated that the phrenic nerve may be a recipient of neurotization by the spinal accessory nerve, which possesses a cranial nerve component that remains intact in these injuries (Tubbs et al., 2008).

Use in Neurotization Procedures

Owing to the relatively large number of efferent fibers it contains, the phrenic nerve has several implications as a motor donor in neurotization surgery (Gu and Ma, 1996). In the setting of brachial plexus injury, particularly of the avulsion type, it may be used to reinnervate the musculocutaneous nerve to restore biceps function (Gu and Ma, 1996). Yet, because of its anatomical contributions from C5, avulsion injury to the upper components of the brachial plexus may damage portions of the phrenic nerve, making it a less viable candidate for this application (Wood and Murray, 2007). Additionally, in laryngeal paralysis, the upper root of a unilateral phrenic nerve may be anastomosed bilaterally via an intermediate free nerve graft to the recurrent laryngeal nerve with the satisfactory restoration of function (Li et al., 2019). Considering its principle physiological role in respiration, some suggest the phrenic nerve may even be a more appropriate donor than the ansa cervicalis for reinnervating laryngeal abductors (Fancello et al., 2017). However, regardless of the application, there always exists a risk of inducing respiratory dysfunction when the phrenic nerve is used as a donor in neurotization procedures, and preservation of diaphragmatic function must be prioritized at all times (Socolovsky et al., 2015).

REFERENCES

Afifi, A.M., Carbullido, M.K., Israel, J.S., Sanchez, R.J., Albano, N.J., 2019. Alternative approach for occipital headache surgery: the use of a transverse incision and "W" flaps. Plast. Reconstr. Surg. Glob Open 7 (4), e2176. https://doi.org/10.1097/GOX.0000000000002176.

Aguirre, V.J., Sinha, P., Zimmet, A., Lee, G.A., Kwa, L., Rosenfeldt, F., 2013. Phrenic nerve injury during cardiac surgery: mechanisms, management and prevention. Heart Lung Circ. 22 (11), 895–902. https://doi.org/10.1016/j.hlc.2013.06.010.

Alberti, P.W., 1962. The greater auricular nerve. Donor for facial nerve grafts: a note on its topographical anatomy. Arch. Otolaryngol. 76, 422–424. https://doi.org/10.1001/archotol.1962.00740050434007.

Aldoori, M.I., Baird, R.N., 1988. Local neurological complication during carotid endarterectomy. J. Cardiovasc. Surg. 29 (4), 432–436.

Altafulla, J., Iwanaga, J., Lachkar, S., et al., 2019. The great auricular nerve: anatomical study with application to nerve grafting procedures. World Neurosurg. 125, e403–e407. https://doi.org/10.1016/j.wneu.2019.01.087.

Aoki, H., Tokunaga, Y., 1965. A new approach to the treatment of glossopharyngeal neuralgia, using the great auricular nerve block. Folia Psychiatr. Neurol. Jpn. 19 (4), 346–354. https://doi.org/10.1111/j.1440-1819.1965.tb01219.x.

Aynehchi, B.B., McCoul, E.D., Sundaram, K., 2010. Systematic review of laryngeal reinnervation techniques. Otolaryngol.

Head Neck Surg. 143 (6), 749–759. https://doi.org/10.1016/j.otohns.2010.09.031.

Bendon, C.L., Giele, H.P., 2014. Second toe metatarsophalangeal joint transfer for sternoclavicular joint reconstruction. J. Hand Surg. Am. 39 (7), 1327–1332. https://doi.org/10.1016/j.jhsa.2014.03.027.

Benkhatar, H., Levy, O., Goemaere, I., Borderie, V., Laroche, L., Bouheraoua, N., 2018. Corneal neurotization with a great auricular nerve graft: effective reinnervation demonstrated by in vivo confocal microscopy. Cornea 37 (5), 647–650. https://doi.org/10.1097/ico.0000000000001549.

Bitner, D.P., Uzbelger Feldman, D., Axx, K., Albandar, J.M., 2015. Description and evaluation of an intraoral cervical plexus anesthetic technique. Clin. Anat. 28 (5), 608–613. https://doi.org/10.1002/ca.22543.

Blake, P., Burstein, R., 2019. Emerging evidence of occipital nerve compression in unremitting head and neck pain. J. Headache Pain 20 (1), 76. https://doi.org/10.1186/s10194-019-1023-y.

Brennan, P.A., Elhamshary, A.S., Alam, P., Anand, R., Ammar, M., 2017. Anastomosis between the transverse cervical nerve and marginal mandibular nerve: how often does it occur? Br. J. Oral Maxillofac. Surg. 55 (3), 293–295. https://doi.org/10.1016/j.bjoms.2016.08.025.

Brennan, P.A., Mak, J., Massetti, K., Parry, D.A., 2019. Communication between the transverse cervical nerve (C2,3) and marginal mandibular branch of the facial nerve: a cadaveric and clinical study. Br. J. Oral Maxillofac. Surg. 57 (3), 232–235. https://doi.org/10.1016/j.bjoms.2018.10.289.

Cesmebasi, A., Muhleman, M.A., Hulsberg, P., et al., 2015. Occipital neuralgia: anatomic considerations. Clin. Anat. 28 (1), 101–108. https://doi.org/10.1002/ca.22468.

Chen, F., Wen, J., Li, P., et al., 2018. Crutchlike incision along the mastoid groove and above the occipital artery protects the lesser occipital nerve and occipital artery in microvascular decompression surgery. World Neurosurg. 120, e755–e761. https://doi.org/10.1016/j.wneu.2018.08.162.

Dehn, T.C., Taylor, G.W., 1983. Cranial and cervical nerve damage associated with carotid endarterectomy. Br. J. Surg. 70 (6), 365–368. https://doi.org/10.1002/bjs.1800700619.

Doi, K., Sakai, K., Kuwata, N., Ihara, K., Kawai, S., 1991. Reconstruction of finger and elbow function after complete avulsion of the brachial plexus. J. Hand Surg. Am. 16 (5), 796–803. https://doi.org/10.1016/s0363-5023(10)80138-8.

Doi, K., Sakai, K., Kuwata, N., Ihara, K., Kawai, S., 1995. Double free-muscle transfer to restore prehension following complete brachial plexus avulsion. J. Hand Surg. Am. 20 (3), 408–414. https://doi.org/10.1016/S0363-5023(05)80097-8.

Domet, M.A., Connor, N.P., Heisey, D.M., Hartig, G.K., 2005. Anastomoses between the cervical branch of the facial nerve and the transverse cervical cutaneous nerve. Am. J. Otolaryngol. 26 (3), 168–171. https://doi.org/10.1016/j.amjoto.2004.11.018.

Drlicek, G., Riegler, G., Pivec, C., et al., 2020. High-resolution ultrasonography of the transverse cervical nerve. Ultrasound Med. Biol. 46 (7), 1599–1607. https://doi.org/10.1016/j.ultrasmedbio.2020.02.003.

Dubuisson, D., 1995. Treatment of occipital neuralgia by partial posterior rhizotomy at C1-3. J. Neurosurg. 82 (4), 581–586. https://doi.org/10.3171/jns.1995.82.4.0581.

Ducic, I., Hartmann, E.C., Larson, E.E., 2009. Indications and outcomes for surgical treatment of patients with chronic migraine headaches caused by occipital neuralgia. Plast. Reconstr. Surg. 123 (5), 1453–1461. https://doi.org/10.1097/PRS.0b013e3181a0720e.

Duvall, J.R., Garza, I., Kissoon, N.R., Robertson, C.E., 2020. Great auricular neuralgia: case series. Headache 60 (1), 247–258. https://doi.org/10.1111/head.13690.

Fancello, V., Nouraei, S.A.R., Heathcote, K.J., 2017. Role of reinnervation in the management of recurrent laryngeal nerve injury: current state and advances. Curr. Opin. Otolaryngol. Head Neck Surg. 25 (6), 480–485. https://doi.org/10.1097/MOO.0000000000000416.

Fiacchini, G., Cerchiai, N., Trico, D., et al., 2018. Frey syndrome, first bite syndrome, great auricular nerve morbidity, and quality of life following parotidectomy. Eur. Arch. Oto-Rhino-Laryngol. 275 (7), 1893–1902. https://doi.org/10.1007/s00405-018-5014-4.

Gu, Y.D., Ma, M.K., 1996. Use of the phrenic nerve for brachial plexus reconstruction. Clin. Orthop. Relat. Res. (323), 119–121. https://doi.org/10.1097/00003086-199602000-00016.

Hartl, D.M., Brasnu, D.F., 2000. Recurrent laryngeal nerve paralysis: current concepts and treatment: part I-phylogenesis and physiology. Ear Nose Throat J. 79 (11), 858. https://doi.org/10.1177/014556130007901109.

Huang, D., Deng, Y., Cheng, J., Bong, Y.R., Schwass, M., Policinski, I., 2020. Comparison of patient reported outcomes following clavicle operative fixation using supraclavicular nerve sparing and supraclavicular nerve sacrificing techniques- a cohort study. Injury. https://doi.org/10.1016/j.injury.2020.10.100.

Humphrey, C.D., Kriet, J.D., 2008. Nerve repair and cable grafting for facial paralysis. Facial Plast. Surg. 24 (2), 170–176. https://doi.org/10.1055/s-2008-1075832.

Ihara, K., Doi, K., Sakai, K., Kuwata, N., Kawai, S., 1996. Restoration of sensibility in the hand after complete brachial plexus injury. J. Hand Surg. Am. 21 (3), 381–386. https://doi.org/10.1016/S0363-5023(96)80348-0.

Jones, M.R., Urits, I., Ehrhardt, K.P., et al., 2019. A comprehensive review of trigeminal neuralgia. Curr. Pain Headache Rep. 23 (10), 74.

Jowett, N., Pineda Ii, R., 2019. Corneal neurotisation by great auricular nerve transfer and scleral-corneal tunnel incisions for neurotrophic keratopathy. Br. J. Ophthalmol. 103 (9), 1235–1238. https://doi.org/10.1136/bjophthalmol-2018-312563.

Jupiter, J.B., Leibman, M.I., 2007. Supraclavicular nerve entrapment due to clavicular fracture callus. J. Shoulder Elbow Surg. 16 (5), e13–e14. https://doi.org/10.1016/j.jse.2006.09.015.

Kawashima, S., Kohno, T., Fujimori, S., et al., 2015. Phrenic nerve reconstruction in complete video-assisted thoracic surgery. Interact. Cardiovasc. Thorac. Surg. 20 (1), 54–59. https://doi.org/10.1093/icvts/ivu290.

Kikuta, S., Jenkins, S., Kusukawa, J., Iwanaga, J., Loukas, M., Tubbs, R.S., 2019. Ansa cervicalis: a comprehensive review of its anatomy, variations, pathology, and surgical applications. Anat. Cell Biol. 52 (3), 221–225. https://doi.org/10.5115/acb.19.041.

Kim, S., Feldman, D.U., Yang, J., 2016. A systematic review of the cervical plexus accessory innervation and its role in dental anesthesia. J. Anesth. Hist. 2 (3), 79–84. https://doi.org/10.1016/j.janh.2016.04.010.

Koshima, I., Nanba, Y., Tsutsui, T., Takahashi, Y., Itoh, S., 2004. New one-stage nerve pedicle grafting technique using the great auricular nerve for reconstruction of facial nerve defects. J. Reconstr. Microsurg. 20 (5), 357–361. https://doi.org/10.1055/s-2004-829998.

Labronici, P.J., Segall, F.S., Martins, B.A., et al., 2013. Clavicle fractures - incidence of supraclavicular nerve injury. Rev. Bras. Ortop. 48 (4), 317–321. https://doi.org/10.1016/j.rboe.2012.09.009.

Lee, M., Brown, M., Chepla, K., et al., 2013. An anatomical study of the lesser occipital nerve and its potential compression points: implications for surgical treatment of migraine headaches. Plast. Reconstr. Surg. 132 (6), 1551–1556. https://doi.org/10.1097/PRS.0b013e3182a80721.

Lee, J.H., Oh, T.S., Park, S.W., Kim, J.H., Tansatit, T., 2017. Temple and postauricular dissection in face and neck lift surgery. Arch. Plast. Surg. 44 (4), 261–265. https://doi.org/10.5999/aps.2017.44.4.261.

Lefkowitz, T., Hazani, R., Chowdhry, S., Elston, J., Yaremchuk, M.J., Wilhelmi, B.J., 2013. Anatomical landmarks to avoid injury to the great auricular nerve during rhytidectomy. Aesthetic Surg. J. 33 (1), 19–23. https://doi.org/10.1177/1090820x12469625.

Li, M., Chen, S., Wang, W., et al., 2014. Effect of duration of denervation on outcomes of ansa-recurrent laryngeal nerve reinnervation. Laryngoscope 124 (8), 1900–1905. https://doi.org/10.1002/lary.24623.

Li, M., Zheng, H., Chen, S., Chen, D., Zhu, M., 2019. Selective reinnervation using phrenic nerve and hypoglossal nerve for bilateral vocal fold paralysis. Laryngoscope 129 (11), 2669–2673. https://doi.org/10.1002/lary.27768.

Marcuzzo, A.V., Šuran-Brunelli, A.N., Dal Cin, E., et al., 2020. Surgical anatomy of the marginal mandibular nerve: a systematic review and meta-analysis. Clin. Anat. 33 (5), 739–750. https://doi.org/10.1002/ca.23497.

McKinney, P., Katrana, D.J., 1980. Prevention of injury to the great auricular nerve during rhytidectomy. Plast. Reconstr. Surg. 66 (5), 675–679. https://doi.org/10.1097/00006534-198011000-00001.

Mehta, A., Birch, R., 1997. Supraclavicular nerve injury: the neglected nerve? Injury 28 (7), 491–492. https://doi.org/10.1016/s0020-1383(97)00041-7.

Mucci, S.J., Dellon, A.L., 1997. Restoration of lower-lip sensation: neurotization of the mental nerve with the supraclavicular nerve. J. Reconstr. Microsurg. 13 (3), 151–155. https://doi.org/10.1055/s-2007-1000241.

Nandra, K.S., Harari, M., Price, T.P., Greaney, P.J., Weinstein, M.S., 2017. Successful reinnervation of the diaphragm after intercostal to phrenic nerve neurotization in patients with high spinal cord injury. Ann. Plast. Surg. 79 (2), 180–182. https://doi.org/10.1097/SAP.0000000000001105.

Nathe, T., Tseng, S., Yoo, B., 2011. The anatomy of the supraclavicular nerve during surgical approach to the clavicular shaft. Clin. Orthop. Relat. Res. 469 (3), 890–894. https://doi.org/10.1007/s11999-010-1608-x.

Ostrowska, M., de Carvalho, M., Apr 2012. Prognosis of phrenic nerve injury following thoracic interventions: four new cases and a review. Clin. Neurol. Neurosurg. 114 (3), 199–204. https://doi.org/10.1016/j.clineuro.2011.12.016.

Paniello, R.C., Feb 2004. Laryngeal reinnervation. Otolaryngol. Clin. N. Am. 37 (1), 161–181. https://doi.org/10.1016/S0030-6665(03)00164-6. vii-viii.

Pantaloni, M., Sullivan, P., 2000. Relevance of the lesser occipital nerve in facial rejuvenation surgery. Plast. Reconstr. Surg. 105 (7), 2594–2599. https://doi.org/10.1097/00006534-200006000-00051 discussion 2600-3.

Peled, Z.M., Pietramaggiori, G., Scherer, S., 2016. Anatomic and compression topography of the lesser occipital nerve. Plast. Reconstr. Surg. Glob Open 4 (3), e639. https://doi.org/10.1097/GOX.0000000000000654.

Poletti, C.E., 1983. Proposed operation for occipital neuralgia: C-2 and C-3 root decompression. Case report. Neurosurgery 12 (2), 221–224. https://doi.org/10.1227/00006123-198302000-00017.

Raikos, A., English, T., Yousif, O.K., Sandhu, M., Stirling, A., 2017. Topographic anatomy of the great auricular point: landmarks for its localization and classification. Surg. Radiol. Anat. 39 (5), 535–540. https://doi.org/10.1007/s00276-016-1758-y.

Ricoy, J., Rodríguez-Núñez, N., Álvarez-Dobaño, J.M., Toubes, M.E., Riveiro, V., Valdés, L., 2019. Diaphragmatic dysfunction. Pulmonology 25 (4), 223–235. https://doi.org/10.1016/j.pulmoe.2018.10.008.

Rowland, A.L., 1955. Treatment of tic douloueux by block or section of the great auricular nerve. AMA Arch. Otolaryngol. 61 (5), 549–553. https://doi.org/10.1001/archotol.1955.00720020566005.

Schauber, M.D., Fontenelle, L.J., Solomon, J.W., Hanson, T.L., 1997. Cranial/cervical nerve dysfunction after carotid endarterectomy. J. Vasc. Surg. 25 (3), 481–487. https://doi.org/10.1016/s0741-5214(97)70258-1.

Seruya, M., Patel, K.M., Keating, R.F., Rogers, G.F., 2013. Supraclavicular nerve graft interposition for reconstruction of pediatric brachial plexus injuries. Plast. Reconstr. Surg. 131 (3), 467e–468e. https://doi.org/10.1097/PRS.0b013e31827c7313.

Sharma, V.S., Stephens, R.E., Wright, B.W., Surek, C.C., 2017. What is the lobular branch of the great auricular nerve? Anatomical description and significance in rhytidectomy. Plast. Reconstr. Surg. 139 (2), 371e–378e. https://doi.org/10.1097/prs.0000000000002980.

Shinohara, S., Yamada, T., Ueda, M., et al., 2017. Phrenic nerve reconstruction and bilateral diaphragm plication after lobectomy. Ann. Thorac. Surg. 104 (1), e9–e11. https://doi.org/10.1016/j.athoracsur.2017.01.101.

Sieg, E.P., Payne, R.A., Hazard, S., Rizk, E., 2016. Evaluating the evidence: is phrenic nerve stimulation a safe and effective tool for decreasing ventilator dependence in patients with high cervical spinal cord injuries and central hypoventilation? Childs Nerv. Syst. 32 (6), 1033−1038. https://doi.org/10.1007/s00381-016-3086-2.

Simó, R., Nixon, I.J., Rovira, A., et al., 2020. Immediate intraoperative repair of the recurrent laryngeal nerve in thyroid surgery. Laryngoscope. https://doi.org/10.1002/lary.29204.

Socolovsky, M., di Masi, G., Bonilla, G., Domínguez Paez, M., Robla, J., Calvache Cabrera, C., 2015. The phrenic nerve as a donor for brachial plexus injuries: is it safe and effective? Case series and literature analysis. Acta Neurochir. 157 (6), 1077−1086. https://doi.org/10.1007/s00701-015-2387-7 discussion 1086.

Som, P.M., Smoker, W.R., Reidenberg, J.S., Bergemann, A.D., Hudgins, P.A., Laitman, J., 2011. Embryology and Anatomy of the Neck. Head and Neck Imaging. Elsevier Health Sciences, pp. 2117−2179. Chap. 34.

Taraquois, R., Joly, A., Sallot, A., Kun Darbois, J.D., Laure, B., Pare, A., 2016. Inferior alveolar nerve reconstruction after segmental resection of the mandible. Rev. Stomatol. Chir. Maxillofac. Chir. Orale 117 (6), 438−441. https://doi.org/10.1016/j.revsto.2016.06.006. Rehabilitation sensitive du nerf alveolaire inferieur apres mandibulectomie interruptrice.

Tubbs, R.S., Salter, E.G., Oakes, W.J., 2006. Anomaly of the supraclavicular nerve: case report and review of the literature. Clin. Anat. 19 (7), 599−601. https://doi.org/10.1002/ca.20208.

Tubbs, R.S., Loukas, M., Salter, E.G., Oakes, W.J., 2007a. Wilhelm erb and erb's point. Clin. Anat. 20 (5), 486−488. https://doi.org/10.1002/ca.20385.

Tubbs, R.S., Salter, E.G., Wellons, J.C., Blount, J.P., Oakes, W.J., 2007b. Landmarks for the identification of the cutaneous nerves of the occiput and nuchal regions. Clin. Anat. 20 (3), 235−238. https://doi.org/10.1002/ca.20297.

Tubbs, R.S., Pearson, B., Loukas, M., Shokouhi, G., Shoja, M.M., Oakes, W.J., 2008. Phrenic nerve neurotization utilizing the spinal accessory nerve: technical note with potential application in patients with high cervical quadriplegia. Childs Nerv. Syst. 24 (11), 1341−1344. https://doi.org/10.1007/s00381-008-0650-4.

Tubbs, R.S., Fries, F.N., Kulwin, C., Mortazavi, M.M., Loukas, M., Cohen-Gadol, A.A., 2016. Modified skin incision for avoiding the lesser occipital nerve and occipital artery during retrosigmoid craniotomy: potential applications for enhancing operative working distance and angles while minimizing the risk of postoperative neuralgias and intraoperative hemorrhage. J. Clin. Neurosci. 32, 83−87. https://doi.org/10.1016/j.jocn.2016.03.015.

Wang, K., Dowrick, A., Choi, J., Rahim, R., Edwards, E., 2010. Post-operative numbness and patient satisfaction following plate fixation of clavicular fractures. Injury 41 (10), 1002−1005. https://doi.org/10.1016/j.injury.2010.02.028.

Weisberger, E.C., Kincaid, J., Riteris, J., 1998. Cable grafting of the spinal accessory nerve after radical neck dissection. Arch. Otolaryngol. Head Neck Surg. 124 (4), 377−380. https://doi.org/10.1001/archotol.124.4.377.

Werner, C., D'Antoni, A.V., Iwanaga, J., Watanabe, K., Dumont, A.S., Tubbs, R.S., 2020. A comprehensive review of the great auricular nerve graft. Neurosurg. Rev. 1−9.

Wolford, L., Rodrigues, D., 2011. Autogenous grafts/allografts/conduits for bridging peripheral trigeminal nerve gaps. In: Atlas of the Oral and Maxillofacial Surgery Clinics of North America. Elsevier, pp. 91−107.

Wood, M.B., Murray, P.M., 2007. Heterotopic nerve transfers: recent trends with expanding indication. J. Hand Surg. Am. 32 (3), 397−408. https://doi.org/10.1016/j.jhsa.2006.12.012.

You, J.M., Wu, Y.S., Wang, Y., 2018. Comparison of postoperative numbness and patient satisfaction using minimally invasive plate osteosynthesis or open plating for acute displaced clavicular shaft fractures. Int. J. Surg. 56, 21−25. https://doi.org/10.1016/j.ijsu.2018.06.007.

Zeng, H., Zhan, T., He, R., Xiong, H., Zheng, Y., Yang, H., 2020. Modified postauricular incision for preservation of the lesser occipital nerve and the great auricular nerve in ear surgery. ORL J. Otorhinolaryngol. Relat. Spec. 82 (3), 150−162. https://doi.org/10.1159/000506209.

Index

Note: Page numbers followed by "f" indicate figures, "t" indicate tables.

CPI Antony Rowe
Eastbourne, UK
May 05, 2021

List of contributors

Joseph V. Bonventre
Brigham and Women's Hospital, Boston, MA, United States; Harvard Medical School, Boston, MA, United States; Harvard Stem Cell Institute, Cambridge, MA, United States

Katja Breitkopf-Heinlein
Heidelberg University, Mannheim, Germany

Keith R. Brennan
University of Manchester, Manchester, United Kingdom

Esther L. Calderon-Gierszal
Department of Urology, University of Illinois at Chicago, Chicago, IL, United States

Jamie A. Davies
University of Edinburgh, Edinburgh, United Kingdom

Mona Elhendawi
The University of Edinburgh, Edinburgh, United Kingdom; Mansoura University, Mansoura, Egypt

Nurfarhana Ferdaos
University of Edinburgh, Edinburgh, United Kingdom; Universiti Teknologi MARA, Selangor, Malaysia

Haristi Gaitantzi
Heidelberg University, Mannheim, Germany

Andrew P. Gilmore
University of Manchester, Manchester, United Kingdom

Tomohiro Ito
National Institute for Environmental Studies, Tsukuba, Japan

Melanie L. Lawrence
University of Edinburgh, Edinburgh, United Kingdom

Weijia Liu
The University of Edinburgh, Edinburgh, United Kingdom

John O. Mason
University of Edinburgh, Edinburgh, United Kingdom

Richard J. McMurtrey
Institute of Neural Regeneration & Tissue Engineering, Highland, UT, United States

Christopher G. Mills
University of Edinburgh, Edinburgh, United Kingdom

Ryuji Morizane
Brigham and Women's Hospital, Boston, MA, United States; Harvard Medical School, Boston, MA, United States; Harvard Stem Cell Institute, Cambridge, MA, United States

Gail S. Prins
Department of Urology, University of Illinois at Chicago, Chicago, IL, United States

Eva Rath
Technical University of Munich, Freising, Germany

Hideko Sone
National Institute for Environmental Studies, Tsukuba, Japan

Charles H. Streuli
University of Manchester, Manchester, United Kingdom

Heyuan Sun
University of Manchester, Manchester, United Kingdom

Jun Sun
University of Illinois at Chicago, Chicago, IL, United States

Jack Williams
University of Manchester, Manchester, United Kingdom

Tin-Tin Win-Shwe
National Institute for Environmental Studies, Tsukuba, Japan

Amber M. Wood
University of Manchester, Manchester, United Kingdom

Yang Zeng
National Institute for Environmental Studies, Tsukuba, Japan

Tamara Zietek
Technical University of Munich, Freising, Germany

Acknowledgments

The Editors of this book acknowledge gratefully the helpful comments of their laboratory colleagues. While working on this book, ML was supported by MRC grant MR/K010735/1, and Kidney Research UK grant RP_002_20160223.

Disclaimer

The practical instructions in this book are intended for use by qualified researchers who are able to make their own assessment of risk. Neither the publisher nor the editors accept responsibility for any injury or loss resulting from use of the protocols. Please note that this book has an international scope, and its authors operate under a range of legal systems: readers must ensure that any protocol they wish to follow is acceptable under their own national system of legal and ethical codes with respect to the use of material from humans or from nonhuman animals.

Introduction

Organoids and mini-organs: Introduction, history, and potential

1

Jamie A. Davies

University of Edinburgh, Edinburgh, United Kingdom

CHAPTER OUTLINE

INTRODUCTION

It is important to begin this book with a definition of terms, because the word "organoid" has been coined several times in the history of biomedicine, and has been used to convey at least three distinct meanings. In the 20th century, "organoid" was sometimes used as a synonym for "organelle" (e.g., Duryee and Doherty, 1954), a sub-cellular structure: this use is now obsolete. In oncology, "organoid" is sometimes used as an adjective to imply a tumor with a complex, tissue-like structure, for example a gland-like carcinoma or a teratoma: this use remains current (e.g., Nesland et al., 1985; Heller et al., 1991), if somewhat obscure. Neither of these meanings is relevant to this book. Here, "organoid" is being used in its most common modern sense, to refer to a three-dimensional assembly that contains cells of more than one type, arranged with realistic histology, at least at the micro-scale. An organoid might be made from cells of humans or other animals, and these might be differentiated cells, stem cells, or a mixture of the two.

Organoids and Mini-Organs. DOI: http://dx.doi.org/10.1016/B978-0-12-812636-3.00001-8

Interest in organoids has increased significantly in the 21st century (Fig. 1.1), fueled on the one hand by rapid developments in stem cell derivation to provide human progenitor cells, and on the other by a strengthening desire to refine, reduce or replace the use of animals in research (reviewed by Davies, 2012). Organoids are being produced for basic research into development and neoplasia, for industrial and medical applications such as toxicology, and—ultimately—for transplantation. At the end of 2013, *The Scientist* named organoids as one of its "advances of the year" (Grens, 2013), not because the technology was new, but because it had suddenly become much more pervasive and visible thanks to some high-profile research papers. About a year and a half later, and for much the same reason, *Nature* published an overview of the potential of the technology (Willyard, 2015). Organoids have now been developed to represent many different parts of the body, for many different reasons, with applications expected to grow still further over the next few years.

Being published in a period of such intense research, this book has two purposes. The first is to help newcomers to the field to set up working organoid systems, whether by using the exact techniques of other researchers, or by using these techniques to inspire the creation of novel organoid systems. The second purpose is to help researchers with working organoid systems find inspiration and advice to help them use their organoids as tools to solve a range of biological and medical problems.

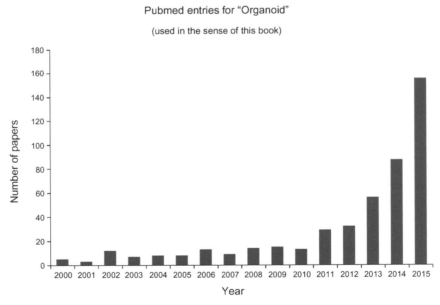

FIGURE 1.1

The rising use of organoids in biological research. The graph shows the number of papers returned from a Pubmed search for "Organoid", and screened manually for "organoid" being used in the sense in which it is used in this book.

ORIGINS OF ORGANOIDS

Organoids have been an important area of research for much longer than most recent reviews imply, particularly the annoyingly large number of reviews that appear to have been written for the sole purpose of portraying their authors as founders of a field. The first mammalian organoids were in fact produced over 60 years ago, and organoids have contributed steadily and significantly to developmental cell biology ever since.

Techniques for constructing organoids have their origins in basic research about the nature of biological organization. A good starting point for this brief history would be the work of H.V. Wilson (1910), who showed that, if a sponge is dissociated into its constituent cells, and these cells are reaggregated randomly, they reorganize to make a realistic and viable new sponge (Wilson, 1910). Though not aimed at making organoids in the modern sense, this experiment was an important demonstration that cells of an adult organism can contain sufficient information to specify a multicellular structure, without any need for outside instructions, and without the need for cells to start from some specific anatomical arrangement contingent on their embryological history. This point is critical to organoid production. In the 1950s, several laboratories began to use the same basic method—disaggregation followed by reaggregation—to determine whether the cells of more complex animals such as vertebrates also had the ability to self-organize (this term was already in use) or whether, for these complex animals, the spatial relationships contingent on past developmental history were critical. Early examples of the disaggregation − reaggregation method of organoid construction being applied to higher vertebrates were provided by Moscona (1952) and by Moscona and Moscona (1952), who made suspensions of chick mesonephric kidney cells. The source tissue included both tubular epithelial cells and mesenchymal cells. On reaggregation and incubation, epithelial cells made small clusters that went on to make tubules surrounded by mesenchyme-derived stroma. This arrangement was reminiscent of the small-scale anatomy of normal mesonephroids, although the overall gross-scale organization of the organ was absent: the structure met the modern definition of an "organoid". These experiments demonstrated that at least some of the cells of embryonic chicks, like the cells of sponges, carried sufficient information to organize themselves realistically, even when their original spatial relationships had been erased.

The observation that different types of cells in the suspension (e.g., epithelial, mesenchymal) would separate in the reaggregate raised questions about how cells choose their neighbors. It was already known from culture experiments that similar cells tend to unite even if they come from tissues of different species. In the 1940s, Harris (1943), Medawar (1948), and Grobstein and Younger (1949) all tried coculturing fragments of tissues from different species to explore the mechanisms of transplant rejection (this was before the role of the immune system in the process was well understood). They each showed that fragments of the same tissue from different species could join and behave as one: indeed, in the case of heart muscle, heart-beat synchronized across the interspecies boundary. Moscona (1956) built on these studies of interspecific combinations to ask whether the association of cells was controlled more by their being of the same histological type, or by their coming from the animal. He mixed suspended mouse and chick embryonic liver cells, and showed that they cooperated in making an organoid, epithelia associating with epithelia, and stroma with stroma, regardless of the species of origin. He also mixed different tissues, for example chick kidney and mouse cartilage, and observed that the cells sorted out reasonably well, and each resulting organoid was formed only of cells exhibiting nuclear markers of its own species. The species-specific nuclear morphologies ruled out any possible mechanism of cells trans-differentiating according to their surroundings, and supported instead the idea of cells choosing their neighbors. The author concluded that type specificity was stronger than species specificity in arranging cells, and that cells were already determined to make a particular tissue. The paper also showed an early application of organoids to problems of pathology, when its author mixed mouse melanoma cells with normal chick cells, and saw some evidence of invasive growth ("infiltration" in his words) by the sarcoma cells.

Part of the drive behind these early organoid experiments, acknowledged and discussed by Weiss and Taylor (1960), was to provide a counterbalance to the prevailing view that most embryogenesis was driven by inductive signaling, a mechanism that had obsessed many embryologists since its discovery in the 1920s (Spemann and Mangold, 1924). The ability of mixtures of cells, isolated from their normal anatomical relationships with the rest of the embryo, to self-organize was taken by these authors as an indication that much epigenetic information was held by the cells themselves, and did not rely on inductive instructions from elsewhere. This did not, though, rule out signaling taking place between different cell types within the self-organized aggregate and, in the 1950s, Grobstein's laboratory used the dissociation − reaggregation technique to explore these signals. It was already known, from the experiments of Gruenwald (1937, 1942), that kidney development relies on inductive signaling between the ureteric bud (the progenitor of the urine collecting duct system) and the surrounding metanephrogenic mesenchyme ("Metanephrogenic mesenchyme" is Grobstein's original term that captures the developmental potential of the tissue.). The mesenchyme induces the ureteric bud to grow and branch, while the bud induces the mesenchyme to make nephrons and stroma. Auerbach and Grobstein (1958) made cell suspensions of metanephrogenic mesenchyme, reaggregated them, and cultured them. On its own this reaggregate did nothing but, when placed in contact with inducing tissue, it made tubules. This showed that the disaggregation and reaggregation process did not itself substitute for induction: the "rules" of development in reaggregates apparently remained the same as in the embryo. The researchers also made suspensions of inducing tissue, mixed them with suspensions of metanephrogenic mesenchyme, and cultured the reaggregate. The cell types segregated and inductive signals passed to the mesenchymal cells, inducing them to make nephrons, and indicating that inductive activity is robust to disaggregation and reaggregation. The inducing tissue used for these experiments was spinal cord, because ureteric buds die. Only decades later, when the Auerbach and Grobstein work was revisited, was a method developed to prevent anoikis in the ureteric bud cells of a disaggregate − reaggregate in culture: in the presence of an inhibitor of Rho-activated kinase (ROCK), the ureteric bud cells survive, segregate from the mesenchyme, and make small collecting duct cysts and treelets that induce the metanephrogenic cells to make nephrons, the whole being a renal organoid (Unbekandt and Davies, 2010).

MECHANISMS OF ORGANOID FORMATION

An important question hanging over the work on organoids in the 1940s and 1950s was the mechanism by which cells of a mixed reaggregate sort out into distinct populations. The most determined and effective approach to this was probably that of Malcolm Steinberg, who proposed that the sorting of cells was due to differential adhesion (Steinberg, 1963). His argument rested on essentially thermodynamic grounds: he proposed that cells express adhesion systems on their surfaces, that different adhesion systems adhere with different strengths (i.e., that binding reduces the free energy in the system by different amounts), and that homotypic adhesive systems will adhere more strongly (lower free energy more) than heterotypic ones. Under these assumptions, and allowing cells to move, the lowest energy state would be one in which cells bind to their own kind in preference to remaining mixed: cells mixtures would therefore separate into homogenous populations (Fig. 1.2). What is more, cells of the more adhesive type will be in the core of a reaggregate, and the less adhesive cells will surround them. In this view, the information content of the cells, in terms of their propensity for self-organization, therefore reduces simply to a quantitative measure of their stickiness.

Since Steinberg suggested the differential adhesion hypothesis, measurements of the relative adhesion strengths of different cells, in homotypic and heterotypic contacts, have been made, and these adhesion strengths have been found to be predictive of sorting behavior. In a more direct test, Foty and Steinberg (2005) engineered different clones of a cell line to express different amounts of the same adhesion molecule, and showed that the cells sorted with the more adhesive in the core. This test separated differences in the amount of adhesion from differences in the type of molecule, or the type of cell, and therefore supported the focus on adhesion alone as the critical determinant of sorting behavior. There is now evidence that the precise type of adhesion molecule may actually matter much less than was originally supposed: when cells expressing different cadherin adhesion molecules at the *same* surface concentration are mixed, they may remain mixed, suggesting that quantitative differences in the number of molecules present may

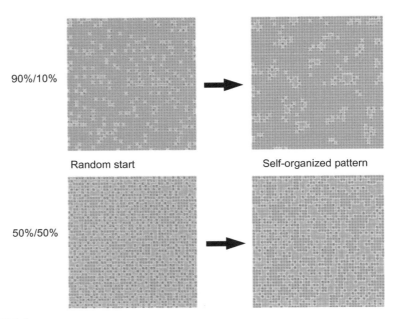

90%/10%

Random start   Self-organized pattern

50%/50%

FIGURE 1.2

Computer simulation of adhesion-mediated phase separation. In each case, homotypic adhesion between green cells and homotypic adhesion between red cells is greater than heterotypic adhesion between red and green cells, and cells are allowed to change positions if this will reduce the free energy of their binding. The result is that randomly-arranged starting populations undergo partial phase separation, but separation cannot complete because islands of one color become separated by the other, and cannot cross without making energetically unfavorable moves. The system therefore remains in a local optimum with a rich alternation of cell types.

be much more important than cadherin type (Duguay et al., 2003). This conclusion is supported by direct measurements of cadherin adhesion on non-living substrates, which show that heterotypic contacts adhere about as well as homotypic ones (Shi et al., 2008).

It is important to note that, despite the strong evidence that sorting behavior can be predicted by adhesion, recent data challenge the view that the underlying mechanism can be explained in terms of simple thermodynamics. In real embryos, thick actin − myosin cables run along the boundary between epithelial cells that express different cadherins. Mutations or knockdown of myosin II prevent the actin − myosin cables forming, and cells start to mix (Monier et al., 2011). This suggests that cells may detect reduced adhesion along a particular interface and actively use actin − myosin to increase surface tension there, reducing the length of the boundary as much as possible, and thus minimizing the area of heterotypic contact. This mechanism is discussed further in Davies (2013); the main point of relevance to this chapter is that sorting is still predictable by adhesion, but uses active cellular mechanisms rather than simple minimization of free energy. In the face of this on-going debate, some authors (e.g., Davies and Cachat, 2016) have moved to using "phase separation" to refer to the sorting of cell types with different homo- and heterotypic interaction properties, as a term that captures the effect while remaining agnostic about the underlying mechanism.

The ability of cells to sort out by adhesion-mediated phase separation is restricted by their capacity to move, and by the system's risk of becoming trapped in a local optimum. Once separation has begun, and clusters of cells of one type form as islands in a sea of the other type, the islands will minimize their boundary area and be relatively rounded. This will be a local optimum, in the sense that any distortion of the boundaries—for example, an invasive tendril growing out from an island—would increase the interfacial area. Without such growth, though, the islands cannot meet and coalesce to reach the global optimum of only one straight boundary (Fig. 1.2). The system is therefore trapped in its local optimum, with a rich alternation of cell types. This restriction has been exploited in the construction of synthetic biological systems that generate de novo patterns using nothing but adhesion-mediated phase separation (Cachat et al., 2016).

The restricted sorting caused by the system becoming trapped in a local optimum is probably critical to the formation of organoids from mixed progenitor cells. For example, in a kidney organoid formed from the kidney progenitor by dissociation and reaggregation, ureteric bud cells that express large quantities of E-cadherin form tight coalescences; islands in a sea of metanephrogenic mesenchyme. Each of these epithelial islands develops into a cyst, and then into a tubule that goes on to branch to make a ureteric bud treelet. Inductive signals from each treelet then organize the surrounding metanephrogenic mesenchyme to make nephrons (Fig. 1.3). An interesting question, still moot, is whether the stability of even mature tissues relies, at least in part, on the system being trapped in a local optimum.

THE PATH TO HUMAN ORGANOIDS

For decades, almost all work and commentary on organoids was done from the point of view of basic developmental biology: organoids were tools that could inform embryologists about cellular mechanisms of development. They had the useful feature that they would allow questions to be asked in a simple system, away from the complexity of the body as a whole. For such uses, animal sources were as useful as human—more so, perhaps, because organoid data could be correlated with in vivo experiments. Occasionally, suggestions for clinically relevant applications were made. In the 1980s, for example, Lauri Saxén suggested the use of organoids as well as intact, cultured embryonic organ rudiments to explore mechanisms of teratogenesis and foetal toxicology (Saxén, 1988). The use of animal organoids for the purposes of studying toxicology would, however, run into the same issues in extrapolating animal data to human that are so problematic in

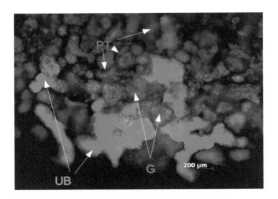

FIGURE 1.3

A kidney organoid produced from human iPS cells, showing a close alternation of different cell types. Ureteric bud cells are stained for Calbdinin-D-28k (green), the proximal tubule part of nephrons are stained with LTL lectin (blue), and glomerular podocytes are stained for WT1 (red).

Image credit: Mona El-Hendawy and author.

standard in vivo animal experiments. For predicting human toxicity, human organoids would obviously be better. In addition, any hope of using organoids as a basis for making transplantable tissues for human clinical use would clearly require human cells as a starting point. For these reasons, interest in making human organoids has steadily grown.

Until the development of ES and iPS cells (see below), production of human organoids depended on the use of fragments of tissue from human foetuses, children or adults. Human keratinocytes, amongst the easier cells to obtain (particularly in countries that practice male circumcision), will form realistically layered epidermal organoids when cultured at an air/medium interface (Noël-Hudson et al., 1995). Mixed with fibroblasts, they organize into a skin organoid that includes a dermis-like layer (Kim et al., 1999). Simple neuronal organoids were constructed in the 1980s and 1990s from foetal brain cells (Lodin et al., 1981), for the purpose of studying the dynamics of virus infection (McCarthy et al., 1991) and neuronal physiology (Aquila-Mansilla and Barnea, 1996; Barnea and Roberts, 1999). Such organoids have also been tested for their ability to integrate into adult animal brains (Bystron et al., 2002). Similarly, human thymocyte aggregates have been used to explore T-cell immunology (Choi et al., 1997).

What made a vast difference to the interest in growing organoids for application was the development of the first human embryonic stem cell (hES cell) lines (Thomson et al., 1998) and, later, human-induced pluripotent stem cell (hiPS cell) lines that can be made from differentiated tissue (Yu et al., 2007). In principle, hiPS cells can be differentiated into any foetal cell type, typically by exposing them to the same sequence of signaling molecules that lead to cells of the same type during normal embryonic development. This created the hope that hiPS cells, perhaps specific to a particular human phenotype, could be turned into the starting material for making organoids, allowing clinically important studies on pathology, toxicology, teratology, etc., to be made on the correct species, and even the correct individual or patient subgroup. It also created the hope that such organoids may be a first step to making new organs for the purposes of transplantation.

Some work in this direction was begun using mouse ES cells, before their human counterparts were available, so that differentiation and culture strategies would be in place for human pluripotent stem cells when they had been developed. Examples of this mouse ES work include the production of gut organoids (Ishikawa et al., 2004), organoids containing kidney components (Kim and Dressler, 2005), cardiac organoids (Guo, 2006), and liver organoids (Mizumoto et al., 2008). Once human ES and iPS cells became available, human organoids began to be produced to represent neural tissue (Schwarts, 2015), prostate (Calderon-Gierszal and Prins, 2015), thyroid (Ma et al., 2015), and kidney (Morizane et al., 2015; Takasato, 2015). For at least some systems, it has been possible to avoid the ESC/iPSC stage by transdifferentiating fibroblasts into the desired organ progenitor cell type; this has, for example, been done for thymus (Bredenkamp et al., 2014).

THE CONSTRUCTION OF ORGANOIDS

As will become apparent in the following chapters, there is more than one way to make organoids. They can be made from stem cells or differentiated cells, and they can be made using only the information in the cells themselves, or with the use of shaped or printed scaffolds.

The simplest types of organoids, at least in terms of starting material, are those that can be made from single cells. An example is the "mini-gut" organoid of Sato et al. (Sato et al., 2009). This is constructed by placing single intestinal stem cells into Matrigel (a laminin-rich gel that is commonly used as an ersatz basement membrane), with some pharmacological support to encourage proliferation and to prevent anoikis. Each intestinal stem cell proliferates to form a small epithelial cyst, which breaks its symmetry to form out-growing buds (Fig. 1.4). Each bud is led by a mixture of cells that have differentiated into Wnt-expressing Paneth cells, and cells remaining in the stem condition. The centripetal gradient in each bud organizes the other epithelium of the bud into organotypic zones of differentiated state.

The gut organoids described above do not represent anything like the complexity of the full organ; in particular they lack stromal components because these have a quite different embryonic origin, and are not made from epithelial stem cells (the epithelium is an endodermal derivative while the stroma come from mesoderm). Where more realistic organoids are wanted, with both epithelial and mesenchymal components, more than one type of stem cell is usually required, although on the positive side, artificial matrix gels may not then be needed.

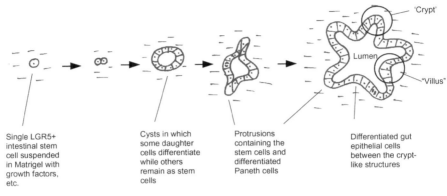

FIGURE 1.4

Production of intestinal organoids by the method of Sato et al. (2009), in which isolated intestinal stem cells are suspended in Matrigel supplemented with appropriate signaling molecules and allowed to proliferate. The cells quickly polarize to make a cyst, and some daughters of the stem cell divisions remain as stem cells while others differentiate, breaking the symmetry of the system. Parts of the epithelium containing stem cells protrude into the Matrigel to form crypt-like structures, while the intervening zones contain differentiated cells similar to those in a villus.

Where stem cells are obtained directly from foetuses, it may be possible to dissect out regions of foetal tissue that already contain all of the stem cell types required, because they were already correctly placed to produce the organ. This was the approach taken by Unbekandt and Davies (2010) to produce renal organoids. Where stem cells are to be made from ES or iPS cell lines, producing all of the organ-specific stem cells can be more complicated. They can either each be made by a specific differentiation protocol and combined, or in some cases produced by a protocol in which iPS cells are differentiated along pathways with ambiguous specification cues that create a mixed population. An excellent example of this approach is provided by Takasato et al. (2015), who showed that the length of a Wnt-agonist phase of a differentiation protocol towards kidneys would bias cells to producing either ureteric bud-type stem cells (the progenitors for collecting duct), or metanephrogenic mesenchyme-type stem cells (the progenitors for nephrons and stroma). The length of treatment could be optimized to produce a mix of each type of stem cell, resulting in a realistic and useful renal organoid with both collecting ducts and nephrons.

ORGANOIDS AS TOOLS FOR CLINICAL RESEARCH

The current surge in interest in organoids has been driven mainly by the clinical sciences, and organoid technology is now being applied to drug development, toxicology, oncology, microbiology, and regenerative medicine.

The classical research-and-development pathway for therapeutic molecules (drugs, antibodies, etc.) proceeds from the identification of candidate compounds in in vitro systems and simple cell culture, to testing for safety and efficacy in non-human animals, to phase I trials (small group; safety) in humans, then via phase II trials (medium group; safety and efficacy), and phase III trials (large group; efficacy, rare side effects, etc.) trials, to widespread clinical use. A source of great frustration to industrial pharmacologists is that compounds that appear to be safe in animal models can show unexpected toxicities to humans. This typically results in withdrawal of the drug, and means that vast amounts of money and researcher time are effectively wasted. Presumably, there are also compounds that are abandoned because they fail toxicity tests in non-human animals that would in fact be perfectly safe and useful in humans. The need to carry the costs of work wasted in this way makes drug development (and drugs themselves) very expensive, and holds back the progress of medicine. Drug developers, therefore, have a very strong need for human-based systems in which drug efficacy and toxicity can be assessed. Human cell lines, which have of course been available for decades, are relatively poor predictors (e.g., Jenkinson et al., 2012) and, while primary cells in simple culture can be a little better (Brown et al., 2008), they are still limited by the absence of normal tissue interactions and geometry, and usually by short life. There has been great hope that three-dimensional organoids might provide better proxies for human beings (see Eglen and Randle, 2016, for a short review).

While safety testing of lead compounds can be done in a relatively slow and labor-intensive way (there being a relatively small number of compounds at this stage of the development cycle), the earlier phases of identifying compounds requires techniques that can efficiently screen tens of thousands of compounds. There are hopes that human-derived organoids can be used there too, and a significant effort is being applied to development of automatic imaging and analysis techniques, by which organoids can be used for high-throughput compound screens (reviewed by Li et al., 2016).

The use of human organoids in toxicology is not limited to pharmacology: environmental toxicants can also be studied this way. A recent example is the use of human embryonic stem cell-derived prostate organoids to investigate the effects of bisphenol-A on the development of prostate organoids. Bisphenol A is an oestrogen-mimicking environmental pollutant that leaches from many plastics and can be detected in the body fluids of most humans in the developed world. Calderon-Gierszal and Prins (2015, 2017) showed that the compound significantly affected the development of prostate organoids, affecting in particular the balance between stem cell differentiation and self-renewal. Similarly, neural organoids ("neurospheres") are being used to study neurotoxicity (Betts, 2010; Zeng et al., 2017).

Human organoids have begun to be used in cancer research, and provide a useful half-way point between simple cell lines (which are easy to use but of limited realism, especially for studying aspects such as invasion and the tumor microenvironment), and *in vivo* animal studies, which have the advantage of complexity, including the presence of the immune and vascular systems, but tell us more about animal oncology than human. Organoids can be established from patient biopsy material, whether normal or transformed. In at least some cases (colon, pancreas), normal tissue organoids, as well as tumors, grow very well and can be propagated apparently indefinitely (Vela and Chen, 2015). This overcomes the classic restriction of cell line studies, that neoplastic cell lines long outlive normal cells from the same patient, so the opportunities for comparative "control" experiments are quickly lost. What is more, in organoids that contain neoplasms, the balance between different clones seems to be preserved better than in two-dimensional culture (reviewed by Hwang et al., 2016). In principle, this allows aspects of tumor biology, such as dependence on specific growth factors, to be explored when multiple neoplastic cells are interacting with normal tissues. In addition, CRISPR/Cas9 gene editing technology is now allowing researchers to make mutations, similar to those described above for mice, in human cells to study the effects of specific combinations of gene losses or oncogenic mutations on human tumor progression (Matano et al., 2015).

The role of loss of specific tumor suppressor genes in the progression from a normal cell to a full-blown metastatic cancer has been explored using organoids made from mice in which the tumor suppressor genes have been flanked with recombinase-dependent recombination sites. These organoids can then be infected by low concentrations of viral vectors carrying the recombinase to create a clone of cells lacking the tumor suppressors in an otherwise isogenic organoid environment. An example is provided by Nadauld et al. (2014), who wished to test the hypothesis that loss of Cdh1, Trp53, and TGFBR2 genes promotes neoplastic change in gastric epithelium. They made mice in which Cdh1 and Trp53 genes were surrounded by lox-P sites, made gastric organoids from them, and infected these organs with adenovirus carrying either GFP-labeled cre recombinase or an inert control. They also used RNA interference to knockdown TGFBR2. Loss of only cdh1 and Trp53 did not result in a cancer-like transformation, but additional loss of TGFBR2 resulted in severe dysplasia, and an appearance reminiscent of gastric cancer. Li et al. (2014) used a similar approach to study the effects of oncogene activation, by using floxed "stop" sequences upstream of oncogenes and adenovirus-vectored cre to un-"stop" them (this unstopping approach is much safer than building viruses for direct transduction of active oncogenes). Some organoids exhibited dysplasia in organoid culture, and a larger set were tumorigenic when grafted into animal hosts. Different combinations of knockout and induced-oncogenes were also used by the authors to explore multi-hit models of tumor progression, and to identify a micro-RNA as a particularly critical oncogene.

The ability of researchers to propagate organoids long-term has also opened up the possibility of keeping biobanks of matched normal and neoplastic tissues for research that can be correlated with clinical outcome (van der Wetering et al., 2015). There is even discussion of direct trials of drug options being conducted on organoids from a specific patient real-time, before the patient himself is treated (Hwang et al., 2016). It has to be noted, however, that culture conditions are still critical, and early-stage neoplasms often grow faster in organoid culture than do late-stage ones, suggesting that some models may turn out to be disappointingly unrealistic (reviewed by Sachs and Clevers, 2014).

Organoids can also be used to study the mechanisms of action of infectious agents. At the time this chapter was written, Brazil was at the center of a major epidemic of Zika virus, and there seemed to be a correlation between Zika infection of a mother and microcephaly of her offspring. An early demonstration of the effect of Zika on the developing human brain was provided by Garcez et al. (2016) and Qian et al. (2016), who made brain-specific organoids (Fernados and Mason, 2017) from human iPS cells, and used them to show that Zika virus infection of the cultures directly affected cell proliferation and death, neural progenitor cells being particularly affected. This reduced the volume of brain tissue produced compared to controls. These experiments were an important demonstration that the virus affects developing brain directly, in a system that required no extrapolation from experimental animal to human. Similarly, human gut organoids, in this case derived from biopsies, have been used to study infections by rotavirus and have enabled researchers to study interferon responses and responses to antiviral compounds (Yin et al., 2015). In this case, the use of human rather than mouse organoids resulted in much more realistic rates of virus replication.

Organoids can be used to study bacterial infections, as well as viral (Sun, 2017). For example, Bartfeld et al. (2015) produced human stomach organoids from surgical biopsy material and micro-injected them with *Helicobacter pylori* (a bacterium associated with stomach ulcers and other chronic diseases of the gut wall). This allowed them to study transcriptional responses of the host tissue. It also allowed them to use subcomponents of the bacteria, such as pure LPS or bacterial strains missing components such as flagella, to determine which parts of the bacteria were responsible for which host responses. The ability of the researchers to direct the organoid system to produce different types of stomach components (pits, glands, etc.) also allowed them to determine which type of host tissue was most responsive to each bacterial stimulus. This resolution would have been very difficult to achieve, in the absence of confounding indirect effects, in any other experimental system.

Not all bacteria are a problem: normal people have approximately 10 times as many bacterial cells as human cells, and most are harmless commensals or helpful symbionts. Recent years have brought a greatly increased appreciation of the important role of the gut microbiome, in particular, in regulating immunity, inflammation, and disease (Boulangé et al., 2016; Yarandi et al., 2016; Elgin et al., 2016). The survival and behavior of microbes, symbionts, and pathogens alike, depend in part on interactions with molecules carried on, or secreted from, the apical surfaces of gut cells. Similarly, the gut can respond to the presence of microbe-derived signals. Organoids allow researchers to study gut — microbe interactions, and to gain clinically useful understanding in a much more realistic setting than traditional microbial culture systems can offer (Lukovac et al., 2014; Van Limbergen et al., 2015; Kitamura et al., 2015).

Organoids are also used for regenerative medicine. The challenge of producing complex transplantable organs is discussed in the next section of this chapter, but organoids of the complexity already discussed can still be used for the purposes of regeneration. An example of the introduction of organoid-derived stem cells to promote regeneration is provided by Pringle et al. (2016), who produced salivary organoids from human salivary gland biopsies, and passaged these to high cell numbers. They then injected cell suspensions made from these organoids into immunodeficient mice whose own salivary glands had been damaged by radiation. The human cells engrafted and significantly restored normal salivary gland function. One interesting approach that has worked unexpectedly well is the engraftment of complete organoids, rather than cell suspensions, into damaged host tissue. This approach relies on the organoid and host cells to reorganize to achieve integration, and stem (or at least proliferation-competent) cells from the organoid to repair the host tissue. An example is provided by the transfer of labeled gut organoids to mouse gut lining damaged by ulcerative colitis: normal-looking colon tissue was regenerated, and it consisted of labeled, and therefore organoid-derived, cells (Yui et al., 2012).

FROM ORGANOIDS TO MINI-ORGANS

For many in the field, the ultimate goal of stem cell-based tissue engineering is to produce engineered transplantable organs as complete replacements for human clinical use. In most cases, the function of an organ depends on its large-scale anatomy, as well as on its micro-scale arrangements of cells, and the organoid level of organization will not be enough. Lungs will not work unless the airways connect properly back to a trachea, and blood flows past alveoli; kidneys will not work unless nephrons are organized properly with relation to a normo-osmotic cortex and a hyper-osmotic medulla, are connected to a drainage system that leads to a ureter, and are provided with a proper blood circulation; colonic transplants will not work unless they have a lumen continuous with the small intestine and anus, and are connected to both blood and enteric nervous systems to allow absorption and peristalsis, and so on.

The ability of cells to make organoids is a vivid testament to the information content borne by cells themselves, but the limitations of the technique may help to identify what needs to be added. Most organs have asymmetric progenitors and develop in an asymmetric environment, in the sense that signals and mechanical forces are not the same in all directions. These asymmetries may well be what provides the information in normal embryos that is missing in organoid systems: if this is so, adding appropriate asymmetries when constructing organoids may result in more realistic large-scale patterning, and make a transition from orga-noids to mini-organs. Lawrence et al. (2017) explore this idea in the context of the kidney, in which micro-manipulation to create two specific asymmetries can turn a typical organoid with a jumble of nephrons and short collecting ducts into a structure in which nephrons are properly arranged around a single collecting duct tree that drains to a single ureter. The structure is not yet a mini-organ (it has neither a vascular nor a nervous system, for example), but it does demonstrate one possible route that can be taken from organoids towards mini-organs.

A completely different strategy for making mini-organs, or even full-sized ones, is to apply cells to a scaffold; either a decellularized matrix from a natural organ, or a printed scaffold. Use of scaffolds lies outside the scope of this book, but it is worth discussing it briefly here so that readers can find recent references should they wish to explore further. In the scaffold-driven approach, the self-organizing abilities of cells are used to allow them to find appropriate locations on the scaffold, based on its micro-scale properties (e.g., the precise matrix molecules on it), and then to adhere and make a normal tissue. The scaffold itself imposes large-scale order. This approach works well enough to have been used clinically for connective tissues such as tendon (Lovati et al., 2016), and structures as large as trachea have been produced and transplanted successfully to human patients (Macchiarini et al., 2004). Even decellularized hearts have been recellularized and transplanted ectopically into animal hosts to assess cell survival and vascularization; obviously, the host heart remained in place to keep the animal alive (Kitahara et al., 2016). For organs with very complex internal tubular anatomy and intimate relationships between vasculature and epithelial tubules, such as lung and kidney, preliminary results have been interesting (e.g., Song et al., 2013), but it is generally acknowledged that the path to a fully functional organ made by recellularization still poses very significant challenges (Stabler et al., 2015; Petrosyan et al., 2016).

LIMITATIONS OF ORGANOIDS

Organoids are useful, but are not a panacea. Organoids growing in vitro lack blood flow, even if they form a vascular system (and many do not even do that, having no vasculogenic cells). Transplanting the organoid into a living host often entices host vasculature to invade and produce a realistic blood supply: indeed, systems such as this can be used to study mechanisms of angio- and vasculogenesis in organoids (Risau et al., 1988). A standard site for organoid transplant is under the renal capsule of a host. For example, Xinaris et al. (2012) transplanted renal organoids into this site, which was already known to vascularize intact kidney rudiments (Preminger et al., 1980), and showed that they became vascularized and capable of filtering blood. Intestinal villus organoids grafted under the renal capsule show a proliferative response to host gut resection, suggesting that humoral growth-promoting factors reach the organoids: indeed, the system may be a useful tool for identifying such factors (Sinagoga and Wells, 2015). The use of in vivo experiments on animals can be avoided by grafting the organoid onto the chorioallantoic membrane of chick or quali embryos, a technique developed for tumor vasculogensis by Murphy (1912): this allows easy access and observation, although the technique is restricted to the window of a few days when the host vasculature is developed enough to be useful, but the chick has not become so mature that its movements are disruptive to the experiment. All of these techniques are labor-intensive, and result in variable vascularization.

Another problem with ES and iPS cell-derived organoids is one of immaturity: as a generalization, organoids from these sources show characteristics of foetal organs, rather than their mature equivalents. Interestingly, some organoids, such as gut villi, can gain a more mature phenotype on long-term passage in culture (reviewed by Sinagoga and Wells, 2015). This suggests that time itself, rather than, or as well as, hormonal and environmental signals, may be important in maturation. If it is, this could be a problem for the goal of engineering transplantable organs from iPS cells in a reasonably short time.

FINAL REMARKS

Following many decades of work, organoid technology has reached a stage of increasingly rapid adoption across a range of biomedical disciplines. It opens new areas of research, particularly where it is essential to perform experiments directly on human tissues, or to gain good access to a complex multicellular system for imaging. It is not, however, a solution to every problem: organoids are not completely realistic, and almost always lack some aspect of their *in vivo* counterparts, and they may be better models for foetal tissues than for adult. The chapters that follow provide excellent advice, from international experts, on how to set up and use organoid systems. Anyone wishing to adapt organoid technology for their own research problems should find these chapters very useful but, as always, when adapting techniques in science, beware the unknown unknowns!

ACKNOWLEDGMENTS

The author acknowledges funding from MRC (MR/K010735/1) and Kidney Research UK (RP_002_20160223) for funding organoid work described in this chapter.

REFERENCES

Aquila-Mansilla, N., Barnea, A., 1996. Human fetal brain cells in aggregate culture: a model system to study regulatory processes of the developing human neuropeptide Y (NPY)-producing neuron. Int. J. Dev. Neurosci. 14, 531–539.

Auerbach, R., Grobstein, C., 1958. Inductive interaction of embryonic tissues after dissociation and reaggregation. Exp. Cell. Res. 1958, 384–397.

Barnea, A., Roberts, J., 1999. An improved method for dissociation and aggregate culture of human fetal brain cells in serum-free medium. Brain. Res. Brain. Res. Protoc. 4, 156—164.

Bartfeld, S., Bayram, T., van de Wetering, M., Huch, M., Begthel, H., Kujala, P., et al., 2015. In vitro expansion of human gastric epithelial stem cells and their responses to bacterial infection. Gastroenterology. 148, 126—136.

Betts, K.S., 2010. Growing knowledge: using stem cells to study developmental neurotoxicity. Environ. Health. Perspect. 118 (10), A432—A437, 2010 Oct.

Boulangé, C.L., Neves, A.L., Chilloux, J., Nicholson, J.K., Dumas, M.E., 2016. Impact of the gut microbiota on inflammation, obesity, and metabolic disease. Genome Med. 20, 42.

Brown, C.D., Sayer, R., Windass, A.S., Haslam, I.S., De Broe, M.E., D'Haese, P.C., et al., 2008. Characterisation of human tubular cell monolayers as a model of proximal tubular xenobiotic handling. Toxicol. Appl. Pharmacol. 233, 428—438.

Bredenkamp, N., Ulyanchenko, S., O'Neill, K.E., Manley, N.R., Vaidya, H.J., Blackburn, C.C., 2014. An organized and functional thymus generated from FOXN1-reprogrammed fibroblasts. Nat. Cell Biol. 16, 902—908.

Bystron, I.P., Smirnov, E.B., Otellin, V.A., Wierzba-Bobrowicz, T., Dymecki, J., 2002. Suspensional reaggregates of human foetal neocortex and tegmentum as objects of neurotransplantation. Folia. Neuropathol. 40, 75—85.

Cachat, E., Liu, W., Martin, K.C., Yuan, X., Yin, H., Hohenstein, P., et al., 2016. 2- and 3-dimensional synthetic large-scale de novo patterning by mammalian cells through phase separation. Sci. Rep. 6, 20664.

Calderon-Gierszal, E.L., Prins, G.S., 2015. Directed differentiation of human embryonic stem cells into prostate organoids in vitro and its perturbation by low-dose bisphenol a exposure. PLoS. ONE. 10, e0133238.

Calderon-Gierszal, E.L., Prinz, G.S., 2017. Prostate organoids: directed differentiation from embryonic stem cells. Chapter 5 of this book.

Choi, E.Y., Park, W.S., Jung, K.C., Chung, D.H., Bae, Y.M., Kim, T.J., et al., 1997. Thymocytes positively select thymocytes in human system. Hum. Immunol. 54, 15—20.

Davies, J.A., 2012. Replacing Animal Models: A Practical Guide to Creating and Using Culture-Based Biomimetic Alternatives. Wiley-Blackwell, Hoboken, NJ.

Davies, J.A., 2013. Mechanisms of Morphogenesis. Elsevier, Amsterdam, pp. 277—279.

Davies, J.A., Cachat, E., 2016. Synthetic biology meets tissue engineering. Biochem. Soc. Trans. 44, 696—701.

Duguay, D., Foty, R.A., Steinberg, M.S., 2003. Cadherin-mediated cell adhesion and tissue segregation: qualitative and quantitative determinants. Dev. Biol. 253, 309—323.

Duryee, W.R., Doherty, J.K., 1954. Nuclear and cytoplasmic organoids in the living cell. Ann. N. Y. Acad. Sci. 58, 1210—1231.

Eglen, R.M., Randle, D.H., 2015. Drug discovery goes three-dimensional: goodbye to flat high-throughput screening? Assay Drug Dev. Technol. 2015 13 (5), 262—265.

Elgin, T.G., Kern, S.L., McElroy, S.J., 2016. Development of the Neonatal Intestinal Microbiome and Its Association With Necrotizing Enterocolitis. Clin. Ther. 38, 706—715.

Fernados, N., Mason, J., 2017 Cerebral organoids: building brains from stem cells. Chapter 8 of this book.

Foty, R.A., Steinberg, M.S., 2005. The differential adhesion hypothesis: a direct evaluation. Dev. Biol. 278, 255−263.

Garcez, P.P., Loiola, E.C., Madeiro da Costa, R., Higa, L.M., Trindade, P., Delvecchio, R., et al., 2016. Zika virus impairs growth in human neurospheres and brain organoids. Science. 2016 352 (6287), 816−818. Available from: http://dx.doi.org/10.1126/science.aaf6116.

Grens, K., 2013. 2013's Big advances in science. The Scientist. Retrieved 26 December 2013.

Grobstein, C., Younger, J.S., 1949. Combination of tissues from different species in flask cultures. Science 110, 501−503.

Gruenwald, P., 1937. Zur Entwicklungsmechanik des Urogenitalsystems beim Huhn. Arch. f. Entw.- mechan. d. Org. 136, 786−813.

Gruenwald, P., 1942. Experiments on distribution and activation of the nephrogenic potency in the embryonic mesenchyme. Physiol. Zool. 15, 396−409.

Guo, X.M., Zhao, Y.S., Chang, H.X., Wang, C.Y., LL, E., Zhang, X.A., Duan, C.M., et al., 2006. Creation of engineered cardiac tissue in vitro from mouse embryonic stem cells. Circulation 113, 2229−2237.

Ishikawa, T., Nakayama, S., Nakagawa, T., Horiguchi, K., Misawa, H., Kadowaki, M., et al., 2004. Characterization of in vitro gutlike organ formed from mouse embryonic stem cells. Am. J. Physiol. Cell Physiol. 286, C1344−C1352.

Jenkinson, S.E., Chung, G.W., van Loon, E., Bakar, N.S., Dalzell, A.M., Brown, C.D., 2012. The limitations of renal epithelial cell line HK-2 as a model of drug transporter expression and function in the proximal tubule. Pflugers. Arch. 464 (6), 601−611, 2012 Dec.

Kim, D., Dressler, G.R., 2005. Nephrogenic factors promote differentiation of mouse embryonic stem cells into renal epithelia. J. Am. Soc. Nephrol. 2005 16 (12), 3527−3534.

Kitahara, H., Yagi, H., Tajima, K., Okamoto, K., Yoshitake, A., Aeba, R., et al., 2016. Heterotopic transplantation of a decellularized and recellularized whole porcine heart. Interact. Cardiovasc. Thorac. Surg. 22, 571−579.

Harris, M., 1943. The compatibility of rat and mouse cells in mixed tissue cultures. Anat. Rec. 87, 107−117.

Heller, D.S., Frydman, C.P., Gordon, R.E., Jagirdar, J., Schwartz, I.S., 1991. An unusual organoid tumor. Alveolar soft part sarcoma or paraganglioma? Cancer 67, 1894−1899.

Hwang, C.I., Boj, S.F., Clevers, H., Tuveson, D.A., 2016. Preclinical models of pancreatic ductal adenocarcinoma. J. Pathol. 238 (2), 197−204, 2016 Jan.

Kim, B.M., Suzuki, S., Nishimura, Y., Um, S.C., Morota, K., Maruguchi, T., et al., 1999. Cellular artificial skin substitute produced by short period simultaneous culture of fibroblasts and keratinocytes. Br. J. Plast. Surg. 52, 573−578.

Kitamura, Y., Murata, Y., Park, J.H., Kotani, T., Imada, S., Saito, Y., et al., 2015. Regulation by gut commensal bacteria of carcinoembryonic antigen-related cell adhesion molecule expression in the intestinal epithelium. Genes. Cells. 20, 578−589.

Lawrence, M.L., Mills, C.G., Davies, J.A., 2017. From organoids to mini-organs: a case study in the kidney. Chapter 9 of this book.

Li, X., Nadauld, L., Ootani, A., Corney, D.C., Pai, R.K., Gevaert, O., et al., 2014. Oncogenic transformation of diverse gastrointestinal tissues in primary organoid culture. Nat. Med. 20 (7), 769−777, 2014 Jul.

Li, L., Zhou, Q., Voss, T.C., Quick, K.L., LaBarbera, D.V., 2016. High-throughput imaging: Focusing in on drug discovery in 3D. Methods. 96, 97−102, 2016 Mar 1.

Lodin, Z., Fleischmannová, V., Hájková, B., Faltin, J., Hartman, J., 1981. Reaggregation of human, chick, and human embryonic brain cells. Factors influencing the formation of a histiotypic unit. Z. Mikrosk. Anat. Forsch. 95, 701−720.

Lovati, A.B., Bottagisio, M., Moretti, M., 2016. Decellularized and engineered tendons as biological substitutes: a critical review. Stem Cells Int 2016, 7276150. Available from: http://dx.doi.org/10.1155/2016/7276150.

Lukovac, S., Belzer, C., Pellis, L., Keijser, B.J., de Vos, W.M., Montijn, R.C., et al., 2014. Differential modulation by *Akkermansia muciniphila* and *Faecalibacterium prausnitzii* of host peripheral lipid metabolism and histone acetylation in mouse gut organoids. MBio 5 (4), 2014 Aug 12 pii: e01438-14.

Ma, R., Morshed, S.A., Latif, R., Davies, T.F., 2015. Thyroid cell differentiation from murine induced pluripotent stem cells. Front. Endocrinol. (Lausanne). 2015 6 (56).

Macchiarini, P., Walles, T., Biancosino, C., Mertsching, H., 2004. First human transplantation of a bioengineered airway tissue. J. Thorac. Cardiovasc. Surg. 128, 638−641.

Matano, M., Date, S., Shimokawa, M., Takano, A., Fujii, M., Ohta, Y., et al., 2015. Modeling colorectal cancer using CRISPR-Cas9-mediated engineering of human intestinal organoids. Nat. Med. 21, 256−262.

McCarthy, M., Resnick, L., Taub, F., Stewart, R.V., Dix, R.D., 1991. Infection of human neural cell aggregate cultures with a clinical isolate of cytomegalovirus. J. Neuropathol. Exp. Neurol. 50, 441−450.

Medawar, P.B., 1948. Tests by tissue culture methods on the nature of immunity to transplanted skin. J. Cell Sci. 89, 239−252.

Mizumoto, H., Aoki, K., Nakazawa, K., Ijima, H., Funatsu, K., Kajiwara, T., 2008. Hepatic differentiation of embryonic stem cells in HF/organoid culture. Transplant Proc. 2008 40 (2), 611−613.

Monier, B., Pélissier-Monier, A., Sanson, B., 2011. Establishment and maintenance of compartmental boundaries: role of contractile actomyosin barriers. Cell Mol Life Sci. 68 (11), 1897−1910. Available from: http://dx.doi.org/10.1007/s00018-011-0668-8.

Morizane, R., Lam, A.Q., Freedman, B.S., Kishi, S., Valerius, M.T., Bonventre, J.V., 2015. Nephron organoids derived from human pluripotent stem cells model kidney development and injury. Nat. Biotechnol. 33, 1193−1200.

Moscona, A., 1952. Cell suspensions from organ rudiments of chick embryos. Exp. Cell Res. 3, 535−539.

Moscona, A., 1956. The development in vigtro of chimeric aggregates of dissociated embryonic chick and mouse cells. PNAS 43, 184−194.

Moscona, A., Moscona, H., 1952. The dissociation and aggregation of cells from organ rudiments of the early chick embryo. J. Anat. 86, 287−301.

Murphy, J.B., 1912. Transplantability of malignant tumors to the embryos of a foreign species. JAMA 59, 874−875.

Nadauld, L.D., Garcia, S., Natsoulis, G., Bell, J.M., Miotke, L., Hopmans, E.S., et al., 2014. Metastatic tumor evolution and organoid modeling implicate TGFBR2 as a cancer driver in diffuse gastric cancer. Genome. Biol. 15 (8), 428, 2014 Aug 27.

Nesland, J.M., Sobrinho-Simões, M.A., Holm, R., Johannessen, J.V., 1985. Organoid tumor in the thyroid gland. Ultrastruct. Pathol. 9, 65−70.

Noël-Hudson, M.S., Dusser, I., Collober, I., Muriel, M.P., Bonté, F., Meybeck, A., et al., 1995. Human epidermis reconstructed on synthetic membrane: influence of experimental conditions on terminal differentiation. In. Vitro. Cell. Dev. Biol. Anim. 31, 508−515.

Petrosyan, A., Zanusso, I., Lavarreda-Pearce, M., Leslie, S., Sedrakyan, S., De Filippo, R. E., et al., 2016. Decellularized renal matrix and regenerative medicine of the kidney: a different point of view. Tissue. Eng. Part. B. Rev. 22 (3), 183−192, 2016 Jun.

Preminger, G.M., Koch, W.E., Fried, F.A., Mandell, J., 1980. Utilization of the chick chorioallantoic membrane for in vitro growth of the embryonic murine kidney. Am. J. Anat. 1980 159 (1), 17−24.

Pringle, S., Maimets, M., van der Zwaag, M., Stokman, M.A., van Gosliga, D., Zwart, E., et al., 2016. Human salivary gland stem cells functionally restore radiation damaged salivary glands. Stem Cells 34 (3), 640−652, 2016 Mar.

Qian, X., Nguyen, H.N., Song, M.M., Hadiono, C., Ogden, S.C., Hammack, C., et al., 2016. Brain-region-specific organoids using mini-bioreactors for modeling ZIKV exposure. Cell. 2016 Apr 21. pii: S0092-8674(16)30467-6. http://dx.doi.org/10.1016/j.cell.2016.04.032.

Risau, W., Sariola, H., Zerwes, H.G., Sasse, J., Ekblom, P., Kemler, R., et al., 1988. Vasculogenesis and angiogenesis in embryonic-stem-cell-derived embryoid bodies. Development. 1988 102 (3), 471−478.

Sachs, N., Clevers, H., 2014. Organoid cultures for the analysis of cancer phenotypes. Curr. Opin. Genet. Dev. 24, 68−73, 2014 Feb.

Sato, T., Vries, R.G., Snippert, H.J., van de Wetering, M., Barker, N., Stange, D.E., et al., 2009. Single Lgr5 stem cells build crypt-villus structures in vitro without a mesenchymal niche. Nature. 459 (7244), 262−265, May 14.

Saxen, L., 1988. Organogenesis of the Kidney. Cambridge University Press, Cambridge, United Kingdom.

Schwartz, M.P., Hou, Z., Propson, N.E., Zhang, J., Engstrom, C.J., Santos Costa, V., et al., 2015. Human pluripotent stem cell-derived neural constructs for predicting neural toxicity. Proc. Natl. Acad. Sci. U.S.A. 2015 112 (40), 12516−12521.

Shi, Q., Chien, Y.H., Leckband, D., 2008. Biophysical properties of cadherin bonds do not predict cell sorting. J. Biol. Chem. 283 (42), 28454−28463.

Sinagoga, K.L., Wells, J.M., 2015. Generating human intestinal tissues from pluripotent stem cells to study development and disease. EMBO J. 2015 34 (9), 1149−1163.

Song, J.J., Guyette, J.P., Gilpin, S.E., Gonzalez, G., Vacanti, J.P., Ott, H.C., 2013. Regeneration and experimental orthotopic transplantation of a bioengineered kidney. Nat. Med. 19, 646−651.

Spemann, H., Mangold, H., 1924. Induction of embryonic primordia by implantation of organizers from a different species. Roux's Arch. Entw. Mech. 100, 599−638.

Stabler, C.T., Lecht, S., Mondrinos, M.J., Goulart, E., Lazarovici, P., Lelkes, P.I., 2015. Revascularization of decellularized lung scaffolds: principles and progress. Am. J. Physiol. Lung. Cell. Mol. Physiol. 309, L1273−L1285.

Steinberg, M.S., 1963. Reconstruction of tissues by dissociated cells. Some morphogenetic tissue movements and the sorting out of embryonic cells may have a common explanation. . Science 141, 401−408.

Sun, J., 2017. Intestinal organoids in studying host-bacterial interactions. Chapter 14 of this book.

Takasato, M., Er, P.X., Chiu, H.S., Maier, B., Baillie, G.J., Ferguson, C., et al., 2015. Kidney organoids from human iPS cells contain multiple lineages and model human nephrogenesis. Nature. 526, 564−568.

Thomson, J.A., Itskovitz-Eldor, J., Shapiro, S.S., Waknitz, M.A., Swiergiel, J.J., Marshall, V.S., et al., 1998. Embryonic stem cell lines derived from human blastocysts. Science. 282, 1145−1147.

Unbekandt, M., Davies, J.A., 2010. Dissociation of embryonic kidneys followed by reaggregation allows the formation of renal tissues. Kidney. Int. 77, 407—416.

van de Wetering, M., Francies, H.E., Francis, J.M., Bounova, G., Iorio, F., Pronk, A., et al., 2015. Prospective derivation of a living organoid biobank of colorectal cancer patients. Cell. 2015 161 (4), 933—945. Available from: http://dx.doi.org/10.1016/j.cell.2015.03.053.

Van Limbergen, J., Geddes, K., Henderson, P., Russell, R.K., Drummond, H.E., Satsangi, J., et al., 2015. Paneth cell marker CD24 in NOD2 knockout organoids and in inflammatory bowel disease (IBD). Gut. 64 (2), 353—354, 2015 Feb.

Vela, I., Chen, Y., 2015. Prostate cancer organoids: a potential new tool for testing drug sensitivity. Expert. Rev. Anticancer. Ther. 15, 261—263.

Weiss, P., Taylor, A.C., 1960. Reconstitution of complete organs from single-cell suspensions of chick embryos in advanced stages of differentiation. PNAS 46, 1177—1185.

Willyard, C., 2015. The boom in mini stomachs, brains, breasts, kidneys and more. Nature 523 (7562), 520—522, 2015 Jul 30 http://dx.doi.org/10.1038/523520a.

Wilson, H.V., 1910. Development of sponges from dissociated tissue cells. Bull. US Bureau Fisheries 1910, 1—30.

Xinaris, C., Benedetti, V., Rizzo, P., Abbate, M., Corna, D., Azzollini, N., et al., 2012. In vivo maturation of functional renal organoids formed from embryonic cell suspensions. J. Am. Soc. Nephrol. 23, 1857—1868.

Yarandi, S.S., Peterson, D.A., Treisman, G.J., Moran, T.H., Pasricha, P.J., 2016. Modulatory Effects of Gut Microbiota on the Central Nervous System: How Gut Could Play a Role in Neuropsychiatric Health and Diseases. J Neurogastroenterol Motil. 22, 201—212.

Yin, Y., Bijvelds, M., Dang, W., Xu, L., van der Eijk, A.A., Knipping, K., et al., 2015. Modeling rotavirus infection and antiviral therapy using primary intestinal organoids. Antiviral. Res. 123, 120—131.

Yu, J., Vodyanik, M.A., Smuga-Otto, K., Antosiewicz-Bourget, J., Frane, J.L., Tian, S., et al., 2007. Induced pluripotent stem cell lines derived from human somatic cells. Science. 318, 1917—1920.

Yui, S., Nakamura, T., Sato, T., Nemoto, Y., Mizutani, T., Zheng, X., et al., 2012. Functional engraftment of colon epithelium expanded in vitro from a single adult Lgr5$^+$ stem cell. Nat. Med. 8, 618—623.

Zeng, Y., Win-Shwe, T-T., Itoh, T, Sone, H., 2017. A 3D neurosphere system using human stem cells for nanotoxicology studies. Chapter 11 of this book.

FURTHER READING

Cachat, E., Liu, W., Hohenstein, P., Davies, J.A., 2014. A library of mammalian effector modules for synthetic morphology. J. Biol. Eng. 8, 26. Available from: http://dx.doi.org/10.1186/1754-1611-8-26.

Eglen, R.M., Randle, D.H., 2015. Drug Discovery Goes Three-Dimensional: Goodbye to Flat High-Throughput Screening?. Assay. Drug. Dev. Technol. 13 (5), 262—265, 2015 Jun.

Grobstein, C., 1955. Inductive interaction in the development of the mouise metanephros. J. Exp. Zool. 130, 319—340.

Constructing Organoids

II

Elements of organoid design

2

Richard J. McMurtrey

Institute of Neural Regeneration & Tissue Engineering, Highland, UT, United States

CHAPTER OUTLINE

INTRODUCTION

The ability to study and treat a wide variety of neurological conditions still poses a tremendous challenge to modern medicine, which has few if any options for repairing neural tissue or restoring function in disrupted neural circuitry. The discovery of underlying pathological mechanisms of neurological diseases is typically limited by the inability to study the disease in living human neural tissues or realistic neural environments, and animal models have been particularly insufficient for the study of distinctly human diseases. Neural organoids, however, enable the formation of complex neural tissues from human stem cells, and provide a tremendous tool for using patient-derived stem cells to create realistic neural tissues, under controlled conditions, for detailed study of numerous undetermined mechanisms of development and disease. These include pharmacologic or toxicologic drug effects in tissues, and novel regenerative medicine applications.

Neural organoids are generally created by suspending stem cells in biomaterial scaffolds and directing cell differentiation to neuroglial lineages, such that the resulting construct replicates features of innate neural tissue (see Chapter 8: Cerebral organoids: building brains from stem cells and Chapter 11: A 3D neurosphere system using human stem cells for nanotoxicology studies). Neuronal cells possess, at least to some extent, the ability to pattern themselves within a homogenous biomaterial scaffold (Lancaster et al., 2013), but it is also possible to guide

Organoids and Mini-Organs. DOI: http://dx.doi.org/10.1016/B978-0-12-812636-3.00002-X

their cellular architecture with more complex configurations of patterned topographical and biochemical cues within the tissue construct (McMurtrey, 2014). Alternatively, it is possible to forego biomaterial scaffolding that guides cellular migration and self-organization, and instead simply grow conglomerate multicellular spheroids (Paşca et al., 2015). The architecture and differentiation of cells can be guided both by intrinsically programmed cell signaling cues, and by external signaling cues in the biomaterial scaffolding and media formulations.

By directing differentiation towards certain fates, neural organoids can replicate basic features of the cerebral cortex, hippocampus, cerebellum, spinal cord, retina, and other neural tissues (Lancaster et al., 2013; Meinhardt et al., 2014; Muguruma et al., 2015), and cerebral organoids have already been used to model conditions of microcephaly, autism, lissencephaly, neurodegenerative diseases, infection by Zika virus, as well as to investigate normal tissue development (Lancaster et al., 2013; Meinhardt et al., 2014; Muguruma et al., 2015; Bershteyn et al., 2017; Mariani et al., 2015; Choi et al., 2014; Dang et al., 2016; Mullard, 2015; Kelava and Lancaster, 2016 Jun 2; Wang et al., 2016). Cerebral organoids can recapitulate neurodevelopment in structural features, as well as in epigenomic expression patterns (Luo et al., 2016). Similarly, organoids may also be produced as representations of other organ types, including cardiac, pulmonary, gastrointestinal, hepatic, pancreatic, or renal tissues.

While neural organoids have demonstrated the ability to form numerous types of cell identities and tissue structures, the results particular to each organoid and each batch of organoids can be quite variable. Current organoid protocols currently do not provide comprehensive control over differentiation, regionalization, or cellular subspecialization, and organoids often form several types of cellular compositions and structures. This is probably due to minor variations in cell signaling cues, stem cell states, metabolic rates, growth patterns, concentration gradients through the constructs, materials, and environmental conditions (for example, oxygen and carbon dioxide levels, atmospheric pressure, pH, etc.), and such variation is perhaps not surprising, considering the comprehensive differentiation potential of pluripotent stem cells. It is, therefore, essential to understand how each design feature of an organoid will influence cellular identities, tissue architecture, and the ultimate function of the synthetic tissue. As described in this chapter, three-dimensional (3D) biomaterial constructs can contain an entire collection of stem cells, molecular cues, diffusion gradients, and topographic scaffolding, and an understanding of how all these components interact will help achieve fine control of cellular identities and tissue formation, and help expand capabilities to regenerate complex tissues.

ELEMENTS OF DESIGN

Design considerations will depend substantially on the intended purpose and the desired tissue type, and the following sections cover both physical and biochemical components of design, as each of these can influence the identity, differentiation, and patterning of stem cells. The biochemical factors involved in growth and differentiation of stem cell-derived tissues, whether provided in the media, in biomaterial scaffolding, or from the direct production by cells, are classically known to influence cell identity and development through a network of cell signaling and gene expression networks, both in vivo and in vitro. Physical cues such as biomaterial scaffolding, topography, biomechanics, and diffusion gradients have also been shown to influence cell differentiation, and the formation and patterning of tissue architecture (McMurtrey, 2014; Aurand et al., 2012; McMurtrey, 2016a). Cells must encode extraordinary instructional processes that ultimately create the structure and organization of the human body, and the mechanisms whereby genetic fonts encode living tomes of extravagant and expansive form are indeed wondrous. Future research must further explore optimal combinations of biomaterial compositions, structural arrangements, molecular signaling factors, patterned scaffolding, culture media, and cellular compositions that can recapitulate developmental events and tissue architectures.

THE ROLE OF DIFFUSION IN ORGANOID DEVELOPMENT

The advent of 3D cell culture capabilities has enabled the formation of novel tissue structures that represent innate tissue architectures and functions. This phenomenon is a result of more realistic interactions between cells and extracellular matrix molecules in a 3D environment than can exist in a two-dimensional (2D) environment, and it is also due to the fact that diffusion limitations arise in 3D tissues that are not present in 2D surface cultures. These diffusion limitations cause delayed nutrient transport into the tissue, and give rise to important spatial concentration gradients within the tissue, including gradients of extrinsic factors (such as gases and nutrients, which are generally highest at the surface of the construct or nearest the nutrient source, and lowest at the central density of cells or at the farthest point from the nutrient source), or gradients of intrinsic factors (such as cell-secreted biochemical signaling molecules and transcription factors, which are generally highest at the central density of cells). These nutrient gradients may include molecules like glucose, oxygen, amino acids, fatty acids, or vitamins, and any metabolic consumption of these nutrients further decreases their availability to cells, and significantly alters the shape of the concentration gradient in the tissue (see Fig. 2.1) (McMurtrey, 2016b). The mass transport limitation of nutrients is one of the principal reasons why 3D tissue size is diffusion-limited, and why implanted tissue structures often suffer cell death during culture or implantation into the body.

Diffusional gradients are also known to play critical roles in innate development, which are vitally important for cell differentiation or maintenance of potency, and for influencing the metabolic state of the cells, as well as essential for axis patterning, self-organization, and regionalization of tissue architecture. Little is known about the cellular programming of shape formation in tissues, but

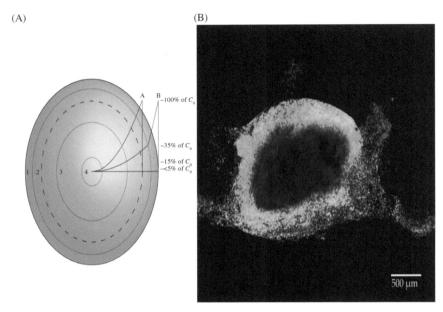

FIGURE 2.1

(A) An example of a concentration gradient of metabolized gas or nutrient through an organoid, including how the gradient of a nutrient changes based on the distribution of cells within the organoid. Curve A represents the nutrient concentration supplied in the media (at a concentration of C_o) and diffusing through an organoid with a homogenous distribution of cells that metabolize the nutrient at a constant rate. This makes a growth limitation on the organoid, where any expansion beyond a maximal diameter (shown by the dashed line) would cause lack of nutrient to the central cells. Curve B shows how the nutrient gradient changes when 85% of the cells in the organoid are placed in only the outer half-volume of the sphere. This results in ~30% increase in maximal diameter of the sphere, which may explain, at least in part, benefits of neurons migrating to an outer cortex of neuroepithelium in the brain during development. (B) A cerebral organoid generated from human iPSCs showing a cortical layer of differentiated neurons (green stain = TUJ1 βIII-tubulin, blue stain = Hoechst nuclear stain).

Figures used with permission from McMurtrey, R.J., 2016b. Analytic models of oxygen and nutrient diffusion, metabolism dynamics, and architecture optimization in three-dimensional tissue constructs with applications and insights in cerebral organoids. Tissue Eng. Part C 22(3), 221–249.

it was recognized many years ago that cells are capable of detecting and responding to the spatiality, directionality, and even the steepness or slope of local concentration gradients in developing insect tissues (Lawrence, 1992). While many of these developmental processes are only partially understood, and remain to be elucidated, it is clear that diffusion dynamics are critical to numerous cell and tissue functions. An understanding of these processes will enable more precisely engineered constructs, with more defined and controllable concentrations of gases, nutrients, signaling factors, and other substances within the construct.

There are several examples of how diffusion phenomena can affect living organisms. It is known that specific concentrations of gases and nutrients can control epigenetic states of stem cells, and likewise these epigenetic states can control metabolic dynamics, nutrient consumption, and cell differentiation. Stem cells tend to prefer anaerobic (glycolytic) metabolism (including primed pluripotent stem cells (PSCs), neural stem cells (NSCs), mesenchymal stem cells (MSCs), and hematopoietic stem cells (HSCs)), while mature cells tend to favor aerobic (oxidative) metabolism, and epigenetic and metabolic states have direct effects on stem cell maintenance and differentiation (Teslaa and Teitell, 2015; Ito and Suda, 2014). The metabolic state is not just a passive consequence, but is in fact a programmed part of the "stemness" state, whether in embryonic stem cells or stem cells reprogrammed from somatic cells (Ezashi et al., 2005; Varum et al., 2011; Mathieu et al., 2014). Reciprocally, environmental limitations in gases and nutrients can upregulate glycolytic processes, and influence stem cell state and reprogramming efficiency. These effects are mediated through numerous signaling pathways, including hypoxia-inducible factors (HIFs), AMP-kinase (AMPK), and the mammalian target of rapamycin complex (mTORC), the downstream targets of which include the same genes as are targeted in stem cell maintenance and reprogramming: *OCT4*, *WNT*, *NANOG*, *KLF4*, *MYC*, *NOTCH*, *SOX2*, *LIN28*, and others. These data suggest that stem cells are more likely to be located at more hypoxic regions in tissues, such as at the central region of spherical organoids. Oxygen levels have also been shown to determine neuronal fates during differentiation (Xie et al., 2014; Ortega et al., 2016; Gustafsson et al., 2005). Thus, environmental concentrations of oxygen, glucose, and other nutrients, metabolites, and factors can play a direct role in stem cell states and localized cellular identities (McMurtrey, 2016b).

The "shape" of a diffusion gradient (meaning the variation in the local concentration of diffusant) through the tissue is dependent on several factors, including the concentration of the diffusant substance, and its production rate over time, whether the diffusant substance is metabolized, and whether this follows zero-order, first-order, or other kinetics, the diffusivity in the matrix or tissue environment, the distribution of cells in the tissue, how the diffusant crosses the interface between media and tissue, the boundary conditions of the diffusant at interfaces between different tissue compartments or between tissue and environment, whether the diffusant can primarily move in one-, two-, or three-dimensions, and whether the diffusant is available in unlimited supply (such as ambient oxygen), or in only limited supply (such as glucose in a static culture well).

Equations that relate these factors and express them as functions showing the predicted diffusion gradient have been derived and expressed in analytic form (McMurtrey, 2016b, 2017). In general, it can be stated that unmetabolized diffusant substances in limited supply and diffusing through an unlimited homogenous medium will exhibit Gaussian-shaped curves in space, declining in concentration farther from the source, regardless of whether the diffusion occurs in one-, two-, or three-dimensions. Similarly, unmetabolized diffusants with relatively unlimited supply will exhibit concentration curves in the shape of the complementary error function ("erfc") in one dimension, in the shape of the Bessel function (first kind, zero order) for two-dimensional (cylindrical) diffusion, and in a hyperbolic curve in three-dimensional (spherical) diffusion. The same conditions with zero-order kinetic metabolism of the diffusant produce a parabolic decline in concentration through space, regardless of whether it diffuses in one-, two-, or three-dimensions, while the same conditions with first-order metabolism produce a hyperbolic sine curve in concentration through space. Thus, differential effects will be exerted on cells based on their position within the organoid, and the local concentration gradient.

COMPARTMENTALIZATION OF MOLECULAR GRADIENT SOURCES

Remarkably, cells possess all the machinery for survival, differentiation, axis patterning, tissue organization, and ultimately for establishing functional networks of memory and thought. "Algorithms" in cells enable carefully timed secretions of signaling cues and transcription factors that communicate with adjacent cells to guide axis patterning, cell specialization, tissue architecture, and organ shape. Numerous intercellular signaling factors are known to guide neural tissue development, many of which form concentration gradients through the tissue. These signals include trophic factors, axonal guidance cues, migratory cues, and many other factors that induce highly specific effects on cell and tissue development.

In many natural tissues, whether mammalian or insect, regional development is mediated by compartmentalized gradients of signaling factors in the organism. While diffusion dynamics can limit mass transport of nutrients, such dynamics can also be desirable and even essential in developmental processes, as they mediate gradients of vital cell signaling cues. The limitations in diffusion produced by biomaterials surrounding cells result in increased internal concentrations of molecular substances secreted by the cells, meaning that bulk cellular constructs and biomaterials naturally mediate endogenously produced molecular gradients. Particularly in nervous system development, local concentration gradients control many aspects of brain and spinal cord regionalization. For example, concentration gradients of sonic hedgehog (SHH), wnt protein (WNT), bone morphogenic protein (BMP), fibroblast growth factor (FGF), retinoic acid (RA), reelin (RELN), chemokine ligands (CXCL), various neurotrophic factors, and many others can control neural tissue development (Muguruma et al., 2015; McMurtrey, 2016a). Thus, 3D cell cultures offer the advantage of mediating preprogrammed intercellular signaling cues and gradients, which further mediate important differentiation and self-organization capabilities.

The same factors that mediate normal development can also be used to guide development in synthetic tissues and cell cultures. It should be recognized, however, that many of these factors do not simply result in a single isolated fate or a single categorical effect, but rather they work together to achieve many complex downstream results, and the timing and concentration of each can produce differential results (McMurtrey, 2016a, 2017). Ventralization of neural tissue can be induced by factors such as sonic hedgehog (SHH), smoothened agonist (SAG), or purmorphamine. Dorsalization can be induced with "wnt" protein (WNT), bone morphogenic protein 4 (BMP4), or cyclopamine. Proteins like WNT, BMP, FGF2, or nodal can induce a caudal fate, while inhibitors of these factors can induce a rostral fate. Inhibitors of BMP (like dorsomorphin, noggin, chordin, or follistatin) and inhibitors of transforming growth factor (TGF)-β (like SB-431542 or lefty) can promote neural differentiation of stem cells. FGF can also inhibit BMP and TGF signaling pathways to induce neuronal fates, but it can also independently promote neural induction and proliferation, as well as promote caudalization or ventralization, depending on timing and conditions (McMurtrey, 2016a; Yan et al., 2016; Bejoy et al., 2016). FGF19 and CXCL12 (SDF1) can be used to induce cerebellar differentiation (Muguruma et al., 2015). Other transcriptional factors can have negative feedback effects on each other, such as Pax6 and Emx2, which guide spatial identities of the cortex. Emx2 promotes the medial caudal region, Pax6 promotes the lateral rostral region, and Emx2 is suppressed by FGF8 while Pax6 is suppressed by SHH signaling.

Similarly, retinoic acid (RA) can induce neural differentiation, with higher concentrations favoring caudalization or posteriorization in neural progenitors. Retinoic acid can also induce activity of SHH, and these two factors work together to produce the floor plate at the ventral portion of the neural tube. Retinoic acid and WNT also interact in ways that alter the assembly of gene promoters, and drive various differentiation signals in stem cells. Both RA and reelin can serve as migration guidance signals for neural stem cells and promote neural migration to the cortex, and these migrations are responsible for filling out the cortical and hippocampal layers, expanding gyri, and creating abundant intracortical connections (McMurtrey, 2016a). Attractive and repulsive neurite guidance molecules like netrins, slits, semaphorins, and ephrins can also be used in the hydrogel to guide neural pathway formations.

The integration of intrinsic or extrinsic factors into organoid constructs can simulate such innate cues. The biochemically-polarized regions are achieved by loading or suspending the designated diffusant molecule in a specific region of the hydrogel architecture in the tissue construct at a specific concentration or specific molar amount within the volume of the designated compartment, and this biochemically-polarized region further provides a higher concentration of the molecular factor in that particular region of the tissue construct. For example, the upper half of an organoid sphere can be imbued with rostral-inducing factors, and the lower half imbued with caudal-inducing factors, or likewise the sphere may be imbued with ventral − dorsal gradients or lateral − medial − lateral gradients.

As further examples, compartmentalization of the biomaterial constructs might be achieved with combinations of small spherical compartments embedded within a larger sphere, or by layer-by-layer assembly of compartments, such as an outer surface layer of hydrogel wrapped around an inner organoid. Such a surface layer could be loaded with a signaling factor such as retinoic acid, which would create a gradient that is high at the external aspect of the sphere, and lower at the internal portion of the sphere, thereby imitating certain neurodevelopmental signals that emerge from the meninges that influence the expansion and migration of neural tissue. Similarly, reelin may be suspended in one half of the outer layer of hydrogel in a spherical tissue construct, while retinoic acid is suspended in the opposite half of the outer layer of the hydrogel compartment in a spherical tissue construct, thereby forming a dually-polarized tissue construct that provides a bidirectional molecular gradient secretion pattern. Additional gradients of molecular factors listed above can also act upon the cells within the hydrogel to produce effects of stem cell maintenance and trophic support, stem cell induction and differentiation, cell growth, cell migration, cell attachment, cell proliferation, cell activity, tissue patterning, and regionalization, or other desired effects of neurulation, corticalization, rostraulization, caudalization, ventralization, or dorsalization.

Thus, innate cellular programs for differentiation and signaling factor release can be recapitulated and further investigated under controlled conditions in synthetic tissue constructs. By activating similar cellular cues and replicating similar polarized regions of molecular factors that form the localized concentration gradients, such compartmental hydrogel configurations could then facilitate formation of complex neuroanatomical structures and their interconnecting neural network structures. Recapitulating these sorts of diffusible differentiation signals and processes in natural 3D culture environments is essential for recapitulating rostral − caudal, ventral − dorsal, and medial − lateral tissue identities of central neural tissue, as well as many more complex architectures (see Fig. 2.2). It is not known to what extent extrinsic signals may override intrinsic cell programming, or how conflicting or complex signals will delineate ultimate tissue fates, but such signals certainly influence and guide the developmental processes. Experimentation with multiple configurations of signaling factors and gradients in organoid constructs will reveal many interesting and useful findings about the role of these factors in development, and will also enable much more targeted and predictable results in cellular subtype differentiation and reproducible formation of specific tissue types. Although these interweaving signaling pathways are highly complex, and although little is still known about many stages and mechanisms of neurodevelopment, carefully designed organoid models will significantly expand the capabilities to engineer specific tissue types, tissue structures, and tissue functions, which will also likely reveal much more insight into these complex processes.

BIOMATERIAL COMPOSITION

Biomaterial hydrogels provide an aqueous medium in a 3D structure that can support cell cultures. Hydrogels may be composed of synthetic polymers, or composed of natural biomaterial substances, such as those found in natural extracellular matrices, including collagen, hyaluronic acid, and Matrigel or Engelbreth − Holm − Swarm sarcoma matrix, and hydrogels may also be composed of any combination of

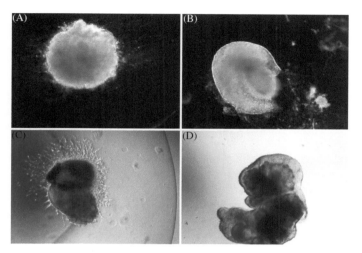

FIGURE 2.2

(A) A cerebral organoid created from human iPSCs differentiated to a neuronal fate shows cellular migration along functionalized nanofilaments in a hydrogel. (B) A cellularized hydrogel rolled with nanofilaments resembles a folded cortical layer or the folding of the hippocampal formation. (C) The choice of biomaterial composition and molecular signaling factors produces different effects on spheroids of differentiating iPSCs – a dual phase spherical hydrogel cultured in neural differentiation media shows prolific neurite outgrowth. (D) An expansive regionalized neuroepithelium is seen as the more translucent layer around the tissue of iPSCs cultured in a biomaterial construct, which will develop into a mini-cortex.

Figures used with permission from McMurtrey, R.J., 2016a. Multi-compartmental biomaterial scaffolds for
patterning neural tissue organoids in models of neurodevelopment and tissue regeneration. J Tissue Eng.
7;7:2041731416671926.

modified natural and synthetic polymers. Natural substances include hyaluronan, chitosan, collagen, gelatin, alginate, agarose, cellulose, heparin, silk, fibrin, fibronectin, vitronectin, laminin, and numerous other types of proteoglycans, glycosaminoglycans, glycoproteins, or amino acid polymers. Hyaluronic acid is one example of a polymer that is found naturally in neural tissue, and thus it has good biocompatibility and can be modified to allow cross-linking or other functionalization. Hyaluronic acid has shown the ability to enhance the survival of neural stem cell implants in the central nervous system (Moshayedi and Carmichael, 2013; Liang et al., 2013). Other polymers like chitosan can also be functionalized with certain chemical moieties to achieve specific functions in a hydrogel scaffold. Synthetic polymers include polylactic acid, polyglycolic acid, polyethylene glycol, polycaprolactone, or many other types, which can also be further modified with functional groups. Traditional cerebral organoids are grown from embryoid bodies implanted into a biomaterial matrix called Matrigel, which is composed of numerous protein types like laminin, collagen, entactin, heparan sulphate proteoglycans, and others. In the future, however, more specific and defined hydrogel polymers may be used to create organoids in a more consistent and targeted manner (as opposed to the varied protein compositions of matrigel traditionally used in organoid culture) (Bento et al., 2016).

Furthermore, a primary goal of tissue engineering is to enhance capabilities for micropatterning the molecular, cellular, and structural features of tissues, and this is best done by considering the full array of complex interacting factors in a tissue (see Fig. 2.3). While diffusive cell-signaling cues can dramatically influence cell patterning, cell patterning can also reciprocally influence the signaling cues, and biomaterial designs can now incorporate molecular signaling gradients that can be predicted by specific physical diffusion models. Importantly, biomaterials also provide a 3D culture environment similar to innate tissue, and they replicate important features and functions of extracellular matrix, such as guiding structural organization of cells, mediating cellular attachment, supporting anchorage-dependent survival, influencing cellular interactions and cellular network formation, replicating

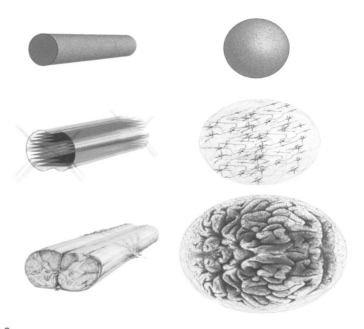

FIGURE 2.3

A general concept of 3D biomaterial scaffolds, within which stem cells can be cultured and differentiated to produce an array of complex cellular identities and tissue structures. These organoid constructs may then be used as models of neurodevelopment, as tools for investigating neurological diseases, or even as future regenerative therapies.

Figure used with permission from McMurtrey, R.J., 2015. Novel advancements in three-dimensional neural tissue engineering and regenerative medicine. Neural Regen. Res. 10(3), 352–354.

biomechanical features of tissues, providing important cues for cell differentiation and other cell signaling functions, preventing the washing away of cells into surrounding fluids, and, as mentioned above, retaining important signaling factors and diffusion gradients in a tissue-like medium. The biomaterials should therefore be chosen and engineered for particular functions, like producing specific desirable hydrogel characteristics for tissue culture, replicating specific components of particular tissue types, driving specific cell lineages, maximizing cell survival, recapitulating innate developmental events, or optimizing integration of synthetic constructs into damaged or diseased tissue.

Functional scaffolding within hydrogels may also be used to create intricate cellular architectures to help replicate complex features of connectivity in natural neural tissue, such as connections between artificial basal ganglia nuclei composed of dopaminergic and cholinergic neurons, between different regions of subtypes of hippocampal neurons, between different cortical layers of neurons, or various ascending, descending, or decussating tracts in the spinal cord. The nanofiber architecture can be assembled prior to embedding in hydrogel, or concurrently at the time of hydrogel polymerization using external scaffolding supports (McMurtrey, 2014). For example, a three-dimensional filament architecture can be assembled on an external scaffolding, and then embedded within a cellularized hydrogel to guide neurite extension in three dimensions, and thereby form a composite structure similar to innately-patterned neural tissue. The fibers may also be functionalized with signaling factors or pharmacological agents that act on receptors of attached cells, or that diffuse into the hydrogel and produce desired effects on cells in a localized manner. By depositing drugs into the fiber polymer solution during their manufacture, the fibers themselves can act as drug-eluting repositories, or compounds can be chemically coupled directly to the fiber polymers for more permanent attachment. The hydrogel itself may also be functionalized with certain molecules or moieties that represent a variety of receptors, guidance molecules, or extracellular matrix groups.

Biomaterials are likely to enhance outcomes of cell therapies in the nervous system, particularly in the central nervous system, where implanted neuroglial cells have difficulty surviving, integrating, and staying at the intended implantation site. Implanting engineered tissues rather than isolated cells is more likely to replicate and restore function of many tissues and organs. If future 3D organoid constructs are intended to be used in a therapeutic manner, the biocompatibility of the scaffolding material must also be taken into consideration. This would likely require the use of xeno-free chemically-defined biomaterials that minimize foreign body reactions, that match structural, mechanical, and molecular features of the innate tissue, and that are safely biodegradable while still supporting cellular integration into the host tissue. For example, hydrogels can be tuned in their stiffness and elastic properties to match the characteristics of particular tissue types. The stiffness or elastic modulus of the hydrogel tissues can be tuned by adjusting the concentration of polymer, by altering the types of polymers used, or by the extent of chemical cross-linking among the polymers. This is important, because these mechanical properties have been shown to influence the differentiation of cells, with softer scaffolds (elastic modulus of 0.1−1 kPa) favoring neuronal fates, and slightly stiffer scaffolds (elastic modulus of 1−10 kPa) favoring astrocytic fates (Aurand et al., 2012). The stiffness of synthetic tissues can also affect their biocompatibility after implantation into the body, where unmatched elastic moduli can either result in disintegration of the implant, or cause increased inflammation and foreign body reactions. The properties of the polymers, and their density and cross-linking, will also affect degradation rates of the implant, which should be tuned to last long enough for appropriate growth and integration into the innate tissue, but not so long that it irritates or interferes with the natural tissue. Certain biomaterials may also be designed to suppress inflammatory reactions through intrinsic signaling mechanisms, or optimize the tissue environment for regenerative capabilities. Additionally, in order to ensure the safety of implantable tissue constructs, it will be important to verify cell identity and cell state in a consistent and thorough manner prior to any implantation of entire tissue constructs.

Nevertheless, recent studies on the use of biomaterials in animal models have already shown several potential therapeutic effects. Polymer matrix scaffolds have been shown to improve mesenchymal stem cell survival and engraftment in a rat model of spinal cord injury, and this also demonstrated improved sensorimotor recovery, and beneficial angiogenic and antiinflammatory effects (Ropper et al., 2017). Biomaterials have also shown the ability to improve implanted cell survival and integration in the nervous system, improve axonal sprouting and regeneration, and enhance neural connectivity through neural lesions (Moshayedi and Carmichael, 2013; Hakim et al., 2015; Lu et al., 2012; Carlson et al., 2016; Cook et al., 2016).

REMAINING CHALLENGES

Organoid designs should aim to expand the library of possible synthetic tissue types and architectures, as well as to improve consistency in the resulting tissues. Further development of complex organoids will be immensely useful as models for numerous diseases, including neurodegeneration, neurogenetic and neurodevelopmental diseases, infectious diseases, cancer and tumor growth, ischemic injuries, traumatic injuries, and others. Organoid designs can also be optimized for use as a high-throughput screening tool for pharmacological agents. In the future, organoids may also serve as potential graft tissues into damaged or degenerated sites of the nervous system for diseases like Parkinson's or Huntington's disease, or for injuries like stroke, traumatic brain injury, or spinal cord injury (Choi et al., 2014; Carballo-Molina et al., 2016; Tang-Schomer et al., 2014; McMurtrey, 2015). Such an approach overcomes many of the shortfalls of traditional cell therapies (such as cell survival, migration, and architecture formation), but would also present new difficulties in producing consistent differentiation of cells and structures of tissues, and therefore much work remains to be done to thoroughly prepare such technologies for therapeutic use.

The ability to accurately and consistently form functional cellular networks also remains a challenge. Synaptic architecture depends on numerous cell types working together, including excitatory and inhibitory neurons and astroglia, but because these cell types arise at different times and at different locations during development, properly inducing these cells to coordinate networks and replicate circuitry of the nervous system is a complicated and unresolved task. Patterned biomaterials and axonal guidance cues may be used in organoid constructs to help unravel these mysteries and investigate mechanisms of synaptogenesis, including how axons and dendrites find appropriate targets among groups of neurons, how synaptic pruning is regulated, and how the synaptic architecture is assembled from initiation to maturity, all in a realistic 3D environment. Synthetic circuitry in organoids could also be used to study neural circuit behaviors and various encoding mechanisms.

Another advancement for neural organoids would be to surmount certain diffusion limitations of nutrients to the tissue. This may be done in part by increasing permeability of the nutrients in the tissue, increasing nutrient supply around the tissue, decreasing thickness or size of the tissue, or minimizing metabolism of the nutrient, although each of these will have particular consequences for the tissue construct. Perfusion of the nutrient through the tissue could ideally be achieved with some form of integrated vascular system, such as a microperfusion system attached to artificial hollow tube filaments, or an actual cellular construction of vessels. Nevertheless, diffusion limitations could also be useful for certain applications like future cell therapies, since stem cells are more likely to survive ischemic insults or implantation into the body when they are cultured under conditions of stress or hypoxic exposure, a phenomenon called "conditioning" (Sart et al., 2014; McMurtrey and Zuo, 2010). The culture of stem cells in oxygen-limited organoid spheres can help condition the cells for subsequent insults, although the full clinical significance of this application has not yet been studied.

Altogether, it is clear that the design of cellular tissue constructs must take into account numerous features, including how each component will affect every other component of the design. All features of the cell types, biomaterials, signaling factors, concentration gradients, and media formulations must be carefully considered in the context of the desired tissue type, the effective function of the tissue, and the intended applications. The nascent field of neural organoid research is only beginning, and, owing to the many new avenues of investigation that it has enabled in regional models of development and pathology in the brain and spinal cord, this field will surely yield many valuable advancements in our ability to better understand and treat numerous neurological conditions.

DECLARATION OF FINANCIAL INTERESTS

The author has no conflicts of interest and no financial disclosures to declare. The author has pending patents in this area of research.

REFERENCES

Aurand, E.R., Lampe, K.J., Bjugstad, K.B., 2012. Defining and designing polymers and hydrogels for neural tissue engineering. Neurosci. Res. 72, 199–213.

Bejoy, J., Song, L., Li, Y., 2016. Wnt-YAP interactions in the neural fate of human pluripotent stem cells and the implications for neural organoid formation. Organogenesis. 12 (1), 1–15.

Bento, A.R., Quelhas, P., Oliveira, M.J., Pêgo, A.P., Amaral, I.F., 2016. Three-dimensional culture of single embryonic stem-derived neural/stem progenitor cells in fibrin hydrogels: neuronal network formation and matrix remodelling. J. Tissue. Eng. Regen. Med..

Bershteyn, M., Nowakowski, T.J., Pollen, A.A., Di Lullo, E., Nene, A., Wynshaw-Boris, A., et al., 2017. Human iPSC-derived cerebral organoids model cellular features of lissencephaly and reveal prolonged mitosis of outer radial Glia. Cell. Stem. Cell. pii: S1934-5909(16)30463-5.

Carballo-Molina, O.A., Sánchez-Navarro, A., López-Ornelas, A., Lara-Rodarte, R., Salazar, P., Campos-Romo, A., et al., 2016. Semaphorin 3C released from a biocompatible hydrogel guides and promotes axonal growth of rodent and human dopaminergic neurons. Tissue. Eng. Part. A. 22 (11–12), 850–861.

Carlson, A.L., Bennett, N.K., Francis, N.L., Halikere, A., Clarke, S., Moore, J.C., et al., 2016. Generation and transplantation of reprogrammed human neurons in the brain using 3D microtopographic scaffolds. Nat Commun. 7, 10862, 17.

Choi, S.H., Kim, Y.H., Hebisch, M., Sliwinski, C., Lee, S., D'Avanzo, C., et al., 2014. A three-dimensional human neural cell culture model of Alzheimer's disease. Nature. 515 (7526), 274–278, 13.

Cook, D.J., Nguyen, C., Chun, H.N., Llorente I, L., Chiu, A.S., Machnicki, M., et al., 2016. Hydrogel-delivered brain-derived neurotrophic factor promotes tissue repair and recovery after stroke. J. Cereb. Blood. Flow. Metab.

Dang, J., Tiwari, S.K., Lichinchi, G., Qin, Y., Patil, V.S., Eroshkin, A.M., et al., 2016. Zika Virus Depletes neural progenitors in human cerebral organoids through activation of the innate immune receptor TLR3. Cell. Stem. Cell. pii: S1934-5909(16)30057-1.

Ezashi, T., Das, P., Roberts, R.M., 2005. Low O2 tensions and the prevention of differentiation of hES cells. Proc. Natl. Acad. Sci. U.S.A. 102 (13), 4783–4788.

Gustafsson, M.V., Zheng, X., Pereira, T., Gradin, K., Jin, S., Lundkvist, J., et al., 2005. Hypoxia requires notch signaling to maintain the undifferentiated cell state. Dev. Cell. 9 (5), 617–628.

Hakim, J.S., Esmaeili Rad, M., Grahn, P.J., et al., 2015. Positively charged oligo[poly(ethylene glycol) fumarate] scaffold implantation results in a permissive lesion environment after spinal cord injury in rat. Tissue. Eng. Part. A. 21 (13–14), 2099–2114.

Ito, K., Suda, T., 2014. Metabolic requirements for the maintenance of self-renewing stem cells. Nat. Rev. Mol. Cell. Biol. 15 (4), 243–256.

Kelava, I., Lancaster, M.A., 2016. Stem cell models of human brain development. Cell. Stem. Cell. 18 (6), 736–748.

Lancaster, M.A., Renner, M., Martin, C.A., Wenzel, D., Bicknell, L.S., Hurles, M.E., et al., 2013. Cerebral organoids model human brain development and microcephaly. Nature. 501 (7467), 373–379, 19.

Lawrence, P., 1992. The Making of a Fly: The Genetics of Animal Design. Blackwell Scientific Publications, Oxford, United Kingdom.

Liang, Y., Walczak, P., Bulte, J.W., 2013. The survival of engrafted neural stem cells within hyaluronic acid hydrogels. Biomaterials. 34, 5521–5529.

Lu, P., Wang, Y., Graham, L., et al., 2012. Long-distance growth and connectivity of neural stem cells after severe spinal cord injury. Cell 150 (6), 1264–1273.

Luo, C., Lancaster, M.A., Castanon, R., Nery, J.R., Knoblich, J.A., Ecker, J.R., 2016. Cerebral Organoids Recapitulate Epigenomic Signatures of the Human Fetal Brain. Cell Rep. 17 (12), 3369–3384, 20.

Mariani, J., Coppola, G., Zhang, P., et al., 2015. FOXG1-dependent dysregulation of GABA/glutamate neuron differentiation in autism spectrum disorders. Cell 162 (2), 375–390.

Mathieu, J., Zhou, W., Xing, Y., Sperber, H., Ferreccio, A., Agoston, Z., et al., 2014. Hypoxia-inducible factors have distinct and stage-specific roles during reprogramming of human cells to pluripotency. Cell. Stem. Cell. 14 (5), 592–605.

McMurtrey, R.J., 2014. Patterned and functionalized nanofiber scaffolds in 3-dimensional hydrogel constructs enhance neurite outgrowth and directional control. J. Neural. Eng. 11, 066009.

McMurtrey, R.J., 2015. Novel advancements in three-dimensional neural tissue engineering and regenerative medicine. Neural Regen. Res. 10 (3), 352–354.

McMurtrey, R.J., 2016a. Multi-compartmental biomaterial scaffolds for patterning neural tissue organoids in models of neurodevelopment and tissue regeneration. J Tissue Eng. 7; 7: 2041731416671926.

McMurtrey, R.J., 2016b. Analytic models of oxygen and nutrient diffusion, metabolism dynamics, and architecture optimization in three-dimensional tissue constructs with applications and insights in cerebral organoids. Tissue Eng. Part C 22 (3), 221–249.

McMurtrey, R.J., 2017. Roles of diffusion dynamics and molecular concentration gradients in cellular differentiation and three-dimensional tissue development. Stem Cells Dev 26 (18), 1293–1303.

McMurtrey, R.J., Zuo, Z., 2010. Isoflurane preconditioning and postconditioning in rat hippocampal neurons. Brain. Res. 1358, 184–190, 28.

Meinhardt, A., Eberle, D., Tazaki, A., Ranga, A., Niesche, M., Wilsch-Bräuninger, M., et al., 2014. 3D reconstitution of the patterned neural tube from embryonic stem cells. Stem Cell Reports 3 (6), 987–999, 9.

Moshayedi, P., Carmichael, S.T., 2013. Hyaluronan, neural stem cells and tissue reconstruction after acute ischemic stroke. Biomatter. 3 (1), e23863.

Muguruma, K., Nishiyama, A., Kawakami, H., Hashimoto, K., Sasai, Y., 2015. Self-organization of polarized cerebellar tissue in 3D culture of human pluripotent stem cells. Cell Rep. 10 (4), 537–550, 3.

Mullard, A., 2015. Stem-cell discovery platforms yield first clinical candidates. Nat. Rev. Drug. Discov. 14 (9), 589–591, 1.

Ortega, J.A., Sirois, C.L., Memi, F., Glidden, N., Zecevic, N., 2016. Oxygen Levels Regulate the Development of Human Cortical Radial Glia Cells. Cereb. Cortex. 2016, 1–17.

Paşca, A.M., Sloan, S.A., Clarke, L.E., Tian, Y., Makinson, C.D., Huber, N., et al., 2015. Functional cortical neurons and astrocytes from human pluripotent stem cells in 3D culture. Nat. Methods. 12 (7), 671−678.

Ropper, A.E., Thakor, D.K., Han, I., Yu, D., Zeng, X., Anderson, J.E., et al., 2017. Defining recovery neurobiology of injured spinal cord by synthetic matrix-assisted hMSC implantation. Proc. Natl. Acad. Sci. U.S.A.

Sart, S., Ma, T., Li, Y., 2014. Preconditioning stem cells for in vivo delivery. Bioresearch Open Access 3, 137−149.

Tang-Schomer, M.D., White, J.D., Tien, L.W., Schmitt, L.I., Valentin, T.M., Graziano, D. J., et al., 2014. Bioengineered functional brain-like cortical tissue. Proc. Natl. Acad. Sci. U.S.A. 111 (38), 13811−13816, 23.

Teslaa, T., Teitell, M.A., 2015. Pluripotent stem cell energy metabolism: an update. EMBO J. 34 (2), 138−153, 13.

Varum, S., Rodrigues, A.S., Moura, M.B., Momcilovic, O., Easley IV, C.A., Ramalho-Santos, J., et al., 2011. Energy metabolism in human pluripotent stem cells and their differentiated counterparts. PLoS One. 6 (6), e20914.

Wang, L., Hou, S., Han, Y.G., 2016. Hedgehog signaling promotes basal progenitor expansion and the growth and folding of the neocortex. Nat. Neurosci. 19 (7), 888−896.

Xie, Y., Zhang, J., Lin, Y., Gaeta, X., Meng, X., Wisidagama, D.R., et al., 2014. Defining the role of oxygen tension in human neural progenitor fate. Stem Cell Rep. 3 (5), 743−757, 11.

Yan, Y., Bejoy, J., Xia, J., Guan, J., Zhou, Y., Li, Y., 2016. Neural patterning of human induced pluripotent stem cells in 3-D cultures for studying biomolecule-directed differential cellular responses. Acta. Biomater. 42, 114−126.

Intestinal organoids: Mini-guts grown in the laboratory

3

Tamara Zietek and Eva Rath
Technical University of Munich, Freising, Germany

CHAPTER OUTLINE

INTRODUCTION

The establishment of a method for long-term in vitro cultivation of intestinal organoids, reported by Sato et al. (2009), has provided a powerful tool for investigating intestinal biology. Intestinal epithelial cells (IEC) have long been recognized as important regulators of metabolic and immune homeostasis, as well as being critical to nutrient absorption (Pitman and Blumberg, 2000; Rath and Haller, 2011), but they have been difficult to study in vitro (Whitehead and Robinson, 2009). Cultivation of primary IEC is only possible for a very limited time-frame, because cells rapidly enter apoptosis. In addition, certain cell types are poorly represented and poorly differentiated in primary cultures, restricting the information that can be obtained. Intestinal epithelial cell lines, as distinct from primary culture, suffer from other major drawbacks: bearing genetic

Organoids and Mini-Organs. DOI: http://dx.doi.org/10.1016/B978-0-12-812636-3.00003-1

modifications or originating from tumor tissue, cell lines provide an inadequate representation of the physiological properties of natural intestinal epithelium. Additionally, most cell lines are restricted to only one subtype of IEC, further limiting the possibility of studying the complex intercellular interactions of epithelial cell biology.

In contrast, intestinal organoids can be kept in culture for years and contain all cell types of the intestinal epithelium, including stem cells, mucin-producing goblet cells, antimicrobial peptide-producing Paneth cells, tuft cells, hormone-producing enteroendocrine cells (EEC), and absorptive enterocytes (Sato et al., 2009). By addition of RANKL, a member of the tumor necrosis factor (TNF) cytokine family, even formation of M cells can be induced in intestinal organoids (de Lau et al., 2012). Furthermore, organoids retain their location-specific function and gene expression throughout long-term culture (Middendorp et al., 2014). By closely reflecting the main characteristics of the mammalian intestinal epithelium, organoids offer many applications in research.

Intestinal organoids are compatible with virtually all methods used to analyze cells and/or tissue samples (Sato and Clevers, 2013a). They are amenable to immunohistochemistry, immunofluorescence, and in situ hybridization (Mahe et al., 2013), gene and protein expression analyses, such as RNAseq and mass spectrometry (VanDussen et al., 2015), live cell imaging (Zietek et al., 2015), and metabolic measurements, e.g., high-resolution respirometry. Also, all standard molecular biological techniques for manipulation can be applied to intestinal organoids. For example, organoids can be transfected with CRISPR/Cas9, DNA, or small interfering RNA, infected with recombinant viruses, and, using the CreERT2 system, "floxed" alleles can be deleted in culture simply by adding tamoxifen to the medium (Berger et al., 2016; Sato and Clevers, 2013a).

The availability of intestinal organoids has promoted stem cell research, as well as molecular research, on gastrointestinal processes and pathologies. As intestinal organoids become more widespread in research, new areas of application are being explored. Representing a reliable model system accurately reflecting in vivo physiology, intestinal organoid culture might also help significantly reducing the number of animals needed for research purposes.

DEVELOPMENT, STRUCTURE AND FUNCTION OF THE NATIVE ORGAN

The intestine is divided functionally and anatomically into the small intestine and the large intestine. The small intestine comprises the duodenum, jejunum, and ileum, whereas the large intestine consists of the cecum (including appendix) and colon, which can be further subdivided into ascending colon, transverse colon, descending colon, and sigmoid colon.

The most prominent role of the intestine is the absorption of nutrients from ingested food, this absorption being mediated by specific nutrient transporters in the brush border membrane of enterocytes (Daniel and Zietek, 2015). Some of these transporters can also transport certain drugs (Daniel and Kottra, 2004).

Functionally, most nutrient and mineral uptake after food ingestion takes place in the small intestine and, consequently, most nutrient transporters are expressed in the duodenum and jejunum (Wuensch et al., 2013; Yoshikawa et al., 2011). Indicating the prominent role of the gut as an immune organ, aggregations of gut associated lymphoid tissue (GALT), the so called Peyer's patches, are found in the ileum. In contrast, the large intestine is responsible for fluid absorption, and harbors the vast majority of the intestinal microbiota.

Almost the complete gastrointestinal tract derives from the embryonic endoderm. During embryonic development, the proximal part of the duodenum (up to the entrance of the bile duct) is formed by the foregut, while the largest proportion of the alimentary canal, from the bile duct to the proximal parts of the transverse colon, is formed by the midgut. Finally, the distal third of the transverse colon, the descending colon, sigmoid colon, and rectum are formed by the hindgut. Embedded in the lining of the gastrointestinal tract, the enteric nervous system (ENS) governs the function of the intestine.

The gastrointestinal wall itself comprises four concentric layers; the mucosa, the submucosa, the muscularis layer, and the serosa (also called the adventitia). The outermost layer, the serosa or adventitia, is formed by connective tissue, and it encloses the muscle layers and the myenteric plexus of the muscularis. Consisting of connective tissue including large blood vessels, lymphatics, and nerves, the submucosa joins the mucosa to the muscle layer, and supports its function. The mucosa, representing the innermost layer of the gastrointestinal tract, is further subdivided into the muscularis mucosae (a thin layer of smooth muscle), the lamina propria (a layer of connective tissue containing many immune cells), and the epithelium (a monolayer of intestinal epithelial cells covering the intestine and forming a barrier between host and lumen). Most digestive, absorptive, and secretory processes are carried out by the IEC.

The morphology of the intestine differs from proximal to distal gut: while the epithelium of the small intestine contains both crypts and villi, with villus length increasing from duodenum to ileum, the colon is villus-free and contains only crypts. Distinct, specialized IEC subtypes are present in the epithelium: stem cells, responsible for the constant renewal of the epithelial layer every 4—5 days; Paneth cells, providing factors to create the stem cell niche at the bottom of the crypt and producing antimicrobial peptides; mucin-producing goblet cells, creating the mucus layer covering the epithelium to additionally create a physical barrier; absorptive enterocytes taking up nutrients and ions; enteroendocrine cells (EEC) secreting different hormones to control bowel movements and regulate metabolism; and taste — chemosensory tuft cells participating in immune responses (Barker, 2014). Of note, different subtypes of IECs are found only in distinct locations of the intestine. For example, different classes of EEC producing different patterns of hormones are found in different places along the gastrointestinal tract. Remarkably, Paneth cells are absent in the colon under normal physiological conditions, indicating differences in stem cell homeostasis between the small intestine and the colonic region. Different populations of stem cells have been proposed for the intestinal epithelium, with crypt base columnar cells (CBCs) and "+4" cells as the most prominent ones (the "+4" designation reflecting the cells' position in the crypt). Yet, the existence of different intestinal stem cell types and a proposed "stem cell hierarchy" are highly controversial (Barker et al., 2012).

In the context of intestinal organoid culture, Leucine-rich repeat-containing G-protein-coupled receptor 5 (Lgr 5), a receptor for R-Spondins, is widely used as marker gene for intestinal stem cells. The stem cell niche is located at the base of the crypts, this base contains both stem cells and Paneth cells. While Paneth cells reside at the crypt bottom, other cells that move upward due to cell division of stem cells are expelled from the crypt, and therefore from the stem cell niche, and they start differentiating. Passing through and contributing to the transit amplifying (TA) zone, cells commit to the secretory or absorptive lineage, and differentiate further into mature cells along the crypt − villus axis. Continuing to move upwards to the villus tip, IECs are finally exfoliated via anoikis (Leushacke and Barker, 2014) after 4−5 days.

An important property of the intestinal epithelium is its close contact to the endogenous luminal microbiota. The importance of this host − microbe interaction is essential for the development and maturation of gut homeostasis, including epithelial cell function, and has been extensively illustrated by comparative studies of germ-free and conventionalized animals. Despite the abundance of bacterial molecules that can potentially activate bacterial molecular pattern receptors and trigger damaging immune responses and inflammation, it is a characteristic feature of the mucosal immune system that protective immune responses against enteropathogenic organisms are allowed to proceed while endogenous microbiota are tolerated. Interestingly, there is accumulating evidence that IEC critically contribute to these processes (Hoffmann et al., 2008). Directly interacting with the microbiota, as well as with immune cells of the lamina propria and with intraepithelial lymphocytes, IEC both sense and determine the composition of the luminal microbiota by producing antimicrobial substances (Clavel and Haller, 2007). In addition, IEC modulate T-cell responses within the lamina propria, e.g., by producing cytokines such as thymic stromal lymphopoietin (TSLP) (Blumberg et al., 2008).

The role of IEC in shaping immune responses, together with the profound impact of gut hormones on the regulation of whole-body metabolism, highlights the diverse functions of the intestine beyond nutrient absorption, and underlines the importance of research to elucidate IEC biology.

THE NEED FOR AN ORGANOID

A satisfactory in vitro model of the intestinal epithelium has been lacking for a long time: neither cell lines nor cultivation of primary cells or tissues resemble the diversity and complexity of the intestine. Additionally, both approaches suffer from substantial drawbacks.

The inherent problem of all lines is their origin from neoplastic tissue, or the genetic modifications introduced to render them cultivable over long time periods. Furthermore, most cell lines are restricted to only one subtype of IEC. Nonetheless, immortalized cell lines are widely used for in vitro research on molecular and cellular processes, because primary IEC culture is possible for only a very limited time frame before apoptosis takes over. Cell lines have the advantage of being well-established, easy to handle, and inexpensive in materials and time. As they are widely used by laboratories all over the world, numerous protocols and experimental results are available in scientific literature. Intestinal epithelial cell lines that are commonly used in gastrointestinal research include the murine duodenal-derived Mode-K cell line, and the colonic Ptk6 cell line, as well as human CaCo-2 cells and the HT-29 cell line. Both human cell lines are colorectal adenocarcinoma cell lines (Fogh et al., 1977), yet CaCo-2 cells are known to exhibit rather a small intestinal phenotype (Pinto et al., 1983; Vincent et al., 1985; Yee, 1997). Due to their tumor-derived nature, phenotypic as well as functional characteristics differ greatly from native human enterocytes (Harwood et al., 2016), indicating the cells to be a rather artificial model system. For example, many small intestinal cell lines do not exhibit typical characteristics of small intestinal enterocytes, such as expression of essential nutrient transporters like the proton-coupled peptide transporter 1 (PEPT1), or the sodium-dependent glucose transporter 1 (SGLT1). Additionally, cell lines show an extremely high variability of experimental outcomes between different laboratories, this problem being particularly acute for CaCo-2 cells (Harwood et al., 2016; Sambuy et al., 2005). Collectively, neither conserving essential epithelial properties nor their region-specific functions, intestinal epithelial cell lines offer only limited possibilities to study complex epithelial cell biology.

Primary intestinal cell cultures derived from isolated intestinal crypts represent another approach to investigate the intestinal epithelium in detail (Reimann et al., 2008). These cultures can be generated from murine and human tissue samples derived from the small or large intestine (Parker et al., 2012), and provide a lot of advantages. They contain different subtypes of intestinal epithelial cells, including absorptive enterocytes and enteroendocrine cells, and conserve their location-specific functions. Cultures can be generated from mice bearing genetic modifications or patients, hence making the primary crypt culture system a good model to study certain aspects of IEC function, e.g., intestinal nutrient sensing and molecular mechanisms underlying the secretion of gastrointestinal hormones (Diakogiannaki et al., 2013; Zietek and Daniel, 2015). In general, these crypt cultures are grown overnight, although under certain conditions they can be kept in culture for a few days. Yet, this system is not suitable for long-term culture, and absorptive enterocytes contained in the culture are poorly differentiated. For example, nutrient transporters cannot be detected at the protein level, and crypt cultures fail to absorb nutrients. Whole-tissue explants are an additional option for cultivation, and constitute a reliable in vitro model that displays properties such as expression and activity of typical nutrient transporters that are found in the small intestine of rodents (Roder et al., 2014). However, tissue explants have poor stability and very limited viability in vitro (maximum of a few hours), so the use of this system is restricted to short-term experiments. It also has to be considered that tissue explants, such as everted gut rings, contain not only IEC, but a number of other cell types and tissues such as muscle, connective tissue, neurons, and macrophages. Depending on the scientific question, this might be a limitation, for example if a researcher wishes to investigate specific processes only in intestinal epithelial cells.

Overall, primary culture of cells or tissue also lacks the possibility of expansion of the sample of interest in vitro. Large numbers of mice are needed for experiments and, in the case of human tissue, availability is a critical issue for scientific questions, being restricted for ethical and organizational reasons.

In conclusion, the limitations of the previously existing in vitro models highlight the potential of intestinal organoid culture as a model system closely reflecting epithelial physiology in a region-specific resolution, and concurrently offering the advantages of easy handling and almost indefinite culture and expansion. Furthermore, organoids can be cryo-conserved over years. Hence, intestinal organoids will allow tackling many of the remaining open questions in the field of intestinal epithelial biology and facilitating research.

DESIGN CONSIDERATIONS

In general, intestinal organoids are used: (1) to model organ development and morphogenesis; (2) to model disease; and (3) for regenerative medicine/personalized medicine. Intestinal organoids can be generated either from single stem cells or from isolated intestinal crypts (Sato et al., 2009). For the murine system, isolation of an appropriate adult intestinal stem cell population for cultivation of organoids largely depends on mice expressing eGFP under the Lgr5 promoter. In the case of the human system, either embryonic stem cells (ESCs) or induced pluripotent stem cells (iPSCs) (Spence et al., 2011) can be used for this purpose. Depending on the experimental method that is used, cultures develop slightly different properties and are sometimes divided into referred to as "organoids" (if grown from stem cells) or "enteroids" if grown from crypts (Wells and Spence, 2014). A nomenclature has been proposed to distinguish between different ex vivo intestinal cultures (Stelzner et al., 2012), but the vast majority of scientific publications simply use the term "organoids" to describe them all.

Establishing intestinal organoid culture from single stem cells is much more complicated and expensive in terms of money, time, and equipment than is the alternative of growing organoids from isolated crypts. The approach of deriving intestinal organoids derived from single stem cells has generally been used for investigation of scientific questions related to stem cell biology, organ development, or morphogenesis. Most of the research that deals with other scientific questions uses the easier approach of deriving organoids from crypts. For example, by using intestinal crypts as a starting material, organoids can be grown from wild-type and genetically manipulated mice, and be used as a sort of "cell line". Also, culturing intestinal organoids from crypts (Sato and Clevers, 2013b) is the best approach for studies on nutrient and drug uptake, as well as incretin hormone secretion (Zietek et al., 2015). Using this method, intestinal organoid cultures can be easily generated within a few hours using standard laboratory equipment. This has been made even easier by the commercial availability of ready-to-use cell culture media for murine small- and large-intestinal organoids.

Intestinal organoids are amenable to all standard molecular biological techniques for manipulation, such as controlled gene expression (Koo et al., 2011), gene knockout, and genetic engineering approaches such as CRISPR/Cas9 technology (Schwank and Clevers, 2016; Schwank et al., 2013). The organoids are compatible with virtually all methods used to analyze cells and/or tissue samples (Sato and Clevers, 2013a) including different approaches for gene- and protein expression analyses (VanDussen et al., 2015), live cell imaging (Zietek et al., 2015), and metabolic measurements (Berger et al., 2016). In summary, intestinal organoid culture can easily be established coming from isolated crypts, closely reflects intestinal physiology, and enables study of a multitude of gastrointestinal processes in a reliable manner.

REMAINING CHALLENGES

Although the cultivation of intestinal organoids has brought enormous benefits to gastrointestinal research and personalized medicine, there are still challenges and hurdles left that need to be overcome. For the generation of murine organoids, tissue availability is not usually a problem, but generation of human intestinal organoids requires both access to the tissue and ethical approval. Tissue is usually obtained fresh from a hospital, and the tissue source needs to be close to the laboratory where organoids are generated. Although resected intestinal tissue can be stored in culture medium for several hours at 4°C prior to organoid generation, the time of storage should be minimized.

The most prominent limitation of organoid technology compared to other mammalian cell culture techniques is the high cost of organoid cultivation. The 3D gel matrix in which intestinal organoids are grown is expensive, as are the growth factors, supplements, and inhibitors that are essential ingredients of the culture medium. In particular, R-Spondin 1, an enhancer of the Wnt signaling pathway, and Noggin, an antagonist of the BMP pathway, are major contributors to the costs. For human intestinal organoid culture, even more additives are required. Also, the preparation of the complete culture medium is time-consuming, as the medium should be prepared fresh before use and not stored longer than a few days. Commercially-available ready-to-use media for intestinal organoid culture are a helpful tool, yet they are neither low-priced nor suitable for all experimental approaches. It is likely, however, that intestinal organoid culture will become less expensive in the near future, thereby allowing a broader scientific community access to this outstanding model system.

It is impressive how organoid cultures conserve the phenotype of the donor from which they are derived. On the other hand, this fact raises a question: What is the "standard, wild-type" representative organoid or donor? Although this has not been investigated in detail yet, it is likely that intestinal organoids derived from different "healthy" human donors who might have been matched by numerous phenotypic parameters will nevertheless display different functional characteristics in vitro. The outcomes of in vitro studies using organoids might vary, reflecting the individual differences of humans and their unique genetic makeup. If intestinal organoid culture is applied by a broad user-community of researchers all over the world, experimental results need to be comparable. So which organoid could serve as the "gold standard", in order to avoid high inter-laboratory variations? This is a critical and important issue that needs to be discussed and clarified by organoid users to further establish this promising in vitro model system.

DETAILED INSTRUCTIONS: HOW TO ISOLATE CRYPTS AND CULTURE INTESTINAL ORGANOIDS

Since Sato et al. (2009) established the protocol for intestinal organoid culture in 2009, several publications have used slight modifications to the method (Mahe et al., 2013; VanDussen et al., 2015; Zietek et al., 2015). These are intended to streamline the protocol, and to reduce costs and effort, for example by reducing the concentrations of certain growth factors, or by using recombinant cell lines to produce Wnt3a-, Noggin-, and R-Spondin 1-conditioned media. Here, we describe protocols for the isolation of small and large intestinal crypts from mouse and human tissue using two different methods. One utilizes EDTA to dissociate crypts from the basal membrane, the other one applies collagenase to digest the intestinal tissues. While the protocol using EDTA is more cost-effective and easy to perform, it requires some experience to identify the fraction that contains most crypts and lowest undesired cell debris. In contrast, the collagenase protocol provides a strict procedure, without the necessity to choose a certain fraction for cultivation. This protocol yields very good numbers of large intestinal crypts, but with an increased risk of contamination by fibroblasts. Mice used for intestinal crypt isolation are typically 6–10 weeks of age, but a substantial number of crypts can also be isolated from older mice. The incubation times given in the protocols are optimized for C57BL6 mice; if other strains are used, incubation times might need to be modified, for example 129SvEv have a more fragile connective tissue than do C57BL6 mice. Human intestinal organoids can be established from different types of tissue resections. Most frequently, samples are derived from surgically resected intestinal tissues, e.g., gastric surgeries (that often involve the removal of parts of the small intestine), resections due to inflammatory or neoplastic diseases, and the adjacent "normal" appearing tissue regions or endoscopic biopsies (Mahe et al., 2015).

ISOLATION OF INTESTINAL CRYPTS USING EDTA SOLUTIONS

Isolation of murine intestinal crypts

The protocol given below is time- and yield-optimized. Due to the omission of repeated washing steps, the fractions gained in the end contain slightly more cell debris. However, the excellent efficiency allows crypts to be isolated, even from small pieces of intestinal tissue (approximately 5 cm) and, during first passaging of organoids, undesired debris is removed any way.

Materials for isolation of murine intestinal crypts:

Equipment:
- scissors, forceps
- sieve, knitting needle
- petri dishes
- 50 mL conical tubes
- 96-well plate (flat bottom)
- 70 μm cell strainer
- centrifuge
- shaker
- pipette tips 1000/100 μL
- microscope

Reagents and Solutions:
- 70% Ethanol
- PBS *without* Ca^{2+}/Mg^{2+}
- 0.5 M EDTA solution
- Penicillin/Streptomycin (AA)

For Organoid Culture:
- Matrigel
- crypt culture medium (see Media composition for intestinal organoid culture)
- 48-well plate

Prepare:
- Matrigel (store at 4°C over night)
- PBS (store at 4°C over night)
- pipette tips 1000/100 μL (store at 4°C over night)
- cool down centrifuge (4°C)
- ice box
- crypt culture medium (CCM); pre-warmed (incubator or room temperature)
- pre-warm 48-well plate in an incubator

Per Mouse/Intestinal Segment:
- 1 × petri dish
- 2 × 50 mL conical tube with 20 mL PBS (supplemented with 1% AA) at 4°C labeled with mouse number
- 4 × 50 mL conical tube with 20 mL PBS at 4°C; labeled with mouse and fraction number
- 2 × 50 mL conical tube (labeled with mouse number)
- 1−2 × 70 μm cell strainer

1. Sacrifice mice according to applicable ethical regulations. Wet the abdomen with 70% ethanol and open the abdominal cavity. Harvest the desired piece of intestine (commonly, the proximal half of the small intestine), removing as much adjacent tissue (blood vessels, fat, connective tissue) as possible (see Fig. 3.1).

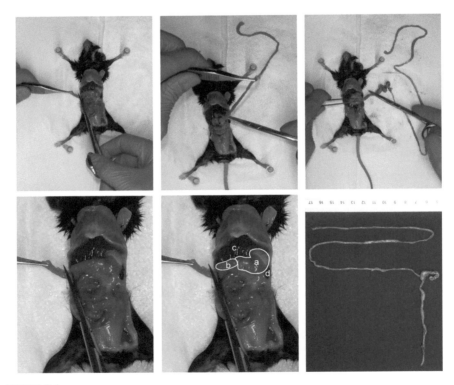

FIGURE 3.1

Upper panel: preparation of the murine intestine. Lower panel: the proximal intestine is cut leaving a piece of the duodenum (b) and the stomach (a) untouched; (c) liver lobes; (d) spleen. Right: small and large intestine prepared.

2. Place the intestinal segments into a petri dish filled with cold PBS and cut the segments to a length of approximately 5–7 cm. If necessary, remove the gut content by squeezing or flushing the segments with cold PBS. Invert the segments using a knitting needle (see Fig. 3.2).

3. Transfer the segments into a 50 mL conical tube filled with 20 mL PBS, and vigorously shake the tube ≈ 10 times.

4. Transfer the segments into a new 50 mL conical tube filled with 20 mL PBS, and place on ice. Add 80 µL of a 0.5M EDTA solution (final concentration = 2 mM). If processing more than one intestinal segment at a time, add EDTA solution at the same time.

5. Incubate at 4°C, gently shaking/rocking for
   30 minutes   for proximal small intestine
   60 minutes   for distal small intestine
   120 minutes   for large intestine.

6. Transfer the segments into a new 50 mL conical tube filled with 20 mL PBS labeled with mouse and fraction number. Vigorously shake the tube ≈ 20 times (fraction 1). Place the tube on ice immediately.

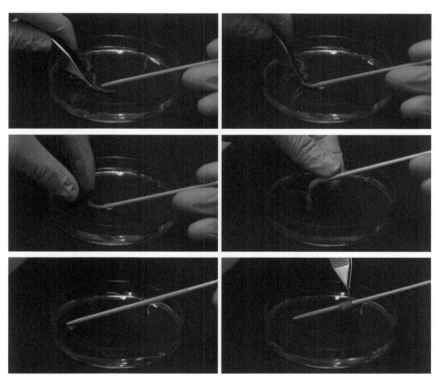

FIGURE 3.2

The procedure of inverting the intestinal segments.

7. Transfer the segments into a new 50 mL conical tube filled with 20 mL PBS, and vigorously shake the tube ≈20 times (fraction 2). Repeat this step to receive 4 fractions.

8. Transfer 100 μL of each fraction into a 96 well-plate for microscopic evaluation. Inspect fractions under the microscope (10 × objective/100 × magnification) to identify fractions enriched in crypts and with low level of debris (see Fig. 3.3).

9. Pass the desired fraction(s) through a 70 μm cell strainer into the appropriately labeled 50 mL conical tube.

10. Spin down the crypts in a centrifuge (300 g, 5 minutes, 4°C). Remove supernatant (the pellet should be quite firm, so the tube can be turned upside down on a sterile paper towel to get rid of remaining PBS).

11. Resuspend the pellet in 10 mL of cold PBS. Use 10 μL of the suspension to count the number of crypts under the microscope, and to estimate the total number of crypts (total number of crypts in 10 mL = numbers of crypts counted in 10 μL × 1000). Take out the correct volume to plate 100−200 crypts per well, and transfer into a labeled 50 mL conical tube.

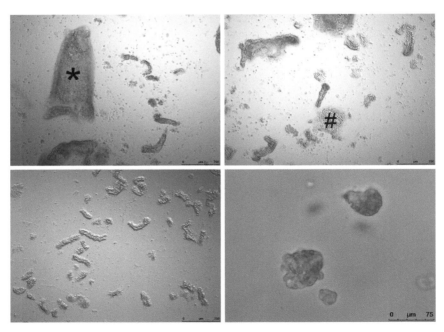

FIGURE 3.3

Different fractions obtained during isolation of murine small intestinal crypts using EDTA. Upper panel: fraction with villi (*) and crypts (left); fraction with mesenchymal cells (#) and crypts (right). Lower panel: fraction enriched with crypts (left); crypts just after embedding in Matrigel (right).

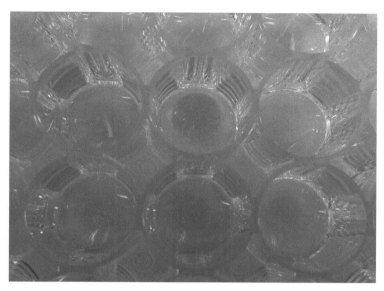

FIGURE 3.4

Organoids embedded in 25 μL of Matrigel in a 48-well plate. Matrigel-droplets should be in the center of the well. The droplets are overlaid with 300 μL of CCM.

12. Spin down the crypts in a centrifuge (300 g, 5 minutes, 4°C). Remove supernatant. Add the desired amount of Matrigel (25 μL/100−200 crypts corresponding to 1 well). Using the chilled pipette tips, carefully pipette up and down 10 times to thoroughly resuspend the pellet. Avoid introducing any bubbles. Keep on ice. It is very important that the Matrigel remains cold.

13. Apply 25 μL of Matrigel suspension per well on the prewarmed 48 well plate using chilled pipette tips. The suspension should be applied on the center of the well, so that it can form a hemispherical droplet. For this purpose, pipette tips with a wider opening can also be used for improved handling (see Fig. 3.4).

14. Incubate the plate at 37°C and allow the Matrigel to solidify for approximately 5−10 minutes. Overlay the Matrigel droplet with 300 μL of crypt culture medium.

Isolation of human intestinal crypts

The protocol given is optimized for a human full-wall intestinal resection, approximately 10 cm^2 in size. Volumes and incubation times might need to be adapted to different sizes of tissue resections.

Equipment:
- scissors, forceps (blunt tip)
- petri dishes
- microscope slides
- 50 mL conical tubes
- 1.5 mL tubes
- 70 μm cell strainer
- 96-well plate (flat bottom)
- centrifuge
- shaker
- pipette tips 1000/100 μL
- microscope

Reagents and Solutions:
- HBSS *without* Ca^{2+}/Mg^{2+}
- 0.5M EDTA solution
- Penicillin/Streptomycin (AA)
- basal culture medium (see Media composition for intestinal organoid culture)

For Organoid Culture:
- Matrigel
- human crypt culture medium (see Media composition for intestinal organoid culture)
- 24-well plate

Prepare:
- Matrigel (store at 4°C over night)
- HBSS (store at 4°C over night)
- pipette tips 1000/100 μL (store at 4°C over night)
- cool down centrifuge (4°C)
- ice box
- human crypt culture medium (hCCM); pre-warmed (incubator or room temperature)
- basal culture medium (BCM); (store at 4°C)
- prewarm 24-well plate in an incubator

Per Intestinal Resection:
- 1 × petri dish
- 2 × 50 mL conical tube with 30 mL HBSS (supplemented with 1% AA) at 4°C; labeled with sample number
- 5 × 50 mL conical tube with 20 mL HBSS at 4°C; labeled with sample and fraction number
- 2 × 50 mL conical tube (labeled with sample number)
- 1−2 × 70 μm cell strainer
  1. Wash the intestinal tissue resection with cold HBSS.
  2. Transfer into a petri dish filled with cold HBSS, and carefully remove the muscle layer and attached connective tissue using scissors and forceps.

3. Discard HBSS and wash the tissue section with new, cold HBSS.
4. Discard HBSS and place the tissue in the petri dish with the luminal side up. Carefully scratch the tissue with gentle pressure using a microscope slide to remove the mucus layer and villi.
5. Transfer the tissue in a 50 mL conical tube filled with 30 mL cold HBSS. Vigorously shake the tube ≈ 10 times. Discard the supernatant.
6. Repeat the washing step (5.) $2-3$ times, until the supernatant remains almost clear.
7. Transfer the tissue in a 50 mL conical tube filled with 30 mL cold HBSS, and place on ice. Add 120 μL of a 0.5M EDTA solution (final concentration = 2 mM). If processing more than one intestinal segment at a time, add EDTA solution at the same time.
8. Incubate at 4°C, gently shaking/rocking for 30 to 60 minutes (small intestine), and 30 to 120 minutes (large intestine).
9. Transfer the tissue into a new 50 mL conical tube filled with 20 mL cold HBSS labeled with sample and fraction number. Vigorously shake the tube $\approx 5-10$ times (fraction 1). Place the tube on ice immediately.
10. Transfer the tissue into a new 50 mL conical tube filled with 20 mL cold HBSS labeled with sample and fraction number. Vigorously shake the tube $\approx 5-10$ times (fraction 2). Repeat this step three more times to receive 5 fractions.
11. Inspect fractions under the microscope according to step 8 of the protocol (isolation of murine intestinal crypts). If the number of crypts appears to be very low, check the supernatant of the chelating step (if numerous crypts are contained, reduce incubation time). If no crypts are lost in this step, the tissue section can be incubated again in HBSS supplemented with 2 mM EDTA at 4°C. Increase time of incubation stepwise ($15-30$ minutes), until a sufficient number of crypts can be harvested.
12. Pass the desired fraction(s) through a 70 μm cell strainer into the appropriately labeled 50 mL conical tube. Spin down the crypts in a centrifuge (350 g, 3 minutes, 4°C). Remove the supernatant and immediately place on ice.
13. Resuspend the pellet in 10 mL of cold basal culture medium. Use 10 μL of the suspension to count the number of crypts under the microscope, and to estimate the total number of crypts (total number of crypts in 10 mL = numbers of crypts counted in 10 μL × 1000). Take out the corresponding volume to plate $50-100$ crypts per well, and transfer into a labeled 50 mL conical tube.
14. Spin down the crypts in a centrifuge (350 g, 3 minutes, 4°C). Remove supernatant. Add the desired amount of Matrigel (50 μL/$50-100$ crypts corresponding to 1 well). Using the chilled pipette tips, carefully pipette up and down 10 times to thoroughly resuspend the pellet. Avoid introducing any bubbles. Keep on ice.
15. Apply 50 μL of Matrigel suspension per well on the pre-warmed 24-well plate using chilled pipette tips. The suspension should be applied on the center of the well, so that it can form a hemispherical droplet. For this

purpose, pipette tips with a wider opening can also be used for an improved handling.

16. Incubate the plate at 37°C and allow the Matrigel to solidify for approximately 10–15 minutes. Overlay the Matrigel droplet with 500 µL of crypt culture medium

ISOLATION OF INTESTINAL CRYPTS USING COLLAGENASE

Isolation of murine intestinal crypts

Equipment:
- scissors, forceps, scalpel
- sieve
- petri dishes
- 50 mL conical tubes
- 15 mL conical tubes
- 96-well plate (flat bottom)
- centrifuge
- water bath
- pipette tips 1000/100 µL
- 10 mL plastic pipette
- microscope
- syringe and 0.22 µm sterile filter
- scale
- 70 µm cell strainer

Reagents and Solutions:
- 70% Ethanol
- DMEM 6546
- Collagenase XI
- PBS *without* Ca^{2+}/Mg^{2+}
- Penicillin/Streptomycin (AA)
- basal culture medium (see Media composition for intestinal organoid culture)

For Organoid Culture:
- Matrigel
- crypt culture medium (see Media composition for intestinal organoid culture)
- 48-well plate

Prepare:
- Matrigel (store at 4°C over night)
- PBS (store at 4°C over night)
- pipette tips 1000/100 µL (store at 4°C over night)
- cool down centrifuge (4°C)
- ice box
- basal culture medium at 4°C (see Cultivation of murine intestinal crypts)

- crypt culture medium (CCM); pre-warmed (incubator or room temperature)
- prewarm 48-well plate in an incubator

Per Mouse/Intestinal Segment:
- 2 × petri dish
- 1−2 × 50 mL conical tube with 20 mL PBS (supplemented with 1% AA) at 4°C labeled with mouse number
- 1−2 × 50 mL conical tube labeled with mouse number
- 6 × 15 mL conical tube labeled with mouse number
- weigh corresponding amount of collagenase XI into a 50 mL conical tube; store at −20°C
- 1 × 70 μm cell strainer

Protocol for isolating small intestinal crypts

1. Prepare the whole small intestine according to step one of protocol Isolation of murine intestinal crypts.
2. Transfer into a petri dish filled with cold PBS. Cut the small intestine into half for easier handling; open the intestinal segments longitudinally using small scissors. Transfer the tissue into a 50 mL conical tube filled with PBS; wash the tissue by vigorously shaking the tube for approximately 5 seconds. This step should be repeated until the intestinal tissue is cleared from mucus and debris (see Fig. 3.5).

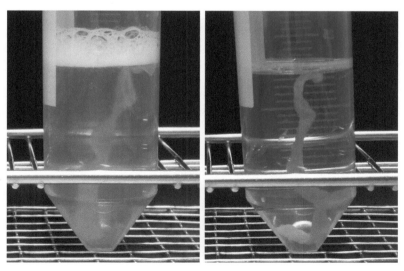

FIGURE 3.5

Isolation of murine small intestinal crypts using collagenase. Washing of intestinal segments in a conical 50 mL tube filled with PBS. Left: after the first washing step; right: after the fourth washing step.

3. Transfer the tissue into a petri dish filled with cold PBS to just cover the bottom. Using forceps and scalpel, cut the tissue in very small pieces (approximately 1 mm^2).

4. Using a 5−10 mL pipette, transfer tissue pieces and PBS into a 15 mL conical tube; fill up to 10 mL with cold PBS. Invert the tube five times, allow the tissue fragments to settle by gravity. Carefully discard the supernatant, and again add 10 mL of cold PBS. Repeat this washing step until the supernatant stays clear (approximately four times).

   a. Prepare the collagenase XI solution by dissolving 14 mg of collagenase XI in prewarmed 40 mL DMEM 6546. Sterile filtrate collagenase XI solution into a 50 mL conical tube and incubate the tube in a water bath at 37°C.

5. Aspire as much of the supernatant as possible; add 10 mL of warm collagenase XI solution. Mix thoroughly.

6. Incubate in a water bath at 37°C for 4.5 minutes. Carefully invert the tube for 30 seconds. Allow the tissue fragments to settle by gravity for 45 seconds. Discard supernatant.

7. Add 10 mL of warm collagenase XI solution. Mix thoroughly, incubate in a water bath at 37°C for 4.5 minutes. Shake the tube for 30 seconds. Allow the tissue fragments to settle by gravity for 45 seconds. Discard supernatant.

8. Add 10 mL of warm collagenase XI solution. Mix thoroughly. Incubate in a water bath at 37°C for 15 minutes, shake for 30 seconds after 4.5 minutes, 9.5 minutes and 14.5 minutes. Allow the tissue fragments to settle by gravity for 45 seconds. Discard supernatant.

9. Add 10 mL of warm collagenase XI solution. Mix thoroughly. Incubate in a water bath at 37°C for 15 minutes, shake for 30 seconds after 4.5 minutes, 9.5 minutes and 14.5 minutes. Allow the tissue fragments to settle by gravity for 45 seconds.

10. Take out supernatant and transfer into a new 15 mL conical tube. Centrifuge at 100 g for 2 minutes at 4°C. Discard supernatant. Resuspend pellet in 10 mL cold PBS.

11. Centrifuge at 100 g for 2 minutes at 4°C. Discard supernatant. Resuspend pellet in 10 mL cold PBS. Pass through a 70 μm cell strainer into an appropriately labeled 50 mL conical tube.

12. Use 10 μL of the suspension to count the number of crypts under the microscope, and to estimate the total number of crypts (total number of crypts in 10 mL = numbers of crypts counted in 10 μL × 1000). Take out the corresponding volume to plate 100−200 crypts per well, and transfer into a labeled 50 mL conical tube.

13. Proceed with steps 12−14 of protocol Isolation of murine intestinal crypts

Protocol for isolating large intestinal crypts

1. Prepare the whole colon according to step one of protocol Isolation of murine intestinal crypts.

2. Perform step 2−4 of protocol for Small intestinal crypt isolation
   a. Prepare the collagenase XI solution by dissolving 16 mg of collagenase XI in 40 mL DMEM 6546. Sterile filtrate collagenase XI solution into a 50 mL conical tube and incubate the tube in a water bath at 37°C.
3. Aspirate as much of the supernatant as possible; add 10 mL of warm collagenase XI solution. Mix thoroughly.
4. Incubate in a water bath at 37°C for 9.5 minutes. Vigorously shake the tube for 30 seconds. Allow the tissue fragments to settle by gravity for 45 seconds. Discard supernatant.
5. Add 10 mL of warm collagenase XI solution. Mix thoroughly, incubate in a water bath at 37°C for 14.5 minutes. Vigorously shake the tube for 30 seconds. Allow the tissue fragments to settle by gravity for 45 seconds. Discard supernatant.
6. Add 10 mL of warm collagenase XI solution. Mix thoroughly. Incubate in a water bath at 37°C for 15 minutes, shake for 30 seconds after 4.5 minutes, 9.5 minutes, and 14.5 minutes. Allow the tissue fragments to settle by gravity for 45 seconds (fraction 1). Transfer the supernatant of fraction 1 into a 15 mL conical tube.
7. Add 10 mL of warm collagenase XI solution to the pellet of fraction 1. Mix thoroughly. Incubate in a water bath at 37°C for 15 minutes, shake for 30 seconds after 4.5 minutes, 9.5 minutes, and 14.5 minutes. Allow the tissue fragments to settle by gravity for 45 seconds (fraction 2).
   a. Meanwhile, centrifuge the supernatant of fraction 1 at 100 g for 2 minutes at 4°C. Discard supernatant. Resuspend the pellet in 10 mL PBS and centrifuge again at 100 g for 2 minutes at 4°C. Discard supernatant and resuspend the pellet in 5 mL PBS. Place the tube on ice.
8. Transfer the supernatant of fraction 2 into a 15 mL conical tube. Centrifuge the supernatant of fraction 2 at 100 g for 2 minutes at 4°C. Discard supernatant. Resuspend the pellet in 10 mL PBS and centrifuge again at 100 g for 2 minutes at 4°C. Discard supernatant and resuspend the pellet in 5 mL PBS.
9. Combine crypt suspensions from fraction 1 and 2 to get 10 mL of crypt suspension. Pass through a 70 μm cell strainer into an accordingly labeled 50 mL conical tube.
10. Use 10 μL of the suspension to count the number of crypts under the microscope, and to estimate the total number of crypts (total number of crypts in 10 mL = numbers of crypts counted in 10 μL × 1000). Take out the corresponding volume to plate 100−200 crypts per well, and transfer into a labeled 50 mL conical tube.
11. Proceed with steps 12−14 of protocol Isolation of murine intestinal crypts.

Isolation of human intestinal crypts

The protocol for isolating human intestinal crypts using collagenase is very similar to those for murine intestinal crypts. Equipment, reagents, solutions, and preparations are the same as given in Isolation of murine intestinal crypts. The protocol is optimized for an initial tissue size of the intestinal resections of approximately 5.5 cm^2.

1. Wash the intestinal tissue resection with cold PBS.
2. Transfer into a petri dish filled with cold PBS and carefully remove the muscle layer and attached connective tissue using scissors and forceps.
3. Discard PBS and wash the tissue section with new, cold PBS. Repeat the washing twice.
4. Perform step 3−5 of protocol for Small intestinal crypt isolation
   Use the following amounts of collagenase XI to prepare the collagenase solution:
   - small intestinal tissue: 15 mg/40 mL DMEM 6546
   - large intestinal tissue: 20 mg/40 mL DMEM 6546
5. Incubate in a water bath at 37°C for 9.5 minutes. Vigorously shake the tube for 30 seconds. Allow the tissue fragments to settle by gravity for 45 seconds (fraction 1). Transfer the supernatant of fraction 1 into a 15 mL conical tube.
6. Add 10 mL of warm collagenase XI solution to the pellet of fraction 1. Mix thoroughly. Incubate in a water bath at 37°C for 9.5 minutes. Vigorously shake the tube for 30 seconds. Allow the tissue fragments to settle by gravity for 45 seconds (fraction 2). Transfer the supernatant of fraction 2 into a 15 mL conical tube.
   a. Meanwhile, centrifuge the supernatant of fraction 1 at 100 g for 2 minutes at 4°C. Discard supernatant. Resuspend the pellet in 10 mL PBS, and centrifuge again at 100 g for 2 minutes at 4°C. Discard supernatant and resuspend the pellet in 5 mL basal culture medium. Place the tube on ice.
7. Add 10 mL of warm collagenase XI solution to the pellet of fraction 2. Mix thoroughly. Incubate in a water bath at 37°C for 9.5 minutes. Vigorously shake the tube for 30 seconds. Allow the tissue fragments to settle by gravity for 45 seconds (fraction 3). Transfer the supernatant of fraction 3 into a 15 mL conical tube.
   a. Meanwhile, centrifuge the supernatant of fraction 2 at 100 g for 2 minutes at 4°C. Discard supernatant. Resuspend the pellet in 10 mL PBS, and centrifuge again at 100 g for 2 minutes at 4°C. Discard supernatant and resuspend the pellet in 5 mL PBS. Place the tube on ice.
8. Add 10 mL of warm collagenase XI solution to the pellet of fraction 3. Mix thoroughly. Incubate in a water bath at 37°C for 9.5 minutes. Vigorously shake the tube for 30 seconds. Allow the tissue fragments to settle by gravity for 45 seconds (fraction 4). Transfer the supernatant of fraction 4 into a 15 mL conical tube.
   a. Meanwhile, centrifuge the supernatant of fraction 3 at 100 g for 2 minutes at 4°C. Discard supernatant. Resuspend the pellet in 10 mL PBS, and centrifuge again at 100 g for 2 minutes at 4°C. Discard supernatant and resuspend the pellet in 5 mL PBS. Place the tube on ice.

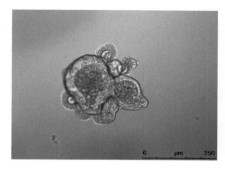 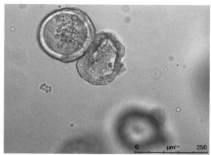

FIGURE 3.6

Murine small intestinal organoids grown for five days in medium containing Wnt3A (right) or not (left). Presence of Wnt3A in the medium leads to more cystic growth.

9. Centrifuge the supernatant of fraction 4 at 100 g for 2 minutes at 4°C. Discard supernatant. Resuspend the pellet in 10 mL PBS and centrifuge again at 100 g for 2 minutes at 4°C. Discard supernatant and resuspend the pellet in 5 mL PBS.

10. Combine supernatants of fractions 1−4 by passing them through a 70 μm cell strainer into a labeled 50 mL conical tube; centrifuge at 350 g, 3 minutes at 4°C.

11. Proceed with steps 13−16 of protocol Isolation of human intestinal crypts.

CULTIVATION OF INTESTINAL ORGANOIDS

The cultivation of murine and human intestinal organoids differs mainly in the composition of the cultivation medium. While murine small intestinal organoids require least supplements, human-derived organoids need several growth factors and inhibitors for proper growth and maintenance, particularly in the first days of culture. Recombinant cell lines producing Wnt3a, Noggin, and R-Spondin1 are commercially available; nevertheless, it is recommended that every batch of conditioned media produced be tested. Supplementation of the medium with Wnt3a inhibits differentiation, increases the proportion of stem cells/proliferating cells, and leads to more cystic growth (see Fig. 3.6). Reduction of Wnt3a, withdrawal of SB202190, or addition of a gamma-secretase inhibitor to block Notch-signaling, all result in preferential differentiation into the different intestinal epithelial cell-lineages. Ready-made media for intestinal organoid culture are commercially available.

Media composition for intestinal organoid culture

Basal culture medium (BCM):

The composition of the basal culture medium for human organoids is identical to that for murine intestinal organoid culture.

BCM	Stock	Dilution	Final Concentration	For 10 mL	
Advanced DMEM/F12				9.7	mL
GlutaMax	200 mM	1:100	2 mM	100	μL
Hepes	1M	1:100	10 mM	100	μL
Penicillin (100 U/mL) and Streptomycin (100 μg/mL) (AA)	100 ×	1:100	1 ×	100	μL

Preparation of supplements for crypt culture medium (CCM):

N-Acetylcystein (NAC)	NAC (MW) = 163.2 g/mol
	500 mM solution = 163 mg in 2 mL PBS
	Sterile filtration, store at −20°C
Recombinant murine EGF	Dissolve in sterile distilled water to a concentration of 100 μg/mL; dilute in sterile 0.1% BSA/PBS to a concentration of 20 μg/mL; store at −80°C
Recombinant murine Noggin	Dissolve in sterile distilled water to a concentration of 100 μg/mL; dilute in sterile 0.1% BSA/PBS to a concentration of 50 μg/mL; store at −80°C
Recombinant human R-Spondin 1	Dissolve in sterile distilled water to a concentration of 200 μg/mL; dilute in sterile 0.1% BSA/PBS to a concentration of 50 μg/mL; store at −80°C
Recombinant murine Wnt3a	Dissolve in sterile distilled water to a concentration of 100 μg/mL; dilute in sterile 0.1% BSA/PBS to a concentration of 50 μg/mL; store at −80°C
Additional Supplements for Human Organoid Culture:	
Nicotinamide	MW = 122.12 g/mol
	1M solution = 500 mg in 4.094 mL sterile PBS
	Store at −80°C
Wnt3a-conditioned medium	Produced by L Wnt-3A (ATCC®) cell line according to the provider's instructions
	Human organoids seem to require non-purified WNT3A, perhaps due to liposomal packaging
Human [Leu15]-Gastrin I	MW = 2080.16 g/mol
	10 μM solution = 100 μg in 4.81 mL sterile 0.1% BSA/PBS; store at −80°C
A83-01 TGFβ kinase/activin receptor-like kinase (ALK 5) inhibitor	MW = 421.52 g/mol
	500 μM solution = 1 mg in 4.74 mL sterile DMSO; Store at −80°C
SB202190 p38 MAP kinase inhibitor	MW = 331.34 g/mol
	30 mM solution = 5 mg in 503 μL sterile DMSO; Store at −80°C
Y-27632 ROCK inhibitor	MW = 320.26 g/mol
	10 mM solution = 1 mg in 312.25 μL sterile PBS; Store at −80°C

(*Continued*)

Continued

LY2157299[a]	MW = 369.4 g/mol
TGF-β receptor type 1 kinase inhibitor	1 mM solution = 1 mg in 2.707 mL sterile DMSO
	Final concentration = 500nM; store at −80°C
Thiazovivin[a]	MW = 311.4 g/mol
ROCK inhibitor	10 mM solution = 1 mg in 321 μL sterile DMSO;
	Final concentration = 2.5 μM; store at −80°C
CHIR99021[a]	MW = 465.3 g/mol
GSK3 inhibitor	10 mM solution = 1 mg in 214.92 μL sterile DMSO;
	Final concentration = 2.5 μM; store at −80°C

[a]*Optional inhibitors.*

Crypt Culture Medium for Murine Intestinal Organoids (CCM):

CCM	Stock	Dilution	Final Concentration	For 3 mL/10 wells	
BCM				2.861	mL
N2 supplement	100×	1:100	1×	30	μL
B27 supplement	50×	1:50	1×	60	μL
N-Acetylcystein	500 mM	1:500	1 mM	6	μL
EGF	20 μg/mL	1:400	50 ng/mL	7.5	μL
Noggin	50 μg/mL	1:500	100 ng/mL	6	μL
R-Spondin 1	50 μg/mL	1:100	500 ng/mL	30	μL
For Murine Large Intestinal Organoid Culture:					
Wnt3a	50 μg/mL	1:500	100 ng/mL	6 μL/ 3 mL	

Crypt Culture Medium for Human Intestinal Organoids (hCCM):

hCCM	Stock	Dilution	Final Concentration	For 5 mL/10 wells	
BCM		1:1		2.395	mL
Wnt3a-conditioned medium				2.323	mL
GlutaMax[a]	200 mM	1:200	1 mM/2 mM	24	μL
Hepes[a]	1M	1:200	5 mM/10 mM	24	μL
AA[a]	100×	1:200	0.5×/1×	24	μL
N2 supplement	100×	1:100	1×	25	μL
B27 supplement	50×	1:100	1×	50	μL
N-Acetylcystein	500 mM	1:1000	1 mM	2.5	μL
Nicotinamide	1M	1:100	10 mM	50	μL
EGF	20 μg/mL	1:400	50 ng/mL	12.5	μL
Noggin	50 μg/mL	1:500	100 ng/mL	10	μL
R-Spondin 1	50 μg/mL	1:100	500 ng/mL	50	μL
Gastrin	10 μM	1:1000	10 nM	5	μL

(Continued)

Continued

hCCM	Stock	Dilution	Final Concentration	For 5 mL/10 wells	
A83-01	500 μM	1:1000	500 nM	5	μL
SB202190	30 mM	1:3000	10 μM	1.67	μL
For the First Two Days of Culture					
Y-27632	10 mM	1:1000	10 μM	5 μL/5 mL	

[a]*These supplements are contained in BCM, and therefore just added for the proportion of Wnt3a-conditioned medium.*

Materials for Cultivation of Intestinal Organoids:

Equipment:
- biosafety cabinet
- incubator (37°C, 5% CO_2, 95% humidity)
- centrifuge (at 4°C)
- 24/48-well plates
- needle (24G) and syringe
- 50 mL conical tubes
- P1000 pipette tips, precooled at 4°C
- P100 pipette tips, precooled at 4°C

or optional:
- P100 pipette tips with a wider opening, precooled at 4°C

Reagents and Solutions:
- Matrigel
- PBS *without* Ca^{2+}/Mg^{2+}, supplemented with 1% AA
- CCM/ hCCM

Intestinal organoid cultivation and passaging/splitting

Intestinal organoids should be provided with new medium 2–3 times per week. The old medium is carefully aspired from the well without touching the Matrigel droplet, and 300/500 μL of new CCM/hCCM is added, respectively. Growth of organoids strongly depends on the density of seeding. If seeded at low densities, organoids grow more slowly. In general also, organoids derived from the large intestine grow more slowly (see Fig. 3.7). Passaging/splitting can therefore be performed every 5–10 days in a ratio of 1:1 to 1:5, depending on growth and density.

Protocol for passaging/splitting of intestinal organoids:

1. Aspire medium
2. Add 500–700 μL of cold PBS to each well and vigorously resuspend the Matrigel droplet using a 1000 μL pipette

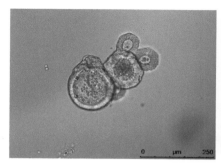 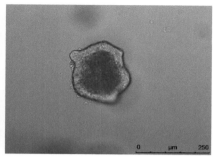

FIGURE 3.7

Murine small intestinal organoids (left) and murine colonic organoids (right) grown for five days in appropriate media. Colonic organoids exhibit a different growth pattern, and an overall slower growth.

    a. optional: instead of PBS, Cell Recovery Solution (CRS) can be used to dissolve the Matrigel. Using 500 μL of (CRS), the droplet is resuspended and the fractions are pooled. The tube is than incubated on ice for 1h and centrifuged as given in step 3.

3. Pool the suspensions of the different wells in a 50 mL conical tube; centrifuge at 350 g, 5 minutes, 4°C. Discard supernatant.

4. Resuspend pellet in 10 mL of cold PBS. Aspire and flush suspension 1−2 times using a syringe with a 24G needle.

5. Centrifuge at 350 g, 5 minutes, 4°C. Discard supernatant. Carefully resuspend with the desired volume of Matrigel (25/50 μL per well); avoid introducing any bubbles. Place on ice.

6. Apply 25 μL/50 μL of Matrigel suspension per well on a pre-warmed 48/24-well plate using chilled pipette tips. The suspension should be applied on the center of the well, so that it can form a hemispherical droplet. For this purpose, pipette tips with a wider opening can also be used for improved handling.

7. Incubate the plate at 37°C and allow the Matrigel to solidify for approximately 5−15 minutes. Overlay the Matrigel droplet with 300 μL/500 μL of CCM/ hCCM.

CRITICAL POINTS

- Working with human (and also murine) tissues, special biosafety precautions are required. Also, ethical approvals have to be obtained for every experiment.
- Working with needles, scalpels, scissors, and other sharp or pointy instruments requires special attention.

- Do not process too many samples at a time. Always keep samples on ice, if applicable.
- Timing is essential for the collagenase XI digestion. Stick to the times given in the protocol.

VERIFICATION

Commonly used methods like quantitative PCR, Western blot, flow cytometry, or immunofluorescence (IF)/immunohistochemistry (IHC) staining can be implemented to analyze intestinal organoids. Organoids can be either used as fresh fixed cells, or can easily be embedded in OCT or paraffin using histogel, allowing the application of a wide range of antibodies. In general, verification of intestinal organoid culture comprises the detection of markers for the different intestinal epithelial cell types (stem cells, Paneth cells, goblet cells, enterocytes, enteroendocrine cells, tuft cells) on mRNA or protein level.

TROUBLESHOOTING

- To increase crypt yield, conical tubes and pipette tips used during the isolation procedure can be coated with BSA. Fill tubes with 1%BSA in PBS, or put tips into a container filled with 1%BSA in PBS and incubate over night at 4°C. Discard the fluid prior to use.
- The Matrigel itself can be supplemented with growth factors, or can be diluted (up to 1:1) with CCM/ hCCM.
- The Matrigel has to be between 4°C and 8°C (4°C is optimal) to allow proper handling. Some fridges do not reach the exact temperature set, resulting in the Matrigel not reaching its fluid state.
- Instead of inverting murine intestinal segments, they can also be cut open and cut into pieces of $2-4$ mm^2.
- Longitudinal opened murine intestinal segments can be gently scratched with a microscope slide to remove the mucus and villi.
- The source of collagenase XI seems to be crucial for the exact incubation times. The efficiency of collagenase also seems to differ between charges. We prefer using collagenase XI from Sigma.
- The pH of the EDTA solution should be pH 8.0, due to solubility reasons.

ACKNOWLEDGMENTS

We would like to thank Eva Martini and Beate Rauscher for help on the protocols, and Johannes Zang for the photo documentation of the mouse preparation.

DECLARATIONS OF FINANCIAL INTERESTS

None.

REFERENCES

Barker, N., 2014. Adult intestinal stem cells: critical drivers of epithelial homeostasis and regeneration. Nat. Rev. Mol. Cell Biol. 15, 19−33.

Barker, N., van Oudenaarden, A., Clevers, H., 2012. Identifying the stem cell of the intestinal crypt: strategies and pitfalls. Cell Stem Cell. 11, 452−460.

Berger, E., Rath, E., Yuan, D., Waldschmitt, N., Khaloian, S., Allgauer, M., et al., 2016. Mitochondrial function controls intestinal epithelial stemness and proliferation. Nat. Commun. 7, 13171.

Blumberg, R.S., Li, L., Nusrat, A., Parkos, C.A., Rubin, D.C., Carrington, J.L., 2008. Recent insights into the integration of the intestinal epithelium within the mucosal environment in health and disease. Mucosal. Immunol. 1, 330−334.

Clavel, T., Haller, D., 2007. Bacteria- and host-derived mechanisms to control intestinal epithelial cell homeostasis: implications for chronic inflammation. Inflamm. Bowel Dis. 13, 1153−1164.

Daniel, H., Kottra, G., 2004. The proton oligopeptide cotransporter family SLC15 in physiology and pharmacology. Pflug Arch. Eur. J. Phys. 447, 610−618.

Daniel, H., Zietek, T., 2015. Taste and move: glucose and peptide transporters in the gastrointestinal tract. Exp. Physiol. 100, 1441−1450.

de Lau, W., Kujala, P., Schneeberger, K., Middendorp, S., Li, V.S., Barker, N., et al., 2012. Peyer's patch M cells derived from Lgr5(+) stem cells require SpiB and are induced by RankL in cultured "miniguts". Mol Cell Biol. 32, 3639−3647.

Diakogiannaki, E., Pais, R., Tolhurst, G., Parker, H.E., Horscroft, J., Rauscher, B., et al., 2013. Oligopeptides stimulate glucagon-like peptide-1 secretion in mice through proton-coupled uptake and the calcium-sensing receptor. Diabetologia. 56, 2688−2696.

Fogh, J., Fogh, J.M., Orfeo, T., 1977. One hundred and twenty-seven cultured human tumor cell lines producing tumors in nude mice. J. Natl. Cancer Inst. 59, 221−226.

Harwood, M.D., Achour, B., Neuhoff, S., Russell, M.R., Carlson, G., Warhurst, G., et al., 2016. In vitro-in vivo extrapolation scaling factors for intestinal P-glycoprotein and breast cancer resistance protein: part I: a cross-laboratory comparison of transporter-protein abundances and relative expression factors in human intestine and Caco-2 Cells. Drug Metab. Dispos. 44, 297−307.

Hoffmann, M., Rath, E., Holzlwimmer, G., Quintanilla-Martinez, L., Loach, D., Tannock, G., et al., 2008. Lactobacillus reuteri 100-23 transiently activates intestinal epithelial cells of mice that have a complex microbiota during early stages of colonization. J. Nutr. 138, 1684−1691.

Koo, B.K., Stange, D.E., Sato, T., Karthaus, W., Farin, H.F., Huch, M., et al., 2011. Controlled gene expression in primary Lgr5 organoid cultures. Nat Methods 9, 81−83.

Leushacke, M., Barker, N., 2014. Ex vivo culture of the intestinal epithelium: strategies and applications. Gut 63, 1345−1354.

Mahe, M.M., Aihara, E., Schumacher, M.A., Zavros, Y., Montrose, M.H., Helmrath, M.A., et al., 2013. Establishment of gastrointestinal epithelial organoids. Curr. Protoc. Mouse Biol. 3, 217−240.

Mahe, M.M., Sundaram, N., Watson, C.L., Shroyer, N.F., Helmrath, M.A., 2015. Establishment of human epithelial enteroids and colonoids from whole tissue and biopsy. J. Vis. Exp..

Middendorp, S., Schneeberger, K., Wiegerinck, C.L., Mokry, M., Akkerman, R.D., van Wijngaarden, S., et al., 2014. Adult stem cells in the small intestine are intrinsically programmed with their location-specific function. Stem Cells. 32, 1083−1091.

Parker, H.E., Wallis, K., le Roux, C.W., Wong, K.Y., Reimann, F., Gribble, F.M., 2012. Molecular mechanisms underlying bile acid-stimulated glucagon-like peptide-1 secretion. Br. J. Pharmacol. 165, 414−423.

Pinto, M., Robineleon, S., Appay, M.D., Kedinger, M., Triadou, N., Dussaulx, E., et al., 1983. Enterocyte-like differentiation and polarization of the human-colon carcinoma cell-line Caco-2 in culture. Biol Cell. 47, 323−330.

Pitman, R.S., Blumberg, R.S., 2000. First line of defense: the role of the intestinal epithelium as an active component of the mucosal immune system. J. Gastroenterol. 35, 805−814.

Rath, E., Haller, D., 2011. Inflammation and cellular stress: a mechanistic link between immune-mediated and metabolically driven pathologies. Eur. J. Nutr. 50, 219−233.

Reimann, F., Habib, A.M., Tolhurst, G., Parker, H.E., Rogers, G.J., Gribble, F.M., 2008. Glucose sensing in L cells: a primary cell study. Cell Metab. 8, 532−539.

Roder, P.V., Geillinger, K.E., Zietek, T.S., Thorens, B., Koepsell, H., Daniel, H., 2014. The role of SGLT1 and GLUT2 in intestinal glucose transport and sensing. PLoS One 9, e89977.

Sambuy, Y., De Angelis, I., Ranaldi, G., Scarino, M.L., Stammati, A., Zucco, F., 2005. The Caco-2 cell line as a model of the intestinal barrier: influence of cell and culture-related factors on Caco-2 cell functional characteristics. Cell Biol. Toxicol. 21, 1−26.

Sato, T., Clevers, H., 2013a. Growing self-organizing mini-guts from a single intestinal stem cell: mechanism and applications. Science 340, 1190−1194.

Sato, T., Clevers, H., 2013b. Primary mouse small intestinal epithelial cell cultures. Methods Mol. Biol. 945, 319−328.

Sato, T., Vries, R.G., Snippert, H.J., van de Wetering, M., Barker, N., Stange, D.E., et al., 2009. Single Lgr5 stem cells build crypt-villus structures in vitro without a mesenchymal niche. Nature 459, 262−265.

Schwank, G., Clevers, H., 2016. CRISPR/Cas9-mediated genome editing of mouse small intestinal organoids. Methods Mol. Biol. 1422, 3−11.

Schwank, G., Koo, B.K., Sasselli, V., Dekkers, J.F., Heo, I., Demircan, T., et al., 2013. Functional repair of CFTR by CRISPR/Cas9 in intestinal stem cell organoids of cystic fibrosis patients. Cell Stem Cell 13, 653−658.

Spence, J.R., Mayhew, C.N., Rankin, S.A., Kuhar, M.F., Vallance, J.E., Tolle, K., et al., 2011. Directed differentiation of human pluripotent stem cells into intestinal tissue in vitro. Nature 470, 105−109.

Stelzner, M., Helmrath, M., Dunn, J.C., Henning, S.J., Houchen, C.W., Kuo, C., et al., 2012. A nomenclature for intestinal in vitro cultures. Am. J. Physiol. Gastrointest. Liver Physiol. 302, G1359−G1363.

VanDussen, K.L., Marinshaw, J.M., Shaikh, N., Miyoshi, H., Moon, C., Tarr, P.I., et al., 2015. Development of an enhanced human gastrointestinal epithelial culture system to facilitate patient-based assays. Gut 64, 911—920.

Vincent, M.L., Russell, R.M., Sasak, V., 1985. Folic acid uptake characteristics of a human colon carcinoma cell line, Caco-2. A newly-described cellular model for small intestinal epithelium. Hum. Nutr. Clin. Nutr. 39, 355—360.

Wells, J.M., Spence, J.R., 2014. How to make an intestine. Development 141, 752—760.

Whitehead, R.H., Robinson, P.S., 2009. Establishment of conditionally immortalized epithelial cell lines from the intestinal tissue of adult normal and transgenic mice. Am. J. Physiol. Gastrointest. Liver Physiol. 296, G455—G460.

Wuensch, T., Schulz, S., Ullrich, S., Lill, N., Stelzl, T., Rubio-Aliaga, I., et al., 2013. The peptide transporter PEPT1 is expressed in distal colon in rodents and humans and contributes to water absorption. Am. J. Physiol-Gastr. L. 305, G66—G73.

Yee, S., 1997. In vitro permeability across Caco-2 cells (colonic) can predict in vivo (small intestinal) absorption in man--fact or myth. Pharm. Res. 14, 763—766.

Yoshikawa, T., Inoue, R., Matsumoto, M., Yajima, T., Ushida, K., Iwanaga, T., 2011. Comparative expression of hexose transporters (SGLT1, GLUT1, GLUT2 and GLUT5) throughout the mouse gastrointestinal tract. Histochem. Cell Biol. 135, 183—194.

Zietek, T., Daniel, H., 2015. Intestinal nutrient sensing and blood glucose control. Curr. Opin. Clin. Nutr. Metab. Care. 18, 381—388.

Zietek, T., Rath, E., Haller, D., Daniel, H., 2015. Intestinal organoids for assessing nutrient transport, sensing and incretin secretion. Sci. Rep. 5, 16831.

Three-dimensional breast culture models

New culture models for analyzing breast development and function

4

Amber M. Wood, Heyuan Sun, Jack Williams, Keith R. Brennan, Andrew P. Gilmore and Charles H. Streuli

University of Manchester, Manchester, United Kingdom

CHAPTER OUTLINE

INTRODUCTION

DEVELOPMENT, STRUCTURE, AND FUNCTION OF THE MAMMARY GLAND

The mammary gland is a milk-producing organ composed of tubular ducts and spherical alveoli, which are surrounded by complex fibroglandular tissue and adipose. The branched, hollow network of epithelial cells is embedded in a stromal matrix containing fibroblasts. Much of mammary gland development occurs following the onset of puberty, when the immature ductal trees extend and branch. In response to hormonal changes during pregnancy, there is a further increase in branching, along with development of spherical alveolar structures (Fig. 4.1). During lactation, the luminal cells of these alveoli differentiate and make milk components, which are secreted into the lumen of the duct and moved to the nipple by contraction of the alveolar basal myoepithelial cells. Following weaning of the infant, the mammary gland undergoes involution, which involves regression

Organoids and Mini-Organs. DOI: http://dx.doi.org/10.1016/B978-0-12-812636-3.00004-3

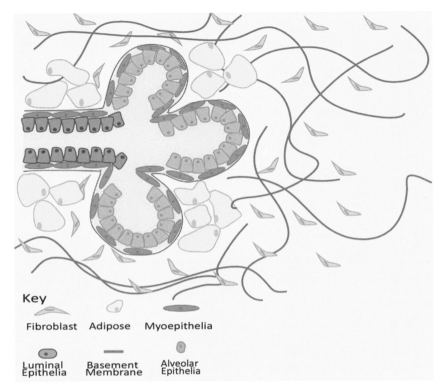

Key

Fibroblast   Adipose   Myoepithelia

Luminal   Basement   Alveolar
Epithelia   Membrane   Epithelia

FIGURE 4.1

Simplified diagram of the differentiated terminal ductal/lobular unit of the mammary gland, composed of hollow alveoli lined with alveolar epithelial cells, and tubular ducts lined with luminal epithelial cells. Surrounding these are the myoepithelial cells, with the ability to contract to force milk to the nipple, and the stroma containing fibroblasts, as well as nerves, blood vessels, and immune cells.

of the differentiated luminal epithelia, in essence returning it to the virgin state (Akhtar et al., 2016).

To understand the mechanisms involved in creating the multi-cellular structures found within the mammary gland, and the way that mammary epithelial cells differentiate to express tissue specific genes, a variety of 3D models have been developed where the cells can be cultured in vitro.

THE NEED FOR THREE-DIMENSIONAL MAMMARY GLAND ORGANOID CULTURES

Determining how the mammary gland forms is important for understanding the development and function of this essential mammalian tissue, as well as the initiation and progression of breast cancer. To date, much of the work examining mammary gland development has focused on the specification, growth, and branching of the ductal epithelium. However, the environment surrounding the cells of the normal mammary gland also has a key role in both tissue development and cellular differentiation. Moreover, changes within this microenvironment contribute to breast cancer progression. Therefore, culture models that closely mimic the in vivo tissue environment are crucial for understanding how the normal mammary gland functions, as well as for understanding the progression of breast cancer.

In vivo, mammary epithelial cells (MECs) contact a discrete basement membrane, not the stromal matrix or the extracellular matrix proteins found in serum. However, historically, most research using MECs has been done either on two-dimensional (2D) plastic, or using protein gels, such as Matrigel, a recombinant basement membrane mix. Although Matrigel can induce in vivo-like behavior in MECs, it cannot develop fully-functioning organ features such as duct structures. Thus, alternative models that are more similar to the tissue environment are required to understand fully the mechanisms involved in breast development and function. These include the 3D culture models that we discuss in this chapter. Also important is the ability to modify these 3D environments to a more tumor-like environment, to reveal how breast cancer develops.

DESIGN CONSIDERATIONS

Extracellular matrix

When designing 3D models for mammary cell culture, the first thing to consider is the composition of the extracellular matrix, as this can dramatically alter the behavior of the cells. The first 3D cell culture models involved gels made of collagen I (Williams et al., 1978). It was demonstrated that primary mouse MECs on floating collagen gels could form tubular structures similar to those seen in vivo. The cells also retained the potential to make their own basement membrane and produce milk, compared to those on attached collagen gels, which formed monolayers and were unable to produce milk (Streuli and Bissell, 1990).

This approach of using 3D mammary cultures was further developed by using matrix isolated from the cell line derived from Engelbreth − Holm − Swarm sarcoma mouse, commercially known as Matrigel (Li et al., 1987). Mammary epithelial cells grown in this environment form rounded, polarized acini (Fig. 4.2), structures similar to those of the alveoli in mammary gland tissue (Aggeler et al., 1991). Matrigel has since become the standard approach for growing MECs in culture. However, Matrigel is a complex mix of components that are poorly defined, and it is not clear how well these mimic the microenvironment of the mammary gland. The primary component, laminin 1, is not the same isoform as found in the basement membrane of the mammary gland. Indeed, MECs grown in Matrigel form their own laminin-containing basement membrane. Thus, what the important component or property of Matrigel is for MEC differentiation is unclear.

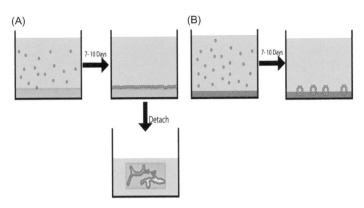

FIGURE 4.2

Mammary epithelial cells grown in 3D protein gels form structures similar to those in mammary gland tissue. (A) The MECs in attached collagen gels form squamous monolayers, while those in detached collagen gels form tubular structures. (B) Those grown in Matrigel form rounded acini.

The composition of the natural mammary gland matrix is much more complex than simply collagen I or basement membrane, and the duct of the mammary gland is also more than a polarized cyst-like structure. Therefore, there is a need for 3D models that have an extracellular matrix composition which is closer to that of the human mammary gland in vivo. The MECs need to be able to form not just acini, but also duct-like structures. One recent publication uses a mix of collagen I, laminin, fibronectin, and hyaluronan (Sokol et al., 2016). Together, these induce primary human MECs to form duct-like structures, which can be traced through the development of immature duct-bud structures to differentiated, milk-producing alveoli. Developments of 3D models that are closer to the in vivo system will improve our understanding of duct development and mammary gland function.

Environmental stiffness

The mechanical stiffness of the cellular microenvironment has a central role in controlling gene expression, thereby determining cell phenotype and differentiation (Gilbert and Weaver, 2016). Notably, while a soft microenvironment is essential for mammary epithelia to form duct-like structures, high extracellular stiffness has been associated with breast cancer (Kai et al., 2016). Furthermore, one of the most significant risk factors for breast cancer development is its mammographic density. Recent studies have shown that regions of high mammographic breast density have a more organized, fibrillar collagenous stroma. These regions are mechanically stiffer than areas of low density, suggesting that increased mechanical stress on MECs may contribute to cancer initiation (McConnell et al., 2016; Boyd et al., 2014). Therefore, tuneable systems can help not only our understanding of the normal mammary gland, but also the disease environment.

The stiffness of 2D cultures can be modified using polyacrylamide based hydrogels (Tse and Engler, 2010). By changing the ratio of acrylamide to bis-acrylamide in these gels, it is possible to change their stiffness. Extracellular matrix proteins can be cross-linked to the hydrogel to generate surfaces coated with specific ECM proteins of differing stiffness. However, care has to be taken to ensure that the coating of the hydrogel with an ECM protein does not alter its stiffness. Our experience coating polyacrylamide-based hydrogels with Matrigel has shown there can be marked changes in stiffness following coating.

A number of ways have been developed to increase the mechanical stiffness of 3D cultures. Traditionally, to mechanically de-stress cells in culture, collagen gels are detached from the well and allowed to float. As the collagen gel no longer has the support of the well, the gel softens and compacts. This method is relatively crude and lacks fine-tuning of the environmental stiffness, transitioning rapidly from a relatively stiff environment to a soft one. Alternative methods to modify ECM stiffness include modifying the concentration of collagen. Although this method has been used to induce a change in phenotype in MECs, it cannot distinguish between the effect of stiffness and that of reduced ligand availability (Provenzano et al., 2009). Collagen I can also be added in varying concentrations to Matrigel, increasing its stiffness. This again introduces variability in ligand availability for the cells, according the proportion of collagen and Matrigel. Moreover, Matrigel and collagen do not mix homogenously, but separate into regions that are either Matrigel- or collagen-rich, with resulting heterogeneity within the culture (Barnes et al., 2014).

An alternative method to increase the stiffness of Matrigel in a more controlled way is through the use of scaffolds. Scaffolds are inert biological or artificial compounds in which the stiffness can be tuned, without having additional effects on the cells. These allow the tuning of the mechanical properties over a range of values, whilst maintaining ligand availability. One example of a scaffold that is currently used with Matrigel is alginate, a polysaccharide derived from algae (Chaudhuri et al., 2014). Alginate is composed of B-D-mannuronate (M) and a-L-guluronate (G), which covalently link together to form G-rich, M-rich, or mixed regions. The G-rich regions bind to divalent ions, such as calcium, to reversibly cross-link them and create a stiffer 3D-network (Fig. 4.3) (Mørch et al., 2006). However, it is worth noting that alginate gels can be added to other mixtures of extracellular matrix proteins, such as collagen I, fibronectin, or Arginylglycylaspartic acid (RGD) peptides (Branco da Cunha et al., 2014; Bidarra et al., 2016). We have used this method to grow MECs in soft and stiff Matrigel. The MECs cultured in soft gels form small rounded acini with lumens, while those grown in stiff gels form irregular shaped, larger clusters.

Tissue shape

A third consideration when generating models of mammary tissue is generating the appropriate structure and shape of the tissue. In the models described in the

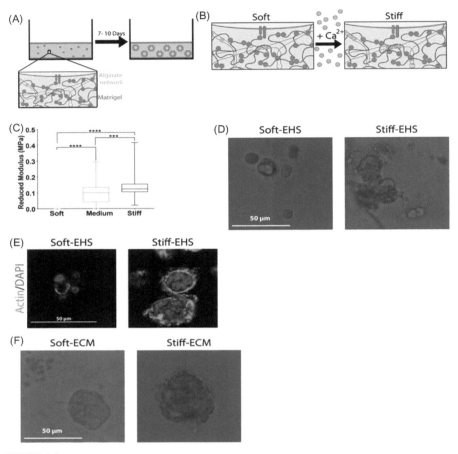

FIGURE 4.3

Alginate-Matrigel gels of different stiffness. (A) Schematic to show that the formation of acini in Alginate-Matrigel gels occurs after 7—10 days. (B) The stiffness of Alginate-Matrigel gels can be increased through the addition of calcium. (C) Atomic force microscopy detects the increase in gel stiffness after calcium addition. (D) Mammary epithelial cells grown in stiff Alginate-Matrigel gels form large and irregular shaped clusters, rather than the rounded, hollow acini when grown in soft gels. (E) Stiffness also disrupts acinar polarity, as seen by actin distribution, whereby actin is localized to the apical surface of acini grown in soft gels, and to the basal surface of those grown in stiff gels. (F) Initial attempts to combine the alginate methodology with a mix of extracellular components (collagen I, laminin, fibronectin, and hyaluronan).

above section, the implanted cells remodel the surrounding matrix to form appropriate structures. However, new 3D printing technologies provide an opportunity to generate a matrix of the appropriate shape, into which cells can be seeded (Li et al., 2014). So far living tissues such as liver, heart, and cartilage have been successfully reconstructed by 3D printers, and are functionally stable for several weeks (Murphy and Atala, 2014; Ma et al., 2016). Consequently, biofabrication using 3D printing has the potential to reconstruct artificial mammary gland environments that can be used for in vitro study of real tissues.

With current aims to reduce the numbers of animals sacrificed for research, 3D printing may eventually allow us to create a human-environment in vitro transplant assay to study the development of the mammary gland, as well as tumor formation. Our understanding of mammary gland biology would also benefit from human-focused in vitro environments, as much research done so far has been based on observations in mouse which although useful, is not the same as the human mammary gland. Our laboratory is currently using a peptide-based gel for printing 3D ECMs. The stiffness of the gels can be tuned by adjusting the pH (Fig. 4.4) (Ulijn and Smith, 2008; Boothroyd et al., 2013). Using this gel, we are now printing structures mimicking mammary tissue, which will provide a better model for studying the cellular response to microenvironmental stiffness.

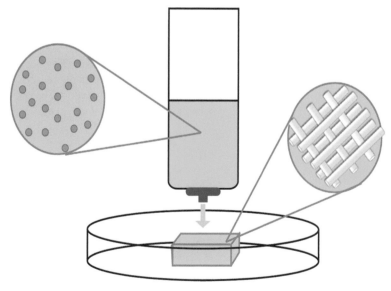

FIGURE 4.4

Three-dimensional printing schematic. Cells are mixed with commercial gel peptide solutions of high or low stiffness, and loaded into a 3D bell plotter. Printing design is programmed in the machine, and gel — cell mix printed onto a dish. Gels are allowed to set before adding medium.

REMAINING CHALLENGES FOR DEVELOPING THREE-DIMENSIONAL MAMMARY EPITHELIAL CELL CULTURE MODELS

Of the methods discussed within this chapter, there are two factors that have not yet been addressed fully. First, the ability to manipulate culture models to mimic the cellular environment observed in cancer needs to be improved. The alginate system has the potential to improve disease models, through the substitution of Matrigel with protein mixes that are more reflective of the disease environment. Alternatively, 3D poly(ethylene) glycol (PEG)-based hydrogels can be used to test ECM ligands and their effect on MEC behavior systematically (Taubenberger et al., 2016). As more information becomes available regarding how the pathological environment changes during disease initiation and progression, these differences can be incorporated into novel 3D models.

Second, the multi-cellularity of breast tissue is important to its function. Current culture models typically use primary luminal epithelial cells or established luminal epithelial cell lines in isolation. However, in vivo luminal epithelial cells are also in contact with myoepithelial cells, and epithelial ducts and alveoli are surrounded by adipose, fibroblasts, and immune cells. Interestingly, heterotypic cultures may prevent primary MECs from becoming senescent, and support the formation of in vivo-like structures (Wang and Kaplan, 2012). Initial attempts to model mammary tissue using multiple cell types have involved cell culture chambers separated by collagen membranes, with fibroblasts in collagen gels in the bottom layer, and epithelial cells on top. It is proposed that this system could be used to explore the interaction of neoplastic cells with the normal mammary environment (Choi et al., 2015). Further development to incorporate immune cells may be beneficial, as these cells are also involved in breast cancer progression (Nagalla et al., 2013; Tabariès et al., 2015).

THREE-DIMENSIONAL GEL SYSTEMS

In order for MECs to behave as they do in their tissue of origin, and for mammary epithelial-derived cancer cells to grow and migrate as they do in vivo, it is crucial to utilize well-tuned 3D culture models. Normal plastic culture dishes are good for initial studies; however, they are inappropriate for understanding MEC function in vivo. When grown in 2D, the cells lose their normal controls of survival, cell cycle, expression of tissue specific genes, and migration. Three-dimensional cultures are therefore critical to provide more normal environments to study all these processes.

Within this chapter, we detail four types of 3D-culture methodology, including traditional collagen or Matrigel gels, and novel methods involving mixes of extracellular matrix components, and the use of scaffolds such as alginate. All four methods allow MECs to form in vivo-like structures. However, by incorporating scaffolds there are more opportunities to manipulate the system to reflect both normal and pathological environments.

DETAILED INSTRUCTIONS

Attached versus floating collagen gels

Materials

Collagen I, from rat tail (Corning; 354236)
   10X DMEM/10XPBS
   0.34 M NaOH (autoclaved)

Procedure

1. On ice, mix 8 volumes of type I Collagen with 1 volume 10X DMEM or 10X PBS
2. Add 1 volume 0.34 M NaOH and mix, avoiding bubbles
3. Transfer gel solution to plate (see Table)
4. Allow the collagen to gel at 37°C for at least 1 hour
5. Remove medium from cells and add trypsin. Incubate at 37°C for sufficient time for cells to detach. Resuspend the cells in complete medium, and spin at 500 rpm for 3 minutes.
6. Remove the medium from the cells and resuspend in 1 mL of complete medium
7. Use 10 μL of cells and dilute 1:10. Count the cells, and calculate the correct number to add per well, appropriate to your cell type
8. Wash the gel twice with complete medium
9. Add cells to gel
10. Refresh medium every 3−4 days
11. Float gel after 24 hours by running a 200 μL tip around the circumference of the gel

Points to note

Dish Diameter	Final Gel Volume
50 mm	3.0 mL
35 mm	1.5 mL
22 mm	0.6 mL

Verifying

Bright-field images may be improved by removing medium first

Cells can be removed from the gel using trypsin for downstream analysis (e.g., cytospinning, protein extraction)

Cells can be lysed directly in the gel for RNA extraction with Trizol (1 mL Trizol per gel)

Gels can be embedded in OCT and cryosectioned for IF.

Common problems

Special care is needed with "floated" gels, because they can be removed inadvertently by vacuum aspiration.

Matrigel

Materials

Matrigel (Corning; 354234)
  Multiwell plates
  Trypsin
  Complete medium

Procedure

1. Work on ice
2. Add appropriate volume of Matrigel to well (see Table)
3. Spread Matrigel around the plate
4. Check the plates are horizontal and allow to set at 37°C for at least 30 minutes
5. Remove medium from cells and add trypsin. Incubate at 37°C for sufficient time for cells to detach. Resuspend the cells in complete medium, and spin at 500 rpm for 3 minutes
6. Remove the medium from the cells and resuspend in 1 mL of complete medium
7. Use 10 μL of cells and dilute 1:10. Count the cells and calculate the correct number to add per well, appropriate to your cell type
8. Add complete medium to well, supplemented with 2% Matrigel
9. Add cells to well
10. Matrigel is stable up to 21 days
11. Refresh medium every 4 days

Points to note

Ensure Matrigel is kept on ice; do not allow it to warm prior to plating it onto the culture dish

Take care when adding solutions to the Matrigel-coated well, so as to avoid disrupting the layer

Density of cells will vary dependant on cell type. We use primary mammary epithelial cells or EpH4s, which are derived from pregnant mouse mammary gland (Fialka et al., 1996) at a density of 1×10^5 cells/mL.

For more invasive cell lines, thicker coats of Matrigel may be required

Multiwell Plate	Matrigel Volume
24-well	50 μL
12-well	100 μL
6-well	250 μL

Verifying

Coverslips can be coated in Matrigel for immunofluorescence
Cells can be lysed directly on Matrigel for RNA and protein extraction

Debugging common problems

Problem	Troubleshooting
Matrigel not spreading evenly on well	Ensure the plate has been cooled prior to adding Matrigel
	Spread Matrigel quickly after adding to well
	Initially coating the well with a thin layer of collagen I can provide a better adhesive layer for the Matrigel
Cells invade through Matrigel and form monolayer on plate	Ensure Matrigel has covered the entire surface of the plate
	Add medium before adding cells
	Make sure cells were not seeded at too high a density
	Take care when changing medium so as to not disrupt the Matrigel layer

Extracellular matrix gels

Materials

13 mm coverslips
24-well plate
Multiwell slide chamber
Collagen I, rat tail, high concentration (Corning; 354249)
Fibronectin, bovine plasma (Sigma; F1141)
Laminin, from Engelbreth − Holm − Swarm mouse (Sigma; L2020)
High MW Hyaluronan (Sigma)
250 mg sterile high MW, high guluronic acid alginate (Novamatrix; SLG100) in 10 mL blank DMEM

Procedure

1. Place a 13 mm coverslip into the well of a 24-well plate or prepare a multiwell slide chamber
2. Prepare the gel mix (see Table; 250 μL final gel volume)
3. Remove medium from cells and add trypsin. Incubate at 37°C for sufficient time for cells to detach. Resuspend the cells in complete medium and spin at 500 rpm for 3 minutes
4. Remove the medium from the cells and resuspend in 1 mL of complete medium
5. Use 10 μL of cells and dilute 1:10. Count the cells and calculate the correct volume containing 2.5×10^5 cells.

6. Add cells to gel mix with (250 μL—cell volume μL—protein volume μL) μL DMEM
7. Pipette the gel onto a coverslip or into a mold
8. Incubate at 37°C for at least 1 hour for the gel to set
9. Float gel in complete medium by carefully detaching from coverslip
10. Refresh medium every 3—4 days

Points to note

Primary cells can be used, ensuring that the volume of cells added is a maximum of 50 μL per gel

The proportion of primary cells that form duct-like structures is very low, and lower primary cell numbers per gel may improve duct-like formation (Sokol et al., 2016)

Gel Component	Final Concentration (mg/mL)
Collagen I	1.7
Fibronectin	0.02
Laminin	0.04
High MW hyaluronan	0.02
Alginate	5

Verifying

Bright-field images may be improved by removing medium first

Cells can be removed from the gel using trypsin for analysis (e.g., cytospinning, protein extraction)

Cells can be lysed directly in the gel for RNA extraction with Trizol (1 mL Trizol per gel)

Gels can be embedded in OCT and cryosectioned for IF.

Alginate-matrigel gels of varying stiffness

Materials

High concentration Matrigel >10 mg/mL (Corning; 354234)

250 mg sterile high MW, high glucuronic acid alginate (Novamatrix; SLG100) in 10 mL blank DMEM

DMEM

1.22 M $CaSO_4$ in ddH_2O (autoclaved)

Trypsin

Complete medium

24-well plate

1 mL syringes

Luer lock couplers

Procedure

1. Protocol is to make a 250 μL gel appropriate for a 24-well plate
2. Coat the wells of a 24-well plate with 40 μL of Matrigel
3. Dilute the 1.22 M $CaSO_4$ to 1:10 in blank DMEM
4. Prepare further dilutions of $CaSO_4$ for each gel stiffness, as used in original publication
5. Prepare gel mixes so that in a final 250 μL gel, the concentration of alginate is 5 mg/mL and the Matrigel is 4.5 mg/mL. Top up to 150 μL with DMEM.
6. Remove medium from cells and add trypsin. Incubate at 37°C for sufficient time for cells to detach. Resuspend the cells in complete medium and spin at 500 rpm for 3 minutes.
7. Remove the medium from the cells and resuspend in 1 mL of complete medium
8. Use 10 μL of cells and dilute 1:10. Count the cells and calculate the correct volume containing 2.5×10^5 cells.
9. Add cells to gel solution with (50 μL—cell volume μl) μl DMEM, and mix well
10. Take 200 μL of gel − cell mix and transfer to a cooled 1 ml syringe
11. To another 1 mL syringe, add 50 μL of $CaSO_4$ solution
12. Join syringes by a luer lock coupler and pump solutions from one syringe to the other approximately six times
13. Draw all the solution into one syringe, detach from the other syringe
14. Slowly push the plunger into the syringe against gravity, then expel the gel mix into a well of a 24-well plate
15. Allow the gel to set for at least 30 minutes, then add 1 mL of complete medium
16. Gels are stable for up to 21 days (e.g., MCF10A acinar formation)
17. Refresh medium every 4 days

Points to note

Ensure all solutions are kept on ice

$CaSO_4$ is made up at a concentration past its saturation point, so make sure to agitate the solution before use

Matrigel can be substituted for alternative proteins such as those found in the Table

Take care not to suck up gels during medium changes

Verifying

Bright-field images may be improved by removing medium first

Cells can be removed from the gel using trypsin for downstream analysis (e.g., cytospinning, protein extraction)

Cells can be lysed directly in the gel for RNA extraction with Trizol (1 mL Trizol per gel)

Gels can be embedded in OCT and cryosectioned for IF.

Debugging common problems

Problem	Troubleshooting
Bubbles	Try and reduce bubbles produced at each step of gel mixing
	Allow gel to rest before mixing by syringe
Difficult to focus on bright-field	Remove medium
Gels are floating	Use trans-well insert to weigh gel down
Lost gel during medium change	Use 1 mL pipette to change and add medium
	Change medium slowly to identify when gel may be being drawn up by pipette
Gel has solidified too early	Work on ice
	Ensure $CaSO_4$ is not added too early
Poor RNA yield	Use Trizol method with LiCl precipitation following Isopropanol step

ACKNOWLEDGMENTS

Core funding for the Wellcome Trust Centre for Cell-Matrix Research (088785/Z/09/Z) from the Welcome Trust, United Kingdom, supported this work. Funding from The Medical Research Council (MRC) and Manchester Alumni Research Impact Scholarship also supported this work. The funders had no role in the decision to publish, or in the preparation of the manuscript.

REFERENCES

Aggeler, J., et al., 1991. Cytodifferentiation of mouse mammary epithelial cells cultured on a reconstituted basement membrane reveals striking similarities to development in vivo. J. Cell. Sci. 99 (Pt 2), 407–417. Available at: http://www.ncbi.nlm.nih.gov/pubmed/1885677 (accessed 14.07.16).

Akhtar, N., et al., 2016. Rac1 controls morphogenesis and tissue-specific function in mammary gland development. Dev. Cell.

Barnes, C., et al., 2014. From single cells to tissues: interactions between the matrix and human breast cells in real time. PLoS. ONE. 9 (4), e93325. Available at: http://www.ncbi.nlm.nih.gov/pubmed/24691468 (accessed 16.06.16).

Bidarra, S.J., et al., 2016. A 3D in vitro model to explore the inter-conversion between epithelial and mesenchymal states during EMT and its reversion. Sci. Rep. 6, 27072. Available at: http://www.nature.com/articles/srep27072 (accessed 01.08.16).

Boothroyd, S., et al., 2013. From fibres to networks using self-assembling peptides. Faraday. Discuss. 166 (0), 195. Available at: http://xlink.rsc.org/?DOI=c3fd00097d (accessed 14.07.16).

Boyd, N.F., et al., 2014. Evidence that breast tissue stiffness is associated with risk of breast cancer. PLoS. ONE. 9 (7), e100937. Available at: http://www.ncbi.nlm.nih.gov/pubmed/25010427 (accessed 15.08.16).

Branco da Cunha, C., et al., 2014. Influence of the stiffness of three-dimensional alginate/collagen-I interpenetrating networks on fibroblast biology. Biomaterials 35 (32), 8927−8936.

Chaudhuri, O., et al., 2014. Extracellular matrix stiffness and composition jointly regulate the induction of malignant phenotypes in mammary epithelium. Nat. Mater. 1−35. Available at: http://www.ncbi.nlm.nih.gov/pubmed/24930031.

Choi, Y., et al., 2015. A microengineered pathophysiological model of early-stage breast cancer. Lab. Chip. 15 (16), 3350−3357. Available at: http://www.ncbi.nlm.nih.gov/pubmed/26158500 (accessed 16.06.16).

Fialka, I., et al., 1996. The estrogen-dependent c-JunER protein causes a reversible loss of mammary epithelial cell polarity involving a destabilization of adherens junctions. J. Cell. Biol. 132 (6), 1115−1132. Available at: http://www.ncbi.nlm.nih.gov/pubmed/8601589 [accessed 09.08.16).

Gilbert, P.M., Weaver, V.M., 2016. *Cellular* adaptation to biomechanical stress across length scales in tissue homeostasis and disease. Semin. Cell. Dev. Biol.

Kai, F., Laklai, H., Weaver, V., 2016. Force Matters: biomechanical regulation of cell invasion and migration in disease. Trends. Cell. Biol.. Available at: http://www.ncbi.nlm.nih.gov/pubmed/27056543 (accessed 05.04.16).

Li, M.L., et al., 1987. Influence of a reconstituted basement membrane and its components on casein gene expression and secretion in mouse mammary epithelial cells. Proc. Natl. Acad. Sci. U.S.A. 84 (1), 136−140. Available at: http://www.ncbi.nlm.nih.gov/pubmed/3467345 (accessed 14.07.16).

Li, X., et al., 2014. 3D-printed biopolymers for tissue engineering application. Int. J. Polym. Sci., 20141−13. Available at: http://www.hindawi.com/journals/ijps/2014/829145/ (accessed 14.07.16).

Ma, X., et al., 2016. Deterministically patterned biomimetic human iPSC-derived hepatic model via rapid 3D bioprinting. Proc. Natl. Acad. Sci. 113 (8), 2206−2211. Available at: http://www.pnas.org/lookup/doi/10.1073/pnas.1524510113 (accessed 14.07.16).

McConnell, J.C., et al., 2016. Increased peri-ductal collagen micro-organization may contribute to raised mammographic density. Breast Cancer Res. BCR 18 (1), 5. Available at: http://www.ncbi.nlm.nih.gov/pubmed/26747277 (accessed 14.07.16).

Mørch, Ý.A., Donati, I., Strand, B.L., 2006. Effect of Ca 2 + , Ba 2 + , and Sr 2 + on Alginate Microbeads. Biomacromolecules. 7 (5), 1471−1480. Available at: http://dx.doi.org/10.1021/bm060010d (accessed 17.03.15).

Murphy, S.V., Atala, A., 2014. 3D bioprinting of tissues and organs. Nat. Biotechnol. 32 (8), 773−785. Available at: http://www.nature.com/doifinder/10.1038/nbt.2958 (accessed 14.07.16).

Nagalla, S., et al., 2013. Interactions between immunity, proliferation and molecular subtype in breast cancer prognosis. Genome Biol. 14 (4), R34. Available at: http://genomebiology.biomedcentral.com/articles/10.1186/gb-2013-14-4-r34 (accessed 1.08.16).

Provenzano, P.P., et al., 2009. Matrix density-induced mechanoregulation of breast cell phenotype, signaling and gene expression through a FAK-ERK linkage. Oncogene 28 (49), 4326−4343. Available at: http://www.pubmedcentral.nih.gov/articlerender.fcgi?artid=2795025&tool=pmcentrez&rendertype=abstract (accessed 11.11.13).

Sokol, E.S., et al., 2016. Growth of human breast tissues from patient cells in 3D hydrogel scaffolds. Breast Cancer Res. BCR 18 (1), 19. Available at: http://www.ncbi.nlm.nih.gov/pubmed/26926363 (accessed 16.06.16).

Streuli, C.H., Bissell, M.J., 1990. Expression of extracellular matrix components is regulated by substratum. J. Cell. Biol. 110 (4), 1405−1415. Available at: http://www.ncbi.nlm.nih.gov/pubmed/2182652 (accessed 14.07.16).

Tabariès, S., et al., 2015. Granulocytic immune infiltrates are essential for the efficient formation of breast cancer liver metastases. Breast Cancer Res. 17 (1), 45. Available at: http://breast-cancer-research.com/content/17/1/45 (accessed 01.08.16).

Taubenberger, A.V., et al., 2016. 3D extracellular matrix interactions modulate tumour cell growth, invasion and angiogenesis in engineered tumour microenvironments. Acta. Biomater. 36, 73−85.

Tse, J.R., Engler, A.J., 2010. Preparation of hydrogel substrates with tunable mechanical properties. Current protocols in cell biology / editorial board, Juan S. Bonifacino … [et al.], Chapter 10(June), p.Unit 10.16. Available at: <http://www.ncbi.nlm.nih.gov/pubmed/20521229> (accessed 21.10.13).

Ulijn, R.V., Smith, A.M., 2008. Designing peptide based nanomaterials. Chem. Soc. Rev. 37 (4), 664−675. Available at: http://www.ncbi.nlm.nih.gov/pubmed/18362975 (accessed 14.07.16).

Wang, X., Kaplan, D.L., 2012. Hormone-responsive 3D multicellular culture model of human breast tissue. Biomaterials. 33 (12), 3411−3420. Available at: http://www.ncbi.nlm.nih.gov/pubmed/22309836 (accessed 16.06.16).

Williams, B.R., et al., 1978. Collagen fibril formation. Optimal in vitro conditions and preliminary kinetic results. J. Biol. Chem. 253 (18), 6578−6585. Available at: http://www.ncbi.nlm.nih.gov/pubmed/28330 (accessed 14.07.16).

Prostate organoids: Directed differentiation from embryonic stem cells

5

Esther L. Calderon-Gierszal and Gail S. Prins

Department of Urology, University of Illinois at Chicago, Chicago, IL, United States

CHAPTER OUTLINE

Organoids and Mini-Organs. DOI: http://dx.doi.org/10.1016/B978-0-12-812636-3.00005-5

INTRODUCTION

The prostate is a male accessory sex gland found in all mammals including monotremes (Davies, 1978; Price, 1963). In man, the prostate contributes 20%−30% of the volume of the seminal plasma (Duncan and Thompson, 2007), where it functions to neutralize the acidic vaginal environment with alkaline secretions, to liquefy the seminal coagulum through proteolytic activity of seminin and prostate specific antigen (PSA), and to provide energy to the sperm cells in the ejaculate (Cunha et al., 1987; Frick and Aulitzky, 1991; Lilja and Abrahamsson, 1988; Mann, 1963; Prins and Lindgren, 2015). In humans, the prostate gland is compact and conical in shape, and is located beneath the bladder where it surrounds the urethra (Fig. 5.1A) (Price, 1963; Timms, 2008).

In 1912, Lowsley provided the first detailed description of the human prostate anatomy by using the newborn prostate to define a lobular model. He divided the prostate into five lobes: an anterior, posterior, middle, and two lateral lobes, by reconstruction of histological serial sections (Lowsley, 1912). Due to its lack of anatomical accuracy for the adult human prostate, Lowsley's neonatal model was replaced by the current human prostate anatomical model established by McNeal in the early 1980s. Using a three-dimensional (3D) model, McNeal described four anatomical zones: central, transition, peripheral, and anterior zones, with the urethra acting as a reference point (McNeal, 1981) (Fig. 5.1A). The central zone

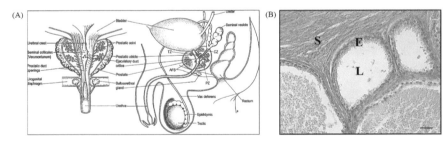

FIGURE 5.1

Human prostate anatomy and architecture. (A) Diagrams of frontal and sagittal sections of adult human prostate indicating its anatomical position and zones: central zone (CZ), peripheral zone (PZ), anterior fibromuscular stroma (AFS), and transition zone (TZ) (Reproduced from Timms, BG (2008) Prostate development: a historical perspective. Differentiation 76: 565−577. With permission). (B) Prostate architecture is shown histologically, and is composed of an epithelial (E), stromal (S), and luminal (L) compartment.

constitutes 25% of the prostate, and is located immediately below the bladder. The transition zone represents approximately 5% of the gland, and it surrounds the proximal urethra up to the verumontanum, where the urethra makes a 70-degree anterior turn. The peripheral zone accounts for 70% of the glandular prostate volume, and it encircles the distal prostatic urethra after the verumontanum. The anterior zone of the prostate is devoid of glandular structures, and contains only fibromuscular stroma. Ejaculatory ducts traverse the prostate between the central and peripheral region, emptying the contents of the vas deferens and seminal vesicle into the urethra at the site of the verumontanum. It is noteworthy that prostate cancer primarily arises from the epithelial cells in the peripheral zone, while benign prostate hyperplasia (BPH) arises from the epithelial cells in the transition zone (McNeal, 1981).

Histologically, the prostate is composed of an epithelial and a stromal compartment (Fig. 5.1B). The epithelial compartment contains three cell types: (1) cuboidal-to-columnar luminal secretory cells that express prostate-specific markers such as NKX3.1, HOXB13, and PSA, as well as cytokeratins 8/18 (CK8/18) and androgen receptor (AR) (Cunha et al., 1987; Prins et al., 1991); (2) nonsecretory basal cells that are located along the basement membrane and express p63 and CK14 (Kurita et al., 2004; Signoretti et al., 2000); and (3) rare neuroendocrine cells that express synaptophysin and chromogranin A (Ousset et al., 2012). The stromal compartment is a collagenous extracellular matrix that is composed of smooth muscle cells, fibroblasts, blood vessels, connective tissue, nerve terminals, and lymph vessels (Cunha et al., 1987). The epithelial − stromal ratio varies among species; for example, humans and primates have approximately equivalent cell numbers in the two compartments, while the adult rat prostate has a ratio of 5:1 (Cunha et al., 1987).

DEVELOPMENT AND STRUCTURE OF THE NATURAL ORGAN

Embryologically, the prostate gland arises from the endoderm-derived urogenital sinus (UGS) which contrasts with the other male accessory sex glands, the vas deferens and seminal vesicles, which are mesodermal in origin (Davies, 1978; Prins and Putz, 2008). Prostate development, support, and growth is dependent upon androgens, which are produced by the fetal testes beginning on the 6th−8th week of gestation in the form of testosterone (T) (Timms, 2008). Importantly, T is enzymatically converted into dihydrotestosterone (DHT) by steroid-5-alpha-reductase, alpha polypeptide 2 (SRD5A2) within prostate cells, and this is essential for proper prostate development (Cunha et al., 1987; Liao, 1968; Timms, 2008). In humans, the anlage of the prostate initiates by the 10th week of gestation, with epithelial buds emerging from the UGS epithelium, elongating and undergoing branching morphogenesis during the second trimester. By the 18th–20th gestational week, secretory cytodifferentiation of the epithelium begins. While human prostate development is complete at birth, the rodent prostate is rudimentary at birth, and undergoes morphogenesis and differentiation during the first 15 days of life (Cunha et al., 1987; Lowsley, 1912; Prins and Putz, 2008; Timms, 2008). Prostatic growth in rodents is an unremitting process that begins *in utero* and continues until sexual maturity (Cunha et al., 1987; Lowsley, 1912; Prins and Putz, 2008; Timms, 2008). In contrast, human prostate growth occurs in two discrete periods, prenatally and pubertally (Cunha et al., 1987).

Although there are species differences, many of the molecular and cellular details of human prostate development have been deduced from detailed studies of the rodent prostate gland. Though prostate development is a continuous process, five distinct stages can be distinguished in the rodent prostate: determination, budding, branching morphogenesis, differentiation, and maturation (Prins and Putz, 2008). While there is no physical evidence of primordium during prostatic determination, this stage is marked by the molecular commitment of certain UGS cells into a prostatic fate. This is followed by initiation that commences as the UGS epithelial cells begin to form buds that grow into the surrounding UGS mesenchyme. In mouse, initiation occurs between embryonic day 16.5 and 17.5 (Sugimura et al., 1986), while in rat it takes place at embryonic day 18.5 (Hayashi et al., 1991). Branching morphogenesis begins postnatally when the elongating UGS epithelial buds contact the prostate mesenchymal pads and form sequential branch points in a proximal-to-distal pattern, adding complexity to the anatomy of the gland (Timms et al., 1994). The branching patterns are lobe-specific and, by postnatal day (PND) 15–30, morphogenesis of the whole complex is complete (Hayashi et al., 1991). Concomitant with branching morphogenesis, epithelial lineage commitment from stem and progenitor cells commences, giving rise to secretory luminal epithelial and nonsecretory basal cells. This androgen-regulated process is initiated by paracrine actions from AR-positive UGS mesenchyme onto adjacent epithelial cells which, in a reciprocal manner, secrete factors such as sonic hedgehog (Shh) and bone morphogenic protein 7 (Bmp7) that drive periductal mesenchyme differentiation into smooth muscle (Cunha, 2008). Epithelial and stromal cytodifferentiation begins between PND 3 and 5 in the rat ventral lobe, and approximately 2 days later in the dorsolateral lobes (Prins and Birch, 1995).

The formation of a lumen in previously solid epithelial cords occurs in a proximal (PND 5) to distal (PND 12) fashion, and is concurrent with epithelial and basal cytodifferentiation. Early epithelial cytodifferentiation in the rat is marked by changing expression patterns of cytokeratins and AR (Hayward et al., 1996a, 1996b, Prins and Birch, 1995), whereas functional differentiation is marked by the synthesis of secretory products in luminal epithelial cells which begins between PND 10 and 20 (Prins and Birch, 1995). Prostatic mesenchymal differentiation occurs postnatally in the rodent, and is concomitant with epithelial differentiation (Prins and Birch, 1995; Prins and Putz, 2008). During the budding stage, mesenchymal cells agglomerate around the tips of UGS epithelial ducts, forming a characteristic pattern along the tip and length of the basement membrane which is associated with spatial-specific expression of growth factors (Timms, 2008). Between PND 3 and 5, condensed mesenchymal cells surrounding the ducts differentiate into a periductal layer of smooth muscle cells, while the interductal cells become mature fibroblasts (Hayward et al., 1996b; Prins and Birch, 1995). The last stage of prostate development is maturation, which is driven by a sharp increase in the levels of circulating androgens at puberty (days 25–40), allowing the prostate to grow to its final adult size and actively synthesize secretory proteins (Cunha et al., 1983; Prins and Putz, 2008).

Although androgens are essential for proper prostate development and growth, other hormones including estrogens and retinoids are also involved in its development and function (Prins and Korach, 2008; Prins and Putz, 2008), as discussed below.

ANDROGEN ACTION

Prostate development and growth in the human and rodent depend on androgens produced by the testes and, to a small degree, the adrenal glands. Testosterone (T) circulates in the blood primarily bound to albumin and sex-hormone-binding globulin (SHBG), with a small fraction present as free T (Feldman and Feldman, 2001). Testosterone enters the prostate cells by diffusion or facilitated uptake, and approximately 90% is rapidly converted to DHT within the prostate by the enzyme SRD5A2 (Liao, 1968; Prins and Putz, 2008). Although T and DHT can both bind and activate AR, DHT has a five-fold higher affinity for the receptor (Feldman and Feldman, 2001). This differential affinity permits amplification of androgen action within the prostate specifically, without requiring increased circulating androgen levels to other organ sites.

Androgen action in the prostate is mediated by classical ligand-induced signaling through its intracellular AR, a nuclear transcription factor member of the steroid − thyroid − retinoid nuclear receptor superfamily (Feldman and Feldman, 2001). Human AR is localized to the q11−q12 region of the X chromosome, and consists of 8 exons that produce a 919 amino acid protein with a molecular weight of 110 kDa (Lonergan and Tindall, 2011). Unliganded AR is found in the cytoplasm bound to heat-shock proteins (HSP), cytoskeletal proteins, and chaperones that prevent the conformational change needed for nuclear translocation and transcriptional activation of AR. Upon ligand binding, the AR undergoes a conformational change, and HSP and other factors dissociate, permitting nuclear localization, dimerization, and binding to androgen response elements (AREs) in the promoter and enhancer regions of target genes, thus activating gene transcription (Feldman and Feldman, 2001; Prins and Lindgren, 2015).

Evidence of the necessity for AR for prostate development was first apparent from the lack of prostate formation in mice and humans with dysfunctional AR (Bardin et al., 1973). Subsequent studies determined that androgen effects on proliferation and differentiation in the developing prostate epithelium are initially elicited by paracrine actions of AR-positive UGM (Cunha et al., 1983). The AR is rapidly induced in the luminal epithelial cells, and is considered an early marker of differentiation. While not required for epithelial proliferation in vivo, epithelial AR is necessary for the expression of secretory genes and their protein products in the murine (Donjacour and Cunha, 1993) and rat models (Prins and Birch, 1995). The importance of AR in the prostate gland was further shown by chemical and surgical castration studies. Castration prior to budding was shown to halt prostate development, while castration at later developmental stages slows but does not stop development (Cunha, 1973). Furthermore, rodent foetal prostate explant cultures retrieved before testicular T was produced were unable to form buds, while cultures collected after testosterone was synthesized produced buds (Aboseif et al., 1997; Lasnitzki and Mizuno, 1977). Together, these results indicate that androgens are necessary for prostate determination and initial budding, but that continued growth, albeit at a reduced rate, can continue in the absence of constant androgenic action.

ESTROGEN ACTION

Although the physiological role of estrogens in the human prostate remains unresolved, high maternal levels of this steroid during the third trimester of pregnancy drive prostatic epithelial squamous metaplasia (SQM), confirming a functional activity of estrogens in this structure during development (Zondek et al., 1986). With aging, elevated estrogens have been correlated with benign prostatic hyperplasia (BPH) and prostatic carcinoma, in human and rodent models (Price, 1963; Prins et al., 2006; Prins and Korach, 2008). Evidence from epidemiological studies has shown a two-fold increase in the risk of developing prostate cancer in African − American men, which correlates with higher maternal levels of estrogens in this population (Henderson et al., 1988; Platz and Giovannucci, 2004). Furthermore, maternal exposure to diethylstilbesterol (DES), a potent estrogen mimic used between the 1940s and 1970s, has been shown to produce high levels of SQM in prostates of newborn males. Although SQM resolved upon DES withdrawal, disorganization of ductal architecture persisted (Yonemura et al., 1995). Studies in the rodent model further support a developmental role of physiological estrogen levels on stromal cell programming (Jarred et al., 2002).

Estrogen is produced within the prostate by the conversion of T into 17β-estradiol by the enzyme aromatase, which is present in stromal cells (Matzkin and Soloway, 1992). Its action, in both human and rodent prostates, is mediated by stromal estrogen receptor α (ERα), epithelial estrogen receptor β (ERβ) and ERα which, like AR, are members of the steroid receptor superfamily of nuclear transcription factors (Prins, 1992; Prins et al., 2001; Prins and Korach, 2008). During development, human fetal prostates express nuclear ERβ in epithelial and basal cells, while ERα is expressed postnatally in the nucleus of periacinar stromal cells (Adams et al., 2002). In rodents, ERα is localized to the mesenchymal cells, and expression declines as morphogenesis takes place (Prins and Birch, 1997). In contrast, ERβ expression rises in the luminal epithelial cells as they differentiate with maximal ERβ levels in the adult rodent prostate (Prins et al., 1998). The ERα and ERβ are encoded by two distinct genes with 9 exons, are composed of 595 and 530 amino acids, respectively, and have molecular weights of 66 and 60−63 kDa respectively (Kuiper et al., 1996; Mosselman et al., 1996; Walter et al., 1985). While there is considerable structural similarity between ERα and ERβ, there are two major differences of note: (1) the amino terminal domain (NTD) of ERβ is approximately 90 nucleotides shorter than that in ERα, which accounts for the 24% homology between their NTDs; and (2) the AF-2 domain in ERβ requires ligand to activate the AF-1 domain, whereas the AF-1 domain in ERα is independent of AF-2 activation (Aranda and Pascual, 2001; Mosselman et al., 1996; Prins and Korach, 2008). Of further note, there is differential affinity for various endogenous and exogenous ligands between these two receptors which accounts for differential estrogenic activities within ER+ cells.

Like AR, unliganded ER is sequestered in the nucleus by a multiprotein inhibitory complex (Le Romancer et al., 2011, Prins and Korach, 2008). Upon ligand binding, classical ER signaling begins by shedding the inhibitory complex, thus changing receptor conformation which permits nuclear localization, homodimerization, and binding to EREs in the promoter regions of target genes, hence activating gene transcription (Aranda and Pascual, 2001; Bjornstrom and Sjoberg, 2005; Le Romancer et al., 2011). There is also evidence for ligand-independent signaling of nuclear ERs via intracellular second messengers, as well as ligand-activated, membrane initiated signaling that can activate many downstream signaling pathways, including Ras/raf/MEK and Akt (Bjornstrom and Sjoberg, 2005; Poulard et al., 2012; Prins et al., 2014; Revankar et al., 2005).

The developing rodent prostate gland expresses ERα in a small proportion of stromal cells, which further declines following morphogenesis and throughout puberty (Prins and Birch, 1997). In humans, however, ERα expression remains constant during foetal development (Shapiro et al., 2005). Work in multiple species suggests that ERα plays a role in the etiology of chronic prostatitis, BPH, prostate cancer, and progression (Prins et al., 2001; Risbridger et al., 2001). On the other hand, epithelial ERβ expression in the rodent is low at birth, increasing as epithelial cytodifferentiation occurs, and reaching maximal expression during puberty. In the human prostate, ERβ expression is observed as early as the 7th week of gestation, and is maintained postnatally for several months before it starts to decline to lower levels in the adult prostate (Adams et al., 2002; Shapiro et al., 2005). Although its role has not been fully established, it has been suggested that ERβ mediates anti-proliferative, anti-inflammatory, and anti-carcinogenic effects

(Ellem and Risbridger, 2009; Hussain et al., 2012). Other estrogen effects include stimulation of prolactin (PRL) release from the pituitary gland, which has been shown to contribute to estrogenic effects in the prostate, as well as inhibition of luteinizing hormone (LH) secretion, and androgen steroidogenesis (i.e., chemical castration) by triggering the negative feedback on the hypothalamic − testicular axis (Huggins and Hodges, 2002; Lee et al., 1981). The latter action was considered the primary action of DES treatment for prostate cancer, a therapy introduced by Charles Huggins in 1950.

RETINOID ACTION

Retinoic acids (RAs) are small lipophilic molecules derived from vitamin A (retinol) that play important roles in development, differentiation, proliferation, and homeostasis of different tissues (Chambon, 1996; Rhinn and Dolle, 2012). The two most common naturally occurring isomers of RA in the prostate are all-trans (ATRA) and 9-cis RA, and they exert their effects by interacting with their receptors (Chambon, 1996; Lohnes et al., 1992). Retinoids have two families of receptors encoded by separate genes, each composed of three isotypes: retinoid acid receptor (RAR) α, β, and γ, and retinoid X receptor (RXR) α, β, and γ. Both families belong to the steroid − thyroid receptor superfamily of nuclear transcription factors, and are differentially expressed during tissue morphogenesis (Chambon, 1996). Both receptor families contain the conserved structural domains present in nuclear receptors: NTD, DBD, hinge region, LBD, and a carboxy-terminal domain (Chambon, 1996; Lohnes et al., 1992). The RAR family of receptors can be activated by almost all RAs including ATRA and 9-cis RA, whereas the RXR family are activated exclusively by 9-cis RA (Chambon, 1996). Following ligand binding, receptors can form homo- or heterodimers on retinoic acid response elements (RAREs) on target gene promoters, thus activating gene transcription (Lohnes et al., 1992). Retinoic acid receptors are present in the developing prostate of humans (Richter et al., 2002), mice (Dolle et al., 1990), and rats (Prins et al., 2002). More specifically, the neonatal rat prostate expresses RARβ in basal epithelial cells, RARγ in periductal stromal cells, and increasing levels of RARα in luminal and smooth muscle cells as they differentiate (Prins et al., 2002).

Some of the first observations that retinoids were important for rat prostate development and homeostasis showed that vitamin A deficiency before prostate budding prevented prostate maturation (Wilson and Warkany, 1948), while deficiency during adulthood caused keratinization of the epithelium (Wolbach and Howe, 1925). Later, studies in the mouse anterior prostate showed that concomitant administration of RA and estrogen inhibited estrogen-induced SQM (Mariotti et al., 1987), which was further confirmed by null RARγ mice studies which exhibited prostatic SQM (Lohnes et al., 1993). Importantly, administration of

ATRA in the culture media of fetal male mice UGS organ cultures showed a stimulatory effect on prostatic bud formation, and increased expression of genes involved in budding including Shh and Bmp4 (Vezina et al., 2008). Interestingly, high or low levels of RA have been shown to inhibit prostate ductal morphogenesis in neonatal mice, and inhibit ductal growth and branching in neonatal rat explants, respectively (Aboseif et al., 1997; Seo et al., 1997). Together, research throughout the years has shown that retinoids at the right doses play an important role in the developing and adult prostate gland.

In addition to hormones, several transcription factors and morphoregulatory genes are also necessary for prostate formation and branching morphogenesis. Importantly, some have been shown to be steroid targets and effectors of steroid-driven prostate morphogenesis. These include the transcription factor Nkx3.1 and the secreted morphogens: Wnts, Fgfs, Bmps, and Egf.

NKX3.1

Nkx3.1 is an androgen regulated (Pu et al., 2007) nuclear transcription factor in the NK homeobox gene family which is expressed in the prostate and bulbourethral gland epithelium (Bieberich et al., 1996). In the mouse, Nkx3.1 was observed at UGS bud sites prior to their emergence in the surrounding mesenchyme, and its epithelial expression continued during budding and branching morphogenesis, suggesting a role in prostate determination (Bieberich et al., 1996). In the rat prostate lobes, a transient peak in Nkx3.1 expression is concomitant with epithelial cytodifferentiation (Prins et al., 2006). Furthermore, its expression presents a gradient pattern with the highest expression at the distal regions (Bieberich et al., 1996). In the absence of Nkx3.1, as seen in null Nkx3.1 mice, the prostate gland exhibits perturbation of normal branching morphogenesis, functional differentiation, and prostatic intraepithelial neoplasia (PIN) during adulthood (Bhatia-Gaur et al., 1999; Kim et al., 2002). Together, the studies suggest a role in branching and differentiation. In human prostate epithelium, loss of NKX3.1 is linked to prostate cancer (Bowen et al., 2000).

FIBROBLAST GROWTH FACTOR-10

Fibroblast growth factor-10 (Fgf10), an androgen-regulated, secreted paracrine factor, exerts its actions on target cells through tyrosine kinase Fgf receptors (FgfR) (Pu et al., 2007; Uematsu, Kan et al., 2000). Developmental studies in the rat ventral lobe and in null Fgf10 mutant mice have unveiled its role in prostate gland initiation, bud outgrowth, and branching morphogenesis (Thomson and Cunha, 1999). Its expression pattern in mesenchymal cells is restricted to the distal ends of the ducts, where it stimulates branching through the proliferation of epithelial cells that express FgfR. Simultaneously, Fgf10 causes the mesenchyme to condense around the distal ends of the elongating ducts (Huang et al., 2005). Renal graft rescue studies of embryonic Fgf10 null mice prostatic rudiments showed insignificant growth and differentiation, suggesting the essential role of Fgf10 on prostate initiation. Importantly, combined exposure to Fgf10 plus testosterone is required to restore prostatic growth in Fgf10 null mice, indicating that Fgf10 is essential, but not sufficient, for bud formation (Donjacour et al., 2003).

Epithelial cells in the distal tips of elongating ducts of the mouse and rat prostate glands express one of the FgfR2 splice variants, FgfR2iiib, which can bind Fgf10 and Fgf7 specifically (Finch et al., 1995). This expression pattern is retained throughout branching morphogenesis, thus stimulating epithelial cell proliferation at the distal tips and driving duct elongation (Huang et al., 2005). Studies utilizing a Mek1/2 inhibitor blocked Fgf10-stimulated branching, indicating that Fgf10-FgfR2iiib actions in the developing prostate are mediated via the ras/raf/Mek/Erk1/2 signaling pathway (Huang et al., 2005). Regulation of Fgf10-induced proliferation has been shown to be controlled by Sprouty proteins, epidermal growth factors (Egfs), and other Fgfs.

BONE MORPHOGENETIC PROTEINS

Bone morphogenetic proteins 4 and 7 (Bmp4 and Bmp7, respectively), members of the Tgfβ gene superfamily, are expressed in the rodent prostate and function by inhibiting prostate growth during development, as shown by murine mutant models in which partial or complete blockade of Bmp4 or Bmp7 caused an increase in branching (Grishina et al., 2005; Lamm et al., 2001; Prins and Putz, 2008). Bmp4 is expressed in the mouse UGM before and during bud initiation, with expression confined to the periductal mesenchyme immediately surrounding the elongating and branching ducts (Lamm et al., 2001; Prins et al., 2006). Bmp4 levels rapidly decline postnatally, thus allowing ductal outgrowth. Bmp7 is similarly expressed in the mouse UGM prior to budding, however, it postnatally localizes to the epithelial cells (Grishina et al., 2005). In the rat prostate, Bmp7 expression is localized to epithelial cells in the distal tips of the gland, rapidly increasing between PND 1 and PND 5 (Huang et al., 2005). Both Bmps signal by binding to their transmembrane Type II receptors, which recruit and phosphorylate Type I receptors, thus activating intracellular pathways involving Smads (Prins and Putz, 2008). Regulation of Bmps is modulated by the endogenous inhibitor, Noggin, which blocks their interaction with receptors by binding to Bmp ligands (Prins and Putz, 2008). In addition, androgens repress Bmp4, which in turn permits bud outgrowth and branching (Pu et al., 2007), while estrogens increase their expression and restrain branching, (Prins et al., 2006) implicating cooperative hormonal regulation of development.

WNTS

The Wnt family of genes encodes secreted glycoproteins that exhibit pleotropic roles ranging from cell proliferation, cell fate, differentiation, migration, and carcinogenesis (Logan and Nusse, 2004). All 19 mammalian Wnt proteins identified to date bind to transmembrane receptors of the Frizzled (Fz) family (Cadigan and Nusse, 1997; Huang et al., 2009). Vertebrate Wnts have been divided into canonical and noncanonical categories, depending on the downstream signaling pathway they activate (Huang et al., 2009). Wnts from the canonical pathway bind to the Fz receptor and low density lipoprotein receptor-related protein 5/6 (LRP5/6) co-receptors, causing phosphorylation of Dishevelled (Dsh) (Bennett et al., 2002; Laudes, 2011; Logan and Nusse, 2004). This inhibits the kinase activity of the Axin/Adenomatus Polyposis Coli (APC)/glycogen synthase kinase-3β (GSK-3β) complex that phosphorylates β-catenin, targeting their proteosomic degradation. Consequently, cytosolic β-catenin accumulates and translocates to the nucleus, where it binds to T cell factor (Tcf)/lymphoid-enhancing factor (Lef) to initiate transcription of Wnt target genes (Bennett et al., 2002; Logan and Nusse, 2004; Ross et al., 2000). Noncanonical Wnts (Brennan and Brown, 2004) bind to the Fz receptor independent from the LRP5/6 co-receptor. The signal is then transduced to Dsh causing its activation, which initiates two downstream pathways: Ca^{++}/Protein kinase C (PKC), and Ras homolog gene family, member A (RhoA)/c-Jun N-terminal kinases (JNK) (Brennan and Brown, 2004; Komiya and Habas, 2008; Laudes, 2011). Importantly, the Wnt signaling pathway is regulated by secreted inhibitors, including secreted Frizzled-related proteins (Sfrp), Wnt inhibitory factors (Wif), and Dickkopf (Dkk) proteins which block the canonical Wnt signaling (Brennan and Brown, 2004; Huang et al., 2009), and by the Wnt activators R-spondins (RSPOs) and Norrin (Cruciat and Niehrs, 2013; Jin and Yoon, 2012).

The canonical Wnts 2, 2b, and 7b, as well as the noncanonical Wnts 4, 5a, and 11, are expressed in the ventral prostate of neonatal rats. Except Wnt7b, all are highly expressed at birth, with declining levels during and after morphogenesis. In contrast, high Wnt7b levels are observed in prostate epithelium upon functional cytodifferentiation (Prins and Putz, 2008). Interestingly, noncanonical Wnt signaling, more specifically Wnt5a, has been reported to inhibit epithelial cell proliferation, ductal growth, and branching morphogenesis in in vivo and ex vivo experiments (Huang et al., 2009). On the other hand, canonical Wnt10b has been shown to be expressed at embryonic day 17 and PND 0 in the bud tips of the ventral, dorsolateral and anterior murine prostatic lobes, implicating it as an early specific prostatic bud marker (Abler et al., 2011; Keil et al., 2012; Mehta et al., 2011). Importantly, human prostate stem-like cells express high levels of WNT10B relative to daughter progenitor cells and differentiated epithelial cells suggesting an important role in stem cell function (Hu et al., 2017).

EPIDERMAL GROWTH FACTOR

Epidermal growth factor (Egf), a secreted peptide, is produced by the luminal epithelial cells in the prostate, and is found at the highest concentration in human prostatic secretions compared to the rest of the body (Kim et al., 1999). Epidermal growth factor exerts its effects by binding to its tyrosine kinase receptor, epidermal growth factor receptor (EgfR). Upon binding, EgfR can homo- or heterodimerize with erbB2 receptors, causing autophosphorylation of its tyrosine residues that in turn activate the phosphatidylinositol 3'-kinase (PI$_3$K), mitogen activated protein kinase (MAPK), or phospholipase C-γ (PLC-γ) signaling cascades (Carpenter and Cohen, 1990; Mimeault et al., 2003). In the developing murine prostate gland, Egf has been shown to mediate its actions through the PLC-γ signaling pathway (Kim et al., 1999). Furthermore, rat UGS explants treated with exogenous Egf showed stimulation of prostate bud formation in the absence of androgens, thus positively regulating prostatic budding (Saito and Mizuno, 1997).

THE NEED FOR AN EMBRYONIC PROSTATE ORGANOID

The importance of the embryonic organoid model detailed herein is multiple, as it is the first prostate in vitro model that: (1) recapitulates human prostate development, as observed in the womb; (2) is derived from normal human embryonic stem cells; (3) replicates human prostate architecture by the presence of an epithelial and stromal compartment; and (4) is functionally differentiated by the expression of PSA. This organoid in a dish can be used to advance and refine our understanding of prostate development, and toxicology, and has direct potential to address causes of prostate disease, disease therapy, and prevention. The step-wise differentiation that gives rise to this model as stem cells differentiate into functional prostate cells can allow the identification of the discrete windows and cell type/lineages from which the prostate develops, and potentially, cancer initiates. Moreover, this model can be used to elucidate the molecular mechanisms and/or epigenetic signatures that change during prostate cancer progression. Finally, this system can be utilized to rapidly screen the efficacy of pharmaceutical agents on human prostatic endpoints.

DESIGN CONSIDERATIONS

To recapitulate prostate development as it occurs *in utero*, activin A was used to induce definitive endoderm differentiation (D'Amour et al., 2005; McCracken et al., 2014; McCracken et al., 2011; Spence et al., 2011), the embryonic origin from which the prostate epithelium arises. Activin A is also known to drive mesoderm differentiation, which can be identified by Brachyury expression. Thus, activin A will prime the cells for later differentiation towards prostate epithelium (endoderm) and stroma (mesoderm).

Studies using embryonic stem cells to derive different tissues, e.g., liver, pancreas, and hindgut, have shown that the precise timing of activation and repression of specific WNTs and FGFs are crucial for tissue specification and patterning (Murry and Keller, 2008). Hence, WNT10B, a secreted canonical WNT, and FGF10 were selected based on relevant scientific evidence (Prins and Putz, 2008). Studies in the mouse have shown that Wnt10b is expressed and secreted by a discrete group of urogenital sinus epithelial cells, that later give rise to prostate buds (Keil et al., 2012; Mehta et al., 2011) and human prostate stem-like cells selectively express high levels of WNT10B (Hu et al., 2017). Fgf10 is expressed and secreted by urogenital mesenchymal cells, and activates its receptor, FGFR2iiic on adjacent epithelial cells. Secretion of this paracrine factor is required for prostatic epithelial budding, ductal elongation, and branching (Huang et al., 2005; Thomson and Cunha, 1999). In our model, we found that the addition of WNT10B and FGF10 for four days was the necessary window to promote prostatic determination (Calderon-Gierszal and Prins, 2015). Shorter culture of definitive endoderm cells in the presence of these morphogens was insufficient to drive a prostatic fate, whereas longer culture reduced organoid formation efficiency. Furthermore, substitution of canonical WNT10B with canonical WNT3A was insufficient to drive prostatic structures, suggesting the essential and specific role of WNT10B in prostate determination.

Normal prostate development, maintenance, and maturation also requires several other factors. Hence, prostate organoid medium was design to provide the optimal combination of these factors, and the adequate ratio of epithelial and stromal medium to support both cell types. It is known that several Wnts are expressed in a spatio-temporal manner in the prostate, thus R-Spondin1, a Wnt agonist, was used to enhance endogenous Wnt signaling (Huang et al., 2009; Jin and Yoon, 2012; Prins and Putz, 2008). Branching morphogenesis is inhibited by BMPs, thus addition of noggin to the medium was necessary to antagonize BMP action (Prins et al., 2006). Epidermal growth factor was also added to the medium, since it has been shown to regulate and promote mesenchymal and epithelial cell proliferation (Kim et al., 1999). ATRA and testosterone were added to drive cytodifferentiation (Prins et al., 2002) and prostate development, respectively. Testosterone was used rather than DHT, since it can be reduced to DHT or aromatized to estradiol-17β which has been also shown to be necessary for prostate development (McPherson et al., 2001). We determined that the combination of these factors was essential to promote prostate organoid growth and maturation as observed in the human male (Figs. 5.2—5.3).

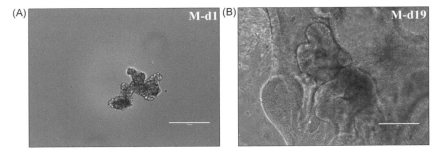

FIGURE 5.2

Prostate organoid development. (A) Phase-contrast images of a representative Matrigel-day 1 (M-d1) cultured organoid; and (B) M-d19 show the entire organoid as it grew in size and complexity over time. Scale bar represents 200 μm.

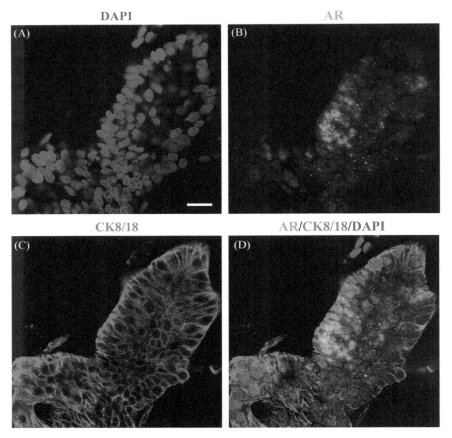

FIGURE 5.3

Confirmation of prostatic nature and cytodifferentiation of prostate organoids. (A) Immunofluorescent analysis by confocal microscopy of representative M-d28 organoid stained with DAPI (blue); (B) luminal cell cytodifferentiation markers AR (green); (C) CK8/18 (red); and (D) merged image reveals cytodifferentiation of organoid. Scale bar represents 20 μm (adapted from Calderon-Gierszal EL, Prins GS (2015).

REMAINING CHALLENGES

To increase the efficiency of prostatic organoid formation in vitro, the following modifications are suggested: (1) testing of different concentrations of morphogens, factors, and testosterone in the prostate organoid medium to identify the minimum necessary factors for growth and support of prostatic organoids; (2) testing of additional secreted morphogens known to be important for prostate development and growth, such as SHH or activation of Notch signaling (Prins and Lindgren, 2015); (3) reduction of the ATRA concentration in a step-wise, time-dependent manner to better mimic physiological levels (Prins and Lindgren, 2015); (4) testing for the lowest concentration of testosterone necessary for prostate support; and (5) testing the utilization of DHT instead of testosterone.

DETAILED INSTRUCTIONS

MATERIALS

Reagents

Cells

- H1 (WA01), or H9 (H9inGFPhES) hESCs (WiCell Research Institute, Madison, WI)

Growth media and supplements

- mTeSR1 medium (StemCell Technologies, cat # 05850)
- DMEM/F12 (Gibco, cat # 11965)
- hES-qualified Matrigel (BD Biosciences, cat # 354277)
- RPMI 1640 medium (Gibco, cat # 11875)
- Defined fetal bovine serum (dFBS; Hyclone, cat # SH30070.01)
- L-glutamine (100X; Invitrogen, cat # 25030-081)
- 100 U/mL penicillin—100 µL/mL streptomycin (Invitrogen, cat # 15140-122)
- BD Matrigel basement membrane matrix growth factor reduced, phenol red-free (BD Biosciences, cat # 356231): order with protein concentration >8 mg/mL
- Prostate epithelial cell growth medium (PrEGM; Lonza, cat # CC-3166)
- Stromal cell basal medium (SCBM; Lonza, cat # CC-3205)
- B27 supplement (50X; Invitrogen, cat # 17504044)
- HEPES buffer (Gibco, cat # 15630)

Enzymes, growth factors, and hormones

- Dispase (StemCell Technologies, cat # 07923)
- Activin A (R&D Systems, cat # 338-AC-050/CF)
- FGF10 (R&D Systems, cat # 345-FG-025/CF)

- WNT10B (R&D Systems, cat # 7196-WN-010/CF)
- Noggin (R&D Systems, cat # 6057-NG-100/CF)
- R-Spondin1 (R&D Systems, cat # 4645-RS-025/CF)
- Epidermal growth factor (EGF; R&D Systems, cat # 236-EG-200)
- All-trans retinoic acid (ATRA) (kindly provided by Dr. Kevin White, University of Chicago. Chicago, IL)
- Testosterone (Sigma-Aldrich Corp., cat # T1500)

Immunostaining reagents

- Goat serum (Vector Laboratories, cat # S-1000)
- Donkey serum (Jackson ImmunoResearch Laboratories Inc., cat # 017-000-001)
- Mouse anti-FOXA2 (Novus Biologicals, cat # H00003170-M12)
- Rabbit anti-Brachyury (Santa Cruz Biotechnology Inc., cat # sc-20109)
- Rabbit anti-AR (Prins et al., 1991)
- Rabbit anti-Vimentin (Epitomics, cat # 2701-1)
- Rabbit anti-TMPRSS2 (Epitomics, cat # 2770-1)
- Guinea pig anti-CK8/18 (ARP American Research Products Inc., cat # 03-GP11)
- Mouse anti-Laminin (LifeSpan BioSciences Inc., cat # LS-C88600)
- Mouse anti-NKX3.1 (Novus Biologicals, cat # NBP1-51609)
- Goat anti-PSA (Santa Cruz Biotechnology Inc., cat # sc-7638)
- Normal rabbit IgG (Kindly provided by Dr. Geoffrey Greene, University of Chicago. Chicago, IL)
- Normal guinea pig IgG (Santa Cruz Biotechnology Inc., cat # sc-2711)
- Normal mouse IgG (Zymed Laboratories Inc., cat # 02-6502)
- Normal goat IgG (Jackson ImmunoResearch Laboratories, cat# 005-000-003)
- Goat anti-rabbit (Invitrogen, cat # A-11034, A-11036)
- Goat anti-guinea pig (Invitrogen, cat # A-11075)
- Goat anti-mouse (Invitrogen, cat # A-11029, A-11031)
- Donkey anti-goat (Invitrogen, cat # A-11057)
- Vectashield mounting medium with DAPI (Vector Laboratories Inc, cat # H-1200)

Essential equipment

- Pulled glass pipettes
- Nunclon delta surface tissue culture dish (4 wells; Nunc, cat # 176740)
    - Critical point: the use of Nunclon dishes is critical, since the coating in the dishes allows the formation of a Matrigel bead necessary for the 3D expansion of the organoids.
- Plastic cover slips (Nunc, cat # 174969)
    - Critical point: hESCs will only attach, grow, and maintain their undifferentiated state by growing on plastic cover slips. The use of plastic cover slips is also necessary for subsequent immunostaining analysis.

Reagent preparation

Matrigel aliquoting and Matrigel-coated plate preparation for hESC

- Thaw hES-qualified Matrigel on ice or at 4° overnight, aliquot Matrigel into chilled microcentrifuge tubes, and store as directed by the manufacturer.
- Coat 6- or 24-well plates per manufacturer's instructions. In brief, thaw Matrigel aliquot on ice, and mix with cold DMEM/F12 medium (final dilution is lot-dependent, thus it is determined by the manufacturer). Medium containing Matrigel must cover the entire surface of the well. Coat plates at room temperature for at least 1 hour before seeding hESC. Plates can be stored for a week at 4°C.
  - Critical point: Matrigel will solidify at room temperature, so it is important to always keep it cold and make sure to add Matrigel to cold medium before coating the plates.

Growth factor and hormone reconstitution

- Reconstitute all growth factors (i.e., activin A, WNT10B, FGF10, R-Spondin1, Noggin, and EGF) as directed per vendor or in 1X PBS
- Reconstitute ATRA in DMSO
- Reconstitute testosterone in 100% ethanol

Matrigel preparation for prostate organoids

- Thaw the bottle of Matrigel basement membrane matrix growth factor reduced, phenol red-free on ice or at 4°C overnight. Once thawed, aliquot Matrigel into prechilled microcentrifuge tubes. To avoid solidification of Matrigel, keep stock and tubes on ice throughout the aliquoting process. For proper storage, follow manufacturer's instructions.
- Thaw Matrigel aliquots on ice or at 4°C overnight. Once thawed, add B27 supplement (final concentration 1X), Noggin (final concentration 100 ng/mL), and EGF (final concentration 100 ng/mL) keeping the tube on ice at all times to avoid solidification. Mix well by carefully pipetting to avoid bubbles. Prostate organoid Matrigel is prepared fresh.

Media preparation

- *Day 1 endoderm differentiation medium*: Mix RPMI 1640 medium, activin A (final concentration 100 ng/mL), L-glutamine (final concentration 2 mM), and 100 U/mL penicillin-100 μL/mL streptomycin. Make fresh daily.
- *Day 2 endoderm differentiation medium*: Mix RPMI 1640 medium, activin A (final concentration 100 ng/mL), 0.2% dFBS (vol/vol), L-glutamine (final concentration 2 mM), and 100 U/mL penicillin-100 μL/mL streptomycin. Make fresh daily.
- *Day 3 endoderm differentiation medium*: Mix RPMI 1640 medium, activin A (final concentration 100 ng/mL), 2% dFBS (vol/vol), L-glutamine (final

concentration 2 mM), and 100 U/mL penicillin-100 μL/mL streptomycin. Make fresh daily.

- *Prostatic fate determination medium*: Mix RPMI 1640 medium, FGF10 (final concentration 500 ng/mL), WNT10B (final concentration 500 ng/mL), 2% dFBS (vol/vol), L-glutamine (final concentration 2 mM), and 100 U/mL penicillin-100 μL/mL streptomycin. Freshly prepared medium is replaced daily for 4 consecutive days.
- *Prostate organoid medium*: Combine 1:2 PrEGM and SCBM. Add L-glutamine (final concentration 2 mM) and 100 U/mL penicillin-100 μL/mL streptomycin, HEPES (final concentration 15 mM), R-Spondin1 (final concentration 500 ng/mL), Noggin (final concentration 100 ng/mL), EGF (final concentration 100 ng/mL), B27 supplement (final concentration 1X), ATRA (final concentration 10 nM), and testosterone (final concentration 1.7 μM). Medium is replaced with freshly prepared medium every 4 days for approximately 30 days (Fig. 5.2A, B).

PROCEDURE

PASSAGING HESC

1. Coat a 24-well plate with Matrigel, as described in the Reagent Preparation section.
2. Passage cells from a 6-well plate that are 85%—90% confluent. If the culture shows less than 20% spontaneous differentiation, these cells/colonies should be manually removed with pulled glass pipettes. Aspirate spent medium and gently wash wells with DMEM/F12.
   a. Critical point: To obtain optimal results in the following steps, the starting density of cells is critical. If more than 20% of cells appear differentiated, the cultures should be terminated.
3. Incubate cells with 1 mg/mL dispase for 5—7 minutes and gently wash cells three times with DMEM/F12.
4. To dislodge colonies and break them into smaller pieces, expel mTeSR1 medium (3 mL per well) while scrapping cells with a serological glass pipette.
   a. Critical point: To avoid spontaneous differentiation, hESC need to be passaged as aggregates and not as single cells.
5. Transfer detached aggregates into 24-well Matrigel-coated plates at a 1:6 ratio. That is, each well from the 6-well plate will be passaged into six wells of a 24-well plate. Each well of the 24-well dish will receive 0.5 mL of medium and hESC.
   a. Critical point: Plastic cover slips can be placed in 24-well plates and coated with Matrigel, as described above.
6. Incubate cells at 37°C, with 5% CO_2 and 95% humidity overnight.

GROWTH OF HESC PRIOR TO DIFFERENTIATION

7. The next day, replenish spent medium with fresh mTeSR1 medium (0.5 mL per well). It is normal to observe extensive floating debris.

    a. Critical point: It is important to obtain uniform distribution of hESC to achieve successful 85%–90% confluent wells.

8. Feed cells and observe colony density daily. Optimal confluency should be reached within 2–4 days.

    a. Critical point: If colonies are too dense or sparse, terminate the cells and start over, as the directed differentiation will be inefficient.

DEFINITIVE ENDODERM AND MESODERM DIFFERENTIATION

9. Once the cells have reached 85%–90% confluence, replenish the spent medium with day 1 endoderm differentiation medium. Monitor changes in cell morphology daily.

10. After 24 hours, replenish the spent medium with day 2 endoderm differentiation medium.

11. After 24 hours, replenish the spent medium with day 3 endoderm differentiation medium. If hESC were seeded in plastic cover slips, carefully remove the cover slips and perform immunostaining for FOXA2 and Brachyury, to confirm definitive endoderm and mesoderm differentiation as described in the Verifying section below.

    a. Critical point: Differentiated cells should be 100% confluent to allow proper prostatic organoid formation.

DIRECTED DIFFERENTIATION INTO PROSTATIC FATE DETERMINATION AND ORGANOID DEVELOPMENT

12. After 24 hours, replace definitive endoderm medium with 0.5 mL of prostatic fate determination medium. Replenish medium every 24 hours for 96 hours.

    a. Critical point: Three-dimensional structures should be observed after ~48 hours in definitive endoderm medium.

13. After carefully detaching 3D structures from the bottom of the wells using a pulled glass pipette, collect them along with any free floating 3D structures using a 200 μL barrier pipette tip. Pool ~20–50 structures into a 1.5 mL microcentrifuge tube, and gently spin at $100 \times g$ for 3 minutes.

14. Transfer 25 μL prostatic fate determination medium + 3D structures into new tubes using a 100 μL barrier pipette tip, and mix with 50 μL cold Matrigel for prostate organoids by gently pipetting up and down to avoid bubbles. Follow Matrigel instructions described in the Reagent Preparation section.

     a. Critical point: Work quickly to avoid Matrigel solidification. The total volume comprising Matrigel + medium containing 3D structures should be 75 μL.

15. Pipette Matrigel-3D structure suspension into the center of one well of a 4-well Nunclon dish.

16. Incubate for 20 minutes at 37°C, 5% CO_2, and 95% humidity, to allow solidification. Gently pipette 0.5 mL prostate organoid medium over the resultant beads so they are completely covered.

17. Freshly prepared media is changed every 4 days. Organoids are grown for ~28−30 days.

CRITICAL POINTS TO NOTE

Although most critical points have been addressed within each step in the materials and procedure sections, below are additional and equivalently important points to note for a successful organoid culture:

1. Only R&D carrier free growth factors were used; growth factors from other vendors have not been tested.

2. Always reconstitute growth factors as instructed by the manufacturer.

3. Growth factors and Matrigel aliquots cannot be reused after thawing.

4. Addition of growth factors needs to be timed precisely to produce efficient cultures and obtain prostate organoids.

VERIFYING

IMMUNOSTAINING TO CONFIRM DEFINITIVE ENDODERM AND MESODERM DIFFERENTIATION

1. Aspirate definitive endoderm medium after the third day of activin A treatment.

2. Wash cells grown on cover slips once with 0.5 mL of 1X PBS.

3. Fix cells with 4% paraformaldehyde for 15 minutes at room temperature (in a fume hood).

4. Wash cells 3 times with 1X PBS, for 5 minutes each wash.

5. Block cells with blocking buffer (1X PBS + 0.5 mL normal serum from the same species as the secondary antibody + 0.3% Triton X-100) for 1 hour at room temperature.

6. Dilute primary antibodies in antibody dilution buffer (1X PBS + 1% BSA + 0.3% Triton-X).

7. Add primary antibodies (mouse anti-FOXA2 1:500, rabbit anti-Brachyury 1:50, normal mouse IgG 1:200, and normal rabbit IgG 1:200).

8. Incubate overnight at 4°C in a humidified box.

9. The next day, wash cells 3 times with 1X PBS, for 5 minutes each wash.
10. Dilute fluorochrome-conjugated secondary antibodies in antibody dilution buffer (goat anti-rabbit 1:200 and goat anti-mouse 1:200).
11. Incubate cover slips with secondary antibodies for 2 hours at room temperature in the dark.
12. Wash cover slips 3 times with 1X PBS, for 5 minutes each wash.
13. Carefully remove cover slips from 24-well plates and mount them on glass slides using Vectashield mounting medium with DAPI.
14. For long-term storage, place slides flat at 4°C, and protect from light.

IMMUNOSTAINING TO CONFIRM PROSTATIC NATURE OF PROSTATE ORGANOIDS

1. Aspirate the prostate organoid medium.
2. Incubate organoids with dispase (1 mg/mL) for 20 minutes at 37°C to partially dissolve the Matrigel.
3. Use 28 gauge $\times$ 1/2″ needles to further dissect individual organoids, and place organoids from the same well into microcentrifuge tubes for the reminder of the procedure.
4. Gently spin them down at $100 \times g$ for 2 minutes.
5. Fix organoids with 4% paraformaldehyde for 20 minutes at room temperature (in a fume hood).
6. Wash organoids 3 times with 1X PBS, for 5 minutes each wash. Gently spin them down at $100 \times g$ for 2 minutes, or allow them to settle to the bottom of the tube by gravity after each wash.
7. Block organoids with blocking buffer (1X PBS + 0.5 mL normal serum from the same species as the secondary antibody + 0.3% Triton X-100) for 1 hour at room temperature. Gently spin at $100 \times g$ for 2 minutes, or allow them to settle to the bottom of the tube by gravity after blocking.
8. Dilute primary antibodies in antibody dilution buffer (1X PBS + 1% BSA + 0.3% Triton-X).
9. Add primary antibodies (rabbit anti-AR 1:100, rabbit anti-vimentin 1:100, rabbit anti-TMPRSS2 1:100, guinea pig anti-CK8/18 1:100, goat anti-PSA 1:100, mouse anti-laminin 1:100, mouse anti-NKX3.1 1:100, normal rabbit IgG 1:200, normal guinea pig IgG 1:300, normal goat IgG 1:100, and normal mouse IgG 1:200).
10. Incubate overnight at 4°C.
11. The next day, wash organoids 3 times with 1X PBS for 5 minutes each wash. Gently spin them at $100 \times g$ for 2 minutes, or allow them to settle to the bottom of the tube by gravity after each wash.
12. Dilute fluorochrome-conjugated secondary antibodies (goat antirabbit 1:200, goat antiguinea pig 1:200, donkey antigoat 1:200, and goat antimouse 1:200) in antibody dilution buffer.

13. Incubate organoids with secondary antibodies for 2 hours at room temperature in the dark.
14. Wash organoids 3 times with 1X PBS for 5 minutes each wash. Gently spin at $100 \times g$ for 2 minutes, or allow them to settle to the bottom of the tube by gravity after each wash.
15. Carefully pipette organoids with a barrier pipette tip onto raised chamber slides, and mount using Vectashield mounting medium with DAPI (Fig. 5.3A–D).
16. For long-term storage, place slides flat at 4°C, protected from light.

DEBUGGING COMMON PROBLEMS

1. hESC colonies are not evenly distributed throughout the wells. To avoid this problem, tap the side of the plate before placing it in the incubator.
2. Matrigel-coating in the dishes is not smooth. Aliquoting Matrigel must always be performed on ice, and using chilled microcentrifuge tubes. Aliquot used for coating must be dissolved in cold mTeSR1 medium. If problems persist, check expiration dates and lot numbers; getting a new bottle will be the best option at this point.
3. Poor definitive endoderm differentiation (determined by FOXA2 and Brachyury immunostaining) can be due to colony overgrowth prior to the induction procedure, or bad activin A. If you suspect overgrowth, start definitive endoderm induction earlier. If bad activin A is suspected, use a fresh aliquot or buy a new reagent.
4. Three-dimensional structures fail to form after 4 days of growth factor treatment. This can occur if the starting hESC density was not adequate (85%–90%), definitive endoderm induction was not optimal (as mentioned in point 3 above), or the activity of the growth factors utilized decreased (try new aliquots).
5. Prostate organoids can fail to expand if the medium is not changed every 3–4 days, or the media is not freshly prepared. This is necessary to ensure the addition of fresh growth factors to the medium.

ACKNOWLEDGMENTS

Immunofluorencence photographs were acquired in the Confocal Microscopy Facility via the Research Resources Center at the University of Illinois at Chicago. This work was supported by grants from the National Institutes of Health, R01-ES015584, R01-ES02207 and RC2-ES018758 and the Michael Reese Research and Education Foundation.

DECLARATION OF FINANCIAL INTERESTS

The authors have no financial interests.

REFERENCES

Abler, L.L., Keil, K.P., Mehta, V., Joshi, P.S., Schmitz, C.T., Vezina, C.M., 2011. A high-resolution molecular atlas of the fetal mouse lower urogenital tract. Dev. Dyn. Offic. Publ. Am. Assoc. Anat. 240, 2364–2377.

Aboseif, S.R., Dahiya, R., Narayan, P., Cunha, G.R., 1997. Effect of retinoic acid on prostatic development. Prostate. 31, 161–167.

Adams, J.Y., Leav, I., Lau, K.M., Ho, S.M., Pflueger, S.M., 2002. Expression of estrogen receptor beta in the fetal, neonatal, and prepubertal human prostate. Prostate. 52, 69–81.

Aranda, A., Pascual, A., 2001. Nuclear hormone receptors and gene expression. Physiol. Rev. 81, 1269–1304.

Bardin, C.W., Bullock, L.P., Sherins, R.J., Mowszowicz, I., Blackburn, W.R., 1973. Androgen metabolism and mechanism of action in male pseudohermaphroditism: a study of testicular feminization. Recent. Prog. Horm. Res. 29, 65–109.

Bennett, C.N., Ross, S.E., Longo, K.A., Bajnok, L., Hemati, N., Johnson, K.W., et al., 2002. Regulation of Wnt signalling during adipogenesis. J. Biol. Chem. 277, 30998–31004.

Bhatia-Gaur, R., Donjacour, A.A., Sciavolino, P.J., Kim, M., Desai, N., Young, P., et al., 1999. Roles for Nkx3.1 in prostate development and cancer. Genes Dev. 13, 966–977.

Bieberich, C.J., Fujita, K., He, W.W., Jay, G., 1996. Prostate-specific and androgen-dependent expression of a novel homeobox gene. J. Biol. Chem. 271, 31779–31782.

Bjornstrom, L., Sjoberg, M., 2005. Mechanisms of estrogen receptor signalling: convergence of genomic and nongenomic actions on target genes. Mol. Endocrinol. (Baltimore, Md) 19, 833–842.

Bowen, C., Bubendorf, L., Voeller, H.J., Slack, R., Willi, N., Sauter, G., et al., 2000. Loss of NKX3.1 expression in human prostate cancers correlates with tumor progression. Cancer. Res. 60, 6111–6115.

Brennan, K.R., Brown, A.M., 2004. Wnt proteins in mammary development and cancer. J. Mammary. Gland. Biol. Neoplasia 9, 119–131.

Cadigan, K.M., Nusse, R., 1997. Wnt signalling: a common theme in animal development. Genes Dev. 11, 3286–3305.

Calderon-Gierszal, E.L., Prins, G.S., 2015. Directed differentiation of human embryonic stem cells into prostate organoids in vitro and its perturbation by low-dose bisphenol a exposure. PLOS One 10 (7), e0133238.

Carpenter, G., Cohen, S., 1990. Epidermal growth factor. J. Biol. Chem. 265, 7709–7712.

Chambon, P., 1996. A decade of molecular biology of retinoic acid receptors. FASEB J. Offic. Publ. Federation Am. Soc. Exp. Biol. 10, 940–954.

Cruciat, C.M., Niehrs, C., 2013. Secreted and transmembrane wnt inhibitors and activators. Cold Spring Harbor Perspect. Biol. 5, a015081.

Cunha, G.R., 1973. The role of androgens in the epithelio-mesenchymal interactions involved in prostatic morphogenesis in embryonic mice. Anat. Rec. 175, 87–96.

Cunha, G.R., 2008. Mesenchymal-epithelial interactions: past, present, and future. Differentiation 76, 578−586.

Cunha, G.R., Chung, L.W.K., Shannon, J.M., Taguchi, O., Fujii, H., 1983. Hormone-induced morphogenesis and growth − role of mesenchymal epithelial interactions. Recent. Prog. Horm. Res. 39, 559−598.

Cunha, G.R., Donjacour, A.A., Cooke, P.S., Mee, S., Bigsby, R.M., Higgins, S.J., et al., 1987. The endocrinology and developmental biology of the prostate. Endocr. Rev. 8, 338−362.

D'Amour, K.A., Agulnick, A.D., Eliazer, S., Kelly, O.G., Kroon, E., Baetge, E.E., 2005. Efficient differentiation of human embryonic stem cells to definitive endoderm. Nat. Biotechnol. 23, 1534−1541.

Davies, J., 1978. Developmental aspects of the male reproductive system. Environ. Health. Perspect. 24, 45−50.

Dolle, P., Ruberte, E., Leroy, P., Morriss-Kay, G., Chambon, P., 1990. Retinoic acid receptors and cellular retinoid binding proteins. I. A systematic study of their differential pattern of transcription during mouse organogenesis. Development 110, 1133−1151.

Donjacour, A.A., Cunha, G.R., 1993. Assessment of prostatic protein secretion in tissue recombinants made of urogenital sinus mesenchyme and urothelium from normal or androgen-insensitive mice. Endocrinology 132, 2342−2350.

Donjacour, A.A., Thomson, A.A., Cunha, G.R., 2003. FGF-10 plays an essential role in the growth of the fetal prostate. Dev. Biol. 261, 39−54.

Duncan, M.W., Thompson, H.S., 2007. Proteomics of semen and its constituents. Proteomics. Clin. Appl. 1, 861−875.

Ellem, S.J., Risbridger, G.P., 2009. The dual, opposing roles of estrogen in the prostate. Ann. N.Y. Acad. Sci. 1155, 174−186.

Feldman, B.J., Feldman, D., 2001. The development of androgen-independent prostate cancer. Nat. Rev. Cancer 1, 34−45.

Finch, P.W., Cunha, G.R., Rubin, J.S., Wong, J., Ron, D., 1995. Pattern of keratinocyte growth factor and keratinocyte growth factor receptor expression during mouse fetal development suggests a role in mediating morphogenetic mesenchymal-epithelial interactions. Dev. Dyn. Offic. Publ. Am. Assoc. Anat. 203, 223−240.

Frick, J., Aulitzky, W., 1991. Physiology of the prostate. Infection. 19 (Suppl 3), S115−S118.

Grishina, I.B., Kim, S.Y., Ferrara, C., Makarenkova, H.P., Walden, P.D., 2005. BMP7 inhibits branching morphogenesis in the prostate gland and interferes with Notch signalling. Dev. Biol. 288, 334−347.

Hayashi, N., Sugimura, Y., Kawamura, J., Donjacour, A.A., Cunha, G.R., 1991. Morphological and functional heterogeneity in the rat prostatic gland. Biol. Reprod. 45, 308−321.

Hayward, S.W., Baskin, L.S., Haughney, P.C., Cunha, A.R., Foster, B.A., Dahiya, R., et al., 1996a. Epithelial development in the rat ventral prostate, anterior prostate and seminal vesicle. Acta Anat. 155, 81−93.

Hayward, S.W., Baskin, L.S., Haughney, P.C., Foster, B.A., Cunha, A.R., Dahiya, R., et al., 1996b. Stromal development in the ventral prostate, anterior prostate and seminal vesicle of the rat. Acta. Anat. 155, 94−103.

Henderson, B.E., Bernstein, L., Ross, R.K., Depue, R.H., Judd, H.L., 1988. The early in utero oestrogen and testosterone environment of blacks and whites: potential effects on male offspring. Br. J. Cancer 57, 216−218.

Hu, W.Y., Hu, D.P., Xie, L., Li, Y., Majumdar, S., Nonn, L., et al., 2017. Isolation and functional interrogation of adult human prostate epithelial cells at single cell resolution. Stem Cell Res 23, 1–12.

Huang, L., Pu, Y., Alam, S., Birch, L., Prins, G.S., 2005. The role of Fgf10 signalling in branching morphogenesis and gene expression of the rat prostate gland: lobe-specific suppression by neonatal estrogens. Dev. Biol. 278, 396–414.

Huang, L., Pu, Y., Hu, W.Y., Birch, L., Luccio-Camelo, D., Yamaguchi, T., et al., 2009. The role of Wnt5a in prostate gland development. Dev. Biol. 328, 188–199.

Huggins, C., Hodges, C.V., 2002. Studies on prostatic cancer: I. The effect of castration, of estrogen and of androgen injection on serum phosphatases in metastatic carcinoma of the prostate. 1941. J. Urol. 168, 9–12.

Hussain, S., Lawrence, M.G., Taylor, R.A., Lo, C.Y., BioResource, A.P.C., Frydenberg, M., et al., 2012. Estrogen receptor beta activation impairs prostatic regeneration by inducing apoptosis in murine and human stem/progenitor enriched cell populations. PLoS. ONE 7, e40732.

Jarred, R.A., McPherson, S.J., Bianco, J.J., Couse, J.F., Korach, K.S., Risbridger, G.P., 2002. Prostate phenotypes in estrogen-modulated transgenic mice. Trends. Endocrinol. Metab. 13, 163–168.

Jin, Y.R., Yoon, J.K., 2012. The R-spondin family of proteins: emerging regulators of WNT signalling. Int. J. Biochem. Cell. Biol. 44, 2278–2287.

Keil, K.P., Mehta, V., Abler, L.L., Joshi, P.S., Schmitz, C.T., Vezina, C.M., 2012. Visualization and quantification of mouse prostate development by in situ hybridization. Differ. Res. Biol. Divers. 84, 232–239.

Kim, H.G., Kassis, J., Souto, J.C., Turner, T., Wells, A., 1999. EGF receptor signalling in prostate morphogenesis and tumorigenesis. Histol. Histopathol. 14, 1175–1182.

Kim, M.J., Bhatia-Gaur, R., Banach-Petrosky, W.A., Desai, N., Wang, Y., Hayward, S.W., et al., 2002. Nkx3.1 mutant mice recapitulate early stages of prostate carcinogenesis. Cancer. Res. 62, 2999–3004.

Komiya, Y., Habas, R., 2008. Wnt signal transduction pathways. Organogenesis 4, 68–75.

Kuiper, G.G., Enmark, E., Pelto-Huikko, M., Nilsson, S., Gustafsson, J.A., 1996. Cloning of a novel receptor expressed in rat prostate and ovary. Proc. Natl. Acad. Sci. U.S.A. 93, 5925–5930.

Kurita, T., Medina, R.T., Mills, A.A., Cunha, G.R., 2004. Role of p63 and basal cells in the prostate. Development (Cambridge, England) 131, 4955–4964.

Lamm, M.L., Podlasek, C.A., Barnett, D.H., Lee, J., Clemens, J.Q., Hebner, C.M., et al., 2001. Mesenchymal factor bone morphogenetic protein 4 restricts ductal budding and branching morphogenesis in the developing prostate. Dev. Biol. 232, 301–314.

Lasnitzki, I., Mizuno, T., 1977. Induction of the rat prostate gland by androgens in organ culture. J. Endocrinol. 74, 47–55.

Laudes, M., 2011. Role of WNT signalling in the determination of human mesenchymal stem cells into preadipocytes. J. Mol. Endocrinol. 46, R65–R72.

Le Romancer, M., Poulard, C., Cohen, P., Sentis, S., Renoir, J.-M., Corbo, L., 2011. Cracking the estrogen receptor's posttranslational code in breast tumors. Endocr. Rev. 32, 597–622.

Lee, C., Prins, G.S., Henneberry, M.O., Grayhack, J.T., 1981. Effect of estradiol on the rat prostate in the presence and absence of testosterone and pituitary. J. Androl. 2, 293–299.

Liao, S., 1968. Evidence for a discriminatory action of androgenic steroids on the synthesis of nucleolar ribonucleic acids in prostatic nuclei. Am. Zool. 8, 233–242.

Lilja, H., Abrahamsson, P.A., 1988. Three predominant proteins secreted by the human prostate gland. Prostate. 12, 29−38.

Logan, C.Y., Nusse, R., 2004. The Wnt signalling pathway in development and disease. Annu. Rev. Cell. Dev. Biol. 20, 781−810.

Lohnes, D., Dierich, A., Ghyselinck, N., Kastner, P., Lampron, C., LeMeur, M., et al., 1992. Retinoid receptors and binding proteins. J. Cell Sci. Suppl. 16, 69−76.

Lohnes, D., Kastner, P., Dierich, A., Mark, M., LeMeur, M., Chambon, P., 1993. Function of retinoic acid receptor gamma in the mouse. Cell 73, 643−658.

Lonergan, P.E., Tindall, D.J., 2011. Androgen receptor signalling in prostate cancer development and progression. J. Carcinog. 10 (20-3163), 83937, Epub 2011 Aug 23.

Lowsley, O.S., 1912. The development of the human prostate gland with reference to the development of other structures at the neck of the urinary bladder. Am. J. Anat. 13, 299−348.

Mann, T., 1963. Biochemistry of the prostate gland and its secretion. Natl. Cancer. Inst. Monogr. 12, 235−246.

Mariotti, A., Durham, J., Frederickson, R., Miller, R., Butcher, F., Mawhinney, M., 1987. Actions and interactions of estradiol and retinoic acid in mouse anterior prostate gland. Biol. Reprod. 37, 1023−1035.

Matzkin, H., Soloway, M.S., 1992. Immunohistochemical evidence of the existence and localization of aromatase in human prostatic tissues. Prostate 21, 309−314.

McCracken, K.W., Howell, J.C., Wells, J.M., Spence, J.R., 2011. Generating human intestinal tissue from pluripotent stem cells in vitro. Nat. Protoc. 6, 1920−1928.

McCracken, K.W., Cata, E.M., Crawford, C.M., Sinagoga, K.L., Schumacher, M., Rockich, B.E., et al., 2014. Modelling human development and disease in pluripotent stem-cell-derived gastric organoids. Nature 516, 400−404.

McNeal, J.E., 1981. The zonal anatomy of the prostate. Prostate 2, 35−49.

McPherson, S.J., Wang, H., Jones, M.E., Pedersen, J., Iismaa, T.P., Wreford, N., et al., 2001. Elevated androgens and prolactin in aromatase-deficient mice cause enlargement, but not malignancy, of the prostate gland. Endocrinology 142, 2458−2467.

Mehta, V., Abler, L.L., Keil, K.P., Schmitz, C.T., Joshi, P.S., Vezina, C.M., 2011. Atlas of Wnt and R-spondin gene expression in the developing male mouse lower urogenital tract. Dev. Dyn. Offic. Publ. Am. Assoc. Anat. 240, 2548−2560.

Mimeault, M., Pommery, N., Henichart, J.P., 2003. New advances on prostate carcinogenesis and therapies: involvement of EGF-EGFR transduction system. Growth factors (Chur, Switzerland) 21, 1−14.

Mosselman, S., Polman, J., Dijkema, R., 1996. ER beta: identification and characterization of a novel human estrogen receptor. FEBS Lett. 392, 49−53.

Murry, C.E., Keller, G., 2008. Differentiation of embryonic stem cells to clinically relevant populations: lessons from embryonic development. Cell 132, 661−680.

Ousset, M., Van Keymeulen, A., Bouvencourt, G., Sharma, N., Achouri, Y., Simons, B.D., et al., 2012. Multipotent and unipotent progenitors contribute to prostate postnatal development. Nat. Cell. Biol. 14, 1131−1138.

Platz, E.A., Giovannucci, E., 2004. The epidemiology of sex steroid hormones and their signalling and metabolic pathways in the etiology of prostate cancer. J. Steroid. Biochem. Mol. Biol. 92, 237−253.

Poulard, C., Treilleux, I., Lavergne, E., Bouchekioua-Bouzaghou, K., Goddard-Leon, S., Chabaud, S., et al., 2012. Activation of rapid oestrogen signalling in aggressive human breast cancers. EmboMol. Med. 4, 1200−1213.

Price, D., 1963. Comparative aspects of development and structure in the prostate. Natl. Cancer. Inst. Monogr. 12, 1−27.

Prins, G.S., 1992. Neonatal estrogen exposure induces lobe-specific alterations in adult rat prostate androgen receptor expression. Endocrinology 130, 3703−3714.

Prins, G.S., Birch, L., 1995. The developmental pattern of androgen receptor expression in rat prostate lobes is altered after neonatal exposure to estrogen. Endocrinology 136, 1303−1314.

Prins, G.S., Birch, L., 1997. Neonatal estrogen exposure up-regulates estrogen receptor expression in the developing and adult rat prostate lobes. Endocrinology 138, 1801−1809.

Prins, G.S., Korach, K.S., 2008. The role of estrogens and estrogen receptors in normal prostate growth and disease. Steroids 73, 233−244.

Prins, G.S., Lindgren, M., 2015. Accessory sex glands in the male. Knobil and Neill's Physiology of Reproduction. Elsevier, pp. 773−804.

Prins, G.S., Putz, O., 2008. Molecular signalling pathways that regulate prostate gland development. Differ. Res. Biol. Divers. 76, 641−659.

Prins, G.S., Birch, L., Greene, G.L., 1991. Androgen receptor localization in different cell types of the adult rat prostate. Endocrinology 129, 3187−3199.

Prins, G.S., Marmer, M., Woodham, C., Chang, W., Kuiper, G., Gustafsson, J.A., et al., 1998. Estrogen receptor-beta messenger ribonucleic acid ontogeny in the prostate of normal and neonatally estrogenized rats. Endocrinology 139, 874−883.

Prins, G.S., Birch, L., Couse, J.F., Choi, I., Katzenellenbogen, B., Korach, K.S., 2001. Estrogen imprinting of the developing prostate gland is mediated through stromal estrogen receptor alpha: studies with alphaERKO and betaERKO mice. Cancer. Res. 61, 6089−6097.

Prins, G.S., Chang, W.Y., Wang, Y., van Breemen, R.B., 2002. Retinoic acid receptors and retinoids are up-regulated in the developing and adult rat prostate by neonatal estrogen exposure. Endocrinology 143, 3628−3640.

Prins, G.S., Huang, L., Birch, L., Pu, Y., 2006. The role of estrogens in normal and abnormal development of the prostate gland. Ann. N.Y. Acad. Sci. 1089, 1−13.

Prins, G.S., Hu, W.Y., Shi, G.B., Hu, D.P., Majumdar, S., Li, G., et al., 2014. Bisphenol A promotes human prostate stem-progenitor cell self-renewal and increases in vivo carcinogenesis in human prostate epithelium. Endocrinology: en20131955.

Pu, Y., Huang, L., Birch, L., Prins, G.S., 2007. Androgen regulation of prostate morphoregulatory gene expression: Fgf10-dependent and -independent pathways. Endocrinology 148, 1697−1706.

Revankar, C.M., Cimino, D.F., Sklar, L.A., Arterburn, J.B., Prossnitz, E.R., 2005. A transmembrane intracellular estrogen receptor mediates rapid cell signalling. Science (New York, NY) 307, 1625−1630.

Rhinn, M., Dolle, P., 2012. Retinoic acid signalling during development. Development (Cambridge, England) 139, 843−858.

Richter, F., Joyce, A., Fromowitz, F., Wang, S., Watson, J., Watson, R., et al., 2002. Immunohistochemical localization of the retinoic Acid receptors in human prostate. J. Androl. 23, 830−838.

Risbridger, G., Wang, H., Young, P., Kurita, T., Wang, Y.Z., Lubahn, D., et al., 2001. Evidence that epithelial and mesenchymal estrogen receptor-alpha mediates effects of estrogen on prostatic epithelium. Dev. Biol. 229, 432−442.

Ross, S.E., Hemati, N., Longo, K.A., Bennett, C.N., Lucas, P.C., Erickson, R.L., et al., 2000. Inhibition of adipogenesis by Wnt signalling. Science (New York, NY) 289, 950−953.

Saito, M., Mizuno, T., 1997. Prostatic bud induction by brief treatment with growth factors. C. R. Seances. Soc. Biol. Fil. 191, 261−265.

Seo, R., McGuire, M., Chung, M., Bushman, W., 1997. Inhibition of prostate ductal morphogenesis by retinoic acid. J. Urol. 158, 931−935.

Shapiro, E., Huang, H., Masch, R.J., McFadden, D.E., Wilson, E.L., Wu, X.R., 2005. Immunolocalization of estrogen receptor alpha and beta in human fetal prostate. J. Urol. 174, 2051−2053.

Signoretti, S., Waltregny, D., Dilks, J., Isaac, B., Lin, D., Garraway, L., et al., 2000. P63 is a prostate basal cell marker and is required for prostate development. Am. J. Pathol. 157, 1769−1775.

Spence, J.R., Mayhew, C.N., Rankin, S.A., Kuhar, M.F., Vallance, J.E., Tolle, K., et al., 2011. Directed differentiation of human pluripotent stem cells into intestinal tissue in vitro. Nature 470, 105−109.

Sugimura, Y., Cunha, G.R., Donjacour, A.A., 1986. Morphogenesis of ductal networks in the mouse prostate. Biol. Reprod. 34, 961−971.

Thomson, A.A., Cunha, G.R., 1999. Prostatic growth and development are regulated by FGF10. Development (Cambridge, England) 126, 3693−3701.

Timms, B.G., 2008. Prostate development: a historical perspective. Differ. Res. Biol. Divers. 76, 565−577.

Timms, B.G., Mohs, T.J., Didio, L.J., 1994. Ductal budding and branching patterns in the developing prostate. J. Urol. 151, 1427−1432.

Uematsu, F., Kan, M., Wang, F., Jang, J.H., Luo, Y., McKeehan, W.L., 2000. Ligand binding properties of binary complexes of heparin and immunoglobulin-like modules of FGF receptor 2. Biochem. Biophys. Res. Commun. 272, 830−836.

Vezina, C.M., Allgeier, S.H., Fritz, W.A., Moore, R.W., Strerath, M., Bushman, W., et al., 2008. Retinoic acid induces prostatic bud formation. Dev. Dyn. Offic. Publ. Am. Assoc. Anat. 237, 1321−1333.

Walter, P., Green, S., Greene, G., Krust, A., Bornert, J.M., Jeltsch, J.M., et al., 1985. Cloning of the human estrogen receptor cDNA. Proc. Natl. Acad. Sci. U.S.A. 82, 7889−7893.

Wilson, J.G., Warkany, J., 1948. Malformations in the genito-urinary tract induced by maternal vitamin A deficiency in the rat. Am. J. Anat. 83, 357−407.

Wolbach, S.B., Howe, P.R., 1925. Tissue changes following deprivation of fat-soluble a vitamin. J. Exp. Med. 42, 753−777.

Yonemura, C.Y., Cunha, G.R., Sugimura, Y., Mee, S.L., 1995. Temporal and spatial factors in diethylstilbestrol-induced squamous metaplasia in the developing human prostate. II. Persistent changes after removal of diethylstilbestrol. Acta. Anat. 153, 1−11.

Zondek, T., Mansfield, M.D., Attree, S.L., Zondek, L.H., 1986. Hormone levels in the foetal and neonatal prostate. Acta. Endocrinol. 112, 447−456.

Kidney organoids

Mona Elhendawi[1,2] and Weijia Liu[1]

[1]*The University of Edinburgh, Edinburgh, United Kingdom* [2]*Mansoura University, Mansoura, Egypt*

CHAPTER OUTLINE

INTRODUCTION

The mammalian kidney is composed of several specialized cell types that work in a highly coordinated way to excrete waste products, to maintain water and electrolyte balance, to control vitamin D metabolism, and to secrete erythropoietin to stimulate erythropoiesis. An average human kidney contains around 1,000,000 nephrons; the functional and structural unit of the kidney (reviewed by Bertram et al., 2011). By the time of birth, nephrogenesis is complete, and any loss or

Organoids and Mini-Organs. DOI: http://dx.doi.org/10.1016/B978-0-12-812636-3.00006-7

damage to the nephrons cannot be replaced by new nephron formation (Hinchliffe et al., 1991; Rumballe et al., 2011).

End-stage renal disease (ESRD) is a serious medical problem, for which current available treatments are restricted to dialysis or, more ideally, renal transplantation (reviewed by Liyanage et al., 2015). Nonetheless, shortage of organ donors and graft rejection are major drawbacks for renal transplantation and, despite the great advances in improving allograft rejection, about one quarter of patients on waiting lists have been suffering from a failed allograft: transplant failure is a frequent cause of either starting dialysis or considering re-transplantation (Mujais and Story, 2006; Yang et al., 2013). Dialysis remains a life-saving treatment for these patients, but it affects quality of life, and it fails to remove large molecular weight and protein-bound waste products, which are removed by natural kidneys (Deltombe et al., 2015).

In 2010, Unbekandt and Davies showed that mouse embryonic kidneys, after being dissociated into single cell suspension and cultured in the presence of Rho-associated coiled-coil kinase inhibitor (ROCK inhibitor) to inhibit dissociation-induced apoptosis, were able to self-organize to form renal structures. Within these, ureteric bud (UB) stem cells developed into multiple collecting duct (CD) trees, around which nephron progenitors condensed and differentiated into nephrons. This technique was modified to include a second step, in which one of the collecting ducts formed in this system was isolated and surrounded with fresh metanephric mesenchyme (MM): the result was kidney tissue arranged much more realistically, around single collecting duct tree (Ganeva et al., 2011) (see Chapter 9: From organoids to mini-organs: A case study in the kidney).

The generation of iPSCs avoids the ethical issues that restrict the use of embryonic pluripotent stem cells, and has strongly encouraged the field of regenerative research (reviewed by Yokoo et al., 2008). Recently, there have been some published protocols using different growth factors for directed differentiation of human-induced pluripotent stem cells (hiPSCs) toward UB and/or MM, and these renal progenitors have been used in generating renal organoids using the idea, described above, of self-organization of the dissociated renal progenitors.

Research groups around the world are currently focusing on different strategies to find new therapeutic modalities for ESRD. These strategies include in situ regeneration of the damaged kidney, recellularization of a decellularized matrix from an adult kidney (Gifford et al., 2015), engineering foetal kidneys from stem cells and allowing them to mature after transplantation into a host (reviewed by Davies and Chang, 2014), and 3D bioprinting (Murphy and Atala, 2014). Each of these approaches has had some success at the level of pilot experiments, and initial results seem to be promising. Any of these strategies still need a cell source for regeneration, and in principle organoids formed from renally-differentiated iPSCs could work as an available source of these cells with the advantage of high-throughput capability. Cultured organoids could also be useful as models for disease modeling, and for screening drugs for nephrotoxicity.

STRUCTURE AND FUNCTION OF THE KIDNEY

In the adult human, the kidneys reside retroperitoneally against the posterior abdominal wall. One side of each kidney has a concave surface called the hilum, which is the point of exit for the ureter and renal vein, and also the point of entry of the renal artery. The kidney is enclosed by a fibrous capsule, beneath which its parenchyma is divided into two zones, the outer cortex surrounding the inner medulla. The human kidney parenchyma is composed of a number of conical lobes, called the renal pyramids. The base of each lobe faces the renal capsule, and the tip region, the papilla, is where the urine flows from the collecting ducts into the corresponding minor calyx. Minor calyces subsequently merge into major calyces that in turn coalesce to form the renal pelvis, which narrows and continues as the ureter.

The healthy adult kidney contains approximately 1,000,000 nephrons, the basic structural and functional units of the kidney. The nephron comprises two major components, the renal corpuscles and the renal tubule. Each renal corpuscle consists of a glomerulus (a tuft of vascular capillaries) surrounded by the expanded proximal end of the nephron, the Bowman's capsule. The renal tubule extends from the capsule, and consists of the proximal convoluted tubule, loop of Henle, which has a descending and an ascending limb, and distal convoluted tubule. The distal convoluted tubule connects to the collecting duct, which develops from the ureteric bud.

Blood enters the glomerulus through an afferent arteriole, and exits via an efferent arteriole. These arterioles can be constricted or relaxed in response to endocrine signals, allowing regulation of the hydrostatic pressure in the glomerulus within close limits. The blood then enters into the peritubular capillaries, which parallel the tubule. This unique structure forms a portal system in which two capillary beds (glomerulus capillaries and peritubular capillaries) are connected by an arteriole, and this connection is important to the functioning of the nephron. The peritubular capillaries then drain into an efferent venule, which combines with efferent venules from other nephrons to flow into the renal vein.

Most functions of the kidney are carried out by the nephron and the cortical part of the collecting duct. Together, these maintain fluid and electrolyte balance in the body through blood filtration. The proximal part of the nephron, in particular, removes liquid waste products generated through metabolism. It is also a mechanism for excreting drugs, such as morphine or penicillin, and for eliminating excess vitamins and other organic substances.

The hydrostatic pressure in the glomerulus drives selective components of blood plasma (water and solutes, but not large proteins) across the filtration barrier into the Bowman's space, and then the ultra-filtrate drains into the proximal convoluted tubule and begins its journey through the nephron. Each portion of the nephron has highly specialized functions arising from the differences in properties of the cells that line the tubule along its length. The proximal tubule is responsible for the reabsorption of all filtered glucose and amino acids, and about two-thirds of filtered water and sodium. Epithelial cells lining the proximal tubule have a dense brush border of microvilli on the apical membranes that greatly increase the area of absorption. The plasma of these cells is packed with mitochondria, which are needed to supply energy for active transport of sodium ions out of the cells. The lumen of the loop of Henle is made up of simple squamous epithelium. Some (about 10%) of the nephrons of the human kidney are the juxtamedullary nephrons, which have long loops of Henle located deeply in the medulla. The descending loop is freely permeable to water and less permeable to ions, while the thin ascending loop is impermeable to water but actively transports salts from the filtrate; this feature is extremely important for establishing an osmotic gradient within the medulla. The distal convoluted tubule is lined with simple cuboidal cells that are shorter than those of the proximal convoluted tubule, and with very few microvilli. Much of the function of the distal tubule is regulated by the endocrine system. Sodium absorption is mediated by aldosterone, the permeability of water increases in the presence of vasopressin, and reabsorption of Ca^{2+} happens in response to parathyroid hormone.

The collecting duct, to which the distal tubules connect, is usually considered to be distinct from the nephron, because it is derived from ureteric bud, in contrast to the nephron which is derived from metanephric mesenchyme. The collecting duct has two main cell types; principal cells and intercalated cells. The more abundant principal cells are specialized to transport water in response to vasopressin (Nielsen and Agre, 1995), while intercalated cells regulate acid − base balance by secreting hydrogen ions and bicarbonate into the collecting duct lumen. After final adjustment in electrolytes and fluid balance, the urine leaves the collecting duct at the renal papilla, and empties into the urinary bladder via the ureter.

NORMAL KIDNEY DEVELOPMENT

Gastrulation in mammals divides the embryo into three germ layers; the ectoderm, the endoderm, and the mesoderm. The intraembryonic mesoderm is further subdivided into paraxial mesoderm, and lateral plate mesoderm, and in between them the intermediate mesoderm (IM); the responsible part of the embryo for the development of all nephric structures. Renal development starts when the IM at its most cranial part condenses and undergoes epithelization to form two nephric ducts (ND; also known as Wolffian ducts or mesonephric ducts) on both sides of the midline. The two tubules continue to grow caudally by mesenchymal-to-epithelial transition of cells at their tips (Saxen, 1987).

Important transcriptional factors for the specification of the ND from the IM, and for its further development and caudal extension, are PAX2, PAX8, and LHX1 (Dressler et al., 1990; Bouchard et al., 2002; Fujii et al., 1994).

The adjacent IM to these ND forms three paired nephric structures in a cranial − caudal succession; the pronephros (the most cranial and the first to appear), the mesonephros, and the metanephros (the most caudal and the last structure to develop). The pronephros is functional in lower vertebrates such as Xenopus embryos (reviewed by Vize et al., 1997) and larval fish (Drummond et al., 1998), but not in amniotes. The mesonephros has been shown to produce urine during embryogenesis in mammals. Both the pronephros and the mesonephros largely degenerate at the end of embryogenesis (in the case of males, some of the mesonephric tubules are modified to become part of the male reproductive system), and only the third pair of kidneys to form, the metanephroi, develop to form the functioning mature kidneys.

Two main progenitors; the ureteric bud (UB) and the metanephric mesenchyme (MM), both originating from the IM, form the mature metanephric kidney. Metanephric kidney development begins in the 5th gestational week in humans, and ends at around the 36th week of gestation. No new nephron formation occurs after birth, but the kidney continues to grow to adult size owing to maturation and growth of the already existing nephrons (Hinchliffe et al., 1991). Fig. 6.1 illustrates metanephric kidney development.

REGULATION OF THE URETERIC BUD OUTGROWTH AND BRANCHING

The UB develops as an outgrowth from the caudal portion of the ND that grows and invades the MM in response to localized signaling (the MM is formed from the posterior IM adjacent to the ND at point of UB outgrowth). The UB starts bifurcation inside the MM, and eventually forms the collecting component of the kidney; the ureter, the renal pelvis, and the collecting duct tree.

Reciprocal signaling between both renal progenitor cell types is crucial for their development and maturation. The MM produces glial cell-derived neurotropic factor (GDNF) which stimulates the tyrosine kinase receptor (RET; expressed in the ND) and the co-receptor GDNF family receptor α1 (GFRα1; expressed in both ND and MM) to induce localized cellular proliferation and migration out of the caudal end of the ND to form the UB (Pachnis et al., 1993; Sainio et al., 1997).

Stringent regulation of the GDNF/RET pathway along the cranial − caudal axis is important to prevent supernumerary and ectopic ureters: several genes have been shown to control the ureteric outgrowth. The transcriptional factors Foxc1 and Foxc2 (Kume et al., 2000), and the Slit2/Robo2 signaling pathway (Grieshammer et al., 2004) prevent cranial expression of *Gdnf* in the MM; deletion of any of these genes results in multiple buds, cranially located to the normal position of the ureter. Other important regulators of the GDNF/RET pathway are BMP4 and Gremlin, with the BMP4 protein secreted from the mesenchyme surrounding the ND to inhibit cranial expansion of the GDNF/RET signaling, and Gremlin secreted from the MM to locally antagonize BMP4 and permit proper ureteric budding (Miyazaki et al., 2000). The protein Sprouty has also been proven to inhibit the ERK − MAP − kinase pathway within the cytoplasm of the

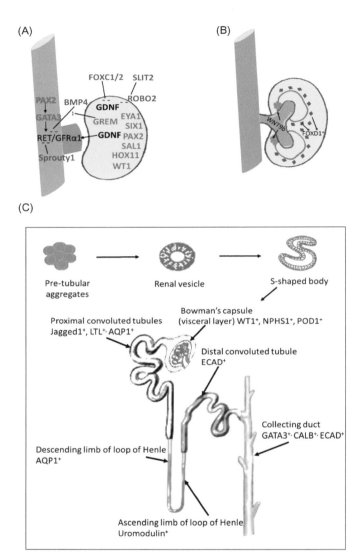

FIGURE 6.1

Illustration of metanephric kidney development. (A) Specification of the metanephric mesenchyme (MM) is marked by the expression of GDNF and the transcriptional regulators EYA1, SIX1, PAX2, SAL1, HOX11, and WT1. The nephric duct expresses the tyrosine kinase receptor RET, which responds to GDNF protein secreted from the metanephric mesenchyme by localized cellular proliferation and migration to form the ureteric bud (UB). The GDNF/RET pathway is tightly regulated along the cranial — caudal axis to prevent supernumerary and ectopic ureters. Enhancers of the GDNF/RET pathway

(*Continued*)

ureteric epithelial cells, thus antagonizing the GDNF/RET pathway, with loss of its function resulting in ectopic ureter (Basson et al., 2005).

The MM expresses different genes, which stimulate the GDNF/RET pathway, including *Eya1*, *Six1*, *Pax2*, *Hox11*, *Wt1*, and *Sall* (reviewed by Dressler, 2006; Davidson, 2009). Deletion of the six alleles of *Hox11* results in failure of expression of *Gdnf* in the MM, and perturbation of UB outgrowth (Wellik et al., 2002). GATA3 is a transcriptional factor expressed in the IM in the presence of PAX2/8 which is important for appropriate RET expression in the ND (Grote et al., 2006). The FGF signaling pathway has also been shown to have a role in patterning UB branching and arborization (Qiao et al., 1999). In 2004, Zhao et al. studied the effect of *Fgfr1* and *Fgfr2* on UB branching and development, and showed that *Fgfr2* mutants failed to develop in a normal way.

MESENCHYME CONDENSATION AND NEPHRON FORMATION

The MM gives rise to three different types of progenitor cells; the nephron progenitor cells (CITED1$^+$, SIX2$^+$) which differentiate into the various cell types of the nephron (Herzlinger et al., 1992; Boyle et al., 2008; Kobayashi et al., 2008), the renal stromal cells (FOXD1$^+$ cells) including mesangial cells, renin producing cells, fibroblasts and pericytes, and the vascular progenitor cells (FLK1$^+$ cells) (Mugford et al., 2008; reviewed by Little and McMahon, 2012).

The invading UB produces inductive signals that stimulate condensation of the nephric progenitors around its growing tips to form the cap mesenchyme (CM). The MM isolated from the UB and cultured in vitro in the absence of extrinsic inducer fail to differentiate, and die by apoptosis. Nevertheless, co-culture of the isolated MM with embryonic spinal cord decreases apoptosis and induces nephron formation (Grobstein, 1953; Grobstein, 1955). However, the exact nature of the inductive signal that the growing UB or the embryonic spinal cord were giving to the MM remained obscure. In 1995, Davies and Garrod (Davies and Garrod, 1995) observed that treatment with lithium chloride, a WNT agonist, could induce tubulogenesis in isolated cultured mouse MM. It was not until 2005 that Carrol et al. identified WNT9b as the specific protein secreted from the UB, that acts through the canonical WNT/β-Catenin pathway to induce MM condensation and initiate nephrogenesis (Carroll et al., 2005).

In response to WNT9b (secreted from the UB) stimulation, the nephron progenitor cells form pre-tubular aggregates close to the ureteric stalk, and begin mesenchymal-to-epithelial transition to form a renal vesicle (RV). The distal end of the renal vesicle then fuses with the ureteric epithelium, forming a

---

◀ are shown in brown, and inhibitors are shown in blue. (B) The UB penetrates the MM and starts bifurcation. WNT9b, secreted from the UB, stimulates the MM to condense and form the cap mesenchyme, which forms aggregates close the ureteric stalk (the pretubular aggregates). (C) Different stages of nephron formation.

comma shaped body that elongates to form S-shaped body. Vascular progenitors expressing FLK1 (vascular endothelial growth factor receptor) then invade the proximal end of the S-shaped body to form the glomerular capillary tuft (reviewed by Schrijvers et al., 2004; Simon et al., 1995; Robert et al., 1996). The S-shaped nephron continues to elongate and differentiate into different specialized cell types forming different parts of the nephron and expressing unique markers:

- Bowman's capsule: at the most proximal end of the nephron, lined with podocytes expressing specific transcriptional factors such as WT1 and podocyte expressed 1 (POD1); transmembrane proteins such as Nephrin (NPHS1), and secreting specific proteins such as VEGF that is thought to recruit endothelial cells (Kreidberg et al., 1993; Ruotsalainen et al., 1999; Kitamoto et al., 1997).
- Proximal convoluted tubule: expressing Jagged1 (JAG1), and AQP1 (Cheng et al., 2003; Barresi et al., 1988; Hennigar et al., 1985; Bauchet et al., 2011).
- Loop of Henle: composed of the thin descending limb expressing AQP1 and the thick ascending limb expressing Tamm-Horsfall protein (Uromodulin) (Bauchet et al., 2011).
- Distal convoluted tubule: the most distal part of nephron that converges with the collecting duct, expressing E-cadherin (ECAD) (Lee et al., 2013).

Notch signaling has been shown to be crucial in patterning cells along the proximal − distal axis of the growing nephrons. In 2003, Cheng et al. used in vitro culture models of mouse embryonic kidney to specifically inhibit Notch signaling using γ secretase inhibitor, and noticed reduced proximal cell fate (podocytes and proximal tubular epithelial cells). Lindström et al., 2015 have shown that a gradient of β-catenin, being highest in the distal end of the nephron and decreasing gradually towards the proximal end, plays a role in patterning the cells along the proximal − distal axis of the nephron, and that loss of the proximal cell fate caused by notch inhibition could be reversed by coinhibiting β-catenin in these cells.

While differentiating to form nephrons, the nephron progenitors maintain a balance between self-renewal and differentiation. This balance is regulated in part by *Six2*, as loss of its function leads to early differentiation of all progenitors and premature cessation of nephrogenesis (Self et al., 2006). Kobayashi et al. (2008) showed in their study that a subpopulation of SIX2$^+$ cells coexpressing WNT4 stops renewing, and begins nephron formation in response to inductive signals from the UB. Absence of WNT4 leads to fewer pre-tubular aggregates, and failure to form epithelial structures (Stark et al., 1994). In contrast, a separate SIX2 positive population coexpressing CITED1 resists the inductive signal, and engages instead in renewal of the stem cell population (Boyle et al., 2008). BMP7-SMAD signaling has been shown to drive the cells into a SIX2$^+$ CITED1$^-$ state to start differentiation (Brown et al., 2013).

Signals from renal stromal cells also have been shown to modulate the balance between self-renewal and differentiation; destroying stroma using diphtheria toxin is associated with thick mesenchymal cap and decreased nephron formation, due to disruption of WNT9b signaling (Das et al., 2013). Mutations in *Foxd1* were also associated with expansion of the progenitors and arrest of differentiation, due to increased levels of proteoglycan decorin (DCN) (normally present at high levels in the medullary interstitium, but not the cortical interstitium) which antagonizes the effect of BMP7 (Fetting et al., 2014).

The fibroblast growth factor (FGF) pathway is another vital signaling pathway in renal development. Deletion of *Fgfr1* and *Fgfr2* in mouse resulted in failure of the MM to respond to inductive signals (Poladia et al., 2006). Another study showed the importance of FGF9 and FGF20 in promoting survival and proliferation of nephron progenitors (Barak et al., 2012).

THE NEED FOR KIDNEY ORGANOIDS

Until recently, research on kidney regeneration and prediction of drug nephrotoxicity have mainly employed 2D culture systems or animal models. While animal models provide information about systemic nephrotoxicity in vivo, the disadvantages include inter-species differences, high cost, and time consumption, with inter-species differences being a particularly serious issue for the pharmacology industry. Culture-based models using human cells are an alternative in principle, but there is a lack of robust in vitro models of human proximal tubules. Primary proximal tubule cells lose their function within hours of isolation, so immortalized human proximal tubule epithelial cell (hPTEC) lines in monolayer culture have been used to model nephrotoxicity. However, some cell lines lack certain anion and cation transporters that are key to drug excretion (Jenkinson et al., 2012), and others have unreliable upregulation of kidney injury biomarkers upon treatment with nephrotoxicants (Huang et al., 2015), making them unsuitable for predictive toxicology. Recently, new hPTEC lines have been developed that exhibit a wider range of functional transporters, and respond to antivirals and environmental carcinogens (Aschauer et al., 2015; Nieskens et al., 2016; Simon-Friedt et al., 2015). Nevertheless, as in vitro cell lines, intrinsically they lack the accuracy in representing the tissue of origin. In addition, 2D culture of single cell types lack the complexity of interactions with other cells and their environment.

There has been an increasing interest in applying 3D printing technology to the biomedical field. While the concept of printing cells accurately layer-by-layer to make a complex tissue may seem promising, substantial challenges emerge in practice. Maintaining viability through the printing process, and achieving the required spatial accuracy, are among the most obvious challenges. Indeed, small errors in accuracy of cell-to-cell interactions are the root of several congenital renal diseases (Kerecuk, Schreuder, and Woolf, 2008). Recent 3D bioprinting attempts with renal cells have only achieved printing of proximal tubule structures (Homan et al., 2016). While this may have the potential to improve the prospect of drug screening, when it comes to modeling human development and disease in vitro, the organization of the body needs to be taken into consideration. Key to the increasing complexity from cells to layered tissues to functioning organs are interactions between individual cells and other types of cells, between cells and their extracellular environment, and even the anatomical relationships between tissue types. The human kidney is a complex organ comprised of a variety of different types of cells and tissues, and kidney function is based on the intricate interplay of a range of highly specialized cells, as well as its three-dimensional structure. Thus, any approach to building the kidney depends on the generation of the correct cell types in sufficient numbers and purity, in the right location. The advantage of organoids is that they use the self-organizing capacity of renal progenitor cells to produce complex tissue that recapitulates structure and function similar to a foetal kidney. Organoids could serve as a platform for high-throughput nephrotoxicity assays, and may be especially useful to predict drug responses in patient subpopulations.

Recent research has shown that fully developed kidneys can be decellularized to provide a complex natural scaffold and extracellular matrix (ECM). When repopulated with embryonic stem cells, the ECM network exerts spatial and organizational influences on cell migration and differentiation (Batchelder et al., 2015). However, a lack of efficient differentiation of the seeded cells into the many normally occurring renal cell types hinders the efficacy of such an approach (McKee and Wingert, 2016). A greater understanding of the specific signaling cues occurring between the renal ECM and seeded cells is likely to be crucial. Related to this pursuit, a kidney organoid serves as a powerful tool for studying renal organogenesis, both during development and in the context of kidney regeneration, to provide valuable insights into the complex pathways of recellularization.

DESIGN CONSIDERATIONS

The collecting duct system and nephrons have distinct temporal − spatial origins. The nephron progenitor, MM, derives from posterior IM, while the collecting duct precursor, UB, derives from anterior IM. Previous attempts to make kidney organoids from pluripotent cells, which paid little attention to this difference, either had very low efficiency (Taguchi et al., 2014), or directed the differentiation of pluripotent stem cells towards only one population; metanephric mesenchyme or ureteric bud (Kang and Han, 2014; Lam et al., 2014; Morizane et al., 2015; Xia et al., 2013).

The protocol we describe here has been adapted from a published study by Takasato et al. (2015). In this study, human-induced pluripotent stem cells are directed through a three-stage differentiation protocol under chemically defined culture conditions (Takasato et al., 2015). The first stage of differentiation is to induce the cells into primitive streak with a high dose of a canonical Wnt signaling agonist, CHIR99021. The second stage is to induce IM from primitive streak by treating the cells with FGF9, which is expressed in IM and supports MM survival in vitro (Barak et al., 2012; Colvin et al., 1999). Cranial − caudal patterning of intermediate mesoderm (in mouse, the cranial − caudal axis is the same as the anterior − posterior axis, hence the names anterior IM and posterior IM) is carefully balanced by adjusting the length of exposure in CHIR and FGF9. At mid-term, cells that have been growing as monolayers are lifted and made into pellets, then cultured at a gas-medium interface. At this point, another pulse of CHIR treatment is given, which actively triggers nephrogenesis and maximizes the number of nephrons produced in three-dimensions. The last stage of differentiation simply withdraws all factors, and allows the cells to further mature and self-organize.

This protocol succeeded in differentiating iPSCs into both renal progenitors (UB and MM) at the same time, recapitulating renal embryogenesis in a more physiologic manner, in which each of the renal progenitors induces development and differentiation of the other. The complex multicellular kidney organoid generated using this method comprises fully segmented nephrons surrounded by endothelia and renal interstitium, and is transcriptionally similar to a first trimester human foetal kidney. In addition, the proximal tubular cells undergo acute apoptosis when exposed to a test nephrotoxicant (Takasato et al., 2015).

The organoid can be further modified using CRISPR/Cas9 gene editing technology to create a disease-specific organoid. For example, knockout of *PKD1* and *PKD2* induces cyst formation in renal tubules, and knockout of podocalyxin causes junctional organization defects in podocyte cells (Freedman et al., 2015). This opens up opportunities for functional studies of human micro-physiology, pathophysiology, and regenerative medicine. The use of hiPSCs as starting material minimizes ethical issues, and enables applications in patient-specific disease modeling and nephrotoxicity screening.

REMAINING CHALLENGES

The generation of kidney organoids has enormous potential benefits for research in kidney regeneration and toxicology. However, there are still challenges that need to be addressed.

The obvious anatomical difference between organoid and native kidney remains as a major challenge. Rather than having nephrons arranged around a single collecting duct tree with a clear exit, the organoid consists of dispersed multiple nonconnected collecting ducts. Also, at present, the organoid in culture reaches up to 8 mm in diameter containing up to 100 nephrons; this is a huge scale-down from an adult kidney, both in size and nephron number. Another limitation of the organoid is vascularization. Although it is reported that an endothelial capillary network was observed in a kidney organoid, a developed peritubular vascular network with glomerular capillaries is still lacking. Sorting different cell types from the organoid, and combining them in the right proportion to engineer a more organized structure could be a way to solve part of the problem.

While there is certainly a long way to go when it comes to generating a functional replacement organ, at the current time, using organoids as a tool for drug screening or disease modeling seems to be more realistic. Nonetheless, meticulous assessment of the functional maturity of different cellular types is still needed.

METHODOLOGY

Reagents:

- Corning Matrigel (BD Biosciences, cat. 354277)
- KnockOut-DMEM (Life Technologies, cat. 10829-018)
- Essential 8 (E8) medium (Life Technologies, cat. A1517001)
- ROCK inhibitor Y-27632 (Tocris, cat. 1254)
- Dulbecco's PBS (DPBS) (Gibco, cat. 14190-094)
- EDTA 0.5 M (Sigma, cat. 03690)
- hiPSC cell line (Lonza Walkersville.inc, clone SFC-AD3-01)
- DMSO (Applichem, cat. A3276)

Equipment:

- 6-well cell culture plates (Geiner Bio-one, Cat. 657160)
- Graduated pipette 1.5 mL, 5 mL, 10 mL
- Pipette controller (Pipetboy, Integra Biosciences)
- Pipetman P3, P20, P200, P1000 (Gilson)
- Pipette tips
- Light microscopy
- Centrifuge
- 15 mL, 50 mL Falcon tubes
- Cryovials
- Nalgene Mr. Frosty Freezing container (Sigma, cat. C1562)
- Biosafety cabinet
- CO_2 incubator

Reagent preparation:

- Matrigel aliquots:
  - Thaw Matrigel on ice at 4°C overnight.
  - Always handle Matrigel on ice and use chilled pipettes and tips to aliquot Matrigel.
  - Aliquot Matrigel according to batch dilution factor into 15 mL Falcon tube.
  - Store the aliquots at −20°C.
- Prepare 10 mM stock solution of ROCK inhibitor (to be used at a final concentration of 10 μM) and store at −80°C.
- Prepare E8 complete medium by adding 50× E8 supplement to E8 basal medium.

COATING PLATES WITH MATRIGEL

1. Thaw Matrigel on ice at 4°C overnight.
2. Dilute Matrigel with cold KO-DMEM using chilled tips, pipette up and down several times without introducing bubbles.
3. Transfer 1 mL of working Matrigel solution per 1 well of a 6-well plate, rock the plate gently, and make sure that all the surface of the well has been covered.
4. Coated plates could be stored sealed at 4°C for up to one week.

THAWING OF HUMAN IPS CELLS

1. Allow Matrigel coated plates to warm at room temperature for 1 hour before use, then aspirate the excess medium and add 1 mL of E8 medium plus ROCK inhibitor.
2. Remove iPSC from liquid nitrogen and thaw quickly in 37°C water bath.
3. Transfer cell suspension to a 15 mL falcon tube with 5 mL of KO-DMEM (dropwise to the wall of the tube to avoid osmotic shock).
4. Centrifuge at ×180 g for 5 minutes.
5. Aspirate the supernatant.
6. Suspend cells in 1 mL of E8 complete media plus ROCK inhibitor.
7. Seed the cells over the surface of the Matrigel-coated wells and transfer them to the incubator.

PASSAGING OF HUMAN IPS CELLS WITH EDTA

Passage the cells when they reach ~80% confluency.

1. Add ROCK inhibitor to the cells 1 hour before passaging.
2. Wash cells once in DPBS.
3. Add 1 mL of 0.5 mM EDTA (in PBS) per one well of a 6-well plate and incubate at 37°C for 5 minutes.
4. Check under the microscope that the periphery of the colonies starts detaching and holes start appearing in the center, then aspirate the EDTA solution.
5. Add 1 mL of complete E8 medium with ROCK inhibitor per well, and dissociate the cells by pipetting up and down.
6. Cells are re-plated on the surface of Matrigel coated plates at a seeding density ranging from 1:5 to 1:10 (meaning that cells from one well are split into 5- to 10-wells) depending on the passage number of the cells, using higher seeding density with lower passages and lower seeding density for higher passages (with higher passages, cells proliferate faster).
7. Change the spent medium daily with a fresh E8 medium.

CYROPRESERVATION OF HUMAN IPSC

Upon receiving the iPSCs, a stock of cryopreserved cells should be kept in liquid nitrogen to ensure enough cells for further experiments.

1. Add ROCK inhibitor to the cells 1 hr before passaging.
2. Follow the same steps as for cell passaging.
3. Re-suspend cells in 0.9 mL of E8 medium plus ROCK inhibitor and transfer to cryovials.
4. Add 0.1 mL of DMSO per cryovial.
5. Store cryovials in freezing container at $-80°C$ overnight.
6. Transfer cryovials to liquid nitrogen the next day.

HIPSCs DIFFERENTIATION

In addition to the reagents and equipment used in maintaining the iPSCs, the following reagents and equipment are required.

Reagents:

- STEMdiff APEL 2 medium (Stemcell Technologies, cat. 05270)
- PFHM-II protein-free hybridoma medium (Gibco, cat. 12040077)
- CHIR99021 (Tocris, cat. 4423)
- Recombinant human FGF9 (R&D systems, cat. 273-F9)
- Heparin (Stemcell Technologies, cat. 07980)
- BSA fraction V (7.5%) (Gibco, cat. 15260-037)

Equipment:

- Cell culture plates; 6-well, 24-well and 96-well plates (the 24-well plates and the 96-well plates ate used for immunostaining)
- Disposable haemocytometer

Reagent preparation:

- Prepare stock APEL medium by supplementing APEL 2 medium with 5% protein-free hybridoma medium.
- Prepare 20 mM stock solution of the CHIR9901 in DMSO and store the aliquots at $-20°C$.
- Prepare 200 µg/mL stock solution of the recombinant human FGF9 in DPBS containing 0.1% BSA and store aliquots at $-20°C$.

Procedure:

1. Coat plates with Matrigel; 1 mL/well for 6-well plates, 0.3 mL/well for 24-well plates, and 50 µL/well for 96-well plates, and incubate at room temperature for 1 hr.
2. Dissociate the iPSCs using the same steps as during regular passaging of the maintenance cells.

3. Transfer the cells into a 15 mL falcon tube and pipette the cell suspension up and down ~20 times using a 5 mL pipette to dissociate the cells into single cells.
4. Seed the cells on the surface of Matrigel coated 6-, 24-, and 96-well plates at a seeding density of 15,000 cells/cm^2, and culture them in E8 complete medium + ROCK inhibitor overnight.
5. Start differentiation on the next morning by removing the spent medium and adding APEL medium containing 8 μM CHIR99021.
6. Change the medium every other day through the whole protocol.
7. After 4 days of CHIR99021 treatment, shift the cells to APEL medium containing 200 ng/mL FGF9 and 1 μg/mL heparin.
8. Continue the FGF9 and heparin treatment for 8 days.
9. On day 13, withdraw all the growth factors, and keep the cells in APEL medium without any growth factors for 5−7 more days.

Notes:

- Cells should reach 50%−60% confluence before starting differentiation.
- Cells tend to detach with the start of CHIR99021 treatment and starting differentiation with fewer cells might lead to cell loss and inability to continue differentiation.

ORGANOID FORMATION AND CULTURE

In addition to the reagents and equipment used in the monolayer culture, the following reagents and equipment are required.

Reagents:

- Antibiotic/Antimycotic (Gibco, cat. 15240-096)
- Trypsin-EDTA (Sigma, cat. T4171)

Equipment:

- Metal grid
- ISOPORE Polycarbonate filter membranes pore size 5 um (Millipore, cat. TMTP02500)
- 30 mm dish (Greiner Bio-one, cat. 627160)
- Micro-centrifuge
- 500 μL Eppendorf tubes
- Flame

Procedure:

For organoid formation, cells are dissociated from monolayers after 7 days of differentiation and cultured in a 3D environment for the rest of the differentiation protocol.

1. Add trypsin-EDTA to the cells (1 mL/well of a 6-well plate and 0.3 mL/well of a 24-well plate) and incubate for 5 minutes.
2. Dissociate the cells by pipetting the trypsin up and down over the wells.

3. Add 1 volume of the trypsin (containing the dissociated cells) to 3 volumes of KO-DMEM medium containing 1% BSA (to dilute and stop the action of the trypsin).
4. Pipette the cell suspension up and down several times, to dissociate the cells into single cells.
5. Spin down the cells at ×180 g for 5 min.
6. Remove the supernatant and re-suspend the cells in APEL medium.
7. Count cells on haemocytometer, then divide the cell suspension into 0.5 mL Eppendorf tubes each containing ∼500,000 cells.
8. Reaggregate the cells by spinning down at ×800 g for 3 min in a micro-centrifuge.
9. Meanwhile, sterilize metal grids on flame and put each of them in a 30 mm dish.
10. Put one of the filter membranes over each metal grid.
11. Transfer the cell pellet onto the surface of the polyester membrane.
12. Treat pellets with CHI99021 (5 μM) in APEL medium for 1 hour then change medium with APEL containing FGF9 (200 ng/mL) and heparin (1 μg/mL), and add antibiotic/antimycotic to the culture medium to prevent infection.
13. Withdraw all growth factors after 5 days of culturing the organoids, and keep them in APEL medium without any growth factors.

Notes:

Change the medium every other day, and pay careful attention to keep the medium level in the culture below the polyester membrane and prevent overflow (the pellets should grow at gas-medium interface).

MONOLAYER IMMUNOSTAINING

Reagents:

- 1 X PBS
- BSA (Sigma, cat. A9647)
- Triton X-100 (Sigma, cat. X100)
- 4% PFA in PBS (Santa Cruz, cat. Sc-281692)

Anti-bodies:

- Oct3/4 (BD Biosciences, cat. 611202)
- Rabbit anti-MIXL1 (GeneTex, cat. GTX60273)
- Rabbit antihuman PAX2 (Biolegend, cat. PRB-276P-200)
- Goat antihuman LHX1 (Santa Cruz Biotechnology, cat. SC-19341)
- Mouse antihuman SIX2 (Abnova, cat. H000-10736-M01)
- Rabbit antihuman Calbindin (Chemicon, cat. AB1778)
- Rabbit antihuman WT1 (Santa Cruz Biotechnology, cat. SC-192)
- Mouse anti-E-cadherin (BD Biosciences, cat. 610181)
- Goat anti-TROP-2 (R&D systems, cat. AF650)
- Sheep anti-NPHS1 (R&D systems, cat. AF4269)
- Rabbit anti-T-Brachyury (Santa Cruz Biotechnology, cat. SC-20109)

- Goat antihuman GATA3 (R&D systems, cat. AF2605)
- Horse AMCA antimouse (Vector Laboratories, cat. C1-2000)
- Donkey antimouse Alexa-488 (Alexa Fluor, cat. A-21202)
- Donkey antirabbit Alexa-594 (Alexa Fluor, cat. A-21207)
- Donkey antigoat Alexa-488 (Alexa Fluor, cat. A-11055)
- Donkey antisheep FITC (Sigma, cat. F7634)
- Vectashield mounting medium (Vector Laboratories, cat. H-1000)

Lectins:

- Fluorescein Lotus lectin (Vector Laboratories, cat. FL-1321)

Equipment:

- Inverted fluorescent microscope (Zeiss Observer D1)

Preparation:

- Prepare 2% BSA solution in PBS.

Procedure:

Perform immunostaining on samples from different stages of the differentiation protocol to confirm stepwise direction of differentiation from pluripotency through the primitive streak, IM stage, and renal differentiation.

1. Aspirate culture medium and wash cells in PBS once, then fix using 4% PFA in PBS for 15 min at room temperature.
2. Wash three times in PBS for 3 minutes each.
3. Use 2% BSA in PBS containing 0.3% Triton X-100 to permeabilize/block the monolayers for 1 hour.
4. Wash cells in PBS three times then incubate with the primary antibodies overnight at 4°C.
5. Wash in PBS three times for 5 minutes each then incubate with secondary antibodies for 1−2 hours at room temperature.
6. Wash in PBS three times for 5 minutes each and image the cells using inverted fluorescence microscope.

Notes:

Working dilutions of the used antibodies are shown in Tables 6.1−6.3, and were prepared using PBS containing 1% BSA.

IMMUNOSTAINING OF THE ORGANOIDS

The same method is used as for staining monolayers, with some differences made for better penetration of the antibodies, and better staining results (since the organoids are thicker than the monolayers):

- Perform the permeabilization/blocking overnight instead of for 1 hour.
- Keep the secondary antibodies overnight at 4°C (rather than 1−2 hours at room temperature).

Table 6.1 List of the Used Primary Antibodies and Their Working Dilutions

Primary Antibodies	Working Dilutions	Company (Cat. Number)	Marker for	Reference
Oct3/4	1:100	BD Biosciences (611202)	Pluripotency	Takahashi and Yamanaka (2006)
Rabbit anti-T Brachyury	1:100	Santa Cruz Biotechnology (SC-20109)	Primitive streak and early stage mesoderm	Rivera-Perez and Magnuson (2005), Beddington et al. (1992)
Rabbit antiMIXL1	1:100	GeneTex (GTX60273)	Primitive streak	Davis et al. (2008)
Rabbit antihuman PAX2	1:200	Biolegend (PRB-276P-200)	IM, UB, MM and renal vesicle	Bouchard et al. (2002), Torres et al. (1995)
Goat anti-human LHX1	1:100	SC (sc-19341)	IM and early renal marker	Tsang et al. (2000)
Mouse anti-human SIX2	1:100	Abnova (H000 10736-M01)	MM and nephrogenic progenitors	Kobayashi et al. (2008), Self et al. (2006)
Rabbit antihuman calbindin	1:200	CHEMICON (AB1778)	Ureteric buds and CD	Davies (1994)
Rabbit antihuman WT1	1:200	Santa Cruz Biotechnology (sc-192)	MM, Cap mesenchyme and podocytes	Kreidberg et al. (1993)
Mouse anti E-cadherin	1:300	BD Bioscience (610181)	Epithelial marker that marks CD and distal convoluted tubules	Lee et al. (2013)
Goat anti-TROP2	1:100	R&D systems (AF650)	Ureteric trunk marker	Tsukahara et al. (2011)
Sheep anti-NPHS1	1:200	R&D systems (AF4269)	Podocyte marker	Ruotsalainen et al. (1999)
Goat antihuman GATA3	1:200	R&D systems (AF2605)	Nephric duct, ureter and collecting ducts	Labastie et al. (1995)

Table 6.2 List of the Used Lectins and Their Working Dilutions

Lectins	Working Dilution	Company (Catalogue Number)	Marker for	Reference
Fluorescein lotus lectin	1:100	Vector laboratories	Proximal convoluted tubules	Barresi et al. (1988) Hennigar et al. (1985)

Table 6.3 List of the Used Secondary Antibodies and Their Working Dilutions

Secondary Antibodies	Working Dilution	Company (Catalogue Number)
Horse AMCA antimouse	1:100	VECTOR (C1-2000)
Donkey antimouse Alexa-488	1:500	Alexa fluor (A-21202)
Donkey antirabbit Alexa-594	1:500	Alexa fluor (A-21207)
Donkey antigoat Alexa-488	1:500	Alexa fluor (A-11055)
Donkey antisheep FITC	1:100	Sigma (F7634)

CRITICAL POINTS

Adding ROCK inhibitor Y-27632 to the culture medium is crucial during freezing and thawing hiPSCs, to achieve maximum cell survival.

During routine passaging of undifferentiated hiPSCs, after EDTA treatment, cells tend to reattach to the plate quickly after adding the E8 medium, to avoid this cells should be detached and collected quickly.

Initial cell density at the start of differentiation is critical for the success of differentiation. Too low density may lead to cell detachment at the beginning stage of differentiation, while too high density may result in growth factors not sufficiently reaching all the cells.

At the point of differentiation when FGF9 was introduced after CHIR treatment (typically starting around Day 4, and may last for 2 days), cells show low adherence and have a tendency to peel off from the culture plate. Very gentle practice is required while changing the medium to minimize the detachment of cells.

VERIFYING

Differentiation Day2:

Morphology: Cells disperse as a monolayer compared to compact colonies when in pluripotent state.

Markers (Primitive streak): T, MIXL1 positive, OCT4 negative. See Fig. 6.2.

Differentiation Day7:

Morphology: Cells become confluent and tightly packed as a sheet.

Markers (Intermediate mesoderm): PAX2, LHX1 positive. See Fig. 6.2.

Differentiation Day18 (end product):

Morphology: The monolayers show tubules and the organoids (typically ~5 mm in diameter) show complex structures inside.

Markers: GATA3, WT1, NPHS1, LTL, JAG1, ECAD, TROP2, CALB, NCAM positive. See Figs. 6.3, 6.4.

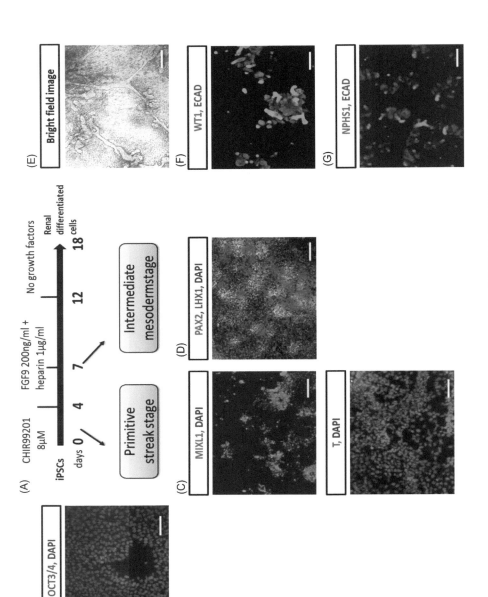

FIGURE 6.2

Monolayer differentiation. (a) Schematic of the differentiation protocol. (b) Undifferentiated iPSCs stained for the pluripotency marker OCT3/4. (c–g) Verification of different steps of differentiation. (c) Immunostaining for 2 days, differentiated cells showing MIXL1+ (top) and T+ (Brachyury) (bottom) cells, both are markers for the primitive streak stage. (d) Immunostaining for 7 days, differentiated cells showing the intermediate mesoderm stage markers; PAX2 (red) and LHX1 (green). (e) Bright-field image for the monolayer after 18 days of differentiation showing branching tubules. (f–g) Immunostaining for 18 days differentiated monolayers; (f) stained for WT1 (MM and podocyte marker, shown in red), and ECAD (distal tubule and collecting duct marker, shown in green). (g) Stained for NPHS1 (podocyte marker, shown in red) and ECAD (green). Scale bar is 200 μM.

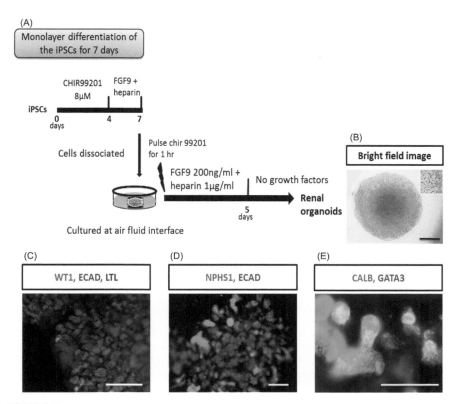

FIGURE 6.3

Organoid formation and differentiation. (a) Schematic of the different steps of culturing organoids. (b) Bright-field image for an organoid after a total of 18 days in culture (7 days as monolayer and 11 days as organoid).The insert is a magnified part of the organoid. Scale bar is 1mm. (b–d) 11 days differentiated organoids (18 days of total culture and differentiation) stained for different renal markers; (b) WT1 (MM and podocyte marker) is shown in red, LTL (proximal tubular marker) is shown in blue, and ECAD (distal tubular and collecting duct marker) is shown in green. (c) NPHS1 (podocyte marker) shown in red and ECAD (in green). (d) CALB (red) and GATA3 (green), both are ureteric bud markers. Scale bar is 200 μM.

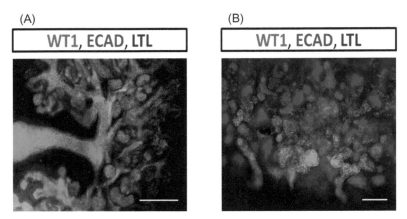

FIGURE 6.4

(A) E11.5 mouse kidney cultured for 7 days and stained for WT1 (red), ECAD (green) and LTL (blue). (B) Renal organoid, after a total of 18 days in culture (7 days as monolayer and 11 days as organoid), stained for the same markers for comparison. Scale bar is 200 μM.

REFERENCES

Aschauer, L., Carta, G., Vogelsang, N., Schlatter, E., Jennings, P., 2015. Expression of xenobiotic transporters in the human renal proximal tubule cell line RPTEC/TERT1. Toxicol. Vitr. 30, 95—105.

Batchelder, C.A., Martinez, M.L., Tarantal, A.F., Shin'oka, T., Imai, Y., et al., 2015. Natural Scaffolds for Renal Differentiation of Human Embryonic Stem Cells for Kidney Tissue Engineering. PLoS One 10, e0143849.

Barak, H., Huh, S.H., Chen, S., Jeanpierre, C., Martinovic, J., Parisot, M., et al., 2012. FGF9 and FGF20 maintain the stemness of nephron progenitors in mice and man. Dev. Cell 22 (6), 1191—1207.

Barresi, G., Tuccari, G., Arena, F., 1988. Peanut and Lotus tetragonolobus binding sites in human kidney from congenital nephrotic syndrome of Finnish type. Histochemistry 89 (2), 117—120.

Basson, M.A., Akbulut, S., Watson-Johnson, J., Simon, R., Carroll, T.J., Shakya, R., et al., 2005. Sprouty1 is a critical regulator of GDNF/RET-mediated kidney induction. Dev Cell 8 (2), 229—239.

Bauchet, A.L., Masson, R., Guffroy, M., Slaoui, M., 2011. Immunohistochemical identification of kidney nephron segments in the dog, rat, mouse, and cynomolgus monkey. Toxicol Pathol. 39 (7), 1115—1128.

Beddington, R.S., Rashbass, P., Wilson, V., 1992. Brachyury — a gene affecting mouse gastrulation and early organogenesis. Dev. Suppl. 166, 157—165.

Bertram, J.F., Douglas-Denton, R.N., Diouf, B., Hughson, M.D., Hoy, W.E., 2011. Human nephron number: implications for health and disease. Pediatr Nephrol. 26 (9), 1529—1533.

Bouchard, M., Souabni, A., Mandler, M., Neubuser, A., Busslinger, M., 2002. Nephric lineage specification by Pax2 and Pax8. Genes Dev. 16, 2958—2970.

Boyle, S., Misfeldt, A., Chandler, K.J., Deal, K.K., Southard-Smith, E.M., Mortlock, D.P., et al., 2008. Fate mapping using Cited1-CreERT2 mice demonstrates that the cap mesenchyme contains self-renewing progenitor cells and gives rise exclusively to nephronic epithelia. Dev Biol. 313 (1), 234–245.

Brown, A.C., Muthukrishnan, S.D., Guay, J.A., Adams, D.C., Schafer, D.A., Fetting, J.L., et al., 2013. Role for compartmentalization in nephron progenitor differentiation. Proc. Natl. Acad. Sci. U.S.A. 110 (12), 4640–4645.

Carroll, T.J., Park, J.S., Hayashi, S., Majumdar, A., McMahon, A.P., 2005. Wnt9b plays a central role in the regulation of mesenchymal to epithelial transitions underlying organogenesis of the mammalian urogenital system. Dev Cell 9 (2), 283–292.

Cheng, H.T., Miner, J.H., Lin, M., Tansey, M.G., Roth, K., Kopan, R., 2003. Gamma-secretase activity is dispensable for mesenchyme-to-epithelium transition but required for podocyte and proximal tubule formation in developing mouse kidney. Development 130 (20), 5031–5042.

Colvin, J.S., Feldman, B., Nadeau, J.H., Goldfarb, M., Ornitz, D.M., 1999. Genomic organization and embryonic expression of the mouse fibroblast growth factor 9 gene. Dev. Dyn. 216, 72–88.

Das, A., Tanigawa, S., Karner, C.M., Xin, M., Lum, L., Chen, C., et al., 2013. Stromal-epithelial crosstalk regulates kidney progenitor cell differentiation. Nat Cell Biol. 15 (9), 1035–1044.

Davidson, A.J., 2009. Mouse kidney development. In: StemBook (Ed.), The Stem Cell Research Community, StemBook.

Davies, J., 1994. Control of calbindin-D28K expression in developing mouse kidney. Dev. Dyn. 199 (1), 45–51.

Davies, J.A., Chang, C.H., 2014. Engineering kidneys from simple cell suspensions: an exercise in self-organization. Pediatr Nephrol. 29 (4), 519–524.

Davies, J.A., Garrod, D.R., 1995. Induction of early stages of kidney tubule differentiation by lithium ions. Dev Biol. 167 (1), 50–60.

Davis, R.P., Ng, E.S., Costa, M., Mossman, A.K., Sourris, K., Elefanty, A.G., et al., 2008. Targeting a GFP reporter gene to the MIXL1 locus of human embryonic stem cells identifies human primitive streak-like cells and enables isolation of primitive hematopoietic precursors. Blood 111 (4), 1876–1884.

Deltombe, O., Van Biesen, W., Glorieux, G., Massy, Z., Dhondt, A., Eloot, S., 2015. Exploring Protein Binding of Uremic Toxins in Patients with Different Stages of Chronic Kidney Disease and during Hemodialysis. Toxins (Basel) 7 (10), 3933–3946.

Dressler, G.R., 2006. The cellular basis of kidney development. Annu Rev Cell Dev Biol. 22, 509–529.

Dressler, G.R., Deutsch, U., Chowdhury, K., Nornes, H.O., Gruss, P., 1990. Pax2, a new murine paired-box-containing gene and its expression in the developing excretory system. Development 109 (4), 787–795.

Drummond, I.A., Majumdar, A., Hentschel, H., Elger, M., Solnica-Krezel, L., Schier, A.F., et al., 1998. Early development of the zebrafish pronephros and analysis of mutations affecting pronephric function. Development 125 (23), 4655–4667.

Fetting, J.L., Guay, J.A., Karolak, M.J., Iozzo, R.V., Adams, D.C., Maridas, D.E., et al., 2014. FOXD1 promotes nephron progenitor differentiation by repressing decorin in the embryonic kidney. Development 141 (1), 17–27.

Freedman, B.S., Brooks, C.R., Lam, A.Q., Fu, H., Morizane, R., et al., 2015. Modelling kidney disease with CRISPR-mutant kidney organoids derived from human pluripotent epiblast spheroids. Nat. Commun. 6, 8715.

Fujii, T., Pichel, J.G., Taira, M., Toyama, R., Dawid, I.B., Westphal, H., 1994. Expression patterns of the murine LIM class homeobox gene lim1 in the developing brain and excretory system. Dev Dyn. 199 (1), 73−83.

Ganeva, V., Unbekandt, M., Davies, J.A., 2011. An improved kidney dissociation and reaggregation culture system results in nephrons arranged organotypically around a single collecting duct system. Organogenesis 7 (2), 83−87.

Gifford, S., Zambon, J.P., Orlando, G., 2015. Recycling organs - growing tailor-made replacement kidneys. Regen Med. 10 (8), 913−915.

Grieshammer, U., Ma, L., Plump, A.S., Wang, F., Tessier-Lavigne, M., Martin, G.R., 2004. SLIT2-mediated ROBO2 signaling restricts kidney induction to a single site. Dev Cell 6 (5), 709−717.

Grobstein, C., 1953. Morphogenetic interaction between embryonic mouse tissues separated by a membrane filter. Nature 172, 869−871.

Grobstein, C., 1955. Inductive interaction in the development of the mouse metanephros. J. Exp. Zool. 130, 319−340.

Grote, D., Souabni, A., Busslinger, M., Bouchard, M., 2006. Pax 2/8-regulated Gata 3 expression is necessary for morphogenesis and guidance of the nephric duct in the developing kidney. Development 133, 53−61.

Hennigar, R.A., Schulte, B.A., Spicer, S.S., 1985. Heterogeneous distribution of glycoconjugates in human kidney tubules. Anat Rec. 211, 376−390.

Herzlinger, D., Koseki, C., Mikawa, T., al-Awqati, Q., 1992. Metanephric mesenchyme contains multipotent stem cells whose fate is restricted after induction. Development 114 (3), 565−572.

Hinchliffe, S.A., Sargent, P.H., Howard, C.V., Chan, Y.F., van Velzen, D., 1991. Human intrauterine renal growth expressed in absolute number of glomeruli assessed by the disector method and Cavalieri principle. Lab Investig. 64 (6), 777−784.

Homan, K.A., Kolesky, D.B., Skylar-Scott, M.A., Herrmann, J., Obuobi, H., et al., 2016. Bioprinting of 3D convoluted renal proximal tubules on perfusable chips. Sci. Rep. 6, 34845.

Huang, J.X., Kaeslin, G., Ranall, M.V., Blaskovich, M.A., Becker, B., Butler, M.S., et al., 2015. Evaluation of biomarkers for in vitro prediction of drug-induced nephrotoxicity: comparison of HK-2, immortalized human proximal tubule epithelial, and primary cultures of human proximal tubular cells. Pharmacol. Res. Perspect. 3, e00148.

Jenkinson, S.E., Chung, G.W., vanLoon, E., Bakar, N.S., Dalzell, A.M., Brown, C.D.A., 2012. The limitations of renal epithelial cell line HK-2 as a model of drug transporter expression and function in the proximal tubule. Eur. J. Physiol. 464, 601−611.

Kang, M., Han, Y.-M., 2014. Differentiation of human pluripotent stem cells into nephron progenitor cells in a serum and feeder free system. PLoS One 9, e94888.

Kerecuk, L., Schreuder, M.F., Woolf, A.S., 2008. Renal tract malformations: perspectives for nephrologists. Nat. Clin. Pract. Nephrol. 4, 312−325.

Kitamoto, Y., Tokunaga, H., Tomita, K., 1997. Vascular endothelial growth factor is an essential molecule for mouse kidney development: glomerulogenesis and nephrogenesis. J. Clin. Investig. 99 (10), 2351−2357.

Kobayashi, A., Valerius, M.T., Mugford, J.W., Carroll, T.J., Self, M., Oliver, G., et al., 2008. Six2 defines and regulates a multipotent self-renewing nephron progenitor population throughout mammalian kidney development. Cell Stem Cell 3 (2), 169−181.

Kreidberg, J.A., Sariola, H., Loring, J.M., Maeda, M., Pelletier, J., Housman, D., et al., 1993. WT-1 is required for early kidney development. Cell 74 (4), 679−691.

Kume, T., Deng, K., Hogan, B.L., 2000. Murine forkhead/winged helix genes Foxc1 (Mf1) and Foxc2 (Mfh1) are required for the early organogenesis of the kidney and urinary tract. Development 127 (7), 1387−1395.

Labastie, M.C., Catala, M., Gregoire, J.M., Peault, B., 1995. The GATA-3 gene is expressed during human kidney embryogenesis. Kidney Int. 47 (6), 1597−1603.

Lam, A.Q., Freedman, B.S., Morizane, R., Lerou, P.H., Valerius, M.T., Bonventre, J.V., 2014. Rapid and efficient differentiation of human pluripotent stem cells into intermediate mesoderm that forms tubules expressing kidney proximal tubular markers. J. Am. Soc. Nephrol. 25, 1211−1225.

Lee, S.Y., Han, S.M., Kim, J.E., Chung, K.Y., Han, K.H., 2013. Expression of E-cadherin in pig kidney. J Vet Sci. 14 (4), 381−386.

Lindström, N.O., Lawrence, M.L., Burn, S.F., Johansson, J.A., Bakker, E.R., Ridgway, R.A., et al., 2015. Integrated β-catenin, BMP, PTEN, and Notch signalling patterns the nephron. Elife. 3, e04000.

Little, M.H., McMahon, A.P., 2012. Mammalian kidney development: principles, progress, and projections. Cold Spring Harb. Perspect. Biol 4 (5), 2012 May 1.

Liyanage, T., Ninomiya, T., Jha, V., Neal, B., Patrice, H.M., Okpechi, I., et al., 2015. Worldwide access to treatment for end-stage kidney disease: a systematic review. Lancet. 385 (9981), 1975−1982.

McKee, R.A., Wingert, R.A., 2016. Repopulating decellularized kidney scaffolds: an avenue for ex vivo organ generation. Materials (Basel) 9, 3.

Miyazaki, Y., Oshima, K., Fogo, A., Hogan, B.L., Ichikawa, I., 2000. Bone morphogenetic protein 4 regulates the budding site and elongation of the mouse ureter. J. Clin. Investig. 105 (7), 863−873.

Morizane, R., Lam, A.Q., Freedman, B.S., Kishi, S., Valerius, M.T., Bonventre, J.V., 2015. Nephron organoids derived from human pluripotent stem cells model kidney development and injury. Nat. Biotechnol. 33, 1193−1200.

Mugford, J.W., Sipilä, P., McMahon, J.A., McMahon, A.P., 2008. Osr1 expression demarcates a multi-potent population of intermediate mesoderm that undergoes progressive restriction to an Osr1-dependent nephron progenitor compartment within the mammalian kidney. Dev. Biol. 324 (1), 88−98.

Mujais, S., Story, K., 2006. Patient and technique survival on peritoneal dialysis in patients with failed renal allograft: a case-control study. Kidney Int. Suppl 103, S133−S137.

Murphy, S.V., Atala, A., 2014. 3D bioprinting of tissues and organs. Nat. Biotechnol. 32 (8), 773−785.

Nielsen, S., Agre, P., 1995. The aquaporin family of water channels in kidney. Kidney Int. 48, 1057−1068.

Nieskens, T.T.G., Peters, J.G.P., Schreurs, M.J., Smits, N., Woestenenk, R., Jansen, K., et al., 2016. A human renal proximal tubule cell line with stable organic anion transporter 1 and 3 expression predictive for antiviral-induced toxicity. AAPS J. 18, 465−475.

Pachnis, V., Mankoo, B., Costantini, F., 1993. Expression of the c-ret proto-oncogene during mouse embryogenesis. Development 119 (4), 1005−1017.

Poladia, D.P., Kish, K., Kutay, B., Hains, D., Kegg, H., Zhao, H., et al., 2006. Role of fibroblast growth factor receptors 1 and 2 in the metanephric mesenchyme. Dev. Biol. 291 (2), 325−339.

Qiao, J., Uzzo, R., Obara-Ishihara, T., Degenstein, L., Fuchs, E., Herzlinger, D., 1999. FGF 7 modulates ureteric bud growth and nephron number in the developing kidney. Development 126 (3), 547−554.

Rivera-Perez, J.A., Magnuson, T., 2005. Primitive streak formation in mice is preceded by localized activation of brachyury and Wnt3. Dev. Biol. 288 (2), 363−371.

Robert, B., St John, P.L., Hyink, D.P., Abrahamson, D.R., 1996. Evidence that embryonic kidney cells expressing flk-1 are intrinsic, vasculogenic angioblasts. Am. J. Physiol. 271 (3 Pt 2), F744−F753.

Rumballe, B.A., Georgas, K.M., Combes, A.N., Ju, A.L., Gilbert, T., Little, M.H., 2011. Nephron formation adopts a novel spatial topology at cessation of nephrogenesis. Dev Biol. 360, 110−122.

Ruotsalainen, V., Ljungberg, P., Wartiovaara, J., Lenkkeri, U., Kestilä, M., Jalanko, H., et al., 1999. Nephrin is specifically located at the slit diaphragm of glomerular podocytes. Proc. Natl. Acad. Sci. U.S.A. 96 (14), 7962−7967.

Sainio, K., Suvanto, P., Davies, J., Wartiovaara, J., Wartiovaara, K., Saarma, M., et al., 1997. Glial-cell-line-derived neurotrophic factor is required for bud initiation from ureteric epithelium. Development 124 (20), 4077−4087.

Saxen, L., 1987. Organogenesis of the kidney. In: Barlow, P.W., Green, P.B., White, C.C. (Eds.), Developmental and Cell Biology Series 19. Cambridge Univ. Press, Cambridge, UK, pp. 1−171.

Schrijvers, B.F., Flyvbjerg, A., De Vriese, A.S., 2004. The role of vascular endothelial growth factor (VEGF) in renal pathophysiology. Kidney Int. 65 (6), 2003−2017.

Self, M., Lagutin, O.V., Bowling, B., Hendrix, J., Cai, Y., Dressler, G.R., et al., 2006. Six2 is required for suppression of nephrogenesis and progenitor renewal in the developing kidney. EMBO J. 25 (21), 5214−5228.

Simon, M., Gröne, H.J., Jöhren, O., Kullmer, J., Plate, K.H., Risau, W., et al., 1995. Expression of vascular endothelial growth factor and its receptors in human renal ontogenesis and in adult kidney. Am. J. Physiol. 268 (2 Pt 2), F240−F250.

Simon-Friedt, B.R., Wilson, M.J., Blake, D.A., Yu, H., Eriksson, Y., Wickliffe, J.K., 2015. The RPTEC/TERT1 cell line as an improved tool for in vitro nephrotoxicity assessments. Biol. Trace Elem. Res. 166, 66−71.

Stark, K., Vainio, S., Vassileva, G., McMahon, A.P., 1994. Epithelial transformation of metanephric mesenchyme in the developing kidney regulated by Wnt-4. Nature. 372 (6507), 679−683.

Taguchi, A., Kaku, Y., Ohmori, T., Sharmin, S., Ogawa, M., Sasaki, H., et al., 2014. Redefining the in vivo origin of metanephric nephron progenitors enables generation of complex kidney structures from pluripotent stem cells. Cell Stem Cell 14, 53−67.

Takahashi, K., Yamanaka, S., 2006. Induction of pluripotent stem cells from mouse embryonic and adult fibroblast cultures by defined factors. Cell 126 (4), 663−676.

Takasato, M., Er, P.X., Chiu, H.S., Maier, B., Baillie, G.J., Ferguson, C., et al., 2015. Kidney organoids from human iPS cells contain multiple lineages and model human nephrogenesis. Nature 526, 564−568.

Torres, M., Gómez-Pardo, E., Dressler, G.R., Gruss, P., 1995. Pax-2 controls multiple steps of urogenital development. Development 121 (12), 4057–4065.

Tsang, T.E., Shawlot, W., Kinder, S.J., Kobayashi, A., Kwan, K.M., Schughart, K., et al., 2000. Lim1 activity is required for intermediate mesoderm differentiation in the mouse embryo. Dev. Biol. 223 (1), 77–90.

Tsukahara, Y., Tanaka, M., Miyajima, A., 2011. TROP2 expressed in the trunk of the ureteric duct regulates branching morphogenesis during kidney development. PLoS One 6 (12), e28607.

Unbekandt, M., Davies, J.A., 2010. Dissociation of embryonic kidneys followed by reaggregation allows the formation of renal tissues. Kidney Int. 77 (5), 407–416.

Vize, P.D., Seufert, D.W., Carroll, T.J., Wallingford, J.B., 1997. Model systems for the study of kidney development: use of the pronephros in the analysis of organ induction and patterning. Dev Biol. 188 (2), 189–204.

Wellik, D.M., Hawkes, P.J., Capecchi, M.R., 2002. Hox11 paralogous genes are essential for metanephric kidney induction. Genes Dev. 16 (11), 1423–1432.

Xia, Y., Nivet, E., Sancho-Martinez, I., Gallegos, T., Suzuki, K., Okamura, D., et al., 2013. Directed differentiation of human pluripotent cells to ureteric bud kidney progenitor-like cells. Nat. Cell Biol. 15, 1507–1515.

Yang, K.S., Kim, J.I., Moon, I.S., Choi, B.S., Park, C.W., Yang, C.W., et al., 2013. The clinical outcome of end-stage renal disease patients who return to peritoneal dialysis after renal allograft failure. Transplant Proc. 45 (8), 2949–2952.

Yokoo, T., Kawamura, T., Kobayashi, E., 2008. Kidney organogenesis and regeneration: a new era in the treatment of chronic renal failure? Clin. Exp. Nephrol. 12 (5), 326–331.

Zhao, H., Kegg, H., Grady, S., Truong, H.T., Robinson, M.L., Baum, M., et al., 2004. Role of fibroblast growth factor receptors 1 and 2 in the ureteric bud. Dev. Biol. 276 (2), 403–415.

Spontaneous self-assembly of liver organoids from differentiated human cells

7

Human liver organoids

Haristi Gaitantzi and Katja Breitkopf-Heinlein

Heidelberg University, Mannheim, Germany

INTRODUCTION

Traditionally, in vitro experimental research has been performed with two-dimensional (2D) monolayer cell cultures. Using primary cells that had been isolated from animals or even human tissue was considered the "gold standard", because it was relatively free from the effects of adaptation to long-term culture, particularly of transformation. With time, the value of results obtained only with such cultures (even with primary cells) has become subject to more and more doubt, and they were often replaced by animal models, mainly mice or rats. While an animal perfectly incorporates systemic aspects and 3D cell − cell communications of the species concerned, it turned out that many of these models do not satisfactorily mimic the corresponding human physiology or disease. The reasons for this are diverse: sometimes (artificial) ways of causing damage to model a disease in an animal lead to disease characteristics that are different from the corresponding human disease. Chronic diseases such as alcoholic liver disease (ALD), for example, develop over long time periods in humans, perhaps several decades. To model such complex long-term processes in animals such as mice,

Organoids and Mini-Organs. DOI: http://dx.doi.org/10.1016/B978-0-12-812636-3.00007-9

with short life times, is obviously difficult. Animal models often reflect only certain aspects or stages of complex diseases, rather than really reproducing the human situation (Teufel et al., 2016; Lin et al., 2014). But, even if the model mimics the disease quite well, there always remains the issue of species differences. The metabolic capacity of murine livers is quite different from that of humans (see e.g., Takahashi et al., 2016; Xie et al., 2013), probably as a consequence of diverse evolutionary adaptations leading to different sets of hepatic enzyme-isoforms and variations.

Therefore, the construction of three-dimensional liver-like structures composed of the diverse hepatic cell types from human sources has become a challenging goal of research by universities, as well as by industry. Such differentiated, tissue-like structures are anticipated to be stable in long-term cultures, with the final goal that they remain vital and functional even after transplantation into a host organism. Even personalized approaches with restitution of organoids from the same donors' cells are already being envisioned, and harbor great potential for future therapies.

DEVELOPMENT, STRUCTURE, AND FUNCTION OF THE NATURAL LIVER

The liver is an organ of great importance to metabolism. As well as being responsible for detoxification of xenobiotics from the blood and converting ammonia into urea, the liver synthesizes albumin and various amino acids, coagulation factors (I, II, V, VII, IX, X, XI, protein C, protein S, and anti-thrombin), and certain hormones. Other functions of the liver include breakdown of insulin and other hormones, storage of nutrients necessary for body health such as glucose, Vitamin A, Vitamin D, iron, and others, and production of immune factors. This wide range of functions performed by a healthy liver means that death is the typical consequence of acute liver failure. There is often no cure for advanced liver disease, making liver transplantation the only option. Liver transplantation is nowadays a routine procedure, with excellent outcomes. However, shortage of donors means that many patients die while waiting for a suitable transplant. In the UK, up to 18% of adults listed for a first elective transplant will die or become too ill for the operation before a graft is available (NHS Blood and Transplant, Liver Activity Report www.odt.nhs.uk).

During embryogenesis, formation of liver tissue is a complex process that is not yet fully understood. The two main liver cell types, hepatocytes and cholangiocytes, derive from endoderm that emerges from the anterior primitive streak of the gastrulating embryo, and is identifiable by the shield stage at embryonic day 7.5 in mouse, and in the third week of human gestation (Gordillo et al., 2015). By mouse embryonic day 9—10 the liver bud containing hepatoblasts forms, and endothelial cells form a necklace around and adjacent to the mouse liver diverticulum. By around embryonic day 18.5 in mouse, and 210 in humans, the hepatoblasts have differentiated into hepatocytes and cholangiocytes. During the last weeks of gestation, inhibition of glycolytic enzymes, coupled with the rise in gluconeogenic enzyme levels, reflects maturation of the liver from a primarily glycolytic role in the first two trimesters to a gluconeogenic role shortly before birth. Hepatocyte maturation continues after birth, with an age-dependent reduction in lipid-to-protein ratio, and increasing membrane cholesterol content that in turn decreases membrane fluidity (Devi et al., 1992).

Fortunately for patients suffering liver damage, the liver is also an organ of extraordinary regeneration capacity. Typically, the adult liver can recover completely from short-term exposure to damaging toxicants. Unlike any other organ, the liver responds to sudden loss of substantial amounts of organ mass by rapidly counterbalancing tissue loss using a complex, but very efficient, process of regrowth up to the original liver mass. Interestingly, this process is not executed by some kind of "outgrowth" at the site of injury, but involves the whole remaining tissue "sensing" the amount of lost material and inducing a controlled proliferation stimulus to many, and perhaps all, remaining cells. This means that loss of half of the liver mass leads to an average of one extra proliferation of each remaining cell, instead of hyper-proliferative activity of the cells at the site of damage. This implies that adult, differentiated liver cells are capable of complete regeneration, seemingly without the need for stem cell involvement.

The adult liver is mainly composed of the following five cell types:

1. *Hepatocytes*: The liver parenchyma mainly consists of hepatocytes, which account for almost 90% of the liver mass (Michalopoulos and DeFrances, 1997), and represent the major functional cell type in healthy liver. In normal adult liver, hepatocytes usually show low rates of proliferation. They are in a differentiated, polarized state, arranged within plates of the thickness of one cell to form an optimal architecture for uptake and release of substances from and to the blood-stream on the one side, and secretion of bile on the other side. Such epithelial polarization is a fundamental property of functional hepatocytes, and it rapidly disappears when primary cells are isolated and cultured as monolayers (Meyer et al., 2015). This dedifferentiation of hepatocytes in vitro most probably results from the loss of necessary three-dimensional cell − cell and cell − matrix interactions. In addition, hepatocytes seem to sense the overall pressure within the liver that is formed by blood flowing in from the intestine via the portal vein and via the hepatic artery delivering the necessary oxygen on the one side, and the efflux of bile on the other side. Changes in pressure, or acute damage, for example due to exposure to hepatotoxic substances, can cause remaining hepatocytes to dedifferentiate. This dedifferentiation includes at least transient arrest of function, increased proliferation, and migration to the site of injury, as well as induction of apoptosis and/or necrosis. Transient dedifferentiation can be considered as a wound-healing response aiming at regeneration of liver functionality.

However, if the injury is too severe, the mature hepatocytes may reach their limit of regenerative capacity, resulting in cellular senescence and arrest of liver regeneration. In that case, another type of quiescent cell, the progenitor cell, which is thought to reside in the canals of Hering, will become activated. These cells can still differentiate into either hepatocytes or cholangiocytes. Therefore, liver regeneration may still be achieved (Riehle et al., 2011).

2. *Hepatic stellate cells (HSC)*: This cell type, also called Ito cell or fat-storing cell, represents the liver pericyte, and in normal liver HSC accounts for 5%−8% of the whole liver cell number. They are located within the space of Disse, between the sinusoidal endothelial cells and the hepatocyte plates. In the healthy liver, HSC are quiescent, storing Vitamin D fat droplets. They become activated by liver damage, and trans-differentiate into fibroblast-like cells, producing scar tissue (mainly collagens) and secreting a diverse set of cytokines. Through these cytokines, they communicate with other hepatic cell types and contribute profoundly to wound-healing processes including fibrosis, inflammation, and regeneration (Hellerbrand, 2013).

3. *Liver sinusoidal endothelial cells (LSEC)*: The extensions of the portal vein and the hepatic artery form a network of so-called sinusoids which criss-cross the whole liver. The architecture of the liver, therefore, forms a kind of sponge with the sinusoids representing the pores, and leading to an expansion of the intrinsic surface area. This allows for an efficient exchange of substances between the blood and the parenchyme. The LSECs line the sinusoid walls to form a loose and easy-to-penetrate barrier (Poisson et al., 2017). In contrast to macrovascular endothelial cells of the large blood vessels, LSECs do not produce a basement membrane under healthy conditions, and they allow even small substance penetration through LSEC-specific formation of fenestrae.

   Another important function of LSECs is that they regulate the hepatic vascular tone so, despite the major changes in hepatic blood flow occurring during digestion, they contribute to the maintenance of a low portal pressure. Interestingly, as a result of direct cellular cross-talk, LSECs can maintain HSC quiescence, thus inhibiting intrahepatic vasoconstriction and fibrosis development. In pathological conditions, LSECs lose their protective properties, and they then promote angiogenesis and vasoconstriction. Similar to hepatocytes, primary isolated LSECs rapidly lose their specialized phenotype when cultured as a monolayer.

4. *Kupffer cells (KC)*: KCs are the resident liver macrophages, the first line of defense against inflammatory agents that reach the liver with the bloodstream. They are located within the sinusoids, loosely attached to the LSEC layer, but also communicating via cellular extensions and secreted factors with other hepatic cell types such as HSC or even hepatocytes (Dixon et al., 2013).

5. *Bile duct epithelial cells (BEC)/cholangiocytes*: Hepatocytes secrete bile salts and detoxification products into the bile canaliculi, which open up into larger

structures and finally unite in the common bile duct. With increase in diameter, the bile ducts gradually become lined by epithelial cells, the cholangiocytes or BECs. In addition to its secretory and excretory functions, the bile duct epithelium also plays an important role in the formation of a barrier to the diffusion of toxic substances from bile into the hepatic interstitial tissue (Rao and Samak, 2013). Bile duct dysfunction, as is seen in some congenital biliary diseases, such as Alagille syndrome and biliary atresia, or bile duct occlusion, lead to the accumulation of bile within the liver. This accumulation (cholestasis) prevents the excretion of detoxification products, and leads ultimately to liver damage.

THE NEED FOR AN ORGANOID/MINI-ORGAN

Liver organoids represent a model that can be used to predict the potential hepatotoxicity of a test substance, e.g., a newly-developed drug. The drug detoxifying enzymes of the liver are quite different in rodents compared to humans, a fact that is reflected in the high tolerance of rats for diverse toxins. This implies that rodent models are a poor choice to be used for determining toxicity of new drugs, or for other approaches like investigating the molecular mechanisms of human liver diseases. The alternative of using human cells in culture harbors a high chance of delivering artifacts that result from nonphysiological culture conditions. This is especially true for 2D (monolayer) cultures. There is widespread use of hepatoma cell lines for toxicity tests as a replacement of primary hepatocytes, but hepatoma cells, being from a cancer, have lost many important features of the primary cells, and may therefore lead to false results. For these reasons, the idea of establishing 3D culture systems composed of several different liver cell types, reflecting faithfully their primary phenotypes, has become an increasingly urgent goal.

In the far future, it might even become possible to grow such organoids in vitro to a size that would allow transplantation, with the goal of supporting a patient's own, damaged liver until a full organ for transplantation becomes available.

DESIGN CONSIDERATIONS

As mentioned above, adult, differentiated liver cells are able to regenerate lost parts of the liver fully, meaning that the regenerative program must always be present, and can become reactivated. If we can manage to activate it in vitro, there would be no need to copy developmental, embryonic processes, or use pluripotent stem cells. Therefore, the idea of our liver organoids was to create an environment in which the cells would spontaneously assemble, and grow into structures which really resemble the normal human liver architecture. Typical spheroids, for example, are cell aggregates that form on nonadhesive surfaces, with randomly distributed cells attaching to each other. Even this already represents the in vivo situation much better than 2D systems but, at least for the liver, it does not get very close to real liver anatomy. The work of Takebe and colleagues, who used stem-cell-derived hepatocytes that spontaneously formed organoids when placed on top of Matrigel (Takebe et al., 2013), served to guide us to develop similar structures using differentiated, adult liver cells.

Since primary human liver cells are of very limited availability, we searched for an alternative which we found in the so-called "upcyte" cells. The upcyte® process involves the stable transfection of primary cells with lentiviral constructs containing sequences leading to expression of growth inducing genes which can be controlled by supplementing or withdrawing certain soluble factors from the growth medium. Stable transfection of primary human hepatocytes, for example, with the human papilloma virus (HPV) genes E6 and E7, was sufficient to induce proliferation of the cells without malignant transformation or fetal reprogramming (Burkard et al., 2012). The transfected cells were selected for low expressing cells, because high over-expression would potentially lead to uncontrolled proliferation. Low expression instead transferred incapability of proliferation in the absence of STAT3 activation. Thus, addition of Oncostatin M (OSM) to the culture medium transiently induces proliferation, whereas its withdrawal allows for redifferentiation of the cells into mature hepatocytes. Second generation upcyte® human hepatocytes can be serially passaged, frozen, and thawed for up to 40 population doublings, without loss of metabolic potential, allowing the production of a total of 10^{13} to 10^{16} cells from a single isolation. Redifferentiated cells show relatively high similarity to primary cells (Levy et al., 2015).

So far, hepatocytes, LSEC and mesenchymal stroma cells (MSC) are available as upcyte® lines, and have been used to generate our first generation of liver organoids (Ramachandran et al., 2015). The "parenchyma" formed within these organoids has already shown important similarities to hepatocytes in vivo, regarding their expression and synthesis of metabolically active enzymes like Cyp450 oxidases, as well as hepatocyte polarization and plate-structure formation (Ramachandran et al., 2015). We have been able to replace the Matrigel by the better-defined and inert matrix, agarose, and to include upcyte® or primary human HSC instead of MSC (see Figs. 7.1–7.3).

REMAINING CHALLENGES

We have already incorporated three important liver cell types: hepatocytes, hepatic stellate cells (HSC), and liver sinusoidal endothelial cells (LSEC). But at least two other cell types are still missing: liver resident macrophages (Kupffer cells), and bile duct epithelial cells (cholangiocytes). Neither of these cell types is yet available

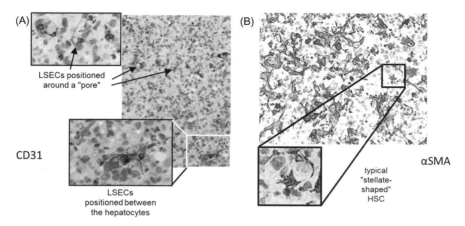

FIGURE 7.1

Immunohistochemical stainings of liver organoids, containing 70% upcyte® hepatocytes, 25% upcyte® LSEC, and 5% upcyte® HSC, 72 h after plating on an agarose matrix. The organoid in (A) was stained for CD31 as general marker of endothelial cells. In (B), expression of α-smooth-muscle-actin (SMA) was determined for the localization of HSC.

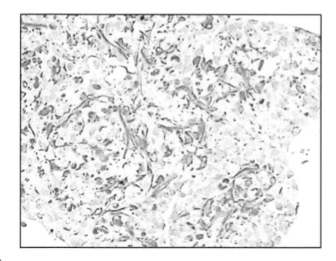

FIGURE 7.2

Immunohistochemical staining of liver organoids, composed and cultured as in Fig. 7.1, but containing primary human HSC instead of upcyte® HSC. The organoid was stained for vimentin, a general mesenchymal marker protein, detecting the HSC in this setting.

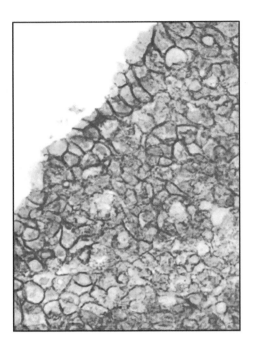

FIGURE 7.3

Immunohistochemical staining of a liver organoid, composed as in Fig. 7.1 after 10 days of culture. The organoid was stained for epithelial cadherin (E-Cadherin), a marker protein for polarized hepatocytes.

as an upcyte® cell line. In the future, we want to include these cell types as well, if not as upcyte® cells, then at least as primary isolated human cells. We have, therefore, begun to establish the isolation procedures for primary hepatocytes, LSEC, HSC, cholangiocytes, and KC from human liver resection samples, and it will be an important task of future studies to construct a human liver organoid with only primary cells from the same donor. Incorporation of KC, or at least blood-derived macrophages, will be another important step towards a system that can also mimic more aspects of the inflammatory response of the liver.

Another remaining challenge is to let "real" sinusoids form inside the organoids. Up to now "spaces" are frequently being formed between the hepatocytes which to some degree resemble sinusoids. We think that these "pores" allow the medium to reach the inside of the organoid, protecting against necrosis in the center. But, while natural sinusoids are lined by LSECs, in our organoids LSECs are located only rarely at the sites of these openings: instead, they are rather evenly distributed throughout the "tissue" (see Fig. 7.1A). The reason for this might be that, so far, we are not able to mimic the physical properties of the hepatic blood flow. We do culture the organoids in a perfusion system, but the sinusoids in vivo are the extensions of the blood vessels themselves, leading to physiological application of flow and pressure especially to the LSEC layer, and to a lower degree also to the hepatocytes behind them. So far, with our system we are not able to reconstruct this physiologic condition of pressure and shear stress, which most likely is the reason why no real sinusoidal spaces, lined with LSEC are forming. More complex setups will be tested in the future, e.g., having the organoid being formed around a pre-existing vascular tree through which the perfusion can be directed.

DETAILED INSTRUCTIONS

(*based on our published protocol*, Ramachandran et al., 2015)

Protocol for 2 organoids (in 2 chambers of the Quasi-vivo® System from Kirkstall with a 24-well plate):

Medium to be mixed with agarose ($\sim$2 mL):

- High Performance medium (Upcyte technologies, Hamburg): 1 mL
- SFM (Serum-free medium; Life technologies): 900 μL
- Fetal calf serum: 100 μL
- Recombinant VEGF to a final concentration of 5 ng/mL
- Recombinant HGF to a final concentration of 5 ng/mL
  - Prewarm this mixture at 37°C

Prepare agarose:

- Add 500 μL water (double-distilled; BBRAUN) to 10 mg agarose (low melting, ultra-pure from Invitrogen)
- Boil in microwave until the fluid clears
- Let cool down a bit, then add the pre-warmed medium (see above); mix well.
- Add 760 μL per chamber (avoid formation of bubbles).
- Let polymerize at 4°C for at least 30 min.

Prepare the medium for the cells ($\sim$3 mL):

- High Performance medium (Upcyte technologies, Hamburg): 1.5 mL
- SFM (Serum-free medium; Life technologies), containing 10% FCS, VEGF (20 ng/mL), HGF (20 ng/mL): 1.5 mL.
- Acetaminophen: 1.5 μL (from a stock of 0.5 M, diluted in ethanol)

Prepare cells (final cell proportions should be roughly: 70% hepatocytes, 25% LSEC, and 5% HSC):

- All cells should have been in culture for at least a few days; do not use freshly thawed cells.
- Dislodge upcyte® hepatocytes with trypsin and count: 3.06 million cells are needed for 2 organoids. Spin down at 90 g for 5 minutes.
- Dislodge upcyte® LSEC with trypsin and count: 1.1 million cells are needed for 2 organoids. Spin down at 720 g for 5 minutes.

- Dislodge upcyte® or primary human HSC with trypsin and count: 220.000 cells are needed for 2 organoids. Spin down at 260 g for 5 minutes.
- Add 320 µL medium drop-wise on top of the polymerized agarose.
- Resuspend the cell pellets one after the other in a total volume of 1.6 mL medium.
- Add 800 µL cell suspension per chamber.
- Incubate at 37°C, 95% O_2, 5% CO_2 over night.
- On the next day, the organoids should have formed spontaneously (Fig. 7.4).
- Connect the organoid-chambers to the perfusion system (Fig. 7.5), and perfuse the chamber(s) with 300 µL/min.
- The medium reservoir containing 25 mL of medium (prepared as described above, but without addition of acetaminophen and with final concentrations of 5 ng/mL VEGF and HGF), is exchanged every 3 days.

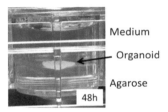

FIGURE 7.4

Liver organoid formed within one well of a 12-well plate 48 h after seeding. The organoid has self-assembled into a sphere, which loosely attaches to the surface of the agarose gel.

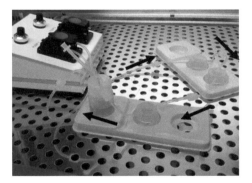

FIGURE 7.5

Three liver organoids cultured with constant perfusion of medium. Several organoids can be cultured "in row", as shown in the picture, or several pump heads can be utilized to generate separated perfusion loops with medium from separate bottles. The arrows indicate the flow direction of the medium.

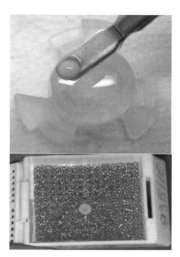

FIGURE 7.6

"Harvesting" of a liver organoid, after 10 days of culture. The organoid was transferred to a histo-cassette for further processing and paraffin block formation.

- After the desired period of time (we tested up to 10 days), the organoids can be harvested by complete transfer to RNA- or protein-lysis buffer, or they can be embedded in paraffin (Fig. 7.6), depending on the desired consecutive method of analysis (e.g., real-time PCR, immunoblot, or immunohistochemistry).

ACKNOWLEDGMENTS

We are thankful to Katharina Schirmer, a former postgraduate of our group, for providing the picture shown in Fig. 7.4.

DECLARATION OF FINANCIAL INTERESTS

Both authors have no conflict of interest to declare.

REFERENCES

Burkard, A., Dähn, C., Heinz, S., Zutavern, A., Sonntag-Buck, V., Maltman, D., et al., 2012. Generation of proliferating human hepatocytes using Upcyte® technology: characterisation and applications in induction and cytotoxicity assays. Xenobiotica. 42, 939−956.

Devi, B.G., Gupta, P.D., Habeebullah, C.M., 1992. Changes in membrane fluidity during human liver development. Biochem. Int. 28, 41−49.

Dixon, L.J., Barnes, M., Tang, H., Pritchard, M.T., Nagy, L.E., 2013. Kupffer cells in the liver. Compr. Physiol. 3, 785−797.

Gordillo, M., Evans, T., Gouon-Evans, V., 2015. Orchestrating liver development. Development 142, 2094−2108.

Hellerbrand, C., 2013. Hepatic stellate cells - the pericytes in the liver. Pflugers Arch. 465, 775−778.

Levy, G., Bomze, D., Heinz, S., Ramachandran, S.D., Noerenberg, A., Cohen, M., et al., 2015. Long-term culture and expansion of primary human hepatocytes. Nat. Biotechnol. 33, 1264−1271.

Lin, S., Lin, Y., Nery, J.R., Urich, M.A., Breschi, A., Davis, C.A., et al., 2014. Comparison of the transcriptional landscapes between human and mouse tissues. Proc. Natl. Acad. Sci. U.S.A. 111, 17224−17229.

Meyer, C., Liebe, R., Breitkopf-Heinlein, K., Liu, Y., Müller, A., Rakoczy, P., et al., 2015. Hepatocyte fate upon TGF-β challenge is determined by the matrix environment. Differentiation 89, 105−116.

Michalopoulos, G.K., DeFrances, M.C., 1997. Liver regeneration. Science 276, 60−66.

Poisson, J., Lemoinne, S., Boulanger, C., Durand, F., Moreau, R., Valla, D., et al., 2017. Liver sinusoidal endothelial cells: Physiology and role in liver diseases. J. Hepatol. 66, 212−227.

Ramachandran, S.D., Schirmer, K., Münst, B., Heinz, S., Ghafoory, S., Wölfl, S., et al., 2015. In vitro generation of functional liver organoid-like structures using adult human cells. PLoS One 10, e0139345.

Rao, R.K., Samak, G., 2013. Bile duct epithelial tight junctions and barrier function. Tissue Barriers 1, e25718.

Riehle, K.J., Dan, Y.Y., Campbell, J.S., Fausto, N., 2011. New concepts in liver regeneration. J. Gastroenterol. Hepatol. 26 (Suppl 1), 203−212.

Takahashi, S., Fukami, T., Masuo, Y., Brocker, C.N., Xie, C., Krausz, K.W., et al., 2016. Cyp2c70 is responsible for the species difference in bile acid metabolism between mice and humans. J. Lipid Res. 57, 2130−2137.

Takebe, T., Sekine, K., Enomura, M., Koike, H., Kimura, M., Ogaeri, T., et al., 2013. Vascularized and functional human liver from an iPSC-derived organ bud transplant. Nature 499, 481−484.

Teufel, A., Itzel, T., Erhart, W., Brosch, M., Wang, X.Y., Kim, Y.O., et al., 2016. Comparison of gene expression patterns between mouse models of nonalcoholic fatty liver disease and liver tissues from patients. Gastroenterology 151, 513−525.

Xie, G., Zhou, D., Cheng, K.W., Wong, C.C., Rigas, B., 2013. Comparative in vitro metabolism of phospho-tyrosol-indomethacin by mice, rats and humans. Biochem. Pharmacol. 85, 1195−1202.

Cerebral organoids: Building brains from stem cells

Nurfarhana Ferdaos[1,2] and John O. Mason[1]

[1]University of Edinburgh, Edinburgh, United Kingdom [2]Universiti Teknologi MARA, Selangor, Malaysia

CHAPTER OUTLINE

INTRODUCTION

Understanding how the mammalian brain develops during embryogenesis is important, because errors during embryogenesis can lead to neurodevelopmental disorders, and may well also contribute to neuropsychiatric conditions that have a developmental component. Improving our understanding of normal brain development will help our understanding of the aetiology. Much of the research aimed at

Organoids and Mini-Organs. DOI: http://dx.doi.org/10.1016/B978-0-12-812636-3.00008-0

unraveling the molecular mechanisms of brain development has focused on the forebrain, as this region is responsible for most higher order cognitive function. As it is very difficult to study human brain development directly, researchers have commonly relied on animal models instead, in particular the mouse. Although it is clearly much simpler than the human brain, the mouse brain is nonetheless a highly complex organ, containing around 70,000,000 neurons, connected in intricate patterns. Embryonic development of the brain is largely under genetic control, and many of the most important regulatory genes and pathways involved are highly conserved between mice and humans. Taken together with the ease with which mice can be genetically modified, this has made the mouse a popular and powerful tool to investigate molecular mechanisms of forebrain development (Andoniadou and Martinez-Barbera, 2013; Southwell et al., 2014). Though many of the mechanisms are conserved between mice and primates, including humans, it is becoming clear that there are differences too, particularly at later stages of development (Florio et al., 2017). Nonetheless, we have learned a great deal from animal models. In particular, it is clear that a complex interplay between transcription factors and signaling molecules regulates the early steps in forebrain development, and that a relatively small number of transcription factors act as high level regulators (Hoch et al., 2009; Hébert, 2013).

Until recently, it had been widely thought that brain development could be studied only in the context of an intact embryo. In the last few years, however, several groups have described methods for growing cerebral organoids — three-dimensional neural tissue that is grown in vitro from pluripotent stem cells, and that closely resembles normal embryonic forebrain (Eiraku et al., 2008; Nasu et al., 2012; Mariani et al., 2012; Lancaster et al., 2013; Kadoshima et al., 2013; Paşca et al., 2015). This exciting breakthrough promises to have a major impact on the study of neural development (Huch and Koo, 2015; Kelava and Lancaster, 2016; Mason and Price, 2016).

A BRIEF OVERVIEW OF MAMMALIAN FOREBRAIN DEVELOPMENT

The forebrain arises at the anterior of the embryo. Initially, the embryonic nervous system consists of the neuroectoderm, a simple epithelial sheet which subsequently folds to form the neural tube in the process of neurulation. The anterior end of the neural tube balloons out, giving rise to the three primary vesicles of the brain: the prosencephalon, mesencephalon, and rhombencephalon, which form the future forebrain, midbrain, and hindbrain respectively (Fig. 8.1). The most rostral part of the prosencephalon becomes divided into: (1) the telencephalon, which gives rise to the cerebral cortex dorsally and the basal ganglia ventrally; and (2) the diencephalon, which gives rise to adult structures including the thalamus. The telencephalon swells rapidly and disproportionately, largely enveloping

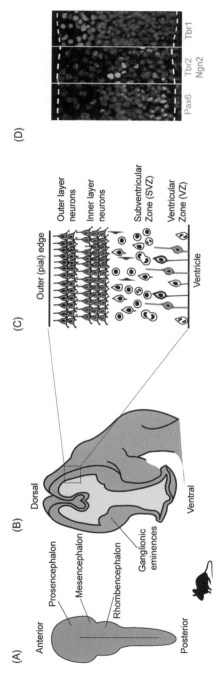

FIGURE 8.1

Embryonic development of the mouse brain. (A) At the neural plate stage, the antero − posterior axis is clearly developed, and the presumptive prosencephalon, mesencephalon, and rhombencephalon can be seen. (B) Structure of the forebrain in a mouse embryo at mid-gestation. Dorsal and ventral telencephalon have clearly differentiated. (C) Organization of cell types in embryonic mouse cortex at mid-gestation. Progenitor cells in the ventricular and subventricular zones divide, giving rise to neurons that subsequently migrate to the pial edge, ultimately generating the characteristic six-layered structure of the adult cerebral cortex. (D) Expression of specific genes identifies cell types in the embryonic cortex. Pax6 is expressed in radial glia in the VZ, Tbr2, and Ngn2 in intermediate progenitor cells in the subventricular zone, and Tbr1 marks early born neurons.

Panels (A) and (B) are modified, with permission, from Price, D.J., Jarman, A.P., Mason, J.O., Kind, P.C., 2010. Building Brains: An Introduction to Neural Development. Wiley-Blackwell, Chichester, UK Price et al. (2010), and panel (D) is modified with permission from Nasu, M., Takata, N., Danjo, T., Sakaguchi, H., Kadoshima, T., Futaki, S., et al., 2012. Robust formation and maintenance of continuous stratified cortical neuroepithelium by laminin-containing matrix in mouse ES cell culture. PLoS ONE. 7(12): e53024.

the diencephalon. It is thought that neural tissue assumes anterior character by default, and that signaling molecules, including Wnts expressed in posterior regions of the embryo, confer more posterior fates on the emerging nervous tissue. In the anterior domain, Wnt signaling is inhibited, allowing forebrain identity to be maintained (Andoniadou and Martinez-Barbera, 2013). Other signaling molecules are also important in the earliest stages of forebrain development, for example FGF signaling is required to activate the transcription factor Foxg1, which is essential for normal development of the forebrain (Xuan et al., 1995; Martynoga et al., 2005). A more detailed discussion of the mechanisms that govern early patterning of the telencephalon is provided in recent reviews by Hoch et al. (2009) and Azzarelli et al. (2015).

The rapid growth of the telencephalon during embryogenesis is driven by the proliferation of progenitor cells. Several types of progenitor cells with specific characteristics have been described. The earliest of these are the neuroepithelial cells (NEC) themselves, which divide rapidly, greatly increasing the size of the progenitor pool. Subsequently, around the onset of neurogenesis (approximately embryonic day (E) 8.5 in the mouse), NECs transform into radial glial cells (RGC). Radial glia are so-called because they express glial markers but they are, in fact, a major group of neural progenitor cells (reviewed by Tan and Shi, 2013). Radial glia undergo a characteristic form of cell division, interkinetic cell migration, in which mitosis occurs at the ventricular edge, and S-phase occurs deeper into the ventricular zone (VZ). Initially, most RGCs undergo symmetric division, giving rise to two RGC daughters. Subsequently, many RGCs divide asymmetrically, giving rise to an RGC and another daughter which could be a neuron, or a more specialized type of neural progenitor or, at late stages of development, a glial cell. Newborn neurons migrate radially, towards the outer (pial) edge of the emerging cerebral cortex. Many of the progeny of asymmetrically dividing RGCs become a distinct type of progenitor, known as an intermediate progenitor cell (IPC). In contrast to RGCs, IPCs divide outside the ventricular zone, in a region known as the subventricular zone. In rodents, most IPCs divide symmetrically, giving rise to two neuronal daughters which then migrate radially towards the pial edge of the cortex (Fig. 8.1). In primates, a variety of IPC types is present, including some types that are thought to contribute significantly to the much larger cortex of primates, and to promote gyrification (Dehay et al., 2015; Florio and Huttner, 2014). Altogether, the population of progenitor subtypes in both rodents and primates is more complex than initially thought. A fuller description of the repertoire of neural progenitor types in the mammalian embryonic cortex and their behaviors is provided by Namba and Huttner (2017). Newborn neurons derived from these progenitors subsequently migrate toward the outer edge of the developing cortex. Those neurons that form the deeper, inner layers are born first, while later born neurons migrate past them to form the outer layers of the cortex, ultimately generating the familiar six-layered structure of mature cerebral cortex (Tan and Shi, 2013).

The progenitor types described above relate only to development of the excitatory, glutamatergic, neurons of the cerebral cortex. The other major class of neurons that contribute to the mature cortex, the GABAergic inhibitory interneurons, are not generated within the cortex itself: rather, they are born in the ventral domain of the telencephalon, in the ganglionic eminences. These neurons then migrate tangentially into the cortex (Gelman and Marin, 2010). Once the two main groups of cortical neurons have reached their final positions, the next step is the formation of synaptic connections between them, initiating the extremely complex process of cortical neuronal circuit formation. While some cortical connections form between cells that are in close proximity to one another, many excitatory cortical neurons transmit signals over long distances, to other parts of the CNS. For example, as the cortex develops, reciprocal connections are formed between neurons in the cortex and in the thalamus. Correct formation of these connections is essential for cortical processing of sensory information, a core component of adult brain function (Leyva-Díaz and López-Bendito, 2013).

THE NEED FOR CEREBRAL ORGANOIDS

Our current understanding of the embryonic development of the mammalian forebrain is based largely on studies in animals, primarily the mouse. While the ultimate goal of much work in this field is to understand human brain development, there are obvious ethical and practical constraints on research using human embryos. Scientists have therefore often relied on alternatives for their studies. Mice are widely used in studies of brain development, in part because the mechanisms that control brain development, particularly at early stages, are thought to be conserved among mammalian species, and in part because of their genetic tractability — it is relatively easy to modify the mouse genome. As much of brain development is under genetic control, exploring the function of specific developmental regulatory genes has been pivotal to our understanding of mechanisms. Tissue-specific inactivation of genes using the cre-*loxP* system is particularly effective (Joyner, 2016). These experiments involve the use of genetic engineering in ES cells to produce a conditional allele of the gene of interest which is then crossed to a strain of mouse that expresses cre recombinase under the control of a tissue-specific promoter, such that the conditional allele becomes inactivated specifically in the tissue of choice. Such experiments usually also include a cre-reporter transgene, to mark cells in which the target gene has been deleted. While transgenic mouse strains have proven to be powerful tools with which to unravel the mechanisms of brain development, they have limitations. Generating embryos with the required combination of transgenic alleles often requires inter-crossing of multiple strains, which can be both time-consuming and costly. It is also important to note that, for ethical reasons, it is desirable to reduce the numbers of animals used in these studies. As cerebral organoids are derived from pluripotent stem cells, they offer the potential to investigate mechanisms controlling early development of the forebrain, without the use of animals.

The recent advent of CRISPR/Cas9-based methods of gene modification represents another major technological breakthrough. This technique greatly increases the ease of generating precise, targeted mutations, both in animals and in stem cells (Doudna and Charpentier, 2014). The combination of CRISPR/Cas9 gene targeting and organoid technology is particularly promising. Multiple genetic modifications can be made simultaneously to a PSC (Wang et al., 2013). Thus, multiple alleles, such as a floxed gene, a cre transgene, and a fluorescent reporter could readily be combined — much more easily than conventional breeding of transgenic strains. CRISPR/Cas9 also makes it easy to envisage high-throughput screens, for example large numbers of mutant cell lines could be made, and tested for their effects on cerebral organoid development, and those showing interesting phenotypes could then be followed up by in vivo studies. New applications for CRISPR/Cas9 continue to emerge, for example Andersson-Rolf et al. (2017) used it as the basis of a new method to create inducible mutations in cultured cells or in mice.

The inaccessibility of the mammalian brain, whether rodent or primate, makes it particularly difficult to study directly during embryogenesis. In most cases, embryonic brains must be removed, fixed, and stained before analysis. One way around this limitation is the use of organotypic cultures, in which slices of embryonic forebrain are maintained in culture over periods of up to a few days. When coupled with live imaging, organotypic cultures have been used to great effect to characterize the behavior and fates of cells within the developing forebrain of both mouse (e.g., Noctor et al., 2004), and human (e.g., Hansen et al., 2010). However, there are some limitations to this method. For example, there is a limit to the length of time for which organotypic explants can be maintained in a healthy condition in culture, and there is a possibility that culture conditions will alter the behavior of cells. The availability of suitable human tissue is also a significant limitation.

As organoids are maintained in culture, they are easily accessible and suitable for live imaging experiments. Individual cells can be visualized in real time, and their behavior tracked in a way that would be impossible in vivo. Nasu et al. (2012) showed that radial glial progenitors in mouse cerebral organoids exhibit the same interkinetic nuclear migration seen in the cortex in vivo. Similarly, Bershteyn et al. (2017) tracked cell divisions and measured cell migration rates in cerebral organoids derived from human iPSCs (induced pluripotent stem cells).

DESIGN CONSIDERATIONS

Embryonic stem (ES) cells can be readily directed to differentiate into specific specialized cell types, including neurons, and have therefore long been attractive as tools to model aspects of brain development. Most historical protocols for neural differentiation of ES cells have involved allowing the cells to form multicellular three-dimensional aggregates known as embryoid bodies, which are subsequently disaggregated to yield two-dimensional cultures of neurons. However, neural differentiation is also highly efficient in the absence of three-dimensional aggregation (Ying et al., 2003), and numerous protocols for efficient two-dimensional differentiation of mouse and human PSCs into neurons in adherent culture have been reported (e.g., Chambers et al., 2009; Gaspard et al., 2008; Shi et al., 2012). Many aspects of normal cortical development are reproduced in these two-dimensional cultures. They contain proliferating progenitor cells that show apico − basal polarity and undergo interkinetic nuclear migration, just like radial glial cortical progenitors in vivo. They grow in rosette-shaped formations which show a degree of spatial organization − rosettes have radial glia-like progenitors close to the center, and differentiated neurons towards the periphery. Neurons produced in this way can integrate into mouse brain after transplantation, and form functional connections (Michelsen et al., 2015) indicating that they are very similar to normal in vivo neurons. Two-dimensional cultures therefore reproduce some early aspects of cortical development well. However, as they lack three-dimensional organization and the tissue architecture of normal cortex, aspects of development which depend upon these cannot be reproduced accurately. It seems likely that three-dimensional organoid cultures should more closely resemble normal embryonic cortex, and therefore make better experimental models.

Pioneering studies from the laboratory of the late Yoshiki Sasai (Watanabe et al., 2005; Eiraku et al., 2008; Nasu et al., 2012) encouraged us to explore the use of cerebral organoids as tools to study mouse forebrain development. Together with a number of studies on human cerebral organoids (Lancaster et al., 2013; Kadoshima et al., 2013; Mariani et al., 2012; Paşca et al., 2015; Qian et al., 2016), these showed that ES cells are able to self-organize into structures that closely resemble the normal embryonic forebrain (Fig. 8.2). Protocols for the production of cerebral organoids from ES cells are remarkably simple, as outlined in Fig. 8.3. This simplicity is consistent with the idea that anterior forebrain fates arise by default, so long as posteriorizing signals (including Wnts) are suppressed (Wilson and Houart, 2004). A few thousand ES cells are allowed to aggregate quickly in a well of a lipid-coated 96-well dish. Culture medium is supplemented with the Wnt inhibitor IWP2, which acts by blocking the secretion of all Wnt proteins from cells within the culture − mouse ES cells are known to express a complex cocktail of Wnt family members (Nordin et al., 2008). The differentiation medium contains two nondefined components, the serum replacement KSR and the extracellular matrix preparation Matrigel (Kleinman and Martin, 2005). These should be batch-tested before use. Nasu et al. (2012) reported improved results using a chemically-defined medium and a laminin/entactin mixture in place of Matrigel, but we have had good results using KSR and Matrigel (Fig. 8.2). Some groups have begun to experiment with synthetic matrices built from chemically-defined components in place of Matrigel, and have reported encouraging results (Meinhardt et al., 2014; Lindborg et al., 2016) but it is not yet clear to what extent these will be able to replace the use of Matrigel in future.

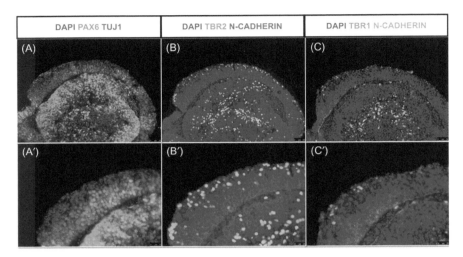

FIGURE 8.2

Cerebral organoids show similar patterns of gene expression to those seen in embryonic cortex. Immunochemical staining of mouse cerebral organoids after 8 days in culture, showing expression of specific markers. Rectangles in top panels indicate areas shown at higher power in the corresponding lower panel. (A, A′) Pax6 (green) is expressed in progenitor cells adjacent to the lumen of the organoid, Tuj1 (red) is expressed in cells at the outer edge. (B, B′) N-cadherin marks the apical edge of the neuroepithelium, adjacent to the lumen, Tbr2 is expressed in the subventricular zone. (C, C′) Tbr1 is expressed in early-born neurons, close to the outer edge of the tissue. Scale bars 100 μm.

Studies on human PSC-derived cerebral organoids have shown that agitation of the growth medium produces good differentiation, most probably by improving nutrient and gas exchange between organoids and the medium (Lancaster et al., 2013; Qian et al., 2016). We do not employ agitation in our current protocol for mouse organoids, which are kept in culture for ∼10−14 days, compared to several months for human cerebral organoids, however, it is clear that there are substantial numbers of necrotic cells in the centers of organoids by around 9−10 days of culture, and it is possible that agitation could produce better results for organoids at or after this stage.

BUILDING BETTER ORGANOIDS

There are three main areas in which future improvements to organoid differentiation could help make them more useful as tools to study mouse brain development − reproducibility, extending differentiation to later stages of brain

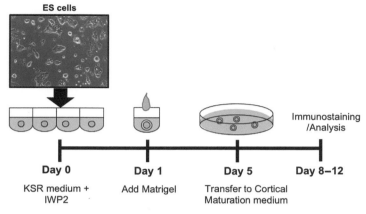

ES cells

Immunostaining /Analysis

Day 0

KSR medium + IWP2

Day 1

Add Matrigel

Day 5

Transfer to Cortical Maturation medium

Day 8–12

FIGURE 8.3

Schematic outline of protocol for generating cerebral organoids from mouse ES cells. Approximately 5000 ES cells are placed in each well of a low-adhesion 96-well plate in medium containing the Wnt inhibitor IWP2. Twenty-four hours later, Matrigel (blue droplet) is added). After 5 days in culture, organoids are transferred to a bacterial grade Petri dish containing cortical maturation medium.

development, and improving the accuracy with which organoids recapitulate normal development.

Reproducibility represents a significant challenge to using cerebral organoids to study forebrain development. There is variation between ES cell lines in the efficiency with which they form cerebral organoids. At this stage, it is unclear how much of this variability reflects inherent biological differences between stem cell lines (possibly affected by culture conditions), and how much of it is a result of variable elements in the differentiation conditions or protocols. This issue is particularly problematic when studying the effect of mutations — obviously it is essential to be confident that any altered cellular behaviors seen in organoids made from mutant cell lines are due to the effects of the mutation, and not to variability between cell lines or culture conditions. One way around this issue is to use CRISPR/Cas9 gene modification to "rescue" the mutation, demonstrating that wild-type behavior is restored (Bershteyn et al., 2017). One of the most likely sources of the variability found in cerebral organoid differentiation is the use of Matrigel which, as noted above, is variable in its precise composition from batch to batch (Kleinman and Martin, 2005). It is likely that defined, synthetic matrices will be developed in future that will remove the necessity to use Matrigel (Lindborg et al., 2016).

At present, mouse cerebral organoids appear to recapitulate early stages of cortical development most faithfully. Long stretches of continuous neuroepithelium form after a few days in culture, but this subsequently breaks down to form smaller spheres (Eiraku et al., 2008). Refinements to the protocol that allow production of organoids that maintain continuous stretches of neuroepithelial tissue for longer should increase their utility as models of forebrain development. Similarly, mouse cerebral organoids contain both early and later born neuronal subtypes, but these do not migrate away from the ventricular zone to form distinct layers, as seen in vivo (Nasu et al., 2012). Interestingly, cerebral organoids grown from human iPSCs can form longer stretches of continuous neuroepithelium and show better migration-dependent separation of neuronal subtypes into layers than is found in mouse organoids. This suggests that protocols used for growing human organoids could indicate ways to improve mouse cerebral organoid differentiation.

We have concentrated our discussion on the development of cerebral cortex tissue from mouse ES cells. As noted above, the two main neuronal subtypes found in the cerebral cortex originate from separate germinal zones — glutamatergic neurons are born dorsally, and GABA-ergic neurons ventrally. Protocols have been described for the separate production of both dorsal and ventral telencephalic organoids, but a more accurate model of cortical development would necessitate production of forebrain organoids that contained both dorsal and ventral telencephalic tissues, juxtaposed in the same configuration as is found in vivo. This could potentially be achieved by localized exposure of regions of the organoids to signals that promote particular fates, perhaps using a microfluidics approach (Bhatia and Ingber, 2014; Nie and Hashino, 2017). This would allow us to use organoids to study additional aspects of forebrain development, such as the mechanisms which control the migration of ventrally-born GABAergic cells into the cortex.

Organoids generated from human PSCs are much larger and more complex than those that have been reported from mouse stem cells to date. Some of these human organoids contain tissues resembling other parts of the brain, such as midbrain and hindbrain, in addition to forebrain, and have therefore been referred to as "minibrains" (Lancaster et al., 2013). Minibrains contain tissue resembling multiple regions of the brain, but these are not organized along dorso — ventral or antero — posterior axes like a normal brain. Nonetheless, this finding clearly holds out the promise that more complex brain-like structures can be grown in vitro, which could allow us to study later stages of neural development, such as the formation of connections between brain regions. For example, if we could grow organoids that contain both telencephalic and diencephalic tissues, they could be used to help determine how reciprocal connections form between the cerebral cortex and the thalamus.

One major constraint on the long-term culture of cerebral organoids and their ability to reach later stages of brain development is their lack of blood vessels. In contrast to embryonic brain tissue, there is no circulation to provide gas exchange, nutrient inflow, or removal of metabolic waste products, placing significant limits on the time for which organoid cultures are viable. These processes can be enhanced to some extent using mechanical agitation of the culture using a spinning bioreactor (Lancaster et al., 2013). This issue has been addressed with other types of organoid which were designed to be transplanted into immunocompromised mice. The investigators included a mixture of endothelial cells and mesenchymal stem cells in their organoids, which served to form blood vessels and promoted efficient vascularization after transplantation (Takebe et al., 2015). It is conceivable that this type of more complex tissue engineering, incorporating multiple cell types, could well lead to improvements in organoid differentiation in the near future.

DETAILED INSTRUCTIONS
OVERVIEW OF THE PROTOCOL

The protocol described here is adapted from the SFEBq protocol developed in the Sasai laboratory (Watanabe et al., 2005; Eiraku et al., 2008; Nasu et al., 2012). We have used this protocol successfully with several lines of mouse ES cell lines, including the Foxg1-venus reporter ES line that expresses fluorescent protein under the control of the forebrain marker gene *Foxg1* (formerly known as *BF-1*) (Eiraku et al., 2008), and our mutant *Pax6*$^{-/-}$ mouse ES cells (Quinn et al., 2010). ES cell lines are routinely cultured on gelatin in medium containing LIF and serum. We have found that differentiation is optimal with cultures of low passage number ES cells that show very low levels of spontaneous differentiation.

In outline, ES cells are allowed to aggregate in nonadherent U-bottomed 96-well plates containing serum-free medium supplemented with the Wnt inhibitor IWP2. The optimum number of cells for aggregation to form organoids varies between ES cell lines. We have found that good results are obtained using 5000 Foxg1-venus cells (Nasu et al., 2012). The cells form uniform spherical aggregates within a few hours of plating. The absence of signaling molecules in the medium permits the default differentiation of the ES cells towards a neural fate, and inhibition of Wnt activity promotes forebrain identity. After 24 hours, Matrigel is added to support the formation of neuroepithelial (NE) structures. After a further four days, organoids are transferred to nonadherent bacterial-grade Petri dishes, and cortical maturation medium is added. Cortical tissue matures progressively over the next few days. The protocol is summarized in Figure 8.3.

DETAILED PROTOCOL FOR THE PREPARATION OF MURINE CORTICAL ORGANOIDS

Day 0: Preparation of single cell suspension and aggregation
1. Allow ES cells to grow to approximately 70%–80% confluence.
2. Aspirate the medium and wash the ES cells twice with prewarmed 1× PBS.
3. Add 1 mL Tryple and incubate at 37°C for a few minutes, to detach the cells from the flask.
4. Dissociate the cells by gentle trituration using a P1000 tip, and transfer the resulting single cell suspension to a 20 mL universal bottle.
5. Add 5 mL ES medium to the cell suspension, and collect the cells by spinning at 250×g, for five minutes.

6. Discard the supernatant and resuspend the cells in 5 mL freshly-prepared KSR medium.
7. Count the total number of cells using a haemocytometer to determine the cell density. Note: the optimum initial cell number for organoid differentiation varies between ES cell lines, and should therefore be determined separately for each cell line. The optimum cell number for Foxg1-venus cells is 5000 cells per well, in 100 μL KSR medium.
8. Once the correct number of cells are prepared and diluted in KSR medium, add IWP2 to a final concentration of 2.5 μM.
9. Aliquot 100 μL of the cell suspension (~5000 cells) into individual wells of 96-well U-bottomed plates.
10. Incubate at 37°C in 5% CO_2.
11. Within a few hours of plating, the cells aggregate to form regular spheres (Fig. 8.4).

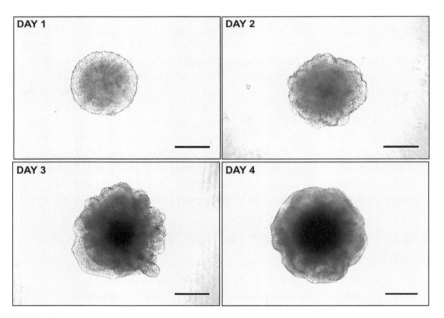

FIGURE 8.4

Phase contrast images showing the appearance of mouse cerebral organoids at different stages of the differentiation process. Organoids are initially spherical, and begin to become more irregular in shape by day 2. Stretches of neuroepithelium become visible as continuous bright areas on the outer edge of the organoids by days 3−4. Scale bars: 200 μm.

Day 1: Adding Matrigel
1. Allow Matrigel to thaw on ice − it solidifies quickly at room temperature, therefore it is important to keep it on ice at all times. Use precooled pipette tips that have been placed in a −20°C freezer for at least one hour to dispense the Matrigel.
2. Add Matrigel directly to each well to a final concentration of 200 µg/mL, and incubate the cells at 37°C in 5% CO_2.

Days 2−5: Cortical maturation
1. After the addition of Matrigel (day two), the spherical aggregates become more irregular in appearance, giving a "bubbly" shape. Bright and continuous NE starts to appear from day three, and continues to grow to day four (Fig. 8.4).
2. On day five, transfer the aggregates into cortical maturation medium, in a 50 mm bacterial-grade Petri dish.
3. It is important to keep the optimum number of organoids (up to ∼16) per Petri dish to avoid fusion of the organoids with one another.
4. Change the cortical maturation medium every other day by carefully removing half of the medium using a P1000 pipette, and replenish with an equal volume of fresh medium.

TROUBLESHOOTING

Although the protocol is generally robust and trouble-free, we have encountered some problems from time to time;

1. Cells fail to aggregate completely, and some dead cells are seen in the 96-well plate.
   Ensure that the starting population of ES cells is healthy, with a minimal appearance of differentiated cells in the culture. Healthy ES cells are an essential prerequisite for successful organoid differentiation.
2. ES cells form multiple small aggregates instead of a single large one.
   This issue can also be a result of suboptimal ES cell cultures, it is important to ensure that ES cells are healthy, and that very few differentiated cells are present. Care should also be taken when seeding cells into the 96-well plates to make sure that the tip does not touch the surface of the plate. The plate has a special coating that prevents the cells from adhering, thus scratches can affect the coating. A variety of suppliers produce suitable plates, we have had good results with PrimeSurface 96-well U-bottom plates supplied by Sumitomo Bakelite.
3. The aggregates do not form bright, radial neuroepithelium on day 3.
   We have found considerable variability between batches of Matrigel. It is important to ensure that the batch used is able to promote efficient neuroepithelial differentiation.

PREPARATION OF ORGANOIDS FOR IMMUNOSTAINING

FIXATION

1. Transfer organoids to 12-well plates using a 1 mL plastic Pasteur pipette. We pool 12 organoids per well.
2. Immerse organoids in 3 mL of 4% paraformaldehyde (PFA) in PBS, and fix for 15−20 minutes at room temperature on a shaking platform. Do not overfix − if fixation is too harsh, this can cause difficulties with subsequent immunochemistry.
3. Remove the PFA by aspiration and discard safely.
4. Rinse organoids three times in 1× PBS, for 10 minutes each.
5. Store in 3 mL of 1× PBS at 4°C until required, or proceed directly to cryoprotection and embedding.

CRYOPROTECTION, EMBEDDING AND CRYOSECTIONING

1. Cryoprotect organoids in 3 mL of 30% sucrose at 4°C overnight.
2. Carefully remove the sucrose solution by aspiration and equilibrate the organoids in 3 mL of embedding medium (50:50 mixture of 30% sucrose: OCT) for 1 hour at 4°C, on a rocking platform.
3. Using a 1 mL Pasteur pipette, transfer up to 12 organoids into an embedding mold.
4. Leave the organoids undisturbed on the bench for 10 minutes, to allow them to settle to the bottom of the molds.
5. Remove the remaining embedding medium by aspiration using a P20 tip, and carefully arrange the organoids to the middle of the mold.
6. Immediately place the mold on dry ice to fix the organoids in position, and quickly fill half of the mold with embedding medium. Leave the mold on dry ice to allow the samples to freeze completely.
7. Store the blocks at −70°C until ready to cryosection.
8. Cryosection at 10 μm in a cryostat chamber, transfer sections onto superfrost slides, and allow to air dry for at least 1 hour.
9. Store slides at −20°C until further use (immunostaining or in situ hybridization).

MEDIA AND REAGENTS

All reagents were obtained from Invitrogen, with the following exceptions:

Growth factor reduced Matrigel (Corning, cat. no. 356231).
IWP2 (Sigma, cat. no. I0536).
Prime Surface 96U Plate (Sumitomo Bakelite, cat. no MS-9096U).
50 mm Petri dish (Fisher Scientific).

KNOCK-OUT SERUM REPLACEMENT (KSR) MEDIUM

Glasgow Minimal Essential Medium (GMEM) (Invitrogen, cat no. 21710-025)
10% Knock-out serum replacement (KSR) (Invitrogen, cat no. 10828010)
1 mM Sodium pyruvate (Invitrogen, cat no. 11360-039)
0.1 mM nonessential amino acids (Invitrogen, cat no. 11140-035)
0.1 mM 2-mercaptoethanol (Invitrogen, cat no. 31350-010)

CORTICAL MATURATION MEDIUM

Dulbecco's Modified Eagle Medium/F12 (Invitrogen, cat no. 21331-020)
1 × Glutamax (Invitrogen, cat no. 35050-038)
1 × N2 (Invitrogen, cat no. 17502-048)

PARAFORMALDEHYDE FIXATIVE REAGENT (4% PFA)

1. Prepare 500 mL 1× PBS and autoclave to sterilize.
2. In a fume hood, add 20 g PFA while the PBS is still hot, fresh from the autoclave.
3. Stir the mixture on a hot plate in a fume hood to dissolve the PFA for 10−15 minutes.
4. Allow the PFA solution to cool to room temperature and store in 50 ml aliquots at −20°C.

CRYOPROTECTION REAGENT (30% SUCROSE)

1. Dissolve 150 g sucrose in 1× PBS to final volume of 500 mL, with moderate heating.
2. Cool and store in aliquots at −20°C.

ACKNOWLEDGMENTS

NF is supported by a PhD studentship from the Ministry of Higher Education, Malaysia (Grant G32486).

REFERENCES

Andersson-Rolf, A., Mustata, R.C., Merenda, A., Kim, J., Perera, S., Grego, T., et al., 2017. One-step generation of conditional and reversible gene knockouts. Nat. Methods 14, 287−289. Available from: http://dx.doi.org/10.1038/nmeth.4156.
Andoniadou, C.L., Martinez-Barbera, J.P., 2013. Developmental mechanisms directing early anterior forebrain specification in vertebrates. Cell Mol. Life. Sci. 70, 3739−3752.

Azzarelli, R., Hardwick, L.J., Philpott, A., 2015. Emergence of neuronal diversity from patterning of telencephalic progenitors. Wiley Interdiscip. Rev. Dev. Biol. 4, 197–214.

Bershteyn, M., Nowakowski, T.J., Pollen, A.A., Di Lullo, E., Nene, A., Wynshaw-Boris, A., et al., 2017. Human iPSC-derived cerebral organoids model cellular features of lissencephaly and reveal prolonged mitosis of outer radial glia. Cell. Stem. Cell. Jan 9. pii: S1934-5909(16)30463-5. Available from: http://dx.doi.org/10.1016/j.stem.2016.12.007. [Epub ahead of print].

Bhatia, S.N., Ingber, D.E., 2014. Microfluidic organs-on-chips. Nat. Biotechnol. 32, 760–772.

Chambers, S.M., Fasano, C.A., Papapetrou, E.P., Tomishima, M., Sadelain, M., et al., 2009. Highly efficient neural conversion of human ES and iPS cells by dual inhibition of SMAD signaling. Nat. Biotechnol. 27, 275–280.

Dehay, C., Kennedy, H., Kosik, K.S., 2015. The outer subventricular zone and primate-specific cortical complexification. Neuron. 85, 683–694.

Doudna, J.A., Charpentier, E., 2014. Genome editing. The new frontier of genome engineering with CRISPR-Cas9. Science 346, 1258096. Available from: http://dx.doi.org/10.1126/science.1258096.

Eiraku, M., Watanabe, K., Matsuo-Takasaki, M., Kawada, M., Yonemura, S., Matsumura, M., et al., 2008. Self-organized formation of polarized cortical tissues from ESCs and its active manipulation by extrinsic signals. Cell. Stem. Cell. 3, 519–532.

Florio, M., Huttner, W.B., 2014. Neural progenitors, neurogenesis and the evolution of the neocortex. Development 141, 2182–2194.

Florio, M., Borrell, V., Huttner, W.B., 2017. Human-specific genomic signatures of neocortical expansion. Curr. Opin. Neurobiol. 42, 33–44.

Gaspard, N., Bouschet, T., Hourez, R., Dimidschstein, J., Naeije, G., van den Ameele, J., et al., 2008. An intrinsic mechanism of corticogenesis from embryonic stem cells. Nature. 455, 351–357.

Gelman, D.M., Marin, O., 2010. Generation of interneuron diversity in the mouse cerebral cortex. Eur. J. Neurosci. 31, 2136–2141.

Hansen, D.V., Lui, J.H., Parker, P.R., Kriegstein, A.R., 2010. Neurogenic radial glia in the outer subventricular zone of human neocortex. Nature. 464, 554–561.

Hébert, J.M., 2013. Only scratching the cell surface: extracellular signals in cerebrum development. Curr. Opin. Genet. Dev. 23, 470–474.

Hoch, R.V., Rubenstein, J.L., Pleasure, S., 2009. Genes and signaling events that establish regional patterning of the mammalian forebrain. Semin. Cell. Dev. Biol. 20, 378–386.

Huch, M., Koo, B.K., 2015. Modeling mouse and human development using organoid cultures. Development 142, 3113–3125.

Joyner, A.L., 2016. From cloning neural development genes to functional studies in mice, 30 years of advancements. Curr. Top. Dev. Biol. 116, 501–515.

Kadoshima, T., Sakaguchi, H., Nakano, T., Soen, M., Ando, S., Eiraku, M., et al., 2013. Self-organization of axial polarity, inside-out layer pattern, and species-specific progenitor dynamics in human ES cell-derived neocortex. Proc. Natl. Acad. Sci. U.S.A. 110, 20284–20289.

Kelava, I., Lancaster, M.A., 2016. Stem Cell Models of Human Brain Development. Cell. Stem. Cell. 18, 736–748.

Kleinman, H.K., Martin, G.R., 2005. Matrigel: basement membrane matrix with biological activity. Semin. Cancer. Biol. 15, 378–386.

Lancaster, M.A., Renner, M., Martin, C.A., Wenzel, D., Bicknell, L.S., Hurles, M.E., et al., 2013. Cerebral organoids model human brain development and microcephaly. Nature 501, 373–379.

Leyva-Díaz, E., López-Bendito, G., 2013. In and out from the cortex: development of major forebrain connections. Neuroscience 254, 26-4.

Lindborg, B.A., Brekke, J.H., Vegoe, A.L., Ulrich, C.B., Haider, K.T., Subramaniam, S., et al., 2016. Rapid induction of cerebral organoids from human induced pluripotent stem cells using a chemically defined hydrogel and defined cell culture medium. Stem Cells Transl. Med. 5, 970–979.

Mariani, J., Simonini, M.V., Palejev, D., Tomasini, L., Coppola, G., Szekely, A.M., et al., 2012. Modeling human cortical development in vitro using induced pluripotent stem cells. Proc. Natl. Acad. Sci. U.S.A. 109, 12770–12775.

Martynoga, B., Morrison, H., Price, D.J., Mason, J.O., 2005. Foxg1 is required for specification of ventral telencephalon and region-specific regulation of dorsal telencephalic precursor proliferation and apoptosis. Dev. Biol. 283, 113–127.

Mason, J.O., Price, D.J., 2016. Building brains in a dish; prospects for growing cerebral organoids from stem cells. Neuroscience 334, 105–118.

Meinhardt, A., Eberle, D., Tazaki, A., Ranga, A., Niesche, M., Wilsch-Bräuninger, M., et al., 2014. 3D reconstitution of the patterned neural tube from embryonic stem cells. Stem Cell Rep. 3, 987–999.

Michelsen, K.A., Acosta-Verdugo, S., Benoit-Marand, M., Espuny-Camacho, I., Gaspard, N., et al., 2015. Area-specific reestablishment of damaged circuits in the adult cerebral cortex by cortical neurons derived from mouse embryonic stem cells. Neuron 85, 982–997.

Namba, T., Huttner, W.B., 2017. Neural progenitor cells and their role in the development and evolutionary expansion of the neocortex. WIREs Dev. Biol. 6, e256.

Nasu, M., Takata, N., Danjo, T., Sakaguchi, H., Kadoshima, T., Futaki, S., et al., 2012. Robust formation and maintenance of continuous stratified cortical neuroepithelium by laminin-containing matrix in mouse ES cell culture. PLoS ONE. 7 (12), e53024.

Nie, J., Hashino, E., 2017. Organoid technologies meet genome engineering. EMBO. Rep. Feb 15 in press http://dx.doi.org/10.15252/embr.201643732.

Noctor, S.C., Martinez-Cerdeno, V., Ivic, L., Kriegstein, A.R., 2004. Cortical neurons arise in symmetric and asymmetric division zones and migrate through specific phases. Nat. Neurosci. 7, 136–144.

Nordin, N., Li, M., Mason, J.O., 2008. Expression profiles of Wnt genes during neural differentiation of mouse embryonic stem cells. Cloning Stem. Cells 10, 37–48.

Paşca, A.M., Sloan, S.A., Clarke, L.E., Tian, Y., Makinson, C.D., Huber, N., et al., 2015. Functional cortical neurons and astrocytes from human pluripotent stem cells in 3D culture. Nat. Methods 12, 671–678.

Price, D.J., Jarman, A.P., Mason, J.O., Kind, P.C., 2010. Building Brains: An Introduction to Neural Development. Wiley-Blackwell, Chichester, UK.

Qian, X., Nguyen, H.N., Song, M.M., Hadiono, C., Ogden, S.C., Hammack, C., et al., 2016. Brain-region-specific organoids using mini-bioreactors for modeling ZIKV exposure. Cell 165, 1238–1254.

Quinn, J.C., Molinek, M., Nowakowski, T.J., Mason, J.O., Price, D.J., 2010. Novel lines of $Pax6^{-/-}$ embryonic stem cells exhibit reduced neurogenic capacity without loss of viability. BMC. Neurosci. 11, 26.

Shi, Y., Kirwan, P., Smith, J., Robinson, H.P., Livesey, F.J., 2012. Human cerebral cortex development from pluripotent stem cells to functional excitatory synapses. Nat. Neurosci. 15, 477−486.

Southwell, D.G., Nicholas, C.R., Basbaum, A.I., Stryker, M.P., Kriegstein, A.R., Rubenstein, J.L., et al., 2014. Interneurons from embryonic development to cell-based therapy. Science 344, 1240622.

Takebe, T., Enomura, M., Yoshizawa, E., Kimura, M., Koike, H., Ueno, Y., et al., 2015. Vascularized and complex organ buds from diverse tissues via mesenchymal cell-driven condensation. Cell. Stem. Cell 16, 556−565.

Tan, X., Shi, S.H., 2013. Neocortical neurogenesis and neuronal migration. Wiley Interdiscip Rev. Dev. Biol. 2, 443−459.

Wang, H., Yang, H., Shivalila, C.S., Dawlaty, M.M., Cheng, A.W., Zhang, F., et al., 2013. One-step generation of mice carrying mutations in multiple genes by CRISPR/Cas-mediated genome engineering. Cell 153, 910−918.

Watanabe, K., Kamiya, D., Nishiyama, A., Katayama, T., Nozaki, S., Kawasaki, H., et al., 2005. Directed differentiation of telencephalic precursors from embryonic stem cells. Nat. Neurosci. 8, 288−296.

Wilson, S.W., Houart, C., 2004. Early steps in the development of the forebrain. Dev. Cell 6, 167−181.

Xuan, S., Baptista, C.A., Balas, G., Tao, W., Soares, V.C., Lai, E., 1995. Winged helix transcription factor BF-1 is essential for the development of the cerebral hemispheres. Neuron 14, 1141−1152.

Ying, Q.L., Stavridis, M., Griffiths, D., Li, M., Smith, A., 2003. Conversion of embryonic stem cells into neuroectodermal precursors in adherent monoculture. Nat. Biotechnol. 21, 183−186.

FURTHER READING

Borello, U., Pierani, A., 2010. Patterning the cerebral cortex: traveling with morphogens. Curr. Opin. Genet. Dev. 20, 408−415.

From organoids to mini-organs: A case study in the kidney

9

Melanie L. Lawrence*, **Christopher G. Mills*** and **Jamie A. Davies**
University of Edinburgh, Edinburgh, United Kingdom

CHAPTER OUTLINE

INTRODUCTION

Organoids are three-dimensional assemblies of cells, containing more than one cell type, that exhibit at least some physiological features of an organ. Typically, organoids arise through the self-organization of their constituent cells without significant outside direction, although imposed changes of the hormonal/growth factor signaling environment are sometimes used if organoids are to be made by directed differentiation of very immature stem cells.

---

*These authors contributed equally to this work.

Organoids and Mini-Organs. DOI: http://dx.doi.org/10.1016/B978-0-12-812636-3.00009-2

The self-organizing potential of organogenic stem cells typically results in production of anatomies that are very realistic at the micro-level, but unrealistic at the macro-level: in other words, someone viewing a small area of organoid through the 60× objective of an optical microscope may well mistake it for a real foetal organ, but someone viewing it through the 5× objective would never be fooled. Whether this lack of realism at the macro level is a problem or not depends on the application. For studies of metabolism, transport, differentiation, and fate choice, the organoid level of organization is often good enough. It has already proved extremely useful in studies on topics as diverse as potency of progenitor cells (Dorrell et al., 2014), cancer development and host-tumor interactions (Weeber et al., 2015; Drost et al., 2016), neurotoxicology (Zeng et al., 2017), nutrient sensing in the gut (Rath and Zietek, 2017), and host−bacterial communication (Sun, 2017). For some potential uses of organs constructed from stem cells, however, most particularly for transplantation to replace damaged natural organs, macroscopic anatomy needs to be correct too.

DEVELOPMENT OF THE NATURAL ORGAN

Development of the mammalian metanephric (permanent) kidney is the result of interaction between two components derived from the embryo's intermediate mesoderm. One of these, the metanephrogenic mesenchyme, is an area of mesenchyme near the caudal end of the intermediate mesoderm that, under a dissecting microscope, can be distinguished from the other mesenchymes that surround it (see Davies, 2002 for review). It can also be distinguished by its expression of Six1 and Gremlin (Nie et al., 2011). The other component is a blind-ended epithelial tubule, the ureteric bud, which branches from the Wolffian duct, a tube running antero-posteriorly along the edge of the intermediate mesoderm. The ureteric bud forms under the influence of GDNF signals produced by the metanephrogenic mesenchyme (Sainio et al., 1997), but only where the thin layer of peri-Wolffian mesenchyme surrounding the duct expresses the BMP antagonist Gremlin, and does not express bud-inhibiting BMP signals (reviewed by Woolf and Davies, 2013) (Fig 9.1A).

Once the ureteric bud has reached the metanephrogenic mesenchyme, it is induced to branch (Fig. 9.1B). There is a naturally unstable feedback loop in the system. Mesenchyme-derived GDNF signals through epithelium-borne Ret receptor, and its GFRα and 2-O-sulphated heparan coreceptors (Trupp et al., 1996; Jing et al., 1996; Davies et al., 2003), to increase local Ret expression, Wnt11 expression, cell proliferation, and thus to promote advance of the ureteric bud tip. The Wnt11 signals to nearby mesenchyme to increase GDNF expression (Majumdar et al., 2003), and the feedback loop between Wnt secretion and GDNF-Ret signaling may even pattern the emergence of new branches by a Turing-type mechanism (Menshykau and Iber, 2013). The older, more distal

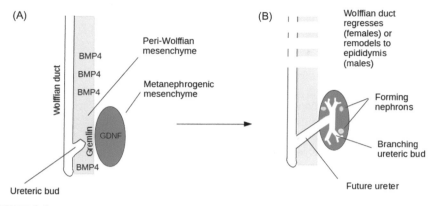

FIGURE 9.1

The early development of the metanephric (permanent) kidney. (A) the metanephrogenic mesenchyme produces GDNF, which promotes ureteric bud emergence, but this is antagonized by BMP4 except in a small region of peri-Wolffian mesenchyme that produces the BMP antagonist Gremlin. (B) Once the ureteric bud enters the metanephrogenic mesenchyme, it is induced by GDNF to branch to form the collecting duct tree. It also induces the mesenchyme to make a population of stem cells around each branch tip, and these stem cells give rise to nephrons. The entire green-colored area, including the ureteric bud inside it, can be cultured ex vivo, and will continue to develop.

regions of the ureteric bud tree mature to form urinary collecting ducts, while the trunk of the tree, still surrounded by peri-Wolffian mesenchyme, matures to become a ureter (reviewed by Woolf and Davies, 2013).

The metanephrogenic mesenchyme condenses around the tips of the ureteric bud to form the cap mesenchyme, a stem cell population that maintains itself and also gives rise, behind the tip region, to differentiating cells (Schreiner, 1902; Reinhoff, 1922). The cells that leave the cap to differentiate, under the influence of Wnt9b produced by the ureteric stalk (Carroll et al., 2005), condense to form a tight aggregate, and undergo a mesenchyme-to-epithelium transition to form a renal vesicle. This vesicle shows, from its earliest formation, proximo-distal polarization, the side nearer the ureteric stalk showing the most distal character in terms of gene expression (Georgas et al., 2009; Lindström et al., 2013). Over the next few days (in mouse: human tissues develop more slowly), the renal vesicle undergoes a series of morphogenetic changes, transforming into a tubule (a nephron) that has distinct "segments"; a Bowman's capsule most proximally, then a proximal tubule, intermediate tubule, and distal tubule that connects to the ureteric bud branch that induced it. The connection happens early, as the renal vesicle transitions to its next stage of development. The development of the nephron does not, however, depend on that connection, and will take place even in mesenchyme induced by chemical mimics of Wnt9b (Davies and Garrod, 1995; Kuure et al., 2007). In addition to the epithelial and epitheliogenic cells already mentioned, the kidney contains FoxD1-positive stem cells that are the precursors of the stroma of the mature organ (reviewed by Fanni et al., 2016).

It follows from the above description that the whole collecting duct system develops as one connected tree, and the position of the nephrons is determined by the branching of that tree. As it matures, the collecting duct system undergoes considerable remodeling, as branch points migrate centripetally in a process of node retraction (Lindström et al., 2015; Fig. 9.2). This has the effect of converting the inner part of the tree from one with a fractal arrangement of regularly-spaced branching points, to one in which the branches of the inner part of the tree radiate from the edge of a central point, a greatly dilated end of the ureter, called the renal pelvis. As this transformation takes place, the earliest-formed nephrons in the center of the kidney die away, leaving only the later-formed ones that are on the outside. The combined action of collecting duct remodeling, and oldest-nephron death, divides the developing organ into two zones; the outer cortex, that contains the last generations of collecting duct branches and also all of the nephrons, and inside this the medulla that contains long, rarely-branched collecting duct tubules radiating away from the pelvis. As this change takes place, the

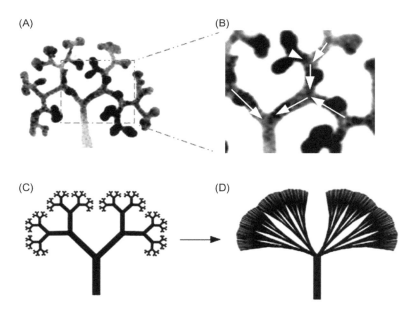

FIGURE 9.2

Remodeling of the collecting duct system by node retraction. (A) The early collecting duct tree has an approximately self-similar (fractal) form. (B) Later, the branch nodes move centripetally to remodel the tree. The effects of this can be seen in the before (C), and after (D), images of computer models of the process.

B. Original movies are available from Lindström et al. (2015).

intermediate tubules of the nephrons extend towards the medulla as loops of Henle (Fig. 9.3).

Although the metanephrogenic mesenchyme seems to contain progenitors capable of differentiating into endothelia, the blood vessels of the kidney develop in an outside-in sequence, possibly using recruitment of endogenous progenitors. Vessels first grow in along the ureteric bud, and form a ring below its first branching point. As the ureteric bud branches, the vessels advance to form a network around the cap mesenchymes, crossing new branch points of the ureteric bud, and thus dividing the cap into two (Munro et al., 2017). In this way, the anatomy of the vascular system also follows that of the ureteric bud/collecting duct tree, though subsequent modeling of both the tree and the larger vessels makes the relationship less apparent in the adult kidney. Cells of the nephrons' Bowman's capsules express VEGF, which attracts endothelial cells to enter and form a glomerulus (Loughna et al., 1997; Akimoto and Hammerman, 2003; Gnudi et al., 2015). Angiopoietins produced by podocytes are also involved with glomerular vascularization (reviewed by Woolf et al., 2009). Similarly, cells of the loop of Henle express angiopoietin-1, which attracts endothelia to form a

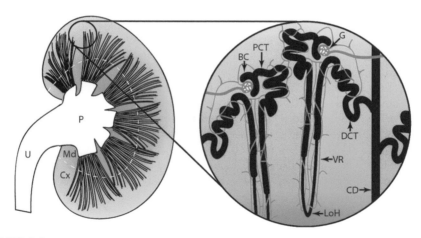

FIGURE 9.3

The anatomy of the adult kidney, with an outer cortex (Cx), an inner medulla (Md), and central pelvis (P) leading to the ureter (U). The detailed view shows the nephron from the glomerulus (G) surrounded by the Bowman's capsule (BC), leading to the proximal convoluted tubule (PCT): all of these are in the cortex. The nephron then leads to the loop of Henle (LoH) which dips into the medulla, and returns to the cortex and the distal convoluted tubule (DCT), which then leads to the collecting duct tree (CD) which will conduct the urine to the renal pelvis. Part of the vasculature is shown, an afferent arteriole entering the glomerulus (G), then leaving to interact with the proximal convoluted tubule and with the loop of Henle via the vasa recta (VR), a vascular structure that passes close to the loop.

second capillary system around them, the vasa recta (Madsen et al., 2010). Later expression of angiopoietin-2, generally an antagonist of endothelial growth, may terminate vasa recta development (Yuan et al., 1999). Nerve projections also enter the kidney, although this has been little studied. While all of these processes continue, stromal cells on the very outside of the kidney form a tough, fibrous capsule.

Shortly after birth in mouse, and by 36 weeks gestation in humans, branching ceases and, soon afterwards, nephron formation ceases as well, apparently because stem cell self-renewal fails to keep up with differentiation (Rumballe et al., 2011). The different timings of these events means that the last generation of nephrons connect to the same last-generation collecting duct branch, forming an "arcade", reminiscent of the arrangement of parallel nephrons draining to one duct that is seen in the mesonephros (Potter, 1972). This effect is particularly pronounced in human kidneys.

DESIGN CONSIDERATIONS

The goal of this work was to take kidney engineering from the organoid stage, in which there is realistic micro-anatomy but no macro-anatomy, to the mini-organ stage, in which both micro- and macro-anatomy are realistic. A discussion of the strategy used to achieve this needs to begin with a review of the method used to make basic organoids.

The first method for making renal organoids from suspensions of *ex fetu* mouse renogenic stem cells was developed by this laboratory in 2010, and consists of a few simple steps (Unbekandt and Davies, 2010). Renogenic stem cells, representing both the ureteric and metanephrogenic mesenchyme tissue types, are isolated, by manual dissection, from E11.5 mouse embryos and disaggregated enzymatically into a suspension of single cells. The cells are then reaggregated in the presence of ROCK inhibitors, which are necessary to protect cells from anoikis. After 24 hours, the ROCK inhibitor is withdrawn, and the reaggregate left to incubate. The E-cadherin-expressing ureteric epithelial cells sort out from the mesenchymal cells, presumably on the basis of adhesion-mediated phase separation (Steinberg 1963; Steinberg and Takeichi, 1994) which, in large populations, is not sufficient to drive full separation, but rather causes alternating zones of the two cell types (Cachat et al., 2016). As a result, the ureteric bud cells form a series of small "cysts" (hollow epithelial spheres) scattered throughout the culture, and these become tubules and eventually small branched trees, presumably under the influence of GDNF made by the mesenchyme. Cap mesenchymes form around the ends of these ureteric tubules, and nephrons form next to them, presumably under the influence of the Wnt9b signaling system that induces nephron formation in natural kidneys. The result is a mass of properly segmented nephrons, expressing appropriate genes and showing appropriate transporter activity, connected to an isolated maturing collecting duct (Fig. 9.4B). The

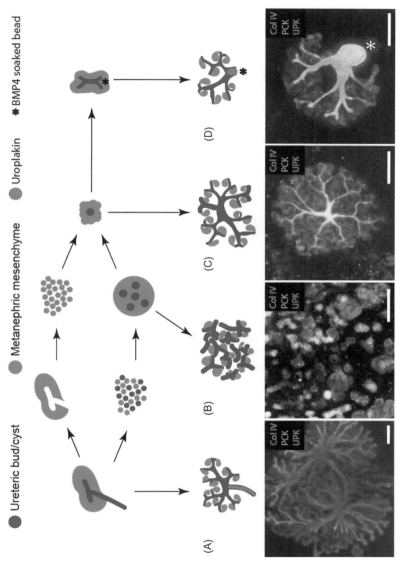

FIGURE 9.4 Illustration of the different renal systems available.

Renal progenitors isolated from E11.5 mouse embryos can be cultured in a number of forms. (A) Intact kidney rudiments develop into flat kidneys in situ, complete with functional nephrons and branching system. The asymmetry of the natural kidney is maintained with the development of a ureter (highlighted by uroplakin, UPK, expression). (B), (C), and (D). Organoids generated from suspensions of renal progenitor cells. Morphological complexity increases from (B) to (D). (B) Simple organoid. Renal progenitors are pelleted and cultured to produce "cysts" characteristic of collecting ducts and nephrons. (C) Advanced organoid. The ureteric "cyst" of a simple organoid is isolated and enveloped with metanephric mesenchyme. A single radial collecting duct system with functional adjacent nephrons develops. (D) Intercepting the advanced organoid early, and applying a BMP4 soaked bead (*) to a branch, results in an asymmetric organoid. Targeted branch swells to form a trunk with no adjacent nephrons. This, together with its expression of uroplakin, suggests a rudimentary urothelium has formed. Col IV, collagen type 4. PCK, pan-cytokeratin. UPK, uroplakin. Scale bar, 200 μM.

micro-anatomy is fine, but the macro-anatomy is hopelessly unrealistic, primarily because the all-around-one-tree arrangement that is at the heart of normal kidney development is absent.

It seemed to us that the critical difference between organ development in the embryo and organoid development in a dish is that organs in the embryo are subject to asymmetries that are absent in culture. In a naturally developing kidney, the presence of just one ureteric bud in one place in the mesenchyme constitutes a critical asymmetry that leads to there being only one collecting duct tree. To recreate one element of this asymmetry, the fact that there is only one ureteric epithelium, we designed a serial reaggregation system. First, a conventional organoid is produced, as above. Then, after 2−3 days of organoid development, one ureteric bud "cyst" is isolated from it by mechanical dissection (the ureteric bud cysts can be distinguished morphologically from the comma-shaped nephron progenitors). This is placed in culture covered with dissected, disaggregated, and reaggregated metanephrogenic mesenchyme, with no additional ureteric bud progenitor cell. The result is the formation of one single ureteric bud tree, which ramifies throughout the culture, and organizes nephron formation around itself (Ganeva et al., 2011). Combining this technique with a shallow-medium culture system that improves maturation of normal kidney rudiments (Sebinger et al., 2010) results in very realistic development of the serial reaggregates. Notably, by about 5 days of culture, the nephron-rich cortex and the medulla become distinct, and nephrons in the cortex send loops of Henle into the medulla (Chang and Davies, 2012).

Manually introducing a single ureteric bud is an example of externally imposed symmetry-breaking. In the basic organoid, ureteric progenitors are dispersed evenly throughout the culture at the beginning, and all places are alike: that is why the maturing organoid fails to reflect large-scale natural anatomy. Placing just one ureteric progenitor "cyst", from an organoid, into mesenchyme breaks this symmetry: all places are no longer alike because, as in the embryo, there is one unique ureteric bud. From this, much more natural large-scale anatomy follows, providing a more realistic organoid and, incidentally, indicating the critical importance of asymmetry to natural renal development. A striking defect that remained was the absence of a ureter. The collecting duct tree was self-contained and had no exit, an arrangement that would of course make this design useless as a functional organ.

Making a ureter would seem to be problematic, because it is not a product of the kidney itself, but rather a product of the ureteric bud shaft that remains outside the kidney proper, and of the peri-Wolffian mesenchyme. There is, however, some evidence that the young ureteric stalk and the young branching region of the ureteric bud are interconvertible. If ureteric stalk is surrounded by metanephrogenic mesenchyme, it branches, induces nephrons, and behaves in all examined ways like the normal ureteric bud in the kidney (Sweeney et al., 2008; Bohnenpoll and Kispert, 2014). Similarly, if the branching parts of the ureteric bud within the kidney are transplanted into the peri-Wolffian mesenchyme, they no longer branch. This strongly suggests that the identity of the young ureteric bud is controlled by signals from the mesenchyme that surrounds it. The peri-Wolffian mesenchyme produces BMP4 and, a few years ago, Doris Herzlinger and her colleagues observed that, if natural embryonic kidneys with their ureters still attached are treated in culture with excess BMP4, ureter markers such as uroplakin extend aberrantly into the oldest parts of the collecting duct system (Brenner-Anantharam et al., 2007). This suggested a method for a second type of symmetry-breaking. This begins with the making of a conventional organoid; one ureteric element is isolated from this and combined with fresh aggregates of metanephrogenic mesenchyme, as described above, to generate a rudiment arranged around one tree. That is the first example of externally imposed symmetry breaking (Fig. 9.4A−C). Then, as this tree begins to grow, a second externally imposed break of symmetry is applied: an affigel bead soaked in BMP4 (or irrelevant protein for a control) is embedded in the culture next to one branch of the tree (Fig. 9.4D). The result of this asymmetric treatment is striking: away from the bead, the ureteric bud branches away and induces nephrons, but the branch next to the bead does not branch or induce nephrons, but instead thickens and expresses the ureter/bladder marker, uroplakin (Fig. 9.4D).

We do not claim, on existing evidence, that what is produced is a complete ureter. The expression of uroplakin, and the anatomical asymmetry of the entire system, does however suggest that our interventions to break symmetry deliberately in a few critical ways have made a culture with a much more realistic macro-anatomy than is present in an organoid. We suggest that this approach, of adding defined symmetry-breaking manipulations to a basic organoid system in a manner that mimics the asymmetries in the embryo, might be a general strategy to move from crude organoids to more realistic mini-organs, not just in the kidney but in other organs too.

REMAINING CHALLENGES

We have already shown that renal organoids can attract and organize a functional exogenous vascular system (Xinaris et al., 2012; Davies and Chang, 2014), so there is a basis for developing this system for use with larger and more mature organoids. The major remaining challenge now is to convert what is a very small (2 mm) and flat organoid into a properly three-dimensional, larger one (though the small, flat ones are easily imaged, and are therefore useful for some studies). There is also the challenge of translating the techniques that have been developed to make mouse renal mini-organoids to the human iPS system which, at present, is stuck at the simple organoid level of organization.

Generating a Murine Renal Organoid (Simple, or Advanced with Single Collecting Duct Tree)

Materials required:

Materials required for all types of renal organoid

Incubator at 37°C with 5% CO_2

MEM: Minimal Essential Medium

KCM: Minimal Essential Medium with 10% FBS, 1% Pen/Strep solution

rKCM: Minimal Essential Medium with 10% FBS, 1% Pen/Strep solution and 1.25 μM of the ROCK inhibitor glycyl-H1152-dihydrochloride

Stainless steel wire mesh

Stainless steel forceps

Polycarbonate membrane 5 μm pores

1 mL syringes

Needles: 25 G 5/8″, 0.5 × 16 mm

Scalpels

90 mm petri dishes

30 mm petri dishes

1.5 mL Eppendorf tubes

0.5 mL Eppendorf tubes

Trypsin-EDTA

Glass pipettes

Cell strainers (40 μm pore size)

P10, P200 pipettes and tips

Materials required for advanced organoid with single collecting duct tree grown in Sebinger culture (in addition to above):

60 mm petri dishes

Autoclaved PBS or water

Nail varnish

60 mm coverslips

Silicone rings (Sarstedt, order number 94.6077.434)

Forceps with rounded ends

PROCEDURE FOR MAKING A SIMPLE MURINE RENAL ORGANOID (REAGGREGATION METHOD)

Before Starting

Prepare conventional cultures fresh on day:

1. Make up 4 mL per culture rKCM
2. Cut out a square roughly 2.5 cm long of stainless steel wire mesh
3. Fashion a stage by removing two lengths of wire from two opposing sides and bending the exposed ends to form legs

4. Make a small hole in the center of the stage by inserting a strong object (we use scissors) and twisting.
5. Autoclave in distilled H_2O: this can be done in batches
6. Transfer immediately and store in 100% methanol or ethanol
7. On day of use, remove a stage from methanol and sterilize by flame until glowing red
8. Place into a 30 mm petri dish, cover and shake vigorously until stage has cooled (prevents the plastic melting)
9. Add rKCM to cover stage
10. Float a polycarbonate membrane on rKCM
11. Gently remove rKCM until it levels with or is just below the stage.
12. Adjust membrane so that it is comfortably sitting on the stage and over the hole
13. Incubate until required.

Embryonic kidney dissections prepared freshly on the day:

1. Isolate uterine horn from timed-mated pregnant mouse at E11.5
2. Place uterine horn in a 90 mm dish with sterile PBS or MEM
3. Using scalpels and forceps, remove embryos from horn and transfer to fresh petri dish with sterile PBS or MEM
4. Cut embryos across the transverse line, keeping the caudal end of the embryo and discarding the cranial end.
5. Remove any intestines or ventral abdominal tissue that may be left
6. Turning the embryos onto their front (ventral side down), remove tail and discard.
7. Using one needle with syringe attached as handle, anchor the cranial end of the remaining embryo, then gently begin to make small cuts along the spine, using a second needle, separating the two sides of the body along the sagittal plane.
8. Once the two sides are separated, turn one side over (ventral side up), and locate the e11.5 kidney (posterior to the nephric duct).
9. Remove from the embryo and place in a small dish with KCM or MEM. If not using immediately, store in incubator in KCM or MEM at 37°C in 5% CO_2 for up to 2 hours.

Procedure

1. Isolate between 6 to 8 murine E11.5 kidney rudiments separated from the Wolffian duct at the intersection of the ureteric stalk and metanephric mesenchyme.
2. Add 200 μL of KCM to a 1.5 mL Eppendorf and set aside
3. Transfer rudiments to 1× Trypsin-EDTA in a 30 mm petri dish and incubate at 37°C for 2 minutes
4. Flame sterilize a glass pipette

5. Using a sterile glass pipette (yellow tips tend to cause sticking to the sides and are best avoided at this stage), carefully remove digested rudiments and transfer to Eppendorf containing KCM to quench trypsin
6. Using a 200 μL pipette, add an additional 200 μL of KCM and homogenize until no structures can be seen under a dissection microscope
7. Place cell strainer in a 30 mm petri dish and transfer cell suspension using a P200 pipette to remove any cell clumps.
8. Repeat previous step using the same cell strainer and dish, but replacing the 200 μL tip
9. Transfer cell suspension to a 0.5 mL Eppendorf using a P200 pipette
10. Centrifuge at 800× g in a table-top centrifuge for 3 minutes
11. Using a P200 pipette, place the tip on the side of the Eppendorf just above the pellet and firmly depress plunger to dislodge pellet (set it to around 40 μL)
12. Gently remove pellet using a fresh sterile glass pipette, and place onto the conventional culture (see "before starting") containing rKCM
13. Replace rKCM with KCM after 16 hours incubation (or overnight)
14. Structures should be visible within 24 hours after initial incubation

GENERATING AN ADVANCED ORGANOID WITH A SINGLE COLLECTING DUCT TREE

1. Generate a reaggregated kidney as above, and use on third day of culture
2. Prepare 2× Trypsin-EDTA
3. Prepare a 90 mm petri dish with KCM and a sterile glass coverslip in bottom of dish
4. Prepare a conventional culture fresh on the day as described in "Before starting", but add KCM rather than rKCM to the level of the top of the grid
5. Dissect 8−10 kidney rudiments per advanced organoid
6. *Optional:* Prepare Sebinger cultures (one for each organoid):

Optional Sebinger Culture Set-up:

1. Place glass coverslips in 1 M HCl in a beaker, heat to 90°C for 1 hour. Rinse thoroughly with distilled water, ensuring all traces of HCl have been removed, then place in fresh distilled water and autoclave.
2. Clean silicone rings well with water and autoclave. If desired, silicone rings can also be kept in 70% ethanol.
3. When ready to set up Sebinger cultures, remove glass coverslips and silicone rings, and dry in an oven at 90°C−100°C until all traces of water are gone.
4. Using nail varnish, stick either the lid or the bottom of a 60 mm dish to the bottom of a 90 mm petri dish. Replace lid on 90 mm petri dish and allow varnish to dry completely.

5. Place dry silicone ring on coverslip, turn over and, using sterile forceps with rounded ends, gently press inner silicone ring edges into coverslip to create a seal.
6. Replace coverslip with silicone ring attached in center of 60 mm petri dish, replace 90 mm dish lid. Use immediately, or wrap in parafilm for use at another time. A visual depiction of this can be found in Sebinger et al. (2010).

Procedure

1. Isolate 8−10 kidney rudiments from E11.5 mouse embryos separated from the Wolffian duct at the intersection of the ureteric stalk and metanephric mesenchyme as described in "Before starting".
2. Incubate isolated rudiments with $2\times$ Trypsin-EDTA for 30−60 seconds.
3. Transfer trypsin treated rudiments to the glass coverslip on bottom of 90 mm petri dish containing KCM.
4. Using two needles (25 G 5/8″, 0.5″16 mm) with 1 mL syringes as handles, strip the metanephric mesenchyme (MM) off the branched ureteric bud (UB) and stalk by placing one needle just under one side of the branch and pulling on the other side with the second needle. Be sure not to remove any UB tips while doing this. Age of the kidney is very important for this stage − more than one branch (T-shape) will make the clean removal of the MM very difficult without contamination with UB cells.
5. Continue to remove the MM in this way until all the 8−10 kidneys have been processed, placing each piece of removed MM together in a clump in the dish.
6. Using a flamed glass pipette, transfer the pooled MM to a 0.5 mL Eppendorf tube containing 200 μL of KCM. Pipette up and down to dissociate the MM.
7. Centrifuge at $800\times g$ in a table-top centrifuge.
8. While the MM is being pelleted, remove the previously-made, 3-day-old reaggregated organoid on polycarbonate filter from the incubator, and place into a fresh 90 mm petri dish with KCM. Isolate a single UB "cyst" from the reaggregate. This is distinguishable by the morphology, which is spherical or slightly branched, but does not contain any evidence of the comma-shaped or S-shaped structure characteristic of the developing nephrons.
9. Carefully transfer the UB "cyst" to the polycarbonate filter in conventional culture previously prepared (on the day).
10. Remove the tube containing the pelleted MM from the centrifuge, and carefully dislodge the pellet from the side using a pipette and a 200 μL tip, and then transfer the pelleted MM using a flamed glass pipette to the isolated UB "cyst" on the polycarbonate filter in conventional culture. If necessary, use the tip of a needle to gently pull the MM pellet to completely surround the UB "cyst".
11. Incubate at 37°C in 5% CO_2 for 20−24 hours.
12. The organoid can continue to be cultured on the polycarbonate membrane for up to 10 days changing media every 2−3 days, or transferred to Sebinger

culture (see "Before starting") after 20−24 hours. Sebinger culture will promote growth of Loops of Henle and more advanced structures.

13. *Optional:* If using Sebinger culture, first add 300 μL KCM to center of silicone ring; gently remove polycarbonate filter with 20−24 h organoid from conventional culture, and place into silicone ring containing KCM; organoid may float off, or may need to be gently scraped off with a needle into the KCM; remove filter and gently submerge early stage organoid; remove media and immediately replace with 85 μL KCM; using a needle or a filter tip, drag the media around the edge of the silicone ring to create a meniscus; using the needle place organoid in center of ring; add 5 mL of sterile PBS or water to 90 mm dish (outermost area outside the 60 mm dish); incubate at 37°C in 5% CO_2 for up to 10 days, changing media every 1−2 days.

GENERATING AN ADVANCED MURINE RENAL ORGANOID WITH MORE ACCURATE MACRO-ANATOMY AND A URETER-LIKE TRUNK

MATERIALS REQUIRED (IN ADDITION TO MATERIALS REQUIRED FOR SIMPLE AND ADVANCED ORGANOIDS ABOVE)

BMP4 solution (5 μg/mL BMP4, 0.1% BSA)
  Affi-beads (BioRad)
  Transwell polyester membrane cell culture inserts
  0.1% BSA

BEFORE STARTING

Construct an advanced organoid with the following amendment:

Isolate a single ureteric bud "cyst" from a simple organoid after 1 day in culture, as opposed to 3 days. Allow cell adhesion to recover for at least 4 hours prior to "cyst" isolation.

PROCEDURE

Proceed from step 11 above.

1. Prepare Transwell by applying 1.5 mL of KCM directly to the well (i.e., under the membrane)
2. Transfer advanced organoid from conventional culture to Transwell, and culture for a further 24 hours day to allow primary branches to develop
3. Fill a 30 mm dish with PBS
4. Add 10 μL of beads

5. Wash (do not worry about loss of beads, there are plenty) with PBS twice
6. Add 5 beads of similar size to a dry 30 mm dish and remove as much PBS as possible
7. Add 40 μL of BMP4 solution (or BSA alone for control beads) to contain beads in a drop, and incubate at room temperature for 1 hour
8. Slowly add PBS to fill dish
9. Remove a single bead with a Gilson, and place on a Transwell membrane with an advanced organoid present
10. Using a hypodermic needle gently push bead (either BMP4-treated or BSA only) to sit in a primary collecting duct branch point
11. Renew with freshly loaded bead daily by needle, being careful not to pierce the membrane or damage the organoid.

Points to note:

- Transferring Transwell inserts to 6-well plates that are not Corning™ may result in media bleeding through, as will using more than 1.5 mL of medium. This may affect the development of the organoid if excessive. Corning™ 6-well plates without the Transwell inserts are available commercially if required.
- The more often the beads are renewed, the more severe the loss of branching and loss of nephron development, but reliability of uroplakin expression increases.

ACKNOWLEDGEMENTS

We are grateful to the British Heart Foundation Centre of Research Excellence (R42477), the Medical Research Council (MR/K010735/1), and the European Union (STEM-BANCC) for funding this work.

DECLARATION OF FINANCIAL INTERESTS

None of the authors has a financial interest in the material described in this Chapter.

REFERENCES

Akimoto, T., Hammerman, M.R., 2003. Microvessel formation from mouse aorta is stimulated in vitro by secreted VEGF and extracts from metanephroi. Am. J. Physiol. Cell Physiol. 284, C1625−C1632.

Bohnenpoll, T., Kispert, A., 2014. Ureter growth and differentiation. Sem. Cell Dev. Biol. 36, 21−30.

Brenner-Anantharam, A., Cebrian, C., Guillaume, R., Hurtado, R., Sun, T.T., Herzlinger, D., 2007. Tailbud-derived mesenchyme promotes urinary tract segmentation via BMP4 signaling. Development. 134, 1967−1975.

Cachat, E., Liu, W., Martin, K.C., Yuan, X., Yin, H., Hohenstein, P., et al., 2016. 2- and 3-dimensional synthetic large-scale de novo patterning by mammalian cells through phase separation. Sci. Rep. 6, 20664.

Carroll, T.J., Park, J.S., Hayashi, S., Majumdar, A., McMahon, A.P., 2005. Wnt9b plays a central role in the regulation of mesenchymal to epithelial transitions underlying organogenesis of the mammalian urogenital system. Dev. Cell 9, 283−292.

Chang, C.H., Davies, J.A., 2012. An improved method of renal tissue engineering, by combining renal dissociation and reaggregation with a low-volume culture technique, results in development of engineered kidneys complete with loops of Henle. Nephron Exp. Nephrol. 121, 79−85.

Davies, J.A., 2002. Morphogenesis of the metanephric kidney. Sci. World J. 2, 1937−1950.

Davies, J.A., Chang, C.H., 2014. Engineering kidneys from simple cell suspensions: an exercise in self-organization. Pediatr. Nephrol. 29 (4), 519−524.

Davies, J.A., Garrod, D.R., 1995. Induction of early stages of kidney tubule differentiation by lithium ions. Dev. Biol. 167 (1), 50−60.

Davies, J.A., Yates, E.A., Turnbull, J.E., 2003. Structural determinants of heparan sulphate modulation of GDNF signalling. Growth Factors 21 (3−4), 109.

Dorrell, C., Tarlow, B., Wang, Y., Canaday, P.S., Haft, A., Schug, J., et al., 2014. The organoid-initiating cells in mouse pancreas and liver are phenotypically and functionally similar. Stem Cell Res. 13, 275−283.

Drost, J., Karthaus, W.R., Gao, D., Driehuis, E., Sawyers, C.L., Chen, Y., et al., 2016. Organoid culture systems for prostate epithelial and cancer tissue. Nat. Protoc. 11, 347−358.

Fanni, D., Gerosa, C., Vinci, L., Ambu, R., Dessì, A., Eyken, P.V., et al., 2016. Interstitial stromal progenitors during kidney development: here, there and everywhere. J Matern. Fetal. Neonatal Med. 29 (23), 3815−3820.

Ganeva, V., Unbekandt, M., Davies, J.A., 2011. An improved kidney dissociation and reaggregation culture system results in nephrons arranged organotypically around a single collecting duct system. Organogenesis 7 (2), 83−87.

Georgas, K., Rumballe, B., Valerius, M.T., Chiu, H.S., Thiagarajan, R.D., Lesieur, E., et al., 2009. Analysis of early nephron patterning reveals a role for distal RV proliferation in fusion to the ureteric tip via a cap mesenchyme-derived connecting segment. Dev. Biol. 332 (2), 273−286.

Gnudi, L., Benedetti, S., Woolf, A.S., Long, D.A., 2015. Vascular growth factors play critical roles in kidney glomeruli. Clin. Sci. (Lond.) 129 (12), 1225−1236.

Jing, S., Wen, D., Yu, Y., Holst, P.L., Luo, Y., Fang, M., et al., 1996. GDNF-induced activation of the ret protein tyrosine kinase is mediated by GDNFR-alpha, a novel receptor for GDNF. Cell 85, 1113−1124.

Kuure, S., Popsueva, A., Jakobson, M., Sainio, K., Sariola, H., 2007. Glycogen synthase kinase-3 inactivation and stabilization of beta-catenin induce nephron differentiation in isolated mouse and rat kidney mesenchymes. J. Am. Soc. Nephrol. 18 (4), 1130−1139.

Lindström, N.O., Hohenstein, P., Davies, J.A., 2013. Nephrons require Rho-kinase for proximal-distal polarity development. Sci. Rep. 3, 2692.

Lindström, N.O., Chang, C.H., Valerius, M.T., Hohenstein, P., Davies, J.A., 2015. Node retraction during patterning of the urinary collecting duct system. J. Anat. 226 (1), 13–21.

Loughna, S., Hardman, P., Landels, E., Jussila, L., Alitalo, K., Woolf, A.S., 1997. A molecular and genetic analysis of renalglomerular capillary development. Angiogenesis 1 (1), 84–101.

Madsen, K., Marcussen, N., Pedersen, M., Kjaersgaard, G., Facemire, C., Coffman, T.M., et al., 2010. Angiotensin II promotes development of the renal microcirculation through AT1 receptors. J. Am. Soc. Nephrol. 21 (3), 448–459.

Majumdar, A., Vainio, S., Kispert, A., McMahon, J., McMahon, A.P., 2003. Wnt11 and Ret/Gdnf pathways cooperate in regulating ureteric branching during metanephric kidney development. Development. 130 (14), 3175–3185.

Menshykau, D., Iber, D., 2013. Kidney branching morphogenesis under the control of a ligand-receptor-based Turing mechanism. Phys. Biol. 10 (4), 046003.

Munro, D.A.D., Hohenstein, P., Davies, J.A., 2017. Cycles of vascular plexus formation within the nephrogenic zone of the developing mouse kidney. Sci. Rep. 7 (1), 3273. Available from: http://dx.doi.org/10.1038/s41598-017-03808-4.

Nie, X., Xu, J., El-Hashash, A., Xu, P.X., 2011. Six1 regulates Grem1 expression in the metanephric mesenchyme to initiate branching morphogenesis. Dev. Biol. 352 (1), 141–151.

Potter, E.L., 1972. Normal and Abnormal Development of the Kidney. Year Book Medical Publishers Inc, Chicago, USA.

Rath, E., Zietek, Y., 2017. Intestinal organoids, a model for biomedical and nutritional research. In: Davies, J.A., Lawrence, M.L. (Eds.), Organoids and Mini-Organs. Elsevier, London.

Reinhoff, W.F., 1922. Development and growth of the metanephros or permanent kidney in chick embryos. Johns Hopkins Hospital Bull. 33, 392–406.

Rumballe, B.A., Georgas, K.M., Combes, A.N., Ju, A.L., Gilbert, T., Little, M.H., 2011. Nephron formation adopts a novel spatial topology at cessation of nephrogenesis. Dev. Biol. 360, 110–122.

Sainio, K., Suvanto, P., Davies, J., Wartiovaara, J., Wartiovaara, K., Saarma, M., et al., 1997. Glial-cell-line-derived neurotrophic factor is required for bud initiation from ureteric epithelium. Development 124, 4077–4087.

Schreiner, K.E., 1902. Ueber die Entwicklung der Amniotenniere. Zeitsch. f. wiss. Zool. Bd71.

Sebinger, D.D., Unbekandt, M., Ganeva, V.V., Ofenbauer, A., Werner, C., Davies, J.A., 2010. A novel, low-volume method for organ culture of embryonic kidneys that allows development of cortico-medullary anatomical organization. PLoSOne 5 (5), e10550.

Steinberg, M.S., 1963. Reconstruction of tissues by dissociated cells. Some morphogenetic tissue movements and the sorting out of embryonic cells may have a common explanation. Science 141, 401–408.

Steinberg, M.S., Takeichi, M., 1994. Experimental specification of cell sorting, tissue spreading, and specific spatial patterning by quantitative differences in cadherin expression. Proc. Natl. Acad. Sci. U.S.A. 91, 206–209.

Sun, J., 2017. Intestinal organoids in studying host-bacterial interactions. In: Davies, J.A., Lawrence, M.L. (Eds.), Organoids and mini-organs. Elsevier, London.

Sweeney, D., Lindström, N., Davies, J.A., 2008. Developmental plasticity and regenerative capacity in the renal ureteric bud/collecting duct system. Development 135, 2505–2510.

Trupp, M., Arenas, E., Fainzilber, M., Nilsson, A.S., Sieber, B.A., Grigoriou, M., et al., 1996. Functional receptor for GDNF encoded by the c-ret proto-oncogene. Nature 381, 785–789.

Unbekandt, M., Davies, J.A., 2010. Dissociation of embryonic kidneys followed by reaggregation allows the formation of renal tissues. Kidney Int. 77 (5), 407–416.

Weeber, F., van de Wetering, M., Hoogstraat, M., Dijkstra, K.K., Krijgsman, O., Kuilman, T., et al., 2015. Preserved genetic diversity in organoids cultured from biopsies of human colorectal cancer metastases. Proc. Natl. Acad. Sci. U.S.A. 112, 13308–13311.

Woolf, A.S., Davies, J.A., 2013. Cell biology of ureter development. J. Am. Soc. Nephrol. 24 (1), 19–25.

Woolf, A.S., Gnudi, L., Long, D.A., 2009. Roles of angiopoietins in kidney development and disease. J. Am. Soc. Nephrol. 20 (2), 239–244.

Xinaris, C., Benedetti, V., Rizzo, P., Abbate, M., Corna, D., Azzollini, N., et al., 2012. In vivo maturation of functional renal organoids formed from embryonic cell suspensions. J. Am. Soc. Nephrol. 23 (11), 1857–1868.

Yuan, H.T., Suri, C., Yancopoulos, G.D., Woolf, A.S., 1999. Expression of angiopoietin-1, angiopoietin-2, and the Tie-2 receptor tyrosine kinase during mouse kidney maturation. J. Am. Soc. Nephrol. 10 (8), 1722–1736.

Zeng, Y., Win-Shwe, T.-T., Itoh, T., Sone, H., 2017. A 3D neurosphere system using human stem cells for nanotoxicology studies. In: Davies, J.A., Lawrence, M.L. (Eds.), Organoids and Mini-Organs. Elsevier, London.

Applications of Organoids

Intestinal organoids: A model for biomedical and nutritional research

10

Eva Rath and Tamara Zietek

Technical University of Munich, Freising, Germany

CHAPTER OUTLINE

INTRODUCTION

Studies on intestinal nutrient and drug absorption, as well as on sensing and gut hormone secretion, are of high relevance to biomedical, pharmacological, and nutritional research. Appropriate in vitro models that would allow a replacement or significant reduction of animal experiments have been lacking to date. Immortalized mammalian cell lines are currently the prime in vitro model used to assess intestinal transport processes, or the secretion of gut hormones in response to luminal stimuli. Although well-established and easy to handle, these cultures do not reflect the complexity of the intestinal epithelium, which has multiple cell types and a region-specific architecture. Primary intestinal cell culture seems a better approach, but it is limited by short-term culture, and enterocytes of such cultures are poorly-differentiated. A few years ago, Sato and colleagues reported for the first time the generation of three-dimensional intestinal organoids cultivated in vitro; so-called "mini-guts" (although they contained only epithelial components) (Sato et al., 2009). Intestinal organoids are generated from isolated intestinal tissue of mice or humans, and can be cultured and multiplied in the laboratory over months. They contain all cell types of the intestinal epithelium, and display the main characteristics of this tissue in the mammalian intestine. As an

Organoids and Mini-Organs. DOI: http://dx.doi.org/10.1016/B978-0-12-812636-3.00010-9

in vitro system, intestinal organoids come closer to normal physiological behavior than rival systems, and are thus useful for a wide variety of applications from gastrointestinal and developmental research to biomedical applications, to pharmacological science and personalized medicine. Even though animal studies cannot be completely replaced by organoid cultures, this novel model system has the potential to significantly reduce the number of in vivo animal experiments, as it gets closer to physiology than any other in vitro model.

The intestine is an organ with numerous physiological functions, and the intestinal epithelium contains different specialized cell subtypes. They include Paneth cells that release antimicrobial compounds, mucus-secreting goblet cells, absorptive enterocytes that are responsible for the uptake of nutrients, and enteroendocrine cells that secrete different hormones into the circulation. The most prominent role of the intestine is nutrition, and the absorption of nutrients from ingested food is mediated by specific nutrient transporters in the brush border membrane of enterocytes (Daniel and Zietek, 2015), some of which can also transport certain drugs (Daniel and Kottra, 2004). Defects in nutrient transporters can lead to disease and malabsorption syndromes, such as the Fanconi − Bickel syndrome (a defect of the glucose/fructose transporter GLUT2) (Santer et al., 2002), or glucose/galactose malabsorption (a deficiency in the sodium-dependent glucose transporter SGLT1) (Wright et al., 2007). The molecular basis of the fructose malabsorption is not clarified yet (Ebert and Witt, 2016), but a contribution of intestinal fructose transporters cannot be excluded (Douard and Ferraris, 2013). However, the intestine is also an endocrine organ that secretes several hormones into the circulation. Depending on which nutrients are present in the intestinal lumen, certain peptide hormones are released from enteroendocrine cells, a process referred to as nutrient sensing (Zietek and Daniel, 2015). Gastrointestinal hormones have numerous physiological and metabolic functions, such as regulation of gastric and intestinal motility, gall bladder contraction, appetite, and fat and carbohydrate metabolism (Svendsen and Holst, 2016). The most prominent ones amongst the gut hormones are the so-called incretin hormones, glucagon-like peptide 1 (GLP-1) and glucose-dependent insulinotropic polypeptide (GIP). These stimulate insulin release from pancreatic beta-cells, regulate blood glucose levels, promote satiety, and protect pancreatic cells from apoptosis (Zietek and Rath, 2016). Incretin-based therapies, mostly GLP-1 mimetics or inhibitors of the GLP-1 degrading enzyme dipeptidyl-peptidase 4 (DPP4), are successfully used for the treatment of metabolic disorders such as type 2 diabetes or obesity (Drucker, 2015).

Different regions of the intestine display different physiological characteristics. The small intestine is divided, from proximal to distal, into the duodenum, jejunum, and ileum. Most nutrient transporters are expressed mainly in the duodenum and jejunum, where they can absorb as many nutrients as possible after food ingestion (Wuensch et al., 2013; Yoshikawa et al., 2011). The function of enteroendocrine cells too, depends on their localization along the gastrointestinal tract—for example, GLP-1-secreting cells are predominantly located in the distal part of the small intestine and in the colon, while the highest density of GIP-expressing cells is found in the proximal small intestine (Habib et al., 2012). Furthermore, intestinal morphology differs from proximal to distal gut: villus length increases from duodenum to ileum, and the colon does not contain any villi, only crypts. As in every organ, the mammalian intestine has its own stem cells. Intestinal stem cells are located in the stem cell niche at the crypt base of the small and large intestine, and all the intestinal epithelial cell types originate from these stem cells (Barker, 2014). While Paneth cells reside at the crypt bottom, absorptive enterocytes, goblet, and enteroendocrine cells start differentiating into mature cells at the crypt − villus boundary, further moving upwards towards the villus tip, where they are finally exfoliated via anoikis (Leushacke and Barker, 2014). This way, human intestinal epithelium is renewed every 4−5 days.

Generally, organoids are used to: (1) model organ development and morphogenesis; (2) model disease; and (3) make tissue for regenerative medicine/personalized medicine. Already, organoid-based research has contributed greatly to elucidating the complex regulation of the intestinal stem cell niche. In particular, the identification of Lgr4 and Lgr5 as receptors of R-Spondins resulted from organoid experiments (de Lau et al., 2011). Organoids can be used to model diseases, either by introducing disease-relevant mutations to characterize the functional consequences, or by deriving organoids from patients to elucidate their disease mechanisms. Recently, intestinal organoids have been drawing increasing attention as diagnostic tools in cystic fibrosis and colorectal cancer (Dekkers et al., 2016a; van de Wetering et al., 2015). Patient-derived intestinal organoids recapitulate epithelial functions, genetic signatures, and, in the case of colorectal cancer, several properties of the original tumor. Therefore, they allow prediction of drug responses in a personalized fashion. In combination with high-throughput drug screens, detection of gene − drug associations will be facilitated (van de Wetering et al., 2015). Intestinal organoids might also become a therapeutic tool, since intestinal organoid transplantation has already been proven feasible (Yui et al., 2012). This opens new possibilities for regenerative medicine and, in combination with editing technology, for gene therapy (Dekkers et al., 2016b). However, the technology for the growth of intestinal organoids is still rapidly progressing. Becoming more and more widespread in research due the availability of protocols and dropping prices for cultivation, new areas of application of this technology are starting to be explored.

In particular, physiological processes involving transporters and receptors, such as nutrient and drug uptake by enterocytes or hormone secretion by enteroendocrine cells, are coming more into focus (Petersen et al., 2014; Schweinlin et al., 2016; Zietek et al., 2015). These processes are of high relevance to malabsorption diseases, drug testing, and metabolic disorders such as obesity or type 2 diabetes. Intestinal organoids, recapitulating essential features of the in vivo tissue architecture, constitute an excellent source of differentiated, fully functional enterocytes. Additionally, they allow enrichment of rare cell types like enteroendocrine cells, which constitute only 1% of the intestinal epithelium under physiological conditions, by the use of certain modulators, e.g., a γ-secretase inhibitor (Petersen et al., 2015). This will have a profound impact on research in these areas by tremendously facilitating experiments.

PROBLEM BEING ADDRESSED HERE

The major and most prominent function of the intestine is probably the absorption of nutrients by absorptive enterocytes. These cells constitute the major fraction of all intestinal epithelial cells that cover our intestinal lumen. Transporters are located in the apical membrane of absorptive enterocytes facing the intestinal lumen, in order to absorb all kinds of nutrients from ingested food (Daniel and Zietek, 2015). Different transporters are responsible for the specific absorption of certain nutrients. Some of them are active transporters using an electrochemical gradient for co-transport of the substrate, such as the proton-coupled peptide transporter PEPT1, or the sodium-dependent glucose transporter SGLT1. Others are passive transporters mediating substrate flux via facilitated diffusion, such as the facilitated glucose transporter 2 (GLUT2), which is located in the basolateral membrane mediating exit of glucose and fructose from the enterocyte into circulation, or the apical fructose transporter GLUT5 (facilitated glucose transporter 5). Some of these transporters also mediate the absorption of orally available drugs (Sugano et al., 2010): an example is the transporter PEPT1, which transports antibiotics of the cephalosporin group (Ganapathy et al., 1995). In order to assess subcellular protein localization, substrate specificities, transport, and inhibition kinetics or molecular regulation of the transporters, an in vitro system is needed that allows the study of these processes in absorptive enterocytes.

In recent years, it has been discovered that intestinal transporters play a dual role in the intestine (Zietek and Daniel, 2015). Next to their transport function in absorptive enterocytes, transporters are also present in the apical membrane of hormone-secreting enteroendocrine cells (Gorboulev et al., 2012), where they serve as sensors to regulate incretin hormone release into circulation (Diakogiannaki et al., 2013; Roder et al., 2014). Previously, a similar function was demonstrated for intestinal receptors as mediators of gut hormone secretion (Reimann et al., 2012). The incretin hormones GLP-1 and GIP are insulinotropic, and hence important regulators of blood glucose levels. Therefore, the novel role of transporters and receptors as sensors in enteroendocrine cells makes them highly interesting targets for the development of incretin-based type 2 diabetes therapies (Gribble and Reimann, 2016; Zietek and Daniel, 2015).

Different in vitro systems are available for use in molecular studies on intestinal transport processes, or for the investigation of nutrient sensing and gut hormone secretion. However, all these models face major drawbacks, and there is a need for a more physiological in vitro model. In particular, when studying nutrient sensing, a model is needed that contains different subtypes of enteroendocrine cells that express different levels of certain gut hormones, as found in the native intestine (Habib et al., 2012). Also, the presence of both absorptive enterocytes and enteroendocrine cells is essential, because gut hormones can act in a paracrine manner by interacting with neighboring cells of the intestinal epithelium (Tolhurst et al., 2012). When studying the biology and functional characteristics of intestinal transporters, it is important to study intracellular signaling pathways as downstream effects of transporter activity. Electrogenic transporters mediate co-transport of nutrients and ions, so transporter activity is coupled to an increase in the intracellular ion concentration (Daniel and Zietek, 2015). An increase in intracellular cation levels caused by transporter activity causes depolarization of the cell membrane. In enteroendocrine cells, which are electrically excitable, this membrane depolarization activates calcium signaling, which triggers release of hormone-containing vesicles (Reimann and Gribble, 2016). Thus, a proper model system for studying underlying mechanisms of nutrient sensing and gut hormone secretion needs to be suitable for studies on intracellular signaling events as well.

NON-ORGANOID APPROACHES

To date, intestinal epithelial cell lines have been the prime in vitro model systems to assess intestinal transport processes, while enteroendocrine cell lines are common models to study the secretion of different gut hormones. An established model for small-intestinal enterocytes is the CaCo-2 cell line (or the CaCo-2 TC7 subclone), derived from a colon adenocarcinoma. This cell line is commonly grown on transwell plates up to 3 or 4 weeks postconfluence for studies on intestinal transport of nutrients, drugs, or other compounds using radio-labeled or fluorescence-labeled substrates (Farrell et al., 2013; Ganapathy et al., 1995; Wang and Li, 2017). The HT-29 cells (and subclones) are a human colon carcinoma cell line well established for research on intestinal transporters, in particular sugar transporters (Delezay et al., 1995; Liu et al., 2016). In order to study the role of transporters in intestinal nutrient sensing, however, other cell lines are required. The most prominent enteroendocrine cell lines used for studies on gut hormone secretion are the murine GLUTag cell line (Emery et al., 2015), the murine STC-1 cell line (Jiang et al., 2016), and the human NCI-H716 cell line (Pais et al., 2014). None of them, however, reflects the complex biology of enteroendocrine cells in vivo (Kuhre et al., 2016). Enteroendocrine cells are distributed throughout the small and large intestine, and their expression patterns of different gut hormones differ highly, depending on their location within the intestinal tract (Habib et al., 2012). For example, the number of GLP-1-secreting cells (often referred to as L-cells) increases gradually from proximal to distal gut, yet GIP-secreting cells (referred to as K-cells) decrease. Thus, enteroendocrine cell lines, which are all tumor-derived, represent very simple and artificial model systems for the investigation of nutrient sensing, gut hormone secretion, and the underlying molecular and regulatory mechanisms. The advantage of mammalian cell lines is that they are well-established by numerous laboratories around the world. There is a lot of scientific data available, as well as established experimental protocols. Furthermore, they are easy to handle and cultivation is cheap. Still, all these cell lines are very simple and artificial model systems. They are mostly tumor-derived, and they represent only one single cell type, not reflecting the complexity of the intestinal mucosa which comprises multiple specialized cell types. Also they are usually grown in two-dimensions, which does not reflect the three-dimensional architecture of the native intestine.

In particular, for studies on nutrient sensing and gut hormone secretion, primary intestinal cell culture is a far better approach, and has been established as a reliable model in the past years (Reimann et al., 2008). Primary cultures grown from isolated intestinal crypts have the advantage that they can be generated from different intestinal segments (Parker et al., 2012), and from mice (wild-type or knockout animals) (Diakogiannaki et al., 2013), or humans (Habib et al., 2013). They comprise absorptive enterocytes, as well as different subtypes of enteroendocrine cells, as found in the native intestine. However, these cultures contain poorly-differentiated enterocytes, and are therefore not suitable for the detection of intestinal transporters and receptors on protein or functional level. They are a short-term culture system not suitable for long-term experiments, and cannot be passaged, which increases the number of laboratory animals needed for culture preparation. The same is the case for isolated intestinal epithelial cells (Grossmann et al., 1998), which comprise all mucosal cell types but display very limited viability in vitro, and do not represent an intact epithelium.

Short-term stability is also a limitation of tissue explants, such as everted gut rings (Roder et al., 2014), or gut sacs from mouse or rat intestine (Praslickova et al., 2012; Surampalli et al., 2016) which are often used for transport studies. Everted gut rings can be either incubated with labeled substrates in vitro, or can be prepared following oral administration of, for example, radio-labeled transporter substrates in rodents (Roder et al., 2014). Everted gut sacs can even be used for flux studies, since the luminal and basolateral compartments can be targeted separately. However, preparation and handling are not trivial, and require some experience. The advantage of tissue explants is that they can be prepared from different intestinal segments, and their region-specific in vivo characteristics are conserved in vitro. The intestinal explant conserves its native architecture, and the mucosa is connected to its surrounding tissue such as submucosa or muscle, and neurons, lymph, blood vessels are included. Depending on the scientific question, this can be an advantage or a disadvantage. Intestinal sensing of nutrients and subsequent gut hormone secretion is sometimes investigated in perfused rodent intestine (Kuhre et al., 2015). The animal is anesthetized and the intestinal lumen is perfused with the putative stimulants ex vivo. The basolateral fluid is collected, and gut hormone contents are analyzed. This technique is not technically easy, and ethical hurdles limit the broad use of this method for studies on nutrient-induced gut hormone release.

A reliable and well-established model used for studies on functional characteristics and regulation of intestinal transporters is heterologous expression in Xenopus laevis oocytes (Hirsch et al., 1996). Following mRNA injection, the protein of interest is expressed in the oocyte, and transport kinetics can be investigated using radio-labeled substrates or electrophysiological approaches in the case of electrogenic transporters (Schulze et al., 2014; Stelzl et al., 2016). This technique is an excellent tool to study functional characteristics of one particular transporter, although the target protein is in an artificial environment and no regulatory factors are present, as they would be in the mammalian cell. In addition, the availability of intact oocytes, and the complicated handling including oocyte injection, are critical issues to be considered when applying this technique. Much easier heterologous expression systems are yeast and E. coli. They enable the generation of recombinant mutants which, once generated, can be cultured or fermented on larger scales, delivering high amounts of protein. Although cheap and easy to handle, these microorganisms are very simplified model systems for the investigation of mammalian proteins, and in particular large membrane proteins. Problems that often occur are misfolding of the protein, or failed membrane insertion. Therefore, these systems are rather more useful for the structural characterization of purified proteins or protein domains (Beale et al., 2015) than for detailed studies on mammalian transporter function and regulation.

Novel and promising approaches that have been established in the very recent past are three-dimensional mammalian cell culture models. Intestinal cell lines such as CaCo-2 or HT-29 are grown on scaffolds, creating a more intestine-like architecture which leads to improved differentiation (Chen et al., 2015). Other three-dimensional models are cultured directly from human small-intestinal epithelial cells and myofibroblasts on coated microporous membranes (Maschmeyer et al., 2015a; Maschmeyer et al., 2015b), and cannot be multiplied in vitro. These models have the potential to be established for transport studies of nutrients or drugs, and cultures grown from human intestinal epithelial cells even comprise different mucosal cell types, but not enteroendocrine cells. The same is the case for three-dimensional bioprinted tissues, another technology that has arisen very recently and has gained enormous attention. This approach is of more value for regenerative medicine and transplantation than for experimental research (Murphy and Atala, 2014). Bioprinting of different tissues, including heart, skin and bones, has been successfully established, but bioprinted intestinal tissues are rare to date and need to be further improved (Wengerter et al., 2016).

DESIGN CONSIDERATIONS

In view of all the limitations of current in vitro models that are used for experimental research in the fields of intestinal transport, sensing, and hormone secretion, the three-dimensional intestinal organoid culture is a model system with great future potential.

It has been demonstrated that intestinal organoids contain all the cell types of the intestinal epithelium (Sato et al., 2009; Spence et al., 2011), including enteroendocrine GIP- and GLP-1-secreting cells (Petersen et al., 2014; Petersen et al., 2015). Organoids can easily be generated from murine or human intestinal tissue, grown in standard cell culture plates, and multiplied in the laboratory over months by passaging. Thus, we recently investigated whether murine intestinal organoids could represent a suitable model system for experimental research on intestinal transport, sensing, and gut hormone secretion (Zietek et al., 2015). Since intestinal nutrient transporters are located specifically in the apical or basolateral membrane, it is essential that the epithelium of the organoids contains polarized enterocytes. Many nutrient transporters such as SGLT1, PEPT1, or GLUT5 are found in the apical membrane facing the intestinal lumen in order to absorb nutrients from ingested food (Daniel and Zietek, 2015). Others, however, like GLUT2 or some amino acid transporters, are located in the basolateral membrane, where they mediate nutrient exit from the enterocyte into the circulation (Roder et al., 2014). It is hence important to ensure proper localization of the transport protein of interest within the intestinal organoid. In the case of studies on incretin hormone secretion, it is essential to verify the presence of enteroendocrine cells in the organoid cultures. This can most easily be done by embedding the organoids in paraffin, and by conducting immunofluorescence. In the case of the transporters (or another intestinal protein), it is recommended that the specificity of staining is verified by using organoid cultures generated from knockout mice lacking the protein of interest. Depending on the target protein, it may be critical to choose the correct part of the intestine when making organoids. This is also relevant to studying gut hormone secretion, because of the differential distribution of enteroendocrine cell subtypes along the intestine. Of note, the yield of crypts, and thus of growing organoids, significantly decreases from proximal to distal small intestine. In the case of studies of nutrient-sensing, a compromise needs to be made if the major location of the investigated sensor protein does not correlate with the maximal density of the enteroendocrine cell subtype of interest.

When it comes to the assessment of transporter activity, regulation, or inhibition, different approaches can be applied, such as the use of fluorescent-labeled, stable isotope-labeled, or radio-labeled transporter substrates. The decision depends on available laboratory equipment, e.g., whether there is access to a radioactive isotope laboratory, or if a mass spectrometry-based platform or fluorescence microscope are available. Radio-labeled transport assays are expensive, but the approach is very sensitive, and labeled substrates are chemically stable. If possible, results obtained from transport and inhibition studies should be verified by the use of intestinal organoids derived from knockout mice. The same applies to experiments on nutrient sensing and gut hormone secretion when a certain sensor protein, an intestinal transporter, or receptor, is investigated. It is important to note that intestinal organoid cultures can also serve as a model for the investigation of intracellular signaling. Fluorescence live-cell imaging is often applied to measure downstream effects of transporter or receptor activities. The substrate flux of proton-coupled transporters, for example, induces a cytosolic acidification that can be visualized by live-cell imaging using fluorescent probes (Chen et al., 2010). In enteroendocrine cells, membrane depolarization following the increase of proton levels induces an elevation of the intracellular calcium concentration, which finally triggers hormone release (Diakogiannaki et al., 2013). This calcium signal, which is also induced by activation of some G-protein-coupled receptors acting as intestinal sensors (Reimann et al., 2012), can be measured by fluorescent live-cell imaging as well.

All these experimental methods for transport (Roder et al., 2014), nutrient-induced hormone secretion (Diakogiannaki et al., 2013), and intracellular signaling (Pais et al., 2014) have been established for other in vitro models, such as two-dimensional mammalian cell cultures or tissue explants. When establishing the use of intestinal organoids for research on gastrointestinal function, we aimed to apply well-established techniques to the three-dimensional organoid cultures. The aim was to keep experimental procedures as simple as possible, so that they can be easily applied by other researchers. The most straightforward approach for all functional studies is simply adding the substrates to the cell culture plate, keeping the organoids in their three-dimensional environment, a dome of laminin-rich gel. However, several issues have to be considered when doing so. In contrast to mammalian cell lines or primary cultures, intestinal organoids are three-dimensional, with a luminal compartment inside and the basolateral membrane on the outside. When adding effectors to the cultures, they first reach the outside of the organoid, which means the basolateral transporters or receptors are always targeted first. As we have demonstrated, molecules of a few kDa in size pass the epithelium of the organoids and enter the organoid lumen (Zietek et al., 2015), either via the paracellular route, or by simple diffusion as the organoid epithelium is leaky to some extent. Anyway, nutrients and small molecules up to a size of 4 kDa reach the inner luminal compartment of the organoid, and consequently are targeting not only the basolateral, but also the apical transporters and receptors. It is, however, not possible in this system to target the apical or basolateral side separately. Ways to exclude the contribution of a certain transporter or receptor would be to use inhibitors, gene knockout, or downregulation of organoids, or employ organoids from knockout mice.

TYPICAL RESULTS

Intestinal organoid cultures for experimental research on functional gastrointestinal processes can most easily be grown from isolated proximal small intestine of mice (Fig. 10.1). Polarization of enterocytes of the intestinal organoid is essential when conducting studies on nutrient transport and sensing, and it can be verified by detection of apical membrane markers such as villin or alkaline phosphatase and basolateral markers such as E-cadhehrin by immunofluorescence (Sato et al., 2009;

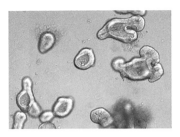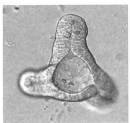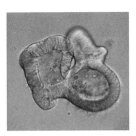

FIGURE 10.1

Organoids grown from murine proximal small intestine, 4 days after 1st passage (wild-type mice). The epithelial layer with a crypt- and villus-like domain, as well as the inner lumen, are clearly visible. At this stage of maturation, organoid cultures are useful for functional studies on intestinal transport, hormone secretion, and intracellular signaling.

Spence et al., 2011; Zietek et al., 2015). Intestinal transporters display proper localization within the organoids: the peptide transporter PEPT1 and the glucose transporter SGLT1 are found in the apical membrane, and the glucose/fructose transporter GLUT2 is found in the basolateral membrane (Zietek et al., 2015), as observed in the native mammalian intestine (Chen et al., 2010; Roder et al., 2014).

Using specific inhibitors (and knockout mice if available), intestinal organoid culture enables the researcher to distinguish between apical and basolateral transport processes (Fig. 10.2). The electrogenic solute carrier SGLT1 is the main apical glucose transporter in the small intestine, while GLUT2 mediates glucose flux at the basolateral membrane via facilitated diffusion. The function of both transporters, and their pharmacological inhibition, can be measured in organoid cultures derived from proximal small intestine (Fig. 10.3). The SGLT1 function can be assessed by uptake of radio-labeled glucose or 1-O-methyl alpha-D-glucopyranoside (α-MDG), a specific nonmetabolizable substrate of SGLT1, and phlorodzin inhibits SGLT1 almost completely. In organoids derived from SGLT1 knockout mice, residual glucose influx via GLUT2 can be observed, and can be inhibited by phloretin. Fructose uptake via GLUT2 and GLUT5 can be detected via radio-labeled transport studies in small-intestinal organoids. Organoids generated from GLUT5 knockout mice still display GLUT2-mediated influx of fructose, which is abolished by phloretin. Transport of short peptides also occurs at the apical and basolateral side of enterocytes. While the apical peptide transporter PEPT1 is well-characterized, not least because it mediates luminal drug absorption (Sugano et al., 2010), the basolateral peptide transport system is less well understood (Berthelsen et al., 2013). Absorption of dipeptides, and of the β-lactam antibiotic cefadroxil by PEPT1, can be measured in intestinal organoids by radio-labeled substrate uptake, and by competitive inhibition studies (Zietek et al., 2015). In organoids derived from PEPT1-deficient mice, remaining dipeptide transport by the basolateral peptide transport system can be observed.

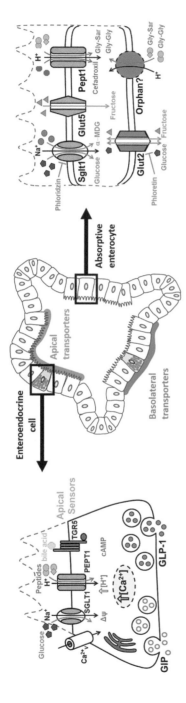

FIGURE 10.2

Scheme demonstrating how organoids are used for in vitro studies on intestinal transport, sensing, and hormone secretion. The three-dimensional organoid (middle) has a polarized epithelial cell monolayer, with intestinal transporters located in the apical membrane (orange) and basolateral membrane (blue). All intestinal epithelial cell subtypes are present, including absorptive enterocytes and enteroendocrine cells with hormone-containing vesicles (red). In absorptive enterocytes (right), active and passive transport of nutrients and drugs by different apical (orange) and basolateral (blue) transporters can be measured, including competitive and noncompetitive inhibition. In enteroendocrine cells (left), nutrient-induced gut hormone secretion can be studied. Apical electrogenic transporters or G-protein-coupled receptors serve as sensors for nutrients or other luminal compounds, and mediate the secretion of incretin hormones induced by an increase in intracellular calcium concentration. Elevation of intracellular calcium or proton levels upon electrogenic transport can be visualized by fluorescent live-cell imaging in all enterocytes. GIP: Glucose-dependent insulinotropic polypeptide; *GLP-1*: Glucagon-like peptide 1; TGR5: bile acid receptor; SGLT1: Sodium-dependent glucose transporter 1; PEPT1: Proton-coupled peptide transporter 1; GLUT2/5: Facilitated glucose transporter 2/5; α-MDG: 1-O-methyl- α-D-glucopyranoside; Gly-Sar: Glycyl-Sarcosin; Gly-Gly: Glycyl-Glycin.

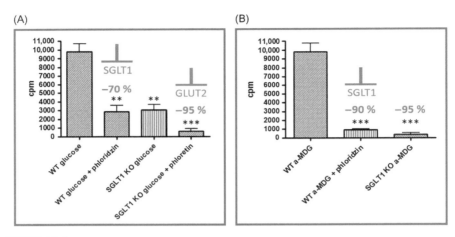

FIGURE 10.3

Sugar transport studies using radio-labeled substrates in murine small-intestinal organoid cultures. (A): Transport of glucose (3 mM) by SGLT1 (sodium-dependent glucose transporter 1) and GLUT2 (facilitated glucose transporter 2) in organoids derived from wild-type (WT) and SGLT1 knockout (KO) mice, including pharmacological inhibition of SGLT1 by phloridzin (1 mM) and of GLUT2 by phloretin (1 mM). (B): SGLT1-specific transport of the nonmetabolizable substrate α-MDG (1-O-methyl-α-D-glucopyranoside, 1 mM) in WT and SGLT1 KO organoids, including inhibition by phloridzin (1 mM). Values on y-axis given as cpm (counts per minute). Data expressed as mean $\pm$ SEM, $n = 3-5$ cultures, statistical analysis using unpaired 2-tailed t-test versus WT glucose or WT α-MDG; **$P < 0.005$; ***$P < 0.001$.

Organoids are therefore a valuable in vitro culture model for studying intestinal nutrient and drug transport, including pharmacological inhibition studies. Three-dimensional organoids can be seeded on transwell plates coated with a porcine small intestinal scaffold, and grown as a two-dimensional monolayer containing different intestinal cell subtypes (Schweinlin et al., 2016). Measurement of paracellular transport of fluorescein and transcellular transport of propranolol has been demonstrated, as well as basolateral efflux of rhodamine123, a substrate of p-glycoprotein (Mdr1). It remains to be evaluated if this model is also suitable for assessing gut hormone secretion and intracellular signaling pathways. Three-dimensional intestinal organoids have been demonstrated to be an excellent model to study intestinal nutrient sensing, gut hormone secretion, and underlying molecular mechanisms (Fig. 10.2) (Zietek et al., 2015). Organoid cultures release the incretin hormones GLP-1 and GIP in response to different secretagogues such as glucose, peptides, and bile acids, and distinct sensor proteins can be verified by use of organoids derived from knockout mice (Fig. 10.4). The GIP- and GLP-1-containing cells can be detected via immunofluorescence in organoids, and are both found in cultures derived from proximal small intestine. GLP-1-secreting L-cells are present in murine and human intestinal

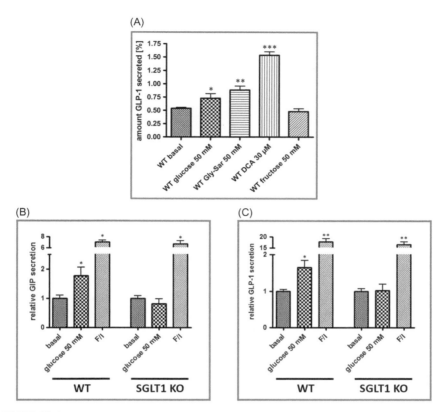

FIGURE 10.4

Nutrient sensing and incretin hormone secretion from murine small-intestinal organoid cultures. (A): GLP-1 (Glucagon-like peptide 1) responses to sugars, to the dipeptide Gly-Sar (Glycyl-Sarcosin), and to the secondary bile acid DCA (deoxycholic acid), measured in organoids derived from wild-type mice. Y-axis displays the amount of GLP-1 secreted by the cultures normalized to the total GLP-1 content (supernatant plus cell lysate). (B), (C): Relative GIP (Glucose-dependent insulinotropic polypeptide) or GLP-1 secretion in response to glucose and F/I (Forskolin/IBMX (3-isobutyl-1-methylxanthine)), measured in organoids generated from wild-type (WT) or SGLT1 knockout (KO) organoids. F/I (10 μM each) is used as a positive control for maximal hormone output. Data expressed as mean ± SEM, $n = 3-6$ cultures, statistical analysis using unpaired 2-tailed t-test versus basal. $*P < 0.05$; $**P < 0.005$; $***P < 0.001$.

organoids, which can be employed to study modulation of L cell development as demonstrated by short-chain fatty acids increasing L-cell number (Petersen et al., 2014). Furthermore, numbers of GIP- and GLP-1-secreting cells were found to be increased upon inhibition of the NOTCH signaling pathway in intestinal organoid cultures (Petersen et al., 2015).

Targeting intestinal sensors in enteroendocrine cells is a promising approach for the treatment of type 2 diabetes, and some sensor proteins have been successfully targeted for the development of synthetic agonists that increase incretin hormone secretion and improve blood glucose control (Watterson et al., 2014). Depending on the type of sensor protein activated by a luminal stimulant, differential signaling cascades are activated in the enteroendocrine cell, finally leading to gut hormone release into the circulation. Elevation of cytosolic calcium concentrations following activation of an intestinal nutrient sensor is a central and common trigger for exocytosis of gut hormone-containing vesicles (Zietek and Daniel, 2015). Thus, when studying the intracellular mechanisms linking luminal nutrient sensing to gut hormone secretion, it is essential to observe changes in intracellular calcium levels. Calcium imaging using fluorescent probes is routinely applied in pharmacological screening to detect activation of receptors by a putative ligand/drug, mainly in cell culture-based assays. Moreover, many transporter activities and intracellular translocation events are regulated by intracellular calcium: PEPT1 activity (Wenzel et al., 2002) and trafficking of GLUT2 (Kellett et al., 2008) are examples. When using intestinal organoids for investigation of nutrient-sensing processes and the underlying signaling mechanisms, it is helpful to use the same model system for calcium imaging (Zietek et al., 2015). Murine organoids loaded with the fluorescent calcium indicator Fura-2-AM display an even intracellular dye distribution in epithelial cells of crypt, as well as villus domains, and a strong, rapid calcium response to glucose via the sensor SGLT1 (Fig. 10.5B). For electrogenic transporters like SGLT1 or PEPT1, membrane depolarization induced by substrate-coupled cation influx is the trigger for opening of voltage-gated L-type calcium currents and subsequent gut hormone release from the enteroendocrine cell (Diakogiannaki et al., 2013). While SGLT1 is sodium-dependent, PEPT1-mediated substrate flux occurs in co-transport with protons, and leads to an acidification of all enterocytes (Chen et al., 2010). Organoids can be easily loaded with the fluorescent proton-indicator BCECF-AM, in order to visualize changes in intracellular proton-levels (Zietek et al., 2015). The dipeptide and PEPT1 substrate glycyl-sarcosine induces a decrease of intracellular proton levels in epithelial cells of murine organoids, including enterocytes of the crypt and villus domains (Fig. 10.5C).

In summary, intestinal organoids have great future potential as a model system for gastrointestinal research, including intestinal nutrient and drug transport, sensing, hormone secretion, and the investigation of underlying intracellular signaling pathways.

REMAINING CHALLENGES

It has been demonstrated that three-dimensional organoid culture is a suitable and versatile model for functional studies on the intestine resembling numerous physiological features of the native organ. Despite all the advantages of this technology,

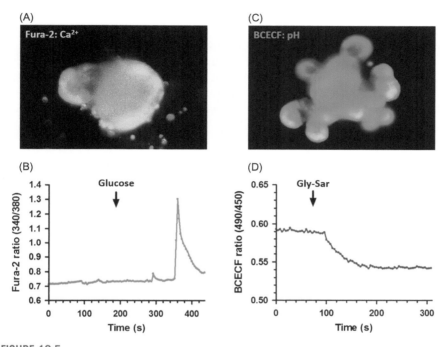

FIGURE 10.5

Fluorescent live cell imaging in small-intestinal organoids derived from wild-type mice. Organoids were loaded with the fluorescent calcium indicator Fura-2 (A), or with the pH indicator BCECF (C). (B): Glucose-induced calcium signal, y-axis displays the Fura-2 fluorescence excitation ratio at 340/380 nm. (D): Intracellular acidification upon treatment with the dipeptide Glycyl-Sarcosin, given as BCECF fluorescence excitation ratio at 490/450 nm. Representative measurements of single organoids.

there are still challenges that need to be addressed in the future. Transport studies can successfully be conducted in intestinal organoids, and specific transporters can be targeted by employing inhibitors and knockout mice. It is, however, not possible to target the apical or basolateral compartments separately, as can be done easily in transwell-based assays. Microinjection of effectors into the lumen of the organoids in order to specifically target the apical proteins is technically challenging. This technique would probably not generate reliable outcomes from transport studies, because the organoid epithelium is not completely tight but in parts leaky *per se*, and it would be additionally damaged by microinjection. An approach based on seeding of three-dimensional organoids on transwell membranes leads to the development of two-dimensional monolayers comprising different enterocytes of the intestinal epithelium (Schweinlin et al., 2016; VanDussen et al., 2015). These cultures are promising models for transport studies, but need further evaluation. The only transporter-mediated substrate flux that has been demonstrated in this system is the efflux of rhodamin123 by p-glycoprotein (Mdr1) (Schweinlin et al., 2016). Furthermore, growth of the cultures requires an extracellular matrix based on a porcine small intestinal scaffold, which is not trivial to prepare, and optimal differentiation needs dynamic culture conditions in a perfusion bioreactor. It would also be of value to verify if this model contains different kinds of hormone-secreting enteroendocrine cells and could be implemented for studies on nutrient sensing and enteroendocrine secretion. The matrices required for growth of three-dimensional organoids, or the two-dimensional transwell-based systems, might be limiting for some compounds. Although many effectors are able to pass these matrices, diffusion of certain compounds could be hindered, due to their steric and/or physiochemical properties. When using the three-dimensional organoid system, it needs to be considered that larger compounds are not able to pass the epithelium of intact organoids, and thus will not reach the inner luminal compartment with apical proteins (when applied from the outside) (Zietek et al., 2015). If using compounds that do not pass the extracellular matrix or do not enter the organoid lumen, organoids can be liberated from the gel matrix and collected in Eppendorf tubes for functional assays (Petersen et al., 2014). Optionally, organoids could then be disrupted (by trituration using a pipette), so that both sides of the epithelium would be exposed to the effector solution.

Most experiments are conducted in small-intestinal organoids from duodenum/proximal jejunum, since they are most easy to grow and give the highest yield. Further functional studies on intestinal organoids derived from different small-intestinal segments and colon are required, as well as comparison of functional properties of murine versus human organoids. Another critical issue is normalization of functional readouts from transport studies. The total amounts of organoids per well can be adjusted by uniform seeding and culturing, and experimental outcomes are stable and reliable with low standard deviation (Fig. 10.3). However, if transport rates between treatments differ only slightly, and assays are sensitive to small changes in transporter activity, careful normalization of substrate transport might be necessary. Total protein content, as often used for normalizing functional readouts from cell culture experiments, is not necessarily recommended for three-dimensional organoid cultures. Residual amounts of the laminin-rich gel matrix, in which organoids are embedded, causes a high background signal in protein quantification assays, while the cellular protein yield from organoids is anyway very low. Normalization to DNA might be a better approach to standardize readouts from transport or other functional studies using three-dimensional organoid cultures.

Further development and improvement of intestinal organoid culture is important, as it currently represents the most physiologically realistic in vitro model for gastrointestinal experimental research. Intestinal organoids will add value to molecular research on diabetes and gastrointestinal disorders, such as malabsorption syndromes. Organoid-based approaches are currently one of the most promising models for pharmacological screening on drug action and bioavailability, including underlying mechanisms.

ACKNOWLEDGMENTS

None.

DECLARATIONS OF FINANCIAL INTERESTS

None.

REFERENCES

Barker, N., 2014. Adult intestinal stem cells: critical drivers of epithelial homeostasis and regeneration. Nat. Rev. Mol. Cell. Biol. 15, 19–33.

Beale, J.H., Parker, J.L., Samsudin, F., Barrett, A.L., Senan, A., Bird, L.E., et al., 2015. Crystal Structures of the Extracellular Domain from PepT1 and PepT2 Provide Novel Insights into Mammalian Peptide Transport. Structure. 23, 1889–1899.

Berthelsen, R., Nielsen, C.U., Brodin, B., 2013. Basolateral glycylsarcosine (Gly-Sar) transport in Caco-2 cell monolayers is pH dependent. J. Pharm. Pharmacol. 65, 970–979.

Chen, M., Singh, A., Xiao, F., Dringenberg, U., Wang, J., Engelhardt, R., et al., 2010. Gene ablation for PEPT1 in mice abolishes the effects of dipeptides on small intestinal fluid absorption, short-circuit current, and intracellular pH. Am. J. Physiol. Gastrointest. Liver. Physiol. 299, G265–G274.

Chen, Y., Lin, Y., Davis, K.M., Wang, Q., Rnjak-Kovacina, J., Li, C., et al., 2015. Robust bioengineered 3D functional human intestinal epithelium. Sci Rep. 5, 13708.

Daniel, H., Kottra, G., 2004. The proton oligopeptide cotransporter family SLC15 in physiology and pharmacology. Pflug Arch Eur J Phys. 447, 610–618.

Daniel, H., Zietek, T., 2015. Taste and move: glucose and peptide transporters in the gastrointestinal tract. Exp. Physiol. 100, 1441–1450.

de Lau, W., Barker, N., Low, T.Y., Koo, B.K., Li, V.S., Teunissen, H., et al., 2011. Lgr5 homologues associate with Wnt receptors and mediate R-spondin signalling. Nature. 476, 293–297.

Dekkers, J.F., Berkers, G., Kruisselbrink, E., Vonk, A., de Jonge, H.R., Janssens, H.M., et al., 2016a. Characterizing responses to CFTR-modulating drugs using rectal organoids derived from subjects with cystic fibrosis. Sci Transl Med 8, 344ra384.

Dekkers, J.F., Gogorza Gondra, R.A., Kruisselbrink, E., Vonk, A.M., Janssens, H.M., de Winter-de Groot, K.M., et al., 2016b. Optimal correction of distinct CFTR folding mutants in rectal cystic fibrosis organoids. Eur. Respir. J. 48, 451–458.

Delezay, O., Baghdiguian, S., Fantini, J., 1995. The development of Na(+)-dependent glucose transport during differentiation of an intestinal epithelial cell clone is regulated by protein kinase C. J. Biol. Chem. 270, 12536–12541.

Diakogiannaki, E., Pais, R., Tolhurst, G., Parker, H.E., Horscroft, J., Rauscher, B., et al., 2013. Oligopeptides stimulate glucagon-like peptide-1 secretion in mice through proton-coupled uptake and the calcium-sensing receptor. Diabetologia. 56, 2688–2696.

Douard, V., Ferraris, R.P., 2013. The role of fructose transporters in diseases linked to excessive fructose intake. J. Physiol. 591, 401–414.

Drucker, D.J., 2015. Deciphering metabolic messages from the gut drives therapeutic innovation: the 2014 Banting Lecture. Diabetes. 64, 317–326.

Ebert, K., Witt, H., 2016. Fructose malabsorption. Mol Cell Pediatr. 3, 10.

Emery, E.C., Diakogiannaki, E., Gentry, C., Psichas, A., Habib, A.M., Bevan, S., et al., 2015. Stimulation of GLP-1 secretion downstream of the ligand-gated ion channel TRPA1. Diabetes. 64, 1202–1210.

Farrell, T.L., Ellam, S.L., Forrelli, T., Williamson, G., 2013. Attenuation of glucose transport across Caco-2 cell monolayers by a polyphenol-rich herbal extract: interactions with SGLT1 and GLUT2 transporters. Biofactors. 39, 448–456.

Ganapathy, M.E., Brandsch, M., Prasad, P.D., Ganapathy, V., Leibach, F.H., 1995. Differential recognition of beta -lactam antibiotics by intestinal and renal peptide transporters, PEPT 1 and PEPT 2. J. Biol. Chem. 270, 25672–25677.

Gorboulev, V., Schurmann, A., Vallon, V., Kipp, H., Jaschke, A., Klessen, D., et al., 2012. Na(+)-D-glucose cotransporter SGLT1 is pivotal for intestinal glucose absorption and glucose-dependent incretin secretion. Diabetes. 61, 187–196.

Gribble, F.M., Reimann, F., 2016. Enteroendocrine Cells: Chemosensors in the Intestinal Epithelium. Annu. Rev. Physiol. 78, 277–299.

Grossmann, J., Maxson, J.M., Whitacre, C.M., Orosz, D.E., Berger, N.A., Fiocchi, C., et al., 1998. New isolation technique to study apoptosis in human intestinal epithelial cells. Am. J. Pathol. 153, 53–62.

Habib, A.M., Richards, P., Cairns, L.S., Rogers, G.J., Bannon, C.A., Parker, H.E., et al., 2012. Overlap of endocrine hormone expression in the mouse intestine revealed by transcriptional profiling and flow cytometry. Endocrinology. 153, 3054–3065.

Habib, A.M., Richards, P., Rogers, G.J., Reimann, F., Gribble, F.M., 2013. Co-localisation and secretion of glucagon-like peptide 1 and peptide YY from primary cultured human L cells. Diabetologia. 56, 1413–1416.

Hirsch, J.R., Loo, D.D., Wright, E.M., 1996. Regulation of Na + /glucose cotransporter expression by protein kinases in Xenopus laevis oocytes. J. Biol. Chem. 271, 14740–14746.

Jiang, S., Zhai, H., Li, D., Huang, J., Zhang, H., Li, Z., et al., 2016. AMPK-dependent regulation of GLP1 expression in L-like cells. J. Mol. Endocrinol. 57, 151–160.

Kellett, G.L., Brot-Laroche, E., Mace, O.J., Leturque, A., 2008. Sugar absorption in the intestine: the role of GLUT2. Annu. Rev. Nutr. 28, 35–54.

Kuhre, R.E., Frost, C.R., Svendsen, B., Holst, J.J., 2015. Molecular mechanisms of glucose-stimulated GLP-1 secretion from perfused rat small intestine. Diabetes. 64, 370–382.

Kuhre, R.E., Wewer Albrechtsen, N.J., Deacon, C.F., Balk-Moller, E., Rehfeld, J.F., Reimann, F., et al., 2016. Peptide production and secretion in GLUTag, NCI-H716, and STC-1 cells: a comparison to native L-cells. J. Mol. Endocrinol. 56, 201–211.

Leushacke, M., Barker, N., 2014. Ex vivo culture of the intestinal epithelium: strategies and applications. Gut. 63, 1345–1354.

Liu, X., Liu, S., Liu, X., Shi, Y., Yang, J., Huang, Z., et al., 2016. Fluorescent 6-amino-6-deoxyglycoconjugates for glucose transporter mediated bioimaging. Biochem. Biophys. Res. Commun.

Maschmeyer, I., Hasenberg, T., Jaenicke, A., Lindner, M., Lorenz, A.K., Zech, J., et al., 2015a. Chip-based human liver-intestine and liver-skin co-cultures--A first step toward systemic repeated dose substance testing in vitro. Eur. J. Pharm. Biopharm. 95, 77–87.

Maschmeyer, I., Lorenz, A.K., Schimek, K., Hasenberg, T., Ramme, A.P., Hubner, J., et al., 2015b. A four-organ-chip for interconnected long-term co-culture of human intestine, liver, skin and kidney equivalents. Lab. Chip. 15, 2688−2699.

Murphy, S.V., Atala, A., 2014. 3D bioprinting of tissues and organs. Nat. Biotechnol. 32, 773−785.

Pais, R., Zietek, T., Hauner, H., Daniel, H., Skurk, T., 2014. RANTES (CCL5) reduces glucose-dependent secretion of glucagon-like peptides 1 and 2 and impairs glucose-induced insulin secretion in mice. Am. J. Physiol. Gastrointest. Liver. Physiol. 307, G330−G337.

Parker, H.E., Wallis, K., le Roux, C.W., Wong, K.Y., Reimann, F., Gribble, F.M., 2012. Molecular mechanisms underlying bile acid-stimulated glucagon-like peptide-1 secretion. Br. J. Pharmacol. 165, 414−423.

Petersen, N., Reimann, F., Bartfeld, S., Farin, H.F., Ringnalda, F.C., Vries, R.G., et al., 2014. Generation of L cells in mouse and human small intestine organoids. Diabetes. 63, 410−420.

Petersen, N., Reimann, F., van Es, J.H., van den Berg, B.M., Kroone, C., Pais, R., et al., 2015. Targeting development of incretin-producing cells increases insulin secretion. J. Clin. Investig. 125, 379−385.

Praslickova, D., Torchia, E.C., Sugiyama, M.G., Magrane, E.J., Zwicker, B.L., Kolodzieyski, L., et al., 2012. The ileal lipid binding protein is required for efficient absorption and transport of bile acids in the distal portion of the murine small intestine. PLoS. ONE. 7, e50810.

Reimann, F., Gribble, F.M., 2016. Mechanisms underlying glucose-dependent insulinotropic polypeptide and glucagon-like peptide-1 secretion. J. Diabetes Investig. 7 (Suppl 1), 13−19.

Reimann, F., Habib, A.M., Tolhurst, G., Parker, H.E., Rogers, G.J., Gribble, F.M., 2008. Glucose sensing in L cells: a primary cell study. Cell Metab. 8, 532−539.

Reimann, F., Tolhurst, G., Gribble, F.M., 2012. G-protein-coupled receptors in intestinal chemosensation. Cell Metab. 15, 421−431.

Roder, P.V., Geillinger, K.E., Zietek, T.S., Thorens, B., Koepsell, H., Daniel, H., 2014. The role of SGLT1 and GLUT2 in intestinal glucose transport and sensing. PLoS. ONE. 9, e89977.

Santer, R., Groth, S., Kinner, M., Dombrowski, A., Berry, G.T., Brodehl, J., et al., 2002. The mutation spectrum of the facilitative glucose transporter gene SLC2A2 (GLUT2) in patients with Fanconi-Bickel syndrome. Hum. Genet. 110, 21−29.

Sato, T., Vries, R.G., Snippert, H.J., van de Wetering, M., Barker, N., Stange, D.E., et al., 2009. Single Lgr5 stem cells build crypt-villus structures in vitro without a mesenchymal niche. Nature. 459, 262−265.

Schulze, C., Bangert, A., Kottra, G., Geillinger, K.E., Schwanck, B., Vollert, H., et al., 2014. Inhibition of the intestinal sodium-coupled glucose transporter 1 (SGLT1) by extracts and polyphenols from apple reduces postprandial blood glucose levels in mice and humans. Mol. Nutr. Food. Res. 58, 1795−1808.

Schweinlin, M., Wilhelm, S., Schwedhelm, I., Hansmann, J., Rietscher, R., Jurowich, C., et al., 2016. Development of an Advanced Primary Human In Vitro Model of the Small Intestine. Tissue. Eng. Part. C. Methods.

Spence, J.R., Mayhew, C.N., Rankin, S.A., Kuhar, M.F., Vallance, J.E., Tolle, K., et al., 2011. Directed differentiation of human pluripotent stem cells into intestinal tissue in vitro. Nature. 470, 105−109.

Stelzl, T., Baranov, T., Geillinger, K.E., Kottra, G., Daniel, H., 2016. Effect of N-glycosylation on the transport activity of the peptide transporter PEPT1. Am. J. Physiol. Gastrointest. Liver. Physiol. 310, G128−G141.

Sugano, K., Kansy, M., Artursson, P., Avdeef, A., Bendels, S., Di, L., et al., 2010. Coexistence of passive and carrier-mediated processes in drug transport. Nat. Rev. Drug. Discov. 9, 597−614.

Surampalli, G., Nanjwade, B.K., Patil, P.A., 2016. Safety evaluation of naringenin upon experimental exposure on rat gastrointestinal epithelium for novel optimal drug delivery. Drug. Deliv. 23, 512−524.

Svendsen, B., Holst, J.J., 2016. Regulation of gut hormone secretion. Studies using isolated perfused intestines. Peptides. 77, 47−53.

Tolhurst, G., Reimann, F., Gribble, F.M., 2012. Intestinal sensing of nutrients. Handb. Exp. Pharmacol. 309−335.

van de Wetering, M., Francies, H.E., Francis, J.M., Bounova, G., Iorio, F., Pronk, A., et al., 2015. Prospective derivation of a living organoid biobank of colorectal cancer patients. Cell. 161, 933−945.

VanDussen, K.L., Marinshaw, J.M., Shaikh, N., Miyoshi, H., Moon, C., Tarr, P.I., et al., 2015. Development of an enhanced human gastrointestinal epithelial culture system to facilitate patient-based assays. Gut. 64, 911−920.

Wang, B., Li, B., 2017. Effect of molecular weight on the transepithelial transport and peptidase degradation of casein-derived peptides by using Caco-2 cell model. Food. Chem. 218, 1−8.

Watterson, K.R., Hudson, B.D., Ulven, T., Milligan, G., 2014. Treatment of type 2 diabetes by free Fatty Acid receptor agonists. Frontiers in endocrinology. 5, 137.

Wengerter, B.C., Emre, G., Park, J.Y., Geibel, J., 2016. Three-dimensional Printing in the Intestine. Clin. Gastroenterol. Hepatol. 14, 1081−1085.

Wenzel, U., Kuntz, S., Diestel, S., Daniel, H., 2002. PEPT1-mediated cefixime uptake into human intestinal epithelial cells is increased by Ca2 + channel blockers. Antimicrob. Agents. Chemother. (Bethesda). 46, 1375−1380.

Wright, E.M., Hirayama, B.A., Loo, D.F., 2007. Active sugar transport in health and disease. J. Intern. Med. 261, 32−43.

Wuensch, T., Schulz, S., Ullrich, S., Lill, N., Stelzl, T., Rubio-Aliaga, I., et al., 2013. The peptide transporter PEPT1 is expressed in distal colon in rodents and humans and contributes to water absorption. Am J Physiol-Gastr L. 305, G66−G73.

Yoshikawa, T., Inoue, R., Matsumoto, M., Yajima, T., Ushida, K., Iwanaga, T., 2011. Comparative expression of hexose transporters (SGLT1, GLUT1, GLUT2 and GLUT5) throughout the mouse gastrointestinal tract. Histochem. Cell. Biol. 135, 183−194.

Yui, S., Nakamura, T., Sato, T., Nemoto, Y., Mizutani, T., Zheng, X., et al., 2012. Functional engraftment of colon epithelium expanded in vitro from a single adult Lgr5 (+) stem cell. Nat. Med. 18, 618−623.

Zietek, T., Daniel, H., 2015. Intestinal nutrient sensing and blood glucose control. Curr. Opin. Clin. Nutr. Metab. Care. 18, 381−388.

Zietek, T., Rath, E., 2016. Inflammation meets metabolic disease: gut feeling mediated by GLP-1. Front. Immunol. 7, 154.

Zietek, T., Rath, E., Haller, D., Daniel, H., 2015. Intestinal organoids for assessing nutrient transport, sensing and incretin secretion. Sci Rep. 5, 16831.

A three-dimensional neurosphere system using human stem cells for nanotoxicology studies

11

Yang Zeng, Tin-Tin Win-Shwe, Tomohiro Ito and Hideko Sone

National Institute for Environmental Studies, Tsukuba, Japan

CHAPTER OUTLINE

INTRODUCTION

The recent development of three-dimensional (3D) culture systems has made it possible to partially recapitulate the complexity of mammalian organogenesis in vitro, and has allowed some transplantable tissues to be made. Culturing human-derived stem cells, such as human embryonic stem cells (hESCs), human-induced pluripotent stem cells (hiPSCs), and human adult stem cells (hAdSCs) in 3D, has opened up new avenues for the exploration of human development, and for regenerative medicine. Organoids are 3D structures derived from iPSCs, hESCA, neonatal tissue stem cells, or AdSCs/adult progenitors, in which cells spontaneously self-organize into properly differentiated functional cell types and specialized progenitors, forming a tissue-like mass that resembles its in vivo counterpart to recapitulate at least some functions of the organ. Neurosphere models have shown great potential as versatile in vitro 3D model systems for developmental neurotoxicity testing (Fritsche and Schreiber, 2011; Hill et al., 2008). Midbrain organoids containing long-lived dopaminergic neurons have been engineered (Tieng et al., 2014). Extracellular signaling pathways trigger human neural

Organoids and Mini-Organs. DOI: http://dx.doi.org/10.1016/B978-0-12-812636-3.00011-0

progenitor cell migration in the system (Moors et al., 2007), and ultrasoft hydro-gels can promote the formation of neurites (axons and dendrites) from neural cells (Palazzolo et al., 2015).

Stem cell models have been used for toxicity screening in the human central nervous system (Hunsberger et al., 2015), and human neural progenitor cells (hNPCs) have great potential for treating neurodegenerative diseases. Moreover, hNPCs can integrate into host tissues, and differentiate into different neuronal subtypes (Cossetti et al., 2012; Ryu et al., 2009). Therefore, hNPCs have been used as a new model system in screening assays for the effects of compounds on the development of the nervous system (Barenys et al., 2016; Breier et al., 2010; Breier et al., 2008; Qin et al., 2012).

To assess the toxicity of nanoparticles, many approaches, including organoid-based and nonorganoid-based in vitro and in vivo models, have been used. We have analyzed the issues involved in using them for toxicity assessments, and have judged the potential advantages and disadvantages of each approach, before considering the design presented here. The following topics will be the focus of this chapter:

- The importance of toxicity assessment and how the problem is being addressed.
- The potential advantages and disadvantages of the organoid-based approach.
- Our current approach.
- Assessment of the effect of nanoparticles on neuronal development using our hNPC-based approach.
- Remaining challenges for future work.

IMPORTANCE OF TOXICITY ASSESSMENTS AND HOW THE PROBLEM IS BEING ADDRESSED

Human exposure to chemicals may be increased because of an expansion of both the variety and quantity of chemicals being used in and released in our environment. It is therefore important to assess the toxicity of chemicals before they reach the public. To assess the effects of chemicals on human and animals, many approaches have been used. Nonorganoid-based in vitro methods can provide assessment of basic parameters such as cell viability, but they cannot simulate the complexity of human and animal bodies. In vivo methods better simulate physiological aspects of chemical exposure, but they also have some limitations. Developmental neurotoxicity (DNT) that occurs with maternal exposure to, for example, methylmercury and thalidomide, have been serious health issues, and it is important that similar effects of future chemicals, including pharmaceuticals, are detected in experimental systems before damage is done to the human population. Rats are widely used as experimental animals for DNT testing. However, this approach is very expensive and time-intensive, and it requires the use of large numbers of animals. Moreover, rat models pose the additional problem of species differences for human extrapolation. To investigate the toxicity of nanoparticles in the human body, we have developed an organoid-based approach for conducting safety studies. Currently, the main challenge to be faced for this approach is the establishment of stable neurosphere models.

THE POTENTIAL ADVANTAGES AND DISADVANTAGES OF THE ORGANOID-BASED APPROACH

Many approaches have been used to assess the toxicity of chemicals. In vivo studies have the advantage of using exposure of intact animals, the internal parts of which are separated from the environment by skin and mucosal tissues. In vivo models are useful for assessing the direct effects of chemicals on animals, which may be similar to the effect on the human body. An example of this in vivo approach is a study of the toxicty of polyamidoamine (PAMAM) dendrimers. In order to determine the effects and biodistribution of these chemicals after intranasal instillation, polyamidoamine (PAMAM) dendrimers were conjugated to fluorophores, and injected intra-nasally into mice, and the biodistribution and effects of PAMAM dendrimers in the mouse brain were then investigated. The findings indicated that PAMAM may have an effect on neuronal differentiation, and that the effect may be associated with oxidative stress and DNA damage (Win-Shwe et al., 2014). However, this was a costly approach, and the mechanism of toxicity in humans may be different from that in animal models. Therefore, to assess the chemical toxicity of PANAM dendrimers in humans, we explored the idea of using a neurosphere model.

Nonorganoid-based in vitro studies have the advantages of being inexpensive and convenient, and have been used for toxicity testing. For example, stem cell models have been used for screening and safety assessment of the central nervous system (Hunsberger et al., 2015; Kolaja, 2014). Rat mesencephalic neural stem cells have been used to study apoptosis (Suzuki and Ishido, 2011), and mouse embryonic stem cells have been used to assess developmental neurotoxicity (Visan et al., 2012), and the changes of gene expression in response to two anticonvulsant drugs (Schultz et al., 2015). Neural progenitor cells have also been used to study adhesion, migration, and developmental neurotoxicity in vitro (Barenys et al., 2016; Gassmann et al., 2010). The neurotoxicity of the PAMAM dendrimer itself has been studied using an hNPC-based cell culture system (Zeng et al., 2016). However, because this simple system lacks sensitivity, no significant difference could be found at low concentrations, in contrast to our newly-established organoid-based approach (Zeng et al., 2016).

The organoid-based approach of making neurospheres has the following advantages: it is convenient; it has an anatomical complexity more similar to in vivo tissue; it improves cell interactions and reflects basic processes of foetal brain development, including proliferation, differentiation, and apoptosis. What is more, development of neurospheres can be controlled by the environment; for example, ultra-soft alginate hydrogels are known to support long-term 3D functional neuronal networks (Palazzolo et al., 2015). Known neurotoxins, such as acrylamide, inhibit neurosphere formation by neural stem cells (Chen et al., 2015). Neurospheres have already been used as models for developmental neurotoxicity testing (Fritsche et al., 2011), and have been useful in comparing human and rat developmental neurotoxicity: differentiating Ntera2/clone D1 (NT2/D1) cell neurospheres have been exposed to human teratogens, to test their developmental neurotoxicity (Hill et al., 2008; Salama et al., 2015).

OUR CURRENT NEUROSPHERE-BASED APPROACH

To establish a model for neurotoxicity assessment of chemicals, PAMAM dendrimer nanoparticles have been used as a test substance in our study. Dendrimers have been proposed for a variety of biomedical applications, and the PAMAM dendrimer is increasingly studied as a model nanomaterial for such uses. The dendritic structure features both modular synthetic control of molecular size and shape, and presentation of multiple equivalent terminal groups. These properties make PAMAM dendrimers highly functional and versatile single-molecule nanoparticles, with a high degree of consistency and low polydispersity.

Recent nanotoxicological studies showed that intravenous administration of amine-terminated PAMAM dendrimers to mice was lethal, causing a disseminated intravascular coagulation-like condition. Our research group recently demonstrated developmental neurotoxicity of PAMAM dendrimer nanoparticles (Zeng et al., 2016). In our study, a 3D neurosphere model based on hNPCs was used to assess the developmental neurotoxicity of PAMAM dendrimers. We investigated the biodistribution of PAMAM dendrimers in the neurosphere, and the effect of PAMAM dendrimer on neurosphere migration and differentiation. We used fluorescence-labeled PAMAM dendrimers to investigate biodistribution in a 3D cell culture model by exposing 3D neurospheres to those dendrimers, and found a time-dependent biodistribution of the dendrimers, which may affect neurosphere migration but not differentiation. To the best of our knowledge, this is the first study that has evaluated the developmental neurotoxicity of PAMAM dendrimer nanoparticles in a 3D cell culture model.

METHOD

We developed a 3D cell culture model for 10 days, to evaluate the neurotoxic effects of PAMAM dendrimers (Zeng et al., 2016; as shown in Fig. 11.1A). Human neural progenitor cells were cultured in NEM (Neural Expansion

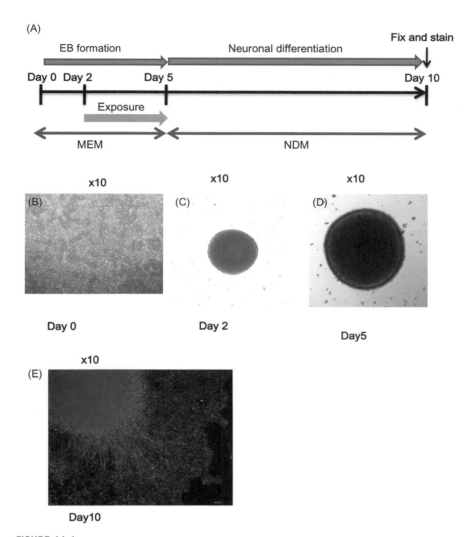

FIGURE 11.1

Experimental time schedules. (A): Cells were seeded on day 0 to form neurospheres and then exposed to chemicals from days 2 to 5. Morphological analysis was conducted on day 10. Morphological photographs for differentiation of hNPCs in the neurosphere assay (B–E). This culture protocol can be used to assess chemicals, including nanoparticles.

Medium, ENStem-A) supplemented with 0.05% b-FGF and 1% L-glutamine on poly-ornithine-coated and laminin-111-coated (Sigma-Aldrich, St. Louis, MO, US) dishes. On day 0 (d0), the cells were transferred to 96-well round bottom plates (Nunc, Falcon), at a density of 6,000 cells per well, to allow neurosphere formation. On day 2 (d2), NEM mixed with PAMAM dendrimers was used to gently replace culture media, and they were then incubated for 72 hours. On day 5 (d5), the neurospheres were gently transferred to a 48-well plate that was pre-coated with laminin-511 and contained neural differentiation media (neurobasal medium, NDM), supplemented with $1 \times B27$, $1 \times N2$, and 10 ng/mL BDNF (brain-derived neurotrophic factor, Invitrogen, Carlsbad, CA). After transfer to the NDM media, spheres grew and neurite cells migrated. After plating for adhesion, polarized individual cells migrated outward from the center of the sphere after 24 hours. After 5 days, the size of the cell body and length of projections increased. After 10 days, cellular projections increased not only in size, but also in density. Individual cells displayed multiple neurite outgrowths and dendritic spines, which are typical characteristics of both immature and mature neuronal phenotypes (Fig. 11.1B−E). The NDM was changed every 3 days, before performing the following assay.

Immunostaining was performed on day 10 (d10). Neurospheres were fixed in 4% paraformaldehyde for 15 minutes, and then treated with 0.1% TritonX-100 for 30 minutes. After incubating with 1% BSA-PBS for 30 minutes at room temperature (RT), cells were incubated with primary antibodies [mouse antimicrotubule-associated protein 2 (MAP2;1:200 dilution; Sigma-Aldrich)] overnight at 4°C. After washing with PBS, the cells were incubated with secondary antibodies (Alexa Fluor 488 donkey antimouse IgG; 1:1,000 dilution) for 1 hour at RT. Following this, the cells were treated with 2 µg/mL Hoechst 33342 solution for 15 minutes at RT. Neurite length per cell and nuclei number were analyzed and calculated using InCell analyzer 1000 (GE Healthcare, Tokyo, Japan). Images were obtained using a 10× objective; furthermore, nine images were acquired for each well, and merged into the one image with image analysis software IN Cell Developer Tool Box 1.7 (GE Healthcare). The area of the sphere, and the elongation of sphere as a marker for neurite migration, were measured using ImageJ, which is an open source image processing program designed for scientific multidimensional images (https://imagej.net/Welcome).

To investigate incorporation and biodistribution of Alexa-labeled PAMAM dendrimers, Alexa568-labeled PAMAM dendrimers at a concentration of 10 µg/mL were incubated with neurospheres in 96-well round bottom plates. The spheres were transferred to a laminin-511-coated glass bottom dish for observation at 24, 48, and 72 hours. Microphotographs showing the incorporation of Alexa568-labeled PAMAM dendrimers were obtained using an Olympus LV1200 high-performance laser scanning microscope (Olympus Optical, Japan). Images for illustration were obtained using 10× or 20× objectives.

To study the mechanism of toxicity, neurospheres were treated with PAMAM dendrimer-NH2 (10 µg/mL) for 72 hours. Four neurospheres each, from the treatment and control groups, were pooled together, and RNAs were isolated from each group. To detect changes in gene expression in neurospheres after PAMAM dendrimer exposure, microarray analyses were performed on two RNA samples (Sureprint G3 Human GE $8 \times 60K$ Ver.2.0 1color 4; Agilent Technologies Inc., Santa Clara, CA, USA). The arrays were hybridized, and scanned in accordance with the manufacturer's directions. The raw data were normalized and filtered by expression to the cut-off low values, and then filtered by flag tag to remove entities that were not detected by GeneSpring GX12.10 software (Agilent Technologies). The microarray data were submitted to Gene Expression Omnibus (GEO) and registered as GSE65875 (http://www.ncbi.nlm.nih.gov/geo/query/acc.cgi?acc=gse65875). Genes with fold changes in $\log_2$ expression values of >1.5 or ≤ 1.5 from each group were selected and combined, to generate a common entity list. Genes from the commonly responsive list were analyzed using single experiment analysis (SEA) of GeneSpring to find matching genes in the WikiPathways. Matched gene entities from the top five pathways were selected. These 12 genes were then analyzed, using the natural language processing (NLP) network analyses of GeneSpring to identify the extent of interactions.

ASSESSMENT OF NANOPARTICLES ON NEURONAL DEVELOPMENT

To study the developmental neurotoxicity of PAMAM dendrimers, neurites in the neurospheres were immunohistochemically stained with anti-MAP2 protein antibody. Typical images of neurite outgrowth and neurospheres are shown in Fig. 11.2(A, B). The effects of PAMAM dendrimers on neurite length per cell, and the number of nuclei that migrated from neural spheres were investigated and quantitatively determined. The dendrimers did not inhibit neurite length per cell at any concentration tested in the present study. To quantify other potential effects of the dendrimers, the central core sizes of the neurosphere without flare areas, which indicated cell proliferations, and with the flare areas, which indicated cell migrations, were measured using ImageJ software. PAMAM dendrimer-NH$_2$ significantly inhibited cell migration in a dose-dependent manner, and the mean area of the extended neurons decreased in comparison with that observed in the controls (Fig. 11.2C). Alexa-PAMAM conjugates at a concentration of $10\,\mu g/mL$ inhibited cell migration, and the extent of inhibition was similar to that observed for PAMAM-NH$_2$ dendrimers. However, Alexa-PAMAM conjugates did not affect migration or differentiation, whereas PAMAM-NH$_2$ dendrimers did, at a concentration of $1\,\mu g/mL$.

To examine the bioincorporation of chemicals in neurospheres, PAMAM dendrimer nanoparticles were conjugated with Alexa 568. Alexa-PAMAM conjugates were incubated with neurospheres for 3 days. A group of neurospheres used as control was treated with PAMAM dendrimers for 3 days, and then treated for

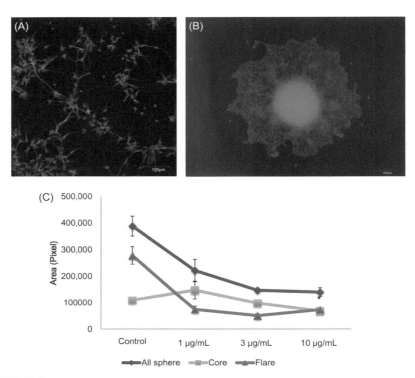

FIGURE 11.2

Photographs and quantified data of neurosphere area after chemical (PAMAM-NH$_2$) treatment were measured using the In-cell analyzer 1000. Morphology of neuronal cells (A), and neurosphere (B), captured with the 20× and 10× optical lens, respectively. Quantified data on the effects on migration of PAMAM-NH$_2$ were acquired using Image J ver4 for measurement of sphere and flare areas (C).

72 hours with the fluorescent agent only. No fluorescent signal was observed in the control group. For the Alexa-PAMAM conjugate-treated group, the Alexa-568 fluorescence signal was only observed on the surface of neurospheres at day 3 (Fig. 11.3A), and an increasing number of Alexa-PAMAM conjugates was observed within the neurospheres at day 5 (Fig. 11.3B). The results showed a time-dependent biodistribution of PAMAM dendrimers, and serve as evidence that Alexa-PAMAM was located in the center of neurospheres after 3 days of exposure, evidence that it was being organized in some way by the cells.

The expression of 50,739 genes was investigated by microarray analysis. Genes that were not detected and with low expression values were filtered out, leaving 25,622 genes. Using fold-changes in log$_2$ expression values of >1.5 or ≤ 1.5, 289 and 171 entities were filtered from two independent experiments, respectively. Thirty-two of these genes were responsive in both experiments.

Day 3   Day 5

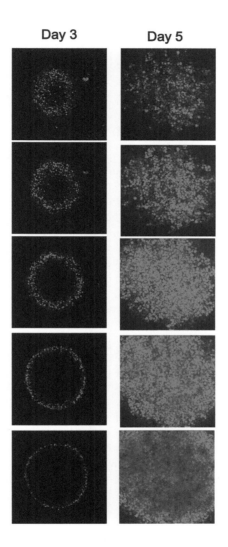

FIGURE 11.3

Distribution images of PAMAM-NH$_2$ dendrimers using a confocal laser microscope. Two-dimensional photographs of sphere cross-sections were acquired at day 3 (A), and day 5 (B), after starting the sphere formation. The top to the bottom in photographs are the top to the middle of sphere. The distance from bottom to the top is 30 μm.

These 32 genes were then analyzed by SEA to find matching genes in WikiPathways. Pathway analysis showed that direct interactions, network targets and regulatory pathways, and Hs_adipogenesis were the most matched pathways. Most of the matched genes, except *CYP26A1*, were downregulated. We then analyzed how the 32 genes interact with each other in NLP. The result revealed four connected components: early growth response gene 1 (EGR1), insulin-like growth factor-binding protein 3 (IGFBP3), tissue factor pathway inhibitor 2 (TFPI2), and adrenomedullin (ADM) were the key nodes.

CHALLENGES FOR FUTURE WORK

Modifications to the culturing protocol may be needed to achieve better stability of spheres in culture, because an opportunity to study long-term exposure is important for toxicological assessment. Potential problems that one may encounter with the protocols described in this manuscript might lie in culturing the neurospheres, choosing neurospheres for the experiments, and subsequent plating processes. The experimenter should ensure that spheres are fed on a regular basis. Neurospheres sorted for the experiments should be round with light- and dark-colored outer and inner regions, respectively. Novice investigators may encounter a problem with irregular migrating areas, or neurospheres that do not attach to the surface under differentiating conditions.

Moreover, this model may not be suitable for other cell lines, or to assess the effects of other chemicals. We will need to determine whether these neurospheres can develop into electro-physiologically competent grafts, for more subtle physiological testing. It will be interesting to explore the advantages and disadvantages of using dendrimers and organoids in the field of neurotoxicology.

In terms of the dendrimer itself, future studies should focus on determining how dendrimer nanoparticles influence plasma proteins in general and procoagulant proteins in particular, as a function of dendrimer generation and chemistry (e.g., charge density, formal charge). Specifically, a focus on how dendrimers influence coagulation factor activation and fibrin polymerization is needed, since dendrimer toxicity may be related to their direct interactions with either blood proteins or cells, or the modulation of complex interactions between both these blood components.

REFERENCES

Barenys, M., Gassmann, K., Baksmeier, C., Heinz, S., Reverte, I., Schmuck, M., et al., 2016. Epigallocatechin gallate (EGCG) inhibits adhesion and migration of neural progenitor cells *in vitro*. Arch. Toxicol. Available from: http://dx.doi.org/10.1007/s00204-016-1709-8.

Breier, J.M., Radio, N.M., Mundy, W.R., Shafer, T.J., 2008. Development of a high-throughput screening assay for chemical effects on proliferation and viability of immortalized human neural progenitor cells. Toxicological Sciences 105 (1), 119—133. Available from: http://dx.doi.org/10.1093/toxsci/kfn115.

Breier, J.M., Gassmann, K., Kayser, R., Stegeman, H., De Groot, D., Fritsche, E., et al., 2010. Neural progenitor cells as models for high-throughput screens of developmental neurotoxicity: State of the science. Neurotoxicol. Teratol. 32 (1), 4—15. Available from: http://dx.doi.org/10.1016/j.ntt.2009.06.005.

Chen, J.H., Lee, D.C., Chen, M.S., Ko, Y.C., Chiu, I.M., 2015. Inhibition of neurosphere formation in neural stem/progenitor cells by acrylamide. Cell. Transplant. 24 (5), 779—796. Available from: http://dx.doi.org/10.3727/096368913X676925.

Cossetti, C., Alfaro-Cervello, C., Donega, M., Tyzack, G., Pluchino, S., 2012. New perspectives of tissue remodelling with neural stem and progenitor cell-based therapies. Cell. Tissue. Res. 349 (1), 321—329. Available from: http://dx.doi.org/10.1007/s00441-012-1341-8.

Fritsche, E., Gassmann, K., Schreiber, T., 2011. Neurospheres as a model for developmental neurotoxicity testing. Methods. Mol. Biol. 758, 99—114. Available from: http://dx.doi.org/10.1007/978-1-61779-170-3_7.

Gassmann, K., Abel, J., Bothe, H., Haarmann-Stemmann, T., Merk, H.F., Quasthoff, K.N., et al., 2010. Species-specific differential AhR expression protects human neural progenitor cells against developmental neurotoxicity of PAHs. Environ. Health. Perspect. 118 (11), 1571—1577. Available from: http://dx.doi.org/10.1289/ehp.0901545.

Hill, E.J., Woehrling, E.K., Prince, M., Coleman, M.D., 2008. Differentiating human NT2/D1 neurospheres as a versatile in vitro 3D model system for developmental neurotoxicity testing. Toxicology 249 (2-3), 243—250. Available from: http://dx.doi.org/10.1016/j.tox.2008.05.014.

Hunsberger, J.G., Efthymiou, A.G., Malik, N., Behl, M., Mead, I.L., Zeng, X., et al., 2015. Induced pluripotent stem cell models to enable in vitro models for screening in the central nervous system. Stem. Cells. Dev. 24 (16), 1852—1864. Available from: http://dx.doi.org/10.1089/scd.2014.0531.

Kolaja, K., 2014. Stem cells and stem cell-derived tissues and their use in safety assessment. J. Biol. Chem. 289 (8), 4555—4561. Available from: http://dx.doi.org/10.1074/jbc.R113.481028.

Moors, M., Cline, J.E., Abel, J., Fritsche, E., 2007. ERK-dependent and -independent pathways trigger human neural progenitor cell migration. Toxicol. Appl. Pharmacol. 221 (1), 57—67. Available from: http://dx.doi.org/10.1016/j.taap.2007.02.018.

Palazzolo, G., Broguiere, N., Cenciarelli, O., Dermutz, H., Zenobi-Wong, M., 2015. Ultrasoft alginate hydrogels support long-term three-dimensional functional neuronal networks. Tissue Eng. Part A 21 (15-16), 2177—2185. Available from: http://dx.doi.org/10.1089/ten.TEA.2014.0518.

Qin, X.Y., Akanuma, H., Wei, F.F., Nagano, R., Zeng, Q., Imanishi, S., et al., 2012. Effect of low-dose thalidomide on dopaminergic neuronal differentiation of human neural progenitor cells: a combined study of metabolomics and morphological analysis. Neurotoxicology 33 (5), 1375—1380. Available from: http://dx.doi.org/10.1016/j.neuro.2012.08.016.

Ryu, J.K., Cho, T., Wang, Y.T., McLarnon, J.G., 2009. Neural progenitor cells attenuate inflammatory reactivity and neuronal loss in an animal model of inflamed AD brain. J. Neuroinflammation 6, Artn39 doi: 10.1186/1742-2094-6-39.

Salama, M., Lotfy, A., Fathy, K., Makar, M., El-Emam, M., El-Gamal, A., et al., 2015. Developmental neurotoxic effects of Malathion on 3D neurosphere system. Appl. Transl. Genom. 7, 13—18. Available from: http://dx.doi.org/10.1016/j.atg.2015.07.001.

Schultz, L., Zurich, M.G., Culot, M., da Costa, A., Landry, C., Bellwon, P., et al., 2015. Evaluation of drug-induced neurotoxicity based on metabolomics, proteomics and electrical activity measurements in complementary CNS *in vitro* models. Toxicol. In. Vitro 30 (1 Pt A), 138−165. Available from: http://dx.doi.org/10.1016/j.tiv.2015.05.016.

Suzuki, J.S., Ishido, M., 2011. Transcriptome of tributyltin-induced apoptosis of the cultured rat mesencephalic neural stem cells. Toxicology 287 (1-3), 61−68. Available from: http://dx.doi.org/10.1016/j.tox.2011.06.001.

Tieng, V., Stoppini, L., Villy, S., Fathi, M., Dubois-Dauphin, M., Krause, K.H., 2014. Engineering of midbrain organoids containing long-lived dopaminergic neurons. Stem. Cells. Dev. 23 (13), 1535−1547. Available from: http://dx.doi.org/10.1089/scd.2013.0442.

Visan, A., Hayess, K., Sittner, D., Pohl, E.E., Riebeling, C., Slawik, B., et al., 2012. Neural differentiation of mouse embryonic stem cells as a tool to assess developmental neurotoxicity *in vitro*. Neurotoxicology 33 (5), 1135−1146. Available from: http://dx.doi.org/10.1016/j.neuro.2012.06.006.

Win-Shwe, T.T., Sone, H., Kurokawa, Y., Zeng, Y., Zeng, Q., Nitta, H., et al., 2014. Effects of PAMAM dendrimers in the mouse brain after a single intranasal instillation. Toxicol. Lett. 228 (3), 207−215. Available from: http://dx.doi.org/10.1016/j.toxlet.2014.04.020.

Zeng, Y., Kurokawa, Y., Zeng, Q., Win-Shwe, T.T., Nansai, H., Zhang, Z., et al., 2016. Effects of polyamidoamine dendrimers on a 3-D neurosphere system using human neural progenitor cells. Toxicol. Sci. 152 (1), 128−144. Available from: http://dx.doi.org/10.1093/toxsci/kfw068.

Zeng, Y., Kurokawa, Y., Win-Shwe, T.T., Zeng, Q., Hirano, S., Zhang, Z., et al., 2016. Effects of PAMAM dendrimers with various surface functional groups and multiple generations on cytotoxicity and neuronal differentiation using human neural progenitor cells. J. Toxicol. Sci. 41 (3), 351−370. Available from: http://dx.doi.org/10.2131/jts.41.351.

FURTHER READING

Moors, M., Rockel, T.D., Abel, J., Cline, J.E., Gassmann, K., Schreiber, T., et al., 2009. Human neurospheres as three-dimensional cellular systems for developmental neurotoxicity testing. Environ. Health. Perspect. 117 (7), 1131−1138, Correction 117(8), A342.

Zeng, Y., Wang, Y., Zeng, Q., Nansai, H., Zhang, Z., Sone, H., 2015. Optimization of neurosphere assays using human neuronal progenitor cells for developmental neurotoxicity testing. Am. J. Tissue Eng. Stem Cell. 2 (1), 7−18.

Organoids for modeling kidney disease

12

Ryuji Morizane[1,2,3] **and Joseph V. Bonventre**[1,2,3]

[1]Brigham and Women's Hospital, Boston, MA, United States [2]Harvard Medical School, Boston, MA, United States [3]Harvard Stem Cell Institute, Cambridge, MA, United States

CHAPTER OUTLINE

INTRODUCTION

Organoids are three-dimensional (3D), organ-like tissues that mimic natural organs, structurally and functionally, in vitro. The following features are generally considered to constitute the main characteristics of organoids: (1) three-dimensional structures; (2) complex multicellular constructs; (3); self-organization; (4) in vitro culture; and (5) recapitulation of developmental programs. There are currently two different sources for generation of organoids: primary tissue or pluripotent stem cells (PSCs) (Fatehullah et al., 2016).

A number of studies have reported generation of organoids from mouse and/or human primary tissues, including lingual (Hisha et al., 2013), salivary gland (Nanduri et al., 2014), esophagus (Sato et al., 2011a; DeWard et al., 2014), stomach (Barker et al., 2010; Stange et al., 2013; Schlaermann et al., 2016; Bartfeld et al., 2015; Wroblewski et al., 2015; Bertaux-Skeirik et al., 2015; Nadauld et al., 2014; Schumacher et al., 2015), intestine (Sato et al., 2011a; Sato et al., 2009; Dekkers et al., 2013; Yin et al., 2014; Drost et al., 2015; Finkbeiner et al., 2015; Finkbeiner et al., 2012; Matano et al., 2015; Fordham et al., 2013; Mustata et al., 2011; Mustata et al., 2013; Sato et al., 2011b; Simmini et al., 2014; van Es et al., 2012; Zhang et al., 2014;

Organoids and Mini-Organs. DOI: http://dx.doi.org/10.1016/B978-0-12-812636-3.00012-2

Horita et al., 2014; Wang et al., 2015; Li et al., 2014; Gracz et al., 2015; Fukuda et al., 2014; Ootani et al., 2009), colon (Sato et al., 2011a; Matano et al., 2015; Jung et al., 2011; Okamoto and Watanabe, 2016; Yui et al., 2012; van de Wetering et al., 2015), liver (Huch et al., 2013b; Huch et al., 2015), pancreas (Huch et al., 2013a; Boj et al., 2015; Greggio et al., 2013), prostate (Karthaus et al., 2014; Gao et al., 2014; Chua et al., 2014), fallopian tube (Kessler et al., 2015), and lung (Mondrinos et al., 2014; Mondrinos et al., 2006). Notably, many primary tissue organoids have been generated from Lgr5+ stem cells from primary tissue using R-spondin, a LGR4/5 ligand (Fatehullah et al., 2016). These organoids were not simply reconstructed by dissociation and reaggregation of the primary tissue, but instead, were generated from the tissue stem cell population.

Human pluripotent stem cells (hPSCs), by virtue of their unlimited self-renewal and ability to generate cells of all three embryonic germ layers, are ideally suited for the generation of functional human kidney cells and tissues (Thomson et al., 1998; Takahashi et al., 2007). There are currently several published studies in which hPSCs have been differentiated into organoids of various tissues including stomach (McCracken et al., 2014; McCracken et al., 2017), intestine (Spence et al., 2011; Cao et al., 2011; Watson et al., 2014), liver (Takebe et al., 2013; Sampaziotis et al., 2015; Ogawa et al., 2015), lung (Dye et al., 2015), brain (Lancaster et al., 2013), anterior pituitary (Ozone et al., 2016), and kidney (Xia et al., 2013; Taguchi et al., 2014; Takasato et al., 2015; Freedman et al., 2015; Morizane et al., 2015; Yamaguchi et al., 2016). Recent advances in directed differentiation protocols toward a kidney lineage have resulted in generation of nephron progenitor cells (NPCs) and kidney (nephron) organoids from human embryonic stem cells (hESCs) and/or human induced pluripotent stem cells (hiPSCs) (Taguchi et al., 2014; Takasato et al., 2015; Morizane et al., 2015; Takasato et al., 2014; Lam et al., 2014).

Both hPSC-derived NPCs and kidney organoids are attractive sources for kidney regeneration. At the same time, kidney organoids can be a novel and useful platform to study kidney diseases in human cells in vitro. There are currently more than 150 inherited kidney diseases (Devuyst et al., 2014). By generating hiPSCs from patients with inherited kidney disease, it is in principle possible to study a disease using kidney organoids derived from patient-derived hiPSCs. Moreover, it is also possible to study inherited kidney diseases by introducing mutations of the target gene with CRISPR/Cas9 genome editing of normal hPSCs (Freedman et al., 2015; Cong et al., 2013; Sterneckert et al., 2014). These approaches enable the analysis of mechanisms of disease due to the mutation, and enable drug screening in vitro, to find new therapeutic approaches (Fig. 12.1).

THE PROBLEM BEING ADDRESSED

Between 9%–14% of the adult population in the United States and other parts of the world suffer from chronic kidney disease (CKD) (Coresh et al., 2007; Ene-Iordache

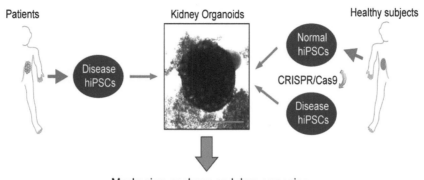

FIGURE 12.1 Kidney organoids and disease modeling for drug screening.

A schematic illustration showing a strategy to model kidney disease with kidney organoids, and to find novel candidates for therapeutics. Disease hiPSCs can be generated from patients with kidney disease, or by genome editing with CRISPR/Cas9 using normal hiPSCs derived from healthy subjects. A scale bar: 500 μm.

et al., 2016). While various kidney diseases have different initiating pathophysiological processes, they result in loss of functional nephrons, and the development of tubulointerstitial fibrosis contributes to the progression of CKD, which eventually often leads to end-stage kidney disease (ESKD). These patients require kidney replacement therapies, such as hemodialysis and kidney transplantation, to survive. Although adult kidneys have an intrinsic capacity to self-repair following injury (Humphreys et al., 2008), the process of nephrogenesis (i.e., the formation of new nephrons) in humans is limited to embryonic development (Little and McMahon, 2012). The establishment of kidney regenerative therapies which recover kidney function is therefore an urgent goal.

Animal models have contributed a great deal to our understanding of kidney physiology and pathophysiology, but models have limitations in translatability to therapies for humans. Recently, the mouse ENCODE Consortium reported that, while there are many similarities, there are important differences between mouse and human genomes (Yue et al., 2014; Stergachis et al., 2014; Cheng et al., 2014; Pope et al., 2014; Vierstra et al., 2014; Lin et al., 2014). They uncovered many DNA variations and differences in gene expression patterns, potentially limiting the usefulness of some disease models in mice to predict natural history or response to therapeutics in human disease. On the other hand, human kidney disease samples are limited in availability and utility for studying disease in vitro. Human kidney cells in culture exhibit dedifferentiated phenotypes, which hinder studies of CKD where kidney tubular dedifferentiation and fibrosis play the important role in pathogenesis.

Pluripotent stem cell-derived kidney organoids offer several advantages to address current issues of kidney research, including an unlimited source of the starting material, no need to acquire primary tissues, and relative ease of genetic modification of progenitor cells. Organoids consist of different cell types in three-dimensional structures. When derived from human cells, organoids can mimic human organs. For this reason, organoids provide a model for the in vitro study of intracellular and inter-compartmental interactions using differentiated human cells in an appropriate nephron and stromal context (Morizane and Bonventre, 2017).

OTHER APPROACHES TO GENERATION OF ORGANOIDS

An important function of kidneys is to produce urine from blood to remove waste products from the body and to maintain balance of fluids, electrolytes, and acid—base status. The main functional unit of kidneys is called a nephron, which consists of a glomerulus and a tubule. The glomerulus filters blood to produce primitive urine, and the tubule reabsorbs most of substances necessary for the body, such as glucose and water. It also controls other important aspects of physiological transport including active secretion. The nephron is derived from nephron progenitor cells (NPCs), which are located at the periphery of kidneys during embryogenesis. The NPCs possess stemness, which allows self-replication and differentiation into the many cell types that form the nephron. Although NPCs no longer exist in adult kidneys, there have been several recent attempts to expand NPCs from mouse or human embryos (Li et al., 2016; Tanigawa et al., 2016; Tanigawa et al., 2015; Brown et al., 2015). Establishment of methods to expand NPCs would provide sources for generation of kidney organoids, mini- kidneys, and ultimately functional bioengineered kidneys. There are, however, ethical concerns regarding the use of human embryos, and also problems of availability. Two studies have demonstrated the possibility of expanding NPCs derived from hPSCs (Li et al., 2016; Tanigawa et al., 2016); however, nephrogenesis from those expanded NPCs has required coculture with mouse embryonic spinal cords (which are surrogate inducers of nephrogenesis), which hinders translation of this technology to therapeutic applications in humans.

One important application of organoids is to model human disease in culture plates. Advantages of organoids relative to animal studies include species of cells and applicability to drug screening. High-throughput screening systems are promising platforms on which to discover novel candidates for therapeutics (Capelle and Arvinte, 2008; Inglese et al., 2007). Although methods to generate organoids need to be refined for high-throughput screening, the organoid is an attractive platform for drug screening, given the use of human tissue and the fact that high-throughput screening cannot be performed with animals.

One drawback of current forms of organoids is that they do not yet mimic the in vivo microphysiological environment. Organoids contain multiple cellular compartments to mimic cellular compartments of organs in vivo, but lack of blood flow in organoids might alter the characteristics of the cells. Some investigators have transplanted organoids to animals to vascularize organoids with blood flow in vivo (Takebe et al., 2013; Takebe et al., 2015; Sharmin et al., 2016), but this approach is not conducive to high-throughput drug screening. Establishment of a microphysiological environment using bioengineering techniques will be required to further expand applications of organoids, and to generate mini-organs in which structures are better modeled, with vasculature bringing blood to the structure and an ability to connect to a urinary exit pathway.

DESIGN CONSIDERATIONS

It has been generally known that metanephric kidneys arise from the intermediate mesoderm; however, the origin of the metanephros has not been clearly defined in human intermediate mesoderm, due to the complexity of kidney development. Three different kidney tissues, namely pronephros, mesonephros, and metanephros, form in humans during embryonic development. Only the metanephros survives and becomes functional kidney, while the pronephros and mesonephros degrade during embryonic development. Taguchi et al. used lineage tracing techniques in mice to identify the precise origin of the metanephros in mouse (Taguchi et al., 2014). They found that the origin of the metanephros was located at the posterior area of the intermediate mesoderm, where Pax2 and Lim1 (known as LHX1 in humans) were not expressed. Pax2 and Lim1 have been used to specify the intermediate mesoderm in mouse embryos (Tsang et al., 2000; Bouchard et al., 2002), and were used as markers of the origin of kidney cells in studies which attempted to induce kidney tubular cells from hPSCs (Xia et al., 2013; Takasato et al., 2014; Lam et al., 2014). Studies from Takasato and our group generated LTL (lotus tetragonolobus lectin) + proximal tubular-like cells from hPSCs via induction of PAX2+LHX1+cells, yet the induction efficiency of SIX2+ nephron progenitor cells (NPCs) from those PAX2+LHX1+ cells was low (~20%) (Takasato et al., 2014; Lam et al., 2014). These findings were consistent with the Taguchi et al. study, which redefined the origin of metanephros in Osr1+Wt1+Pax2-Lim1-posterior intermediate mesoderm in mice. Thus, it was predicted that the induction of OSR1+WT1+PAX2-LHX1- posterior intermediate mesoderm cells from hPSCs would facilitate the differentiation into NPCs, and subsequently metanephros-derived functional kidneys.

To induce the posterior intermediate mesoderm from hPSCs, we mimicked the early patterning of mesoderm from the primitive streak. The primitive streak is a structure that forms in the blastula during early stages of mammalian embryos, and appears as an elongating groove at the caudal or posterior end of the embryo. The cells migrate from the primitive streak anteriorly, and form mesoderm tissues from the paraxial-to-lateral plate mesoderm. Importantly, the cell locations in the primitive streak define the subsequent differentiation into paraxial or lateral plate mesoderm (Iimura and Pourquie, 2006; Sweetman et al., 2008). In other words, the cells located at the anterior part of the primitive streak differentiate into paraxial mesoderm, while the posterior cells in the primitive streak become the lateral plate mesoderm. The intermediate mesoderm lies between the paraxial and lateral plate mesoderm. The progenitor cells of the intermediate mesoderm are located at the center of the primitive streak. The gradient of Wnt3a and BMP4 patterns the anterior − posterior axis of the primitive streak. Higher levels of BMP4 induce the posterior primitive streak (Lengerke et al., 2008; Liu et al., 1999). Hence, we thought that it was required to adjust the BMP4 signal level to induce cells that would mimic those at the center of the primitive streak, the origin of the intermediate mesoderm.

The cells migrate from the primitive streak anteriorly, and form mesoderm tissues from the anterior part of embryos towards the posterior (Deschamps and van Nes, 2005). In other words, the cells that migrate from the primitive streak at earlier stages of embryonic development subsequently differentiate into the more anterior mesoderm, and those that migrate from the late stage of the primitive streak subsequently form the posterior mesoderm. Taguchi et al. also showed consistent results using lineage tracing techniques to track the subsequent differentiation of Brachyury (T)+ primitive streak cells at different stages of embryonic development (Taguchi et al., 2014). They found that T+ primitive streak cells at E7.5 of mouse embryos form the anterior intermediate mesoderm, and subsequently differentiate into Wolffian ducts, while T+ primitive streak cells at E8.5 form the posterior intermediate mesoderm, and differentiate into the metanephric mesenchyme (NPCs). Collectively, to induce the posterior intermediate mesoderm, it would be the most efficient to induce the cells located at the center of the late-stage primitive streak.

Since there are no specific markers to identify those late-stage mid-primitive streak cells during the directed differentiation of hPSCs in vitro, we identified the best timing and treatments of WNT and BMP4 modulators by examining the subsequent differentiation into WT1+HOXD11+ posterior intermediate mesoderm cells made from hPSCs. HOXD11 is also abundantly expressed in the lateral plate mesoderm (Patterson et al., 2001); therefore, we used WT1 and OSR1 to identify the posterior intermediate mesoderm in combination with HOXD11 (Morizane et al., 2015). From our initial screening experiments, we found that longer treatment with CHIR99021 (CHIR, a WNT activator), with subsequent differentiation with activin A, is more likely to induce HOXD11 expression. This finding was consistent with developmental studies using mice, as described above. Longer treatment with CHIR induced the later stage of primitive streak cells, which subsequently form the posterior mesoderm, thus mimicking the anterior − posterior patterning of mesoderm in embryonic development in vivo.

Differentiation from the posterior intermediate mesoderm into SIX2+ NPCs was somewhat understood from previous studies including ours (Taguchi et al., 2014; Takasato et al., 2014; Lam et al., 2014). Barak et al. revealed the important role of Fgf9 and Fgf20 in maintenance of stemness of NPCs in mice and humans (Barak et al., 2012). Reciprocal interaction of the metanephric mesenchyme and ureteric buds is a key component of kidney development (Majumdar et al., 2003). Both the metanephric mesenchyme and ureteric buds produce growth factors and promote the differentiation of each other. Barak et al. showed that reduction of Fgf9 and Fgf20 levels lead to loss of NPCs in mice, indicating critical roles of Fgf signals in NPC differentiation and maintenance. They also demonstrated that Fgf9 is produced by ureteric buds, while Fgf20 is expressed in NPCs. These results therefore suggested that treatment with FGF9 might be required to induce NPCs from the posterior intermediate mesoderm cells derived from hPSCs, unless ureteric bud cells are simultaneously induced by the directed differentiation protocol. In our recent study, we used a low dose of FGF9 (10 ng/ml) to induce SIX2+SALL1+WT1+PAX2+ NPCs from WT1+HOXD11+ posterior intermediate mesoderm cells that had been derived from hPSCs (Morizane et al., 2015), but addition of FGF20 was not required, as predicted by Barak's study (Barak et al., 2012).

NPCs derived from hPSCs would be attractive sources for cell therapies and bioengineered kidney structures. There are currently five studies that induced NPCs from hPSCs (Taguchi et al., 2014; Morizane et al., 2015; Takasato et al., 2014; Kang and Han, 2014; Toyohara et al., 2015). One key difference among these five study protocols is whether or not they specifically induced the posterior intermediate mesoderm cells as progenitors of NPCs. The protocol from Takasato, Kang, or Toyohara attempted to induce PAX2+ or OSR+ IM cells, and resulted in relatively modest efficiency of induction of NPCs (SIX2+ cells: 10−38%) after longer differentiation periods (16−27 days) (Takasato et al., 2014; Kang and Han, 2014; Toyohara et al., 2015). On the other hand, the protocol from Taguchi and ours attempted to induce specifically posterior IM cells. The approaches of Taguchi et al. and ours resulted in higher differentiation efficiency (SIX2+ cells: 62−92%), with shorter differentiation periods (8−14 days). In our study, we evaluated the induction efficiency at each step of differentiation with assays of multiple protein markers by immunostaining in order to follow patterns consistent with in vivo kidney development through the posterior intermediate mesoderm induction. This resulted in a highly efficient (SIX2+ cells: ~75−92%) and rapid (~8−9 days) differentiation protocol to derive SIX2+SALL1+WT1+PAX2+ NPCs from both hESCs and hiPSCs (Morizane et al., 2015; Morizane and Bonventre, 2017).

NPCs are capable of differentiating into nephron epithelial cells, including the Bowman's capsule of the glomerulus and tubule epithelia. There are currently four studies that have demonstrated generation of kidney organoids (Taguchi et al., 2014; Takasato et al., 2015; Freedman et al., 2015; Morizane et al., 2015). Two of those four studies, including ours, first induced NPCs from hPSCs, and then generated kidney organoids from NPCs (Taguchi et al., 2014; Morizane et al., 2015). Taguchi et al. used mouse embryonic spinal cords to stimulate epithelialization of NPCs on a polycarbonate filter, and showed early-stage nephron structures resembling S-shaped bodies which expressed markers for podocytes (WT1 and NPHS1) and tubules (CDH1 and CDH6). The NPC markers, namely SALL1 and PAX2, however, were still expressed in those structures, indicating that immature nephrons were induced using mouse embryonic spinal cords. Their work was the first to demonstrate the differentiation of hPSCs into kidney organoids containing nephron-like structures, yet further refinement of the protocol was required to facilitate applications of hPSCs.

KIDNEY ORGANOID GENERATION FROM hPSCs

One of the most important applications of hPSCs is to model human diseases and perform drug screening using disease hiPSCs or CRISPR-mutants of hPSCs, in order to find candidates for therapeutic drugs (Sterneckert et al., 2014). For this purpose, the organoids have to be generated in small-well culture which is suited for high-throughput screening. Protocols that require coculture with mouse embryonic spinal cord to generate kidney organoids may interfere with the ability to attain uniformity, and hence hinder drug screening. Moreover, use of mouse embryonic spinal cords, with their undefined components, makes it difficult to perform disease modeling and mechanism analyses, since undefined components might affect disease phenotypes in kidney organoids either derived from patients with genetic kidney disease, or from hPSCs genetically engineered to mimic the human disease.

To address these issues, we have developed a differentiation protocol for kidney organoids with fully defined components in small-well culture suitable for 96-well screening dishes. We developed two methods to generate kidney organoids from NPCs. The first is simply to continue differentiation from the NPC stage in regular culture plates as a two-dimensional culture system. This is standard adhesion culture, yet cells spontaneously form multiple layers and three-dimensional structures in culture plates (Morizane et al., 2015). This two-dimensional system is suited for live cell monitoring and immunocytochemical analyses, since the structures are not too thick.

The second approach involved switching to a three-dimensional culture system using ultra-low attachment 96-well round bottom plates. By replating NPCs onto the ultra-low attachment plates, a large number of kidney organoids can be generated in small-well three-dimensional culture. Kidney organoids contain segmented nephrons with characteristics of podocytes (WT1+PODXL+NPHS1+), proximal tubules (LTL+CDH2+AQP1+), loops of Henle (CDH1+UMOD+), and distal convoluted tubules (CDH1+UMOD-) in an organized, continuous arrangement. Since the induction efficiency of NPCs is very high, the reproducibility of kidney organoids in each small well is very high with our differentiation approach, once NPCs are generated at high efficiency. We used fully defined components for the differentiation, and followed in vivo development with high efficiency at each step of differentiation (Fig. 12.2). Our organoid system allows for the study of developmental analyses of kidneys. As one example, we used a Notch inhibitor,

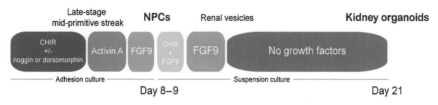

FIGURE 12.2 A differentiation protocol of hPSCs into NPCs and kidney organoids.

Nephron progenitor cells (NPCs) can be induced within 8–9 days of differentiation from human pluripotent stem cells (hPSCs). Subsequent differentiation of NPCs with defined factors generates kidney organoids within 21 days of differentiation. CHIR: CHIR99021. FGF: fibroblast growth factor. Morizane et al. (2015).

> Morizane, R., et al., 2015. Nephron organoids derived from human pluripotent stem cells model kidney development and injury. Nat. Biotechnol.

DAPT, after the induction of renal vesicles, to show involvement of Notch signal in nephron formation. DAPT significantly reduced the induction of LTL+ proximal tubules, indicating that Notch signaling is necessary for proximal tubule differentiation. This result was consistent with previous animal studies (Cheng et al., 2007), indicating that the organoid system will be a useful platform for studies of human kidney developmental disease.

Two other studies, one from our laboratory, did not specifically induce NPCs as a preliminary step of kidney organoid generation, but resulted in generation of kidney organoids (Takasato et al., 2015; Freedman et al., 2015). Freedman et al. in our group took a unique approach to generate kidney organoids (Freedman et al., 2015). Cavitated spheroids were first generated from hPSCs by sandwiching cells between two layers of Matrigel. Those spheroids possessed pluripotency, and the cells expressed pluripotent markers including OCT4, SOX2, TRA1-60, and NANOG, even after several passages. Differentiation from those cavitated spheroids was initiated with CHIR. Then, after 1.5 days treatment of CHIR, the cells were stochastically differentiated for up to 16 days. Although foot processes were not observed by electron microscopy, PODXL+WT1+SYNPO+ podocyte-like cells were induced after the stochastic differentiation. There were also LTL+ tubular structures resembling proximal tubules, yet immaturity markers including LHX1 and PAX2 were still expressed in those LTL+ tubular structures. Nephrotoxic assays were also attempted, and KIM-1 was upregulated in LTL+ tubular structures after 48-hour treatment with 50 μM cisplatin. The nephron-like structures possess some of the characteristics of nephrons in vivo. Importantly, this protocol induced other lineage cells along with nephron-like cells. There were vWF+CD31+ endothelia-like cells and TUJ1+ neuron-like cells induced simultaneously, suggesting multiple lineages, including lateral plate and ectoderm derivatives, can be induced with this approach.

Takasato et al. reported generation of kidney organoids containing multiple lineages (Takasato et al., 2015). Interestingly, this study also did not induce

NPCs as a preliminary stage of kidney organoid generation. Takasato et al. differentiated hiPSCs with CHIR for 4 days, and subsequently treated cells with 200 ng/mL FGF9 for 3 days. After dissociation into single cells, the cells were spun down to form a pellet. The cell pellet was cultured on a Transwell dish with 200 ng/mL FGF9 for 5 days after CHIR pulse treatment. After FGF9 treatment, the cell pellet was cultured without additional growth factors for an additional 13 days, then segmented nephron-like structures were generated. Those structures included WT1+NPHS1+ podocytes, LTL+CUBN+ immature proximal tubules, LTL+CDH1+ mature proximal tubules, CDH1+UMOD+ loops of Henle, and CDH1+GATA3+PAX2+ collecting ducts. Like our study (Freedman et al., 2015), Takasato et al. also observed CD31+ endothelia-like cells in kidney organoids. Nephrotoxic assays were also performed using cisplatin at 5 μM and 20 μM. After 24 hours of treatment with cisplatin, LTL+CDH1- proximal tubules did not appear to respond to either 5 or 20 μM of cisplatin, yet LTL+CDH1+ mature proximal tubules underwent apoptosis identified by cleaved caspase 3 expression.

In conclusion, collectively, four studies have demonstrated generation of kidney organoids with different approaches, yet further studies are required to further characterize the functionalities of kidney organoids, and to explore potential applications. Pronephros and mesonephros contain immature nephrons during embryogenesis in humans. Kidney development is very complicated, and it is difficult to distinguish metanephros functional kidney structures from pro/mesonephros based on only marker analyses.

DISEASE MODELING USING KIDNEY ORGANOIDS

One of the most important applications of hPSCs is to model human diseases in vitro, in order to study mechanisms of the disease and to find new therapeutic approaches. One strength of this application is that a large number of chemicals can be screened in human cells in order to find new candidate therapeutic drugs, an application not possible in animal studies where the sample numbers are limited. Drug-induced kidney injury is one of the major causes of acute and chronic kidney injury (AKI), and also often a cause for termination of clinical trials of new drugs. Kidney organoids can be a novel tool to evaluate nephrotoxicity of drugs as a preclinical trial in a dish.

Mature nephrons express a variety of transporters, and nephrotoxicants are taken up via those transporters. Cisplatin is a clinically used anti-cancer drug, and is known to cause kidney injury (Perazella and Moeckel, 2010). Proximal tubular cells take up cisplatin via organic cation transporters (OCTs) (Ludwig et al., 2004; Yonezawa et al., 2005); therefore, it is also important for nephrotoxic assays that kidney organoids possess mature phenotypes with transporter expression. When organoids that we generated were treated with cisplatin at 5 μM for 24 hours, kidney injury molecule-1 (KIM-1), a well-established injury marker for proximal tubules, was significantly upregulated in LTL+ proximal tubules, discovered by our laboratory (Vaidya et al., 2010; Morizane et al., 2015; Morizane and Bonventre, 2017). We also evaluated γH2AX expression, a DNA damage marker (Chen et al., 2000), to determine whether the injury with cisplatin at 5 or 50 μM was specific to proximal tubules. At a cisplatin concentration of 5 μM, these organoids showed upregulation of γH2AX in LTL+ proximal tubules (Morizane et al., 2015), indicating LTL+ proximal tubules in organoids actively take in cisplatin via OCTs. A cisplatin concentration of 50 μM resulted in global DNA damage in all cell types in kidney organoids. Kidney organoids, therefore, would be a novel tool to evaluate the nephrotoxicity of drugs.

There are currently more than 150 inherited kidney diseases (Devuyst et al., 2014). These diseases account for most children and approximately 10% of adults who have end-stage kidney disease. Yet, there are currently few models that have led to new therapeutics for inherited kidney diseases. Published studies with iPSCs and organoids have focused on polycystic kidney disease (PKD), especially autosomal dominant PKD (ADPKD). Autosomal dominant PKD is the most common inherited kidney disease, and accounts for 7%−10% of all patients on renal replacement therapy worldwide (Ong et al., 2015). Autosomal dominant PKD, however, is a late-onset disease where cysts can be detected by ultrasound in approximately 68% of 30-year-old individuals with ADPKD (Nahm et al., 2002). Hence, it might be difficult to detect cystic phenotypes in kidney organoids derived from patients with ADPKD, yet early phenotypes of ADPKD might be able to be detected in kidney organoids, or even in undifferentiated hiPSCs, since the target genes, PKD1/PKD2, are ciliary proteins expressed in many cell types (Van Adelsberg and Frank, 1995). Our group previously generated hiPSCs from three ADPKD patients with PKD1 mutations, and analyzed protein localization of PKD1 and PKD2 in undifferentiated hiPSCs and hepatoblasts derived from those hiPSCs (Freedman et al., 2013). The expression of PKD2 protein in cilia was reduced in cells from patients with PKD1 mutations, suggesting trafficking of PKD2 to the cilium is mediated by the normal PKD1 protein. This phenomenon might be the cause for cystogenesis in ADPKD patients. Further studies are required to elucidate mechanisms of cystogenesis due to reduced PKD2 expression in the cilium, and why it takes a few decades to form cysts in ADPKD patients.

Another recent study of ADPKD using patient-derived hiPSCs attempted to explore risk factors for intracranial aneurysms (Ameku et al., 2016). The authors established hiPSCs from three ADPKD patients without intracranial aneurysms and four patients with aneurysms, and compared gene expression profiles between those two groups after differentiation into endothelial cells. They found that the expression level of a metalloenzyme gene, matrix metaloproteinase-1 (MMP1), was specifically elevated in hiPSC-derived endothelial cells from ADPKD patients with aneurysms. In addition, they confirmed the positive correlation between the serum MMP1 levels and the development of intracranial aneurysms in 354 ADPKD patients, indicating that high serum MMP1 levels may be a novel risk factor.

In both studies (Freedman et al., 2013; Ameku et al., 2016), however, clinical phenotypes of ADPKD, such as kidney cysts and aneurysms, were not reproduced in culture systems using hiPSCs derived from ADPKD patients. One reason might be that there were inadequate differentiation protocols to generate kidney organoids at that time. In addition, considering the long time course of disease progression of ADPKD, alternative approaches to model ADPKD might need to be developed beyond patient-derived hiPSCs, so that clinical phenotypes can be reproduced in culture systems. In our group's study, we hypothesized that complete knock-out of PKD1 or PKD2 genes might facilitate cystic phenotypes in culture systems. Knock-out lines of PKD1 or PKD2 were created in H9 hESCs using CRISPR/Cas9 genome editing approaches (Freedman et al., 2015). Although the differentiation protocol into kidney organoids that we used might need further refinement, as we discussed above, cyst formation was observed in 6% of kidney organoids derived from CRISPR-mutants, while cyst formation was rarely seen in kidney organoids derived from wild-type H9 cells. One important advantage of this CRISPR approach is that the genetic background will be exactly the same in the nonmutated control parental line. Because of the recent findings that genetic background dominates over variation due to cellular origin or Sendai virus (SeV) infection in hPSCs (Choi et al., 2015), it is desirable to use the same hPSCs with exactly the same genetic background as controls when we analyze phenotypes resulting from CRISPR/Cas9-induced genetic modification. The two approaches are complementary: comparison of hiPSCs from patients with and without the disease, and comparison of wild-type cells and CRISPR/Cas9 mutated cells.

In conclusion, modeling kidney diseases using kidney organoids derived from hPSCs is an attractive approach to study mechanisms of human inherited kidney diseases and drug-induced nephropathy. To optimize this approach, however, differentiation approaches, genetic background, and epigenetic variation should be considered when disease phenotypes are analyzed in kidney organoids.

REMAINING CHALLENGES

Human induced pluripotent stem cells (hiPSCs) can be readily generated from patients with kidney disease, enabling the development of immunocompatible tissues, as well as patient-specific models of kidney disease (Takahashi et al., 2007). One goal of hiPSC studies would be to regenerate kidney function. Kidneys form very complicated structures for their function of maintenance of the internal milieu. There are many challenges to the use of organoids for the generation of functional bioengineered kidney tissue for kidney regenerative therapies and modeling kidney disease. One of the challenges relates to vascularization. Vascularization of kidney organoids will have to be induced in an organized way to direct blood flow from renal arteries and to venous structures. Sharmin et al. demonstrated vascularization of glomeruli when hPSC-derived podocytes were transplanted to a mouse kidney subcapsular space (Sharmin et al., 2015).

Outgrowth of host mouse endothelial cells to transplanted human podocytes was observed, though capillary loops, an important structure of glomeruli to facilitate blood filtration, were rarely formed. Takebe et al. generated kidney buds by mixing human umbilical vein endothelial cells (HUVEC), mesenchymal stem cells (MSCs), and mouse embryonic kidney cells. This group then transplanted kidney buds to a preformed cranial window of a nonobese diabetic/severe combined immunodeficient (NOD/SCID) mouse (Takebe et al., 2015). Vascularized glomerular structures similar to Sharmin's were observed, with outgrowths of host mouse endothelial cells. These in vivo transplantation experiments are encouraging; however, further studies are required to incorporate vascular systems into kidney organoids in vitro, which might facilitate development of functional bioengineered kidneys in the future.

Another challenge involves the egress of formative urine. Current studies suggest the induction of collecting duct cells in organoids (Takasato et al., 2015; Xia et al., 2014); yet, the structures were not organized enough to excrete urine outside the kidney organoids. One approach might be to coculture hPSC-derived NPCs and ureteric buds, in order to recapitulate in vivo kidney development where reciprocal interaction of NPCs and ureteric buds may result in organized branching formation of collecting duct systems. Xia et al. showed the induction of ureteric bud progenitor-like cells from hPSCs (Xia et al., 2014), yet subsequent directed differentiation into ureteric buds and collecting duct cells has not been established. Considering the recent study from Taguchi (Taguchi et al., 2014), the differentiation protocols into ureteric bud lineage cells need to be established independently from NPC differentiation. Establishment of differentiation protocols to produce ureteric bud cells from hPSCs might facilitate generation of organized kidney structures with urinary exit.

One possible approach for generation of functional bioengineered kidneys is to use three-dimensional bioprinting. Lewis' group has developed a bioprinting method to fabricate three-dimensional tissue constructs replete with vasculature, multiple types of cells, and extracellular matrix, and applied this system to kidney cells (Kolesky et al., 2014; Bhunia et al., 2002). Heterogeneous structures are generated in three dimensions by precisely coprinting multiple materials, known as bioinks. The system is capable of perfusing liquid into lumens of vasculature or tubule-like channels, which might be applicable to mimic blood flow and intratubular flow in vascular and tubular channels respectively.

ACKNOWLEDGEMENTS

This study was supported by National Institutes of Health grants R37 DK039773 and R01 DK072381 (to J.V.B.), and UG3 TR002155-01 (to J.V.B. and R.M.) a Grant-in-Aid for a Japan Society for the Promotion of Science (JSPS) Postdoctoral Fellowship for Research Abroad (to R.M.), a ReproCELL Stem Cell Research grant (to R.M.), a Brigham and Women's Hospital Research Excellence Award (to R.M.), a Brigham and Women's Hospital Faculty Career Development Award (to R.M.), and a Harvard Stem Cell Institute Seed Grant (to R.M.).

DECLARATION OF FINANCIAL INTERESTS

J.V.B. is a coinventor on KIM-1 patents that have been licensed by Partners Healthcare to several companies. He has received royalty income from Partners Healthcare. J.V.B. and R.M. are coinventors on patents (PCT/US16/52350) on organoid technologies that are assigned to Partners Healthcare. J.V.B. or his family has received income for consulting from companies interested in biomarkers: Sekisui, Millennium, Johnson & Johnson, and Novartis. J.V.B. is a cofounder, consultant to, and owns equity in, Goldfinch Bio.

REFERENCES

Ameku, T., et al., 2016. Identification of MMP1 as a novel risk factor for intracranial aneurysms in ADPKD using iPSC models. Sci. Rep. 6, 30013.

Barak, H., et al., 2012. FGF9 and FGF20 maintain the stemness of nephron progenitors in mice and man. Dev. Cell 22 (6), 1191−1207.

Barker, N., et al., 2010. Lgr5(+ve) stem cells drive self-renewal in the stomach and build long-lived gastric units in vitro. Cell Stem Cell 6 (1), 25−36.

Bartfeld, S., et al., 2015. In vitro expansion of human gastric epithelial stem cells and their responses to bacterial infection. Gastroenterology 148 (1), p. 126−136, e6.

Bertaux-Skeirik, N., et al., 2015. CD44 plays a functional role in Helicobacter pylori-induced epithelial cell proliferation. PLoS Pathog. 11 (2), e1004663.

Bhunia, A.K., et al., 2002. PKD1 induces p21(waf1) and regulation of the cell cycle via direct activation of the JAK-STAT signaling pathway in a process requiring PKD2. Cell 109 (2), 157−168.

Boj, S.F., et al., 2015. Organoid models of human and mouse ductal pancreatic cancer. Cell 160 (1−2), 324−338.

Bouchard, M., et al., 2002. Nephric lineage specification by Pax2 and Pax8. Genes Dev. 16 (22), 2958−2970.

Brown, A.C., Muthukrishnan, S.D., Oxburgh, L., 2015. A synthetic niche for nephron progenitor cells. Dev Cell 34 (2), 229−241.

Cao, L., et al., 2011. Intestinal lineage commitment of embryonic stem cells. Differentiation 81 (1), 1−10.

Capelle, M.A., Arvinte, T., 2008. High-throughput formulation screening of therapeutic proteins. Drug Discov Today Technol 5 (2−3), e71−e79.

Chen, H.T., et al., 2000. Response to RAG-mediated VDJ cleavage by NBS1 and gamma-H2AX. Science 290 (5498), 1962−1965.

Cheng, H.T., et al., 2007. Notch2, but not Notch1, is required for proximal fate acquisition in the mammalian nephron. Development 134 (4), 801−811.

Cheng, Y., et al., 2014. Principles of regulatory information conservation between mouse and human. Nature 515 (7527), 371−375.

Choi, J., et al., 2015. A comparison of genetically matched cell lines reveals the equivalence of human iPSCs and ESCs. Nat. Biotechnol..

Chua, C.W., et al., 2014. Single luminal epithelial progenitors can generate prostate organoids in culture. Nat. Cell Biol. 16 (10), p. 951−961, 1−4.

Cong, L., et al., 2013. Multiplex genome engineering using CRISPR/Cas systems. Science 339 (6121), 819–823.

Coresh, J., et al., 2007. Prevalence of chronic kidney disease in the United States. JAMA 298 (17), 2038–2047.

DeWard, A.D., Cramer, J., Lagasse, E., 2014. Cellular heterogeneity in the mouse esophagus implicates the presence of a nonquiescent epithelial stem cell population. Cell Rep. 9 (2), 701–711.

Dekkers, J.F., et al., 2013. A functional CFTR assay using primary cystic fibrosis intestinal organoids. Nat. Med. 19 (7), 939–945.

Deschamps, J., van Nes, J., 2005. Developmental regulation of the Hox genes during axial morphogenesis in the mouse. Development 132 (13), 2931–2942.

Devuyst, O., et al., 2014. Rare inherited kidney diseases: challenges, opportunities, and perspectives. Lancet 383 (9931), 1844–1859.

Drost, J., et al., 2015. Sequential cancer mutations in cultured human intestinal stem cells. Nature 521 (7550), 43–47.

Dye, B.R., et al., 2015. In vitro generation of human pluripotent stem cell derived lung organoids. Elife4.

Ene-Iordache, B., et al., 2016. Chronic kidney disease and cardiovascular risk in six regions of the world (ISN-KDDC): a cross-sectional study. Lancet Glob. Health 4 (5), e307–e319.

van Es, J.H., et al., 2012. Dll1 + secretory progenitor cells revert to stem cells upon crypt damage. Nat Cell Biol. 14 (10), 1099–1104.

Fatehullah, A., Tan, S.H., Barker, N., 2016. Organoids as an in vitro model of human development and disease. Nat. Cell Biol. 18 (3), 246–254.

Finkbeiner, S.R., et al., 2012. Stem cell-derived human intestinal organoids as an infection model for rotaviruses. MBio 3 (4), e00159–12.

Finkbeiner, S.R., et al., 2015. Transcriptome-wide analysis reveals hallmarks of human intestine development and maturation in vitro and in vivo. Stem Cell Rep.

Fordham, R.P., et al., 2013. Transplantation of expanded fetal intestinal progenitors contributes to colon regeneration after injury. Cell Stem Cell 13 (6), 734–744.

Freedman, B.S., et al., 2013. Reduced ciliary polycystin-2 in induced pluripotent stem cells from polycystic kidney disease patients with PKD1 mutations. J. Am. Soc. Nephrol. 24 (10), 1571–1586.

Freedman, B.S., et al., 2015. Modelling kidney disease with CRISPR-mutant kidney organoids derived from human pluripotent epiblast spheroids. Nat. Commun. 6, 8715.

Fukuda, M., et al., 2014. Small intestinal stem cell identity is maintained with functional Paneth cells in heterotopically grafted epithelium onto the colon. Genes Dev. 28 (16), 1752–1757.

Gao, D., et al., 2014. Organoid cultures derived from patients with advanced prostate cancer. Cell 159 (1), 176–187.

Gracz, A.D., et al., 2015. A high-throughput platform for stem cell niche co-cultures and downstream gene expression analysis. Nat. Cell Biol. 17 (3), 340–349.

Greggio, C., et al., 2013. Artificial three-dimensional niches deconstruct pancreas development in vitro. Development 140 (21), 4452–4462.

Hisha, H., et al., 2013. Establishment of a novel lingual organoid culture system: generation of organoids having mature keratinized epithelium from adult epithelial stem cells. Sci. Rep. 3, 3224.

Horita, N., et al., 2014. Fluorescent labelling of intestinal epithelial cells reveals independent long-lived intestinal stem cells in a crypt. Biochem. Biophys. Res. Commun. 454 (4), 493−499.

Huch, M., et al., 2013a. Unlimited in vitro expansion of adult bi-potent pancreas progenitors through the Lgr5/R-spondin axis. EMBO J. 32 (20), 2708−2721.

Huch, M., et al., 2013b. In vitro expansion of single Lgr5 + liver stem cells induced by Wnt-driven regeneration. Nature 494 (7436), 247−250.

Huch, M., et al., 2015. Long-term culture of genome-stable bipotent stem cells from adult human liver. Cell 160 (1−2), 299−312.

Humphreys, B.D., et al., 2008. Intrinsic epithelial cells repair the kidney after injury. Cell Stem Cell 2 (3), 284−291.

Iimura, T., Pourquie, O., 2006. Collinear activation of Hoxb genes during gastrulation is linked to mesoderm cell ingression. Nature 442 (7102), 568−571.

Inglese, J., et al., 2007. High-throughput screening assays for the identification of chemical probes. Nat. Chem. Biol. 3 (8), 466−479.

Jung, P., et al., 2011. Isolation and in vitro expansion of human colonic stem cells. Nat Med 17 (10), 1225−1227.

Kang, M., Han, Y.M., 2014. Differentiation of human pluripotent stem cells into nephron progenitor cells in a serum and feeder free system. PLoS One 9 (4), e94888.

Karthaus, W.R., et al., 2014. Identification of multipotent luminal progenitor cells in human prostate organoid cultures. Cell 159 (1), 163−175.

Kessler, M., Hoffmann, K., Brinkmann, V., Thieck, O., Jackisch, S., Toelle, B., et al., 2015. The Notch and Wnt pathways regulate stemness and differentiation in human fallopian tube organoids. Nat. Commun. 6, 8989. Available from: https://doi.org/10.1038/ncomms9989.

Kolesky, D.B., et al., 2014. 3D bioprinting of vascularized, heterogeneous cell-laden tissue constructs. Adv. Mater. 26 (19), 3124−3130.

Lam, A.Q., et al., 2014. Rapid and efficient differentiation of human pluripotent stem cells into intermediate mesoderm that forms tubules expressing kidney proximal tubular markers. J. Am. Soc. Nephrol. 25 (6), 1211−1225.

Lancaster, M.A., et al., 2013. Cerebral organoids model human brain development and microcephaly. Nature 501 (7467), 373−379.

Lengerke, C., et al., 2008. BMP and Wnt specify hematopoietic fate by activation of the Cdx-Hox pathway. Cell Stem Cell 2 (1), 72−82.

Li, X., et al., 2014. Oncogenic transformation of diverse gastrointestinal tissues in primary organoid culture. Nat. Med. 20 (7), 769−777.

Li, Z., et al., 2016. 3D culture supports long-term expansion of mouse and human nephrogenic progenitors. Cell Stem Cell 19 (4), 516−529.

Lin, S., et al., 2014. Comparison of the transcriptional landscapes between human and mouse tissues. Proc. Natl. Acad Sci U.S.A. 111 (48), 17224−17229.

Little, M.H., McMahon, A.P., 2012. Mammalian kidney development: principles, progress, and projections. Cold Spring Harb. Perspect. Biol. 4 (5).

Liu, P., et al., 1999. Requirement for Wnt3 in vertebrate axis formation. Nat. Genet. 22 (4), 361−365.

Ludwig, T., et al., 2004. Nephrotoxicity of platinum complexes is related to basolateral organic cation transport. Kidney Int. 66 (1), 196−202.

Majumdar, A., et al., 2003. Wnt11 and Ret/Gdnf pathways cooperate in regulating ureteric branching during metanephric kidney development. Development 130 (14), 3175–3185.

Matano, M., et al., 2015. Modeling colorectal cancer using CRISPR-Cas9-mediated engineering of human intestinal organoids. Nat. Med. 21 (3), 256–262.

McCracken, K.W., et al., 2014. Modelling human development and disease in pluripotent stem-cell-derived gastric organoids. Nature 516 (7531), 400–404.

McCracken, K.W., et al., 2017. Wnt/beta-catenin promotes gastric fundus specification in mice and humans. Nature.

Mondrinos, M.J., et al., 2006. Engineering three-dimensional pulmonary tissue constructs. Tissue Eng. 12 (4), 717–728.

Mondrinos, M.J., et al., 2014. Engineering de novo assembly of fetal pulmonary organoids. Tissue Eng. Part A 20 (21-22), 2892–2907.

Morizane, R., Bonventre, J.V., 2017. Generation of nephron progenitor cells and kidney organoids from human pluripotent stem cells. Nat. Protoc. 12 (1), 195–207.

Morizane, R., et al., 2013. Kidney specific protein-positive cells derived from embryonic stem cells reproduce tubular structures in vitro and differentiate into renal tubular cells. PLoS One 8 (6), e64843.

Morizane, R., et al., 2015. Nephron organoids derived from human pluripotent stem cells model kidney development and injury. Nat. Biotechnol.

Mustata, R.C., et al., 2011. Lgr4 is required for Paneth cell differentiation and maintenance of intestinal stem cells ex vivo. EMBO Rep. 12 (6), 558–564.

Mustata, R.C., et al., 2013. Identification of Lgr5-independent spheroid-generating progenitors of the mouse fetal intestinal epithelium. Cell Rep. 5 (2), 421–432.

Nadauld, L.D., et al., 2014. Metastatic tumor evolution and organoid modeling implicate TGFBR2 as a cancer driver in diffuse gastric cancer. Genome Biol. 15 (8), 428.

Nahm, A.M., Henriquez, D.E., Ritz, E., 2002. Renal cystic disease (ADPKD and ARPKD). Nephrol. Dial Transplant 17 (2), 311–314.

Nanduri, L.S., et al., 2014. Purification and ex vivo expansion of fully functional salivary gland stem cells. Stem Cell Rep. 3 (6), 957–964.

Ogawa, M., et al., 2015. Directed differentiation of cholangiocytes from human pluripotent stem cells. Nat. Biotechnol. 33 (8), 853–861.

Okamoto, R., Watanabe, M., 2016. Role of epithelial cells in the pathogenesis and treatment of inflammatory bowel disease. J. Gastroenterol. 51 (1), 11–21.

Ong, A.C., et al., 2015. Autosomal dominant polycystic kidney disease: the changing face of clinical management. Lancet 385 (9981), 1993–2002.

Ootani, A., et al., 2009. Sustained in vitro intestinal epithelial culture within a Wnt-dependent stem cell niche. Nat. Med. 15 (6), 701–706.

Ozone, C., et al., 2016. Functional anterior pituitary generated in self-organizing culture of human embryonic stem cells. Nat. Commun. 7, 10351.

Patterson, L.T., Pembaur, M., Potter, S.S., 2001. Hoxa11 and Hoxd11 regulate branching morphogenesis of the ureteric bud in the developing kidney. Development 128 (11), 2153–2161.

Perazella, M.A., Moeckel, G.W., 2010. Nephrotoxicity from chemotherapeutic agents: clinical manifestations, pathobiology, and prevention/therapy. Semin. Nephrol. 30 (6), 570–581.

Pope, B.D., et al., 2014. Topologically associating domains are stable units of replication-timing regulation. Nature 515 (7527), 402−405.

Sampaziotis, F., et al., 2015. Cholangiocytes derived from human induced pluripotent stem cells for disease modeling and drug validation. Nat. Biotechnol. 33 (8), 845−852.

Sato, T., et al., 2009. Single Lgr5 stem cells build crypt-villus structures in vitro without a mesenchymal niche. Nature 459 (7244), 262−265.

Sato, T., et al., 2011a. Long-term expansion of epithelial organoids from human colon, adenoma, adenocarcinoma, and Barrett's epithelium. Gastroenterology 141 (5), 1762−1772.

Sato, T., et al., 2011b. Paneth cells constitute the niche for Lgr5 stem cells in intestinal crypts. Nature 469 (7330), 415−418.

Schlaermann, P., et al., 2016. A novel human gastric primary cell culture system for modelling Helicobacter pylori infection in vitro. Gut 65 (2), 202−213.

Schumacher, M.A., et al., 2015. The use of murine-derived fundic organoids in studies of gastric physiology. J. Physiol. 593 (8), 1809−1827.

Sharmin, S., et al., 2015. Human induced pluripotent stem cell-derived podocytes mature into vascularized glomeruli upon experimental transplantation. J. Am. Soc. Nephrol.

Sharmin, S., et al., 2016. Human induced pluripotent stem cell-derived podocytes mature into vascularized glomeruli upon experimental transplantation. J. Am. Soc. Nephrol. 27 (6), 1778−1791.

Simmini, S., et al., 2014. Transformation of intestinal stem cells into gastric stem cells on loss of transcription factor Cdx2. Nat. Commun. 5, 5728.

Spence, J.R., et al., 2011. Directed differentiation of human pluripotent stem cells into intestinal tissue in vitro. Nature 470 (7332), 105−109.

Stange, D.E., et al., 2013. Differentiated Troy + chief cells act as reserve stem cells to generate all lineages of the stomach epithelium. Cell 155 (2), 357−368.

Stergachis, A.B., et al., 2014. Conservation of trans-acting circuitry during mammalian regulatory evolution. Nature 515 (7527), 365−370.

Sterneckert, J.L., Reinhardt, P., Scholer, H.R., 2014. Investigating human disease using stem cell models. Nat. Rev. Genet. 15 (9), 625−639.

Sweetman, D., et al., 2008. The migration of paraxial and lateral plate mesoderm cells emerging from the late primitive streak is controlled by different Wnt signals. BMC Dev. Biol. 8, 63.

Taguchi, A., et al., 2014. Redefining the in vivo origin of metanephric nephron progenitors enables generation of complex kidney structures from pluripotent stem cells. Cell Stem Cell 14 (1), 53−67.

Takahashi, K., et al., 2007. Induction of pluripotent stem cells from adult human fibroblasts by defined factors. Cell 131 (5), 861−872.

Takasato, M., et al., 2014. Directing human embryonic stem cell differentiation towards a renal lineage generates a self-organizing kidney. Nat. Cell Biol. 16 (1), 118−126.

Takasato, M., et al., 2015. Kidney organoids from human iPS cells contain multiple lineages and model human nephrogenesis. Nature 526 (7574), 564−568.

Takebe, T., et al., 2013. Vascularized and functional human liver from an iPSC-derived organ bud transplant. Nature 499 (7459), 481−484.

Takebe, T., et al., 2015. Vascularized and complex organ buds from diverse tissues via mesenchymal cell-driven condensation. Cell Stem Cell 16 (5), 556−565.

Tanigawa, S., et al., 2015. Preferential propagation of competent SIX2 + nephronic progenitors by LIF/ROCKi treatment of the metanephric mesenchyme. Stem Cell Rep. 5 (3), 435–447.

Tanigawa, S., et al., 2016. Selective in vitro propagation of nephron progenitors derived from embryos and pluripotent stem cells. Cell Rep.

Thomson, J.A., et al., 1998. Embryonic stem cell lines derived from human blastocysts. Science 282 (5391), 1145–1147.

Toyohara, T., et al., 2015. Cell therapy using human induced pluripotent stem cell-derived renal progenitors ameliorates acute kidney injury in mice. Stem Cells Transl. Med. 4 (9), 980–992.

Tsang, T.E., et al., 2000. Lim1 activity is required for intermediate mesoderm differentiation in the mouse embryo. Dev. Biol. 223 (1), 77–90.

Vaidya, V.S., et al., 2010. Kidney injury molecule-1 outperforms traditional biomarkers of kidney injury in preclinical biomarker qualification studies. Nat. Biotechnol. 28 (5), 478–485.

Van Adelsberg, J.S., Frank, D., 1995. The PKD1 gene produces a developmentally regulated protein in mesenchyme and vasculature. Nat. Med. 1 (4), 359–364.

Vierstra, J., et al., 2014. Mouse regulatory DNA landscapes reveal global principles of cis-regulatory evolution. Science 346 (6212), 1007–1012.

Wang, X., et al., 2015. Cloning and variation of ground state intestinal stem cells. Nature 522 (7555), 173–178.

Watson, C.L., et al., 2014. An in vivo model of human small intestine using pluripotent stem cells. Nat. Med. 20 (11), 1310–1314.

van de Wetering, M., et al., 2015. Prospective derivation of a living organoid biobank of colorectal cancer patients. Cell 161 (4), 933–945.

Wroblewski, L.E., et al., 2015. Helicobacter pylori targets cancer-associated apical-junctional constituents in gastroids and gastric epithelial cells. Gut 64 (5), 720–730.

Xia, Y., et al., 2013. Directed differentiation of human pluripotent cells to ureteric bud kidney progenitor-like cells. Nat. Cell Biol. 15 (12), 1507–1515.

Xia, Y., et al., 2014. The generation of kidney organoids by differentiation of human pluripotent cells to ureteric bud progenitor-like cells. Nat. Protoc. 9 (11), 2693–2704.

Yamaguchi, S., et al., 2016. Generation of kidney tubular organoids from human pluripotent stem cells. Sci. Rep. 6, 38353.

Yin, X., et al., 2014. Niche-independent high-purity cultures of Lgr5 + intestinal stem cells and their progeny. Nat. Methods 11 (1), 106–112.

Yonezawa, A., et al., 2005. Association between tubular toxicity of cisplatin and expression of organic cation transporter rOCT2 (Slc22a2) in the rat. Biochem. Pharmacol. 70 (12), 1823–1831.

Yue, F., et al., 2014. A comparative encyclopedia of DNA elements in the mouse genome. Nature 515 (7527), 355–364.

Yui, S., et al., 2012. Functional engraftment of colon epithelium expanded in vitro from a single adult Lgr5(+) stem cell. Nat. Med. 18 (4), 618–623.

Zhang, Y.G., et al., 2014. Salmonella-infected crypt-derived intestinal organoid culture system for host-bacterial interactions. Physiol. Rep. 2 (9).

Intestinal organoids in studying host − bacterial interactions

13

Jun Sun

University of Illinois at Chicago, Chicago, IL, United States

CHAPTER OUTLINE

INTRODUCTION AND THE PROBLEM BEING ADDRESSED

Host − microbial interactions are the interactions that take place between microbes (e.g., bacteria, parasites, viruses) and their host (e.g., humans, animals). The study of host − microbial interactions requires suitable model systems to mimic the in vivo infection. For the past few decades, researchers have employed various in vitro and in vivo experimental models to understand host − microbial interactions. The ultimate aim of these models is to create an environment in vitro that can imitate the real circumstances of the human, to elucidate physiological mechanisms of host responses in health and diseases. These models consist of cell culture lines deriving from human or animal cells (Dingli and Nowak, 2006), selected animals that can be infected with pathogens orally or by inoculation. (Fang et al., 2013), and organoids modeling host − bacterial interactions (Fatehullah et al., 2016). For some infective agents, good model systems are entirely lacking, while for others the systems that exist are far from optimal.

Organoids and Mini-Organs. DOI: http://dx.doi.org/10.1016/B978-0-12-812636-3.00013-4

NONORGANOID-BASED APPROACHES, AND ADVANTAGES AND DISADVANTAGES OF THE ORGANOID-BASED APPROACH IN STUDYING HOST — BACTERIAL INTERACTIONS

The intestinal epithelium is the most rapidly self-renewing tissue in adult mammals, and it includes a range of differentiated cell types, each with its own properties. Most in vitro models used to investigate interactions between *Salmonella* and intestinal epithelial cells fail to recreate the differentiated tissue components and structures observed in the normal intestine. One approach to creating differentiated cells is through a suspension culture technology that uses a rotating wall vessel bioreactor to keep cells in suspension with bubble-free aeration. The three-dimensional (3D) aggregates formed this way are characterized by cell polarity, extracellular matrix production, and organ-specific differentiation. However, this system may lack the normal stem cell niches that are responsible for the renewal of normal intestinal tissues (Zhang et al., 2014).

The newly-developed organoid system acts as a bridge between in vivo and in vitro systems. Ootani and colleagues have reported a complex culture system from minced whole intestinal tissue embedded in a 3D collagen structure with the support of stromal cells (Ootani et al., 2009). Sato and colleagues have established a relatively simple organoid culture system, using Matrigel as an ECM substitute, supplemented with growth factors constituting key endogenous niche signals. The system has been used to create 3D structures with distinct crypt-like and villus-like domains bordering a central lumen containing dead cells extruded from the constantly renewing epithelial layer (Sato et al., 2009). The organoids faithfully recapitulated *in vivo* epithelial architecture, and contained the full complement of stem, progenitor, and differentiated cell types (Fatehullah et al., 2016; Sato et al., 2009). Since then, intestinal organoids have been used in various aspects of basic and clinical research. The system has subsequently been adapted for generating human intestinal organoids, and also for generating organoids from animal models with different genetic modifications.

Today, adult stem cells from many murine and human tissues can be grown in vitro and self-organize into organoids that resemble their in vivo counterpart. Because organoids can be generated from different endodermal organs, or from specific sites of the gut, including the small intestine and colon (Sato et al., 2011a; Yui et al., 2012; Sato et al., 2011b), researchers can study the tissue-specific or site-specific aspects of particular host — pathogen interactions. The accessibility of organoids to observation and manipulation also allows researchers to make discoveries that would be more difficult to make in an animal model. Organoids allow us to address questions of cell and developmental biology, immunology, and pharmacology in unprecedented ways.

Studying tissue patterning and organ morphogenesis has, however, still been hindered by the lack of optimal culture conditions. A highly accurate, reproducible culture model would help to overcome current limitations that hinder the technology's transition from bench to bedside. Ideally, because host cell-to-host cell interactions are relevant to host − microbial interactions, organoids co-cultured with immune cells may be needed for more comprehensive studies.

DESIGN CONSIDERATIONS

Salmonella Typhimurium is a primary enteric pathogen that can infect humans and other animals. Infection begins with the ingestion of contaminated food or water, allowing *Salmonella* to reach the intestinal epithelium, and to cause gastrointestinal disease. In 2014, we reported the use of an organoid culture system to study the pathophysiology of bacterial − epithelial interactions after *S. Typhimurium* infection (Zhang et al., 2014).

We chose to use organoids because they allowed us to study tissue-specific and site-specific host interactions with *Salmonella*. We wished to learn whether this in vitro model system recapitulated a number of observations from in vivo studies of the *Salmonella*-infected intestine: bacterial invasion, altered tight junctions, inflammatory responses, and decreased stem cells during host − bacterial interactions. Our previous study has demonstrated *Salmonella* regulation of intestinal stem cells through the Wnt/beta-catenin pathway (Liu et al., 2010), so we also wanted to examine the direct regulation of stem cell markers in the organoids altered by *Salmonella* infection.

METHOD DESIGNED AND TYPICAL RESULTS

Using crypt-derived mouse intestinal organoids, we were able to visualize the invasiveness of *S. Typhimurium*, and the morphologic changes of the organoids (Zhang et al., 2014). In the organoids, the domains border a central lumen containing dead cells extruded from the constantly renewing epithelial layer. We infected the culture by colonization with pathogenic *Salmonella enterica* serovar Typhimurium 14028S (10^7 CFU). The first 30-min incubation allowed bacteria to contact the surface of the organoid cells. Thirty minutes later, the extracellular bacteria were washed away with Hank's balanced salt solution (HBSS). Then, the infected organoids were incubated in culture media with gentamicin for 1 hour. We found that bacterial infection significantly reduced the growth of organoids, including budding and the total area of the organoid cultures. *S. Typhimurium* entered the epithelial cells of the organoids, and this resulted in disruption of the tight junctions. For example, the tight junction (TJ) protein ZO-1 staining was decreased and disconnected in the Salmonella-infected organoids (Fig. 13.1). Interestingly, the TJ protein Claudin7 did not appear to be affected.

An inflammatory response based on NF-κB pathway activation was examined in the organoids infected with *Salmonella*. *Salmonella*-infected organoids had a significantly decreased total IkBα and increased phospho-IkBα. The phospho-NF-kB

A White field ZO-1(Green)

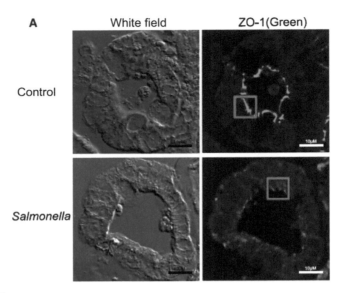

Control

Salmonella

FIGURE 13.1

Salmonella-induced disruption of tight junction protein ZO-1 (Barrandon and Green) in the mouse intestinal organoids (Zhang et al., 2014).

p65 was also increased in the *Salmonella*-infected organoids. By confocal microscopy, we found that NF-kB p65 had translocated into the nucleus in organoids infected with *Salmonella*. As the downstream targets of NF-kB activation, inflammatory cytokines (e.g., IL-2, IL-4, IL-6, and TNF-a) were significantly increased in the infected organoids, compared to the organoids without any infection. Moreover, the ELISA was sensitive enough to detect IL-6 protein in the culture medium 1 hour post *Salmonella* infection. The IL-6 protein was significantly enhanced in the culture medium post 1-, 2-, and 4-hour infection (Zhang et al., 2014). Moreover, our western blot, PCR, and immunofluorescence data demonstrated that stem cell markers (Lgr5 and Bmi1) were significantly decreased by *Salmonella* infection (determined using GFP-labeled Lgr5 organoids).

For the first time, then, we had created an in vitro model system that recapitulated a number of observations from in vivo studies of the *Salmonella*-infected intestine, including *Salmonella* invasion, disrupted tight junction structure, increased inflammatory cytokines, and decreased stem cell markers during host − bacterial interactions. We demonstrated that the *Salmonella*-infected organoid culture system is a new and feasible experimental tool for studying host−bacterial interactions.

Using intestinal organoids (iHOs) derived from human-induced pluripotent stem cells (hIPSCs), Forbester et al. (Forbester et al., 2014; Forbester et al., 2015) established microinjection of *S. Typhimurium* into the lumen of iHOs. RNA sequencing showed 1448 genes to be significantly upregulated in iHOs infected with S. *Typhimurium*, and 577 genes to be significantly downregulated compared to controls. Upregulated genes included those encoding proinflammatory cytokines, including CCL20, IL1B, and IL23A. Utilizing a *S. Typhimurium* mutant strain that lacked the invA component of the SPI-1 type III secretion system, Forbester and colleagues demonstrated that this system could be utilized to functionally assess the pathogenesis of defined mutants (Forbester et al., 2014; Forbester et al., 2015).

Microinjection of organoids with bacteria can mimic bacterial infection in a relatively well-controlled environment, allowing for direct examination of pathogen interactions with epithelial cells in the absence of confounding variables introduced by immune cells or the commensal microbiota. Wilson et al. reported that Paneth cells in organoids from both wild-type mice and Mmp7$^{-/-}$ mice produced granules containing pro-α-defensins. Organoids formed a sealed lumen that contains concentrations of α-defensins capable of restricting growth of *S. Typhimurium* for at least 20 hours postinfection (Wilson et al., 2015).

In addition to pathogenic bacterial studies, organoids can be useful for the commensal bacteria, probiotics, and microbiome studies. For example, region-specific changes in ion composition and pH correlated with region-specific alteration of luminal and mucosal-associated bacteria with general decreases in Firmicutes and increases in Bacteroidetes members (e.g., *Bacteroides thetaiotaomicron*) (Engevik et al., 2013). Inoculation of *Bacterioides thetaiotaomicron* in wild-type and NHE3$^{-/-}$ terminal ileum organoids displayed increased fut2 and fucosylation. These data suggest that *B. thetaiotaomicron* alone is sufficient for the increased fucosylation seen in vivo (Engevik et al., 2013).

REMAINING CHALLENGES

Studying human and bacteria interactions with the host remains severely limited, because of nonexistent or inappropriate animal models and challenge to culture bacteria in vitro, due to strict human − host specificity or physiology. Organoids are one of the most accessible and physiologically relevant models to study the dynamics of host − microbial interaction in a controlled environment. Specifically, human organoids from a susceptible host will be used to test their responses to pathogens, probiotics, and drugs. The progress in generating organoids that faithfully recapitulate the human in vivo tissue composition has extended organoid applications from being just a basic research tool, to a translational platform with a wide range of uses. In combination with genetic, transcriptome, and proteomic profiling, both murine- and human-derived organoids have revealed crucial aspects of development, homeostasis, and diseases. The commercial development of more standardized, validated, organoid culture media and affordable materials will be valuable in ensuring that the organoid system becomes accessible to a wide range of academic and clinical researchers, to further maximize its potential.

ACKNOWLEDGEMENTS

This work was supported by the NIDDK 1R01DK105118-01 and the UIC Cancer Center to Jun Sun.

DECLARATION OF FINANCIAL INTERESTS

No financial interests.

REFERENCES

Dingli, D., Nowak, M.A., 2006. Cancer biology: infectious tumour cells. Nature. 443 (7107), 35–36.

Engevik, M.A., Aihara, E., et al., 2013. Loss of NHE3 alters gut microbiota composition and influences *Bacteroides thetaiotaomicron* growth. Am. J. Physiology-Gastrointestinal Liver Physiol. 305 (10), G697–G711.

Fang, S.B., Kapikian, A.Z., et al., 2013. Human intestinal in vitro organ culture as a model for investigation of bacteriae-host interactions. J. Exp. Clin. Med. 5 (2), 43–50.

Fatehullah, A., Tan, S.H., et al., 2016. Organoids as an in vitro model of human development and disease. Nat. Cell. Biol. 18 (3), 246–254.

Forbester, J.L., Goulding, D., et al., 2014. Intestinal organoids are a novel system to study *Salmonella enterica Serovar Typhimurium* interaction with the intestinal epithelial barrier. Immunology 143, 111–112.

Forbester, J.L., Goulding, D., et al., 2015. Interaction of *Salmonella enterica Serovar Typhimurium* with intestinal organoids derived from human induced pluripotent stem cells. Infect. Immun. 83 (7), 2926–2934.

Liu, X., Lu, R., et al., 2010. Salmonella regulation of intestinal stem cells through the Wnt/beta-catenin pathway. FEBS Lett. 584 (5), 911–916.

Ootani, A., Li, X., et al., 2009. Sustained in vitro intestinal epithelial culture within a Wnt-dependent stem cell niche. Nat. Med. 15 (6), 701–706.

Sato, T., Vries, R.G., et al., 2009. Single Lgr5 stem cells build crypt-villus structures in vitro without a mesenchymal niche. Nature 459 (7244), 262–265.

Sato, T., Stange, D.E., et al., 2011a. Long-term expansion of epithelial organoids from human colon, adenoma, adenocarcinoma, and Barrett's epithelium. Gastroenterology 141 (5), 1762–1772.

Sato, T., van Es, J.H., et al., 2011b. Paneth cells constitute the niche for Lgr5 stem cells in intestinal crypts. Nature 469 (7330), 415–418.

Wilson, S.S., Tocchi, A., et al., 2015. A small intestinal organoid model of non-invasive enteric pathogen-epithelial cell interactions. Mucosal Immunol. 8 (2), 352–361.

Yui, S., Nakamura, T., et al., 2012. Functional engraftment of colon epithelium expanded in vitro from a single adult Lgr5(+) stem cell. Nat. Med. 18 (4), 618–623.

Zhang, Y.G., Wu, S., et al., 2014. Salmonella-infected crypt-derived intestinal organoid culture system for host-bacterial interactions. Physiol. Rep. 2 (9).

FURTHER READING

Barrandon, Y., Green, H., 1987. Three clonal types of keratinocyte with different capacities for multiplication. Proc. Natl. Acad. Sci. U.S.A. 84 (8), 2302−2306.

Klotz, C., Aebischer, T., et al., 2012. Stem cell-derived cell cultures and organoids for protozoan parasite propagation and studying host-parasite interaction. Int. J. Med. Microbiol. 302 (4−5), 203−209.

Ng, S., Schwartz, R.E., et al., 2015. Human iPSC-derived hepatocyte-like cells support plasmodium liver-stage infection in vitro. Stem Cell Reports 4 (3), 348−359.

Four challenges for organoid engineers

14

Jamie A. Davies and Melanie L. Lawrence
University of Edinburgh, Edinburgh, United Kingdom

CHAPTER OUTLINE

INTRODUCTION

Although organoid technology has its roots in experiments carried out over a century ago (see Davies, 2017, for a review), our ability to make organoids from human pluripotent cells is only a few years old and the field, like a young organoid, is at the stage of self-organization with only limited evidence of mature function. In the "future challenges" section of the foregoing chapters, some themes cropped up again and again. One was the need to produce organoids that show improved functional maturation. A second was a need to produce greater numbers of organoids reliably, and a third was the need to produce larger and more anatomically realistic organoids. These challenges represent three areas in which focused efforts may produce great reward. To them, we add a fourth challenge, of a very different nature but equally important in its way.

MAKING ORGANOIDS MORE MATURE

Organoids grown in vitro tend to form tissues that have a foetal level of maturation, as evidenced by physiological studies, and by comparing transcriptomes of the organoid and of natural tissues at different stages of development (Dye et al., 2015; Takasato et al., 2015). For most medical applications, post-natal tissues (paediatric/adult/senescent) are relevant, and the foetal stage is too young. The problem of immaturity is not restricted to human organoids; it is seen in mouse

Organoids and Mini-Organs. DOI: http://dx.doi.org/10.1016/B978-0-12-812636-3.00014-6

organoids, even when they are cultured for a time long enough for the natural foetal organ to mature. There is significant evidence that maturation depends on the organoid's environment (in either the sense of diffusible molecules, vascular and blood cells, or both). For example, Watson et al. (2014) showed that grafting human intestinal organoids into mice results in them acquiring a mature pheno-type, and Dye et al. (2016) showed a similar effect with lung organoids. From this, it may be possible to graft immature, embryonic-like human organoids into a healthy host for maturation, followed by transplantation into an intended recipi-ent. Improvement of the maturation of organoids in vitro will presumably depend on identification of the critical factors present in vivo. Experiments that expose organoids to fractions of the in vivo environment (for example, transplanted within a filter membrane that admits humoral factors but not cells, or cultured in vitro but exposed to flowing blood from a host animal) may be one approach.

MAKING ORGANOIDS IN LARGER NUMBERS

It is often claimed that organoids produced from human iPSCs will offer a system for pharmacological or toxicological screening that is more realistic, and therefore better in terms of predictive value for clinical application, than screening in animal models (Liu et al., 2016). Many screens, especially at the earlier stages of develop-ment, are very high-throughput, and their conversion to being human-based will require organoids to be produced reliably and in large numbers. Some progress is being made at applying the techniques of process engineering to organoid produc-tion to make the goal of high numbers achievable. A very recent example is pro-vided by Arora et al. (2017), who took this approach to improve the production of hindgut organoids. These organoids, which consist of a variety of intestinal epithe-lial cell types, richly and realistically patterned in a villus-like overall architecture, with mesenchymal cells surrounding them, can be produced by exposure of human iPSCs to a sequence of signals that mimic the sequence that would be experienced by hind-guts in an embryo (Spence et al., 2011; McCracken et al., 2011). In the early stages of culture, far more spheroids form than go on to form mature orga-noids, and the low yield of the intended product is a significant challenge to high-throughput production. Arora and colleagues addressed this by constructing a capillary-based sorting system, in which spheroids could be accepted or rejected according to morphological features assessed automatically by computer. Sorting criteria based on size and presence of internal cells raised the fraction of spheroids that formed organoids from 13% to 51%. Clearly, there is still room for improve-ment, but this work illustrates how construction of automated systems can signifi-cantly improve reliability. It also implies that a low initial efficiency of a technique for making a novel organoid does not necessarily mean that the technique will have no practical use: it may be possible to apply engineering techniques to improve it later. Finally, the work illustrates the advantages to be gained by applying interdis-ciplinary approaches to organoid biology.

MAKING LARGER ORGANOIDS

Organoids, as they are made now, are small: typically $100\,\mu m - 1$ mm in diameter. For some applications, especially imaging, small size is an advantage. For others, particularly the aim of making transplantable tissues, small size is a major problem. There have been some attempts to grow larger organoids, simply by increasing culture times, volumes, and oxygenation (e.g., Qian et al., 2016), and these have met with partial success.

An interesting alternative approach to making larger organoids is to make smaller ones and combine them. This approach has been successful in the relatively simple, epithelia-only organoid system of the gut. When grown in Matrigel, intestinal organoids grow as independent, budding cysts (Sato et al., 2009). When grown in a specific collagen-based matrix, however, these organoids coalesce (Sachs et al., 2017). Sachs and colleagues made their culture system by placing cold, unpolymerized collagen with intestinal organoids suspended in it at the bottom of a well, and allowing surface tension to draw the collagen to the edge of the well: they then warmed the collagen to allow it to polymerize, and added medium violently enough to detach the collagen and leave it floating as a ring. Within days, the collagen contracted, causing the ring to contract, bringing the organoids into contact with one another. Where they met, they fused to produce a long tube with a continuous lumen, with crypt-like side-branches, and other features similar to those of normal gut (although, of course, mesenchymal tissue was still absent). In principle, this technique might be applied to other tubular epithelial systems, and perhaps endothelia, as long as the absence of stroma is not important to the experiment. It may not work in more complex organoids in which mesenchymal cells are present, and likely to impede connections of epithelia.

FACING ETHICAL CHALLENGES

Making organoids from iPS cells is often presented as being a way to escape from ethical quandaries, and indeed it does carry far less ethico-legal baggage than working with *ex fetu* human material, or with human embryonic stem cells. Some ethical issues do, however, remain, and they are likely to become more prominent as our ability to make realistic human tissues improves. One issue, which applies to current work and work of the near future, concerns the source of the human iPS cells used to produce organoids, particularly those organoids used to explore mechanisms of disease, or to develop therapies. The need for reliability and standardization drives researchers in the direction of optimizing organoid production from a very small number of iPS cell lines, perhaps only one, that happen to produce excellent yields. Humans are genetically diverse, and the question of the extent to which this diversity should be represented in organoids is an ethical, as well as a practical, question; ethical because it connects with the question "for whom are medicines being developed"? At what point, on the path from exploratory studies towards clinical trials, should diversity be made an expectation? How much diversity is enough?

A quite different ethical issue centers on the transplantation of human organoids into animals for in vivo physiological studies. There may be less concern about some or all of the pancreatic tissue of an animal being of human origin, but how about transplantation of cerebral neurospheres (Fernados and Mason, 2017; Zeng et al., 2017)? The problems raised by human − animal chimaerism were addressed a few years ago by the Academy of Medical Sciences (2011), and UK Home Office codes for approval/ disapproval of this type of project are based largely on that report. A second problem comes from construction of "organoids" that represent the entire early embryo, rather than a specific organ or tissue (Martin et al., 2015). A construction approximating an early mouse embryo has already been assembled from murine stem cells (Harrison et al., 2017). If a human version is constructed, how far should it be allowed to develop?

Application of organoid-based assays to some problems in pharmacology and toxicology may require the development of new regulatory frameworks, so that the assays are seen as valid (better) replacements for animal experiments. This will not be necessary for early stage research, intended simply to identify candidate molecules, but it will be necessary for pre-clinical safety testing. Regulatory acceptance often involves measures of standardization, and this links back to the problems of reliable production mentioned above, and also to the tension between standards and diversity.

Interest in organoids is growing rapidly, and they have the potential to change that way that medical research is done, but their potential will be realized only when the challenges above are overcome. It is our hope that the preceding chapters of this book will give readers help and inspiration to make valuable progress in this direction.

REFERENCES

Academy of Medical Sciences, 2011. Animals Containing Human Material. <https://acmedsci.ac.uk/file-download/35228-Animalsc.pdf>.

Arora, N., Alsous, J.I., Guggenheim, J.W., Mak, M., Munera, J., Wells, J.M., et al., 2017. A process engineering approach to increase organoid yield. Development 144, 1128−1136.

Davies, J.A., 2017. Organoids and mini-organs: introduction, history and potential. Chapter 1 in this book.

Dye, B.R., Hill, D.R., Ferguson, M.A., Tsai, Y.H., Nagy, M.S., Dyal, R., et al., 2015. In vitro generation of human pluripotent stem cell derived lung organoids. Elife. 2015 Mar 24;4. doi: 10.7554/eLife.05098.

Dye, B.R., Dedhia, P.H., Miller, A.J., Nagy, M.S., White, E.S., Shea, L.D., et al., 2016. A bioengineered niche promotes in vivo engraftment and maturation of pluripotent stem cell derived human lung organoids. Elife. 2016 Sep 28;5. pii: e19732. doi: 10.7554/eLife.19732.

Ferdaos, N., Mason, J.O, 2017. Cerebral organoids: building brains from stem cells. Chapter in this book.

Harrison, S.E., Sozen, B., Christodoulou, N., Kyprianou, C., Zernicka-Goetz, M., 2017. Assembly of embryonic and extra-embryonic stem cells to mimic embryogenesis in vitro. Science. Available from: http://dx.doi.org/10.1126/science.aal1810.

Liu, F., Huang, J., Ning, B., Liu, Z., Chen, S., Zhao, W., 2016. Drug discovery via human-derived stem cell organoids. Front. Pharmacol. 7, 334, 2016 Sep 22.

Martin, F., Pera, M.F., de Wert, G., Dondorp, W., Lovell-Badge, R., Mummery, C.L., et al., 2015. What if stem cells turn into embryos in a dish? Nat. Methods 12, 917−919.

McCracken, K.W., Howell, J.C., Wells, J.M., Spence, J.R., 2011. Generating human intestinal tissue from pluripotent stem cells in vitro. Nat Protoc 6 (12), 1920−1928, 2011 Nov 10.

Qian, X., Nguyen, H.N., Song, M.M., Hadiono, C., Ogden, S.C., Hammack, C., et al., 2016. Brain-region-specific organoids using mini-bioreactors for modeling ZIKV exposure. Cell 165, 1238−1254.

Sachs, N., Tsukamoto, Y., Kujala, P., Peters, P.J., Clevers, H., 2017. Intestinal epithelial organoids fuse to form self-organizing tubes in floating collagen gels. Development 144, 1107−1112, 2017.

Sato, T., Vries, R.G., Snippert, H.J., van de Wetering, M., Barker, N., Stange, D.E., et al., 2009. Single Lgr5 stem cells build crypt-villus structures in vitro without a mesenchymal niche. Nature. 459, 262−265.

Spence, J.R., Mayhew, C.N., Rankin, S.A., Kuhar, M.F., Vallance, J.E., Tolle, K., et al., 2011. Directed differentiation of human pluripotent stem cells into intestinal tissue in vitro. Nature 470 (7332), 105−109, 2011 Feb 3.

Takasato, M., Er, P.X., Chiu, H.S., Maier, B., Baillie, G.J., Ferguson, C., et al., 2015. Kidney organoids from human iPS cells contain multiple lineages and model human nephrogenesis. Nature 526, 564−568.

Watson, C.L., Mahe, M.M., Múnera, J., Howell, J.C., Sundaram, N., Poling, H.M., et al., 2014. An in vivo model of human small intestine using pluripotent stem cells. Nat. Med. 20, 1310−1314.

Zeng, Y., Win-Shwe, T.-T., Itoh, T., Sone, H., 2017. A three-dimensional neurosphere system using human stem cells for nanotoxicology studies. Chapter 11 in this book.

Index

Note: Page numbers followed by "f" refer to figures.